The Health and Lifestyle Survey: Seven Years On

# The
# HEALTH
# *and*
# LIFESTYLE
# SURVEY:
## *Seven Years On*

A longitudinal study of a nationwide sample,
measuring changes in physical and mental
health, attitudes and lifestyle.

*Edited by*

**Brian D Cox**

**Felicia A Huppert**

**Margaret J Whichelow**

## Dartmouth
Aldershot · Brookfield USA · Hong Kong · Singapore · Sydney

Published by
Dartmouth Publishing Company Limited
Gower House
Croft Road
Aldershot
Hants GU11 3HR
England

Dartmouth Publishing Company
Old Post Road
Brookfield
Vermont 05036
USA

A CIP catalogue record for this book is available from
the British Library.

ISBN 1 85521 410 5

Design by David Cutting Graphics, Cambridge

Printed in Great Britain by Hartnolls Ltd, Bodmin, Cornwall

# CONTENTS

# CONTRIBUTORS

Brian D Cox  *Survey Director*
>   Department of Community Medicine, University of Cambridge Clinical School,
>   Institute of Public Health, Robinson Way, Cambridge CB2 2SR.

Mildred Blaxter  *Consultant*
>   School of Economic and Social Studies,
>   University of East Anglia, Norwich NR4 7TJ.

Felicia A Huppert
>   Department of Psychiatry, University of Cambridge Clinical School,
>   Addenbrooke's Hospital, Cambridge CB2 2QQ.

Judith Nickson  *Database Manager*
>   Department of Community Medicine, University of Cambridge Clinical School,
>   Institute of Public Health, Robinson Way, Cambridge CB2 2SR.

A Toby Prevost
>   Department of Community Medicine, University of Cambridge Clinical School,
>   Institute of Public Health, Robinson Way, Cambridge CB2 2SR.

Virginia J Swain
>   Department of Community Medicine, University of Cambridge Clinical School,
>   Institute of Public Health, Robinson Way, Cambridge CB2 2SR.

Margaret J Whichelow
>   Department of Community Medicine, University of Cambridge Clinical School,
>   Institute of Public Health, Robinson Way, Cambridge CB2 2SR.

Joyce E Whittington
>   Department of Community Medicine, University of Cambridge Clinical School,
>   Institute of Public Health, Robinson Way, Cambridge CB2 2SR.

# FOREWORD

## Lord Butterfield Kt. O.B.E., D.M., F.R.C.P.,
## Chairman, The Health Promotion Research Trust

It is a pleasure and privilege to be asked to write a Foreword to this work and I begin by congratulating the investigators responsible on their enterprise and success.

It is over 30 years since the leading investigators, Drs Brian Cox and Margaret Whichelow, first left the confines of the laboratories of the Department of Medicine at Guy's Hospital and joined myself and Harry Keen and the rest of us in the 1962 Diabetic Survey, which made its mark at the time and provided Professors Harry Keen and John Jarrett and their colleagues with a powerful base and firm foundation for a good deal of invaluable clinical epidemiological investigation into diabetes and its complications.

Since then, Cox and Whichelow, for some years with me, but more lately with others, have greatly widened these interests to a survey not just confined to diabetes and related topics but the whole range of chronic disease and health matters, concentrating on the attitudes, knowledge and beliefs of the individuals. And they have done this not in a single town but in all parts of the country.

The first major work, carried out in close association with Professor Mildred Blaxter, Mrs Judith Nickson and a multidisciplinary team, and supported by the Health Promotion Research Trust (HPRT) and its staff, particularly the Trust's Research Committee under Miss Eileen Cole aided especially by Professor Arthur Buller, resulted in the now very well known, I am almost tempted to call classic, Health and Lifestyle Survey undertaken eight years ago. It involved 9003 adults selected at random from addresses all over the UK; they were interviewed in 1984-85 in their homes and most were also examined by a nurse.

A particular feature of the study was the decision of HPRT, with the most generous and helpful collaboration of the survey team, to place the raw data of their survey in the computer archives of the ESRC at the University of Essex, so making the results available to whosoever wanted to use them. I am pleased that so many workers have availed themselves of these research facilities in quite separate research studies, over 200 of which have been published.

As the Trustees of HPRT faced the problems of deciding how to conclude their research and dissemination programme after their ten years in existence, it became obvious that a repeat survey of the same people after seven years would be a unique opportunity to add a longitudinal dimension and garner much invaluable information about changes in the health and particularly the health behaviour of a sample of the nation. This would be especially interesting and valuable at this time, following the recent activities of the Government and the Department of Health concerning the Health of the Nation and their emphasis on health promotion and widening the strength of the Health Education Authority.

The earlier HPRT Research Committee concerned with the original survey in the 1980s was re-established and enlarged to include Professor Keatinge of the Department of Physiology, Queen Mary and Westfield College. Drs Cox and Whichelow and the other grantholders, Professor Day and Dr Huppert, in the survey organisation set out to trace as many of the original sample as they could. There have, of course, also been in place since 1986 arrangements to flag members of the original sample for death on the NHS register at OPCS, so that those whose lives had subsequently ended were already recorded.

The results of the repeat survey are set out in this publication and I am sure they will be sought and studied particularly by groups of investigators from many regions and indeed overseas.

In addition, it is my personal hope that the results of both surveys, the original one and this recent follow up, will attract attention and interest among the Regional Directors of Research and Development set up by the Department of Health. They of course have responsibility to identify the health needs of the population.

I believe that the methods and the questionnaire instruments and examination techniques which the survey team evolved and tested in the homes of their subjects have now been exposed to considerable use, and they must be useful starting points for any work that Health Regions or Districts decide to initiate to define the health status of their local populations. And equally or even more important they will provide methods for monitoring the progress of health behaviour and cost reductions consequent upon improvements in lifestyle. This should be of interest to Government, particularly the Treasury.

And finally — as a medical student at Johns Hopkins in Baltimore, MD, USA, graduating nearly fifty years ago, and today as a Consultant in diabetes to the World Health Organization in Geneva — I should mention the international implications of the studies reported here. The philosophies which lie behind the work, the planning, the questionnaire instruments and clinical methods used in the *subjects' own homes* all deserve very warm commendation and attention abroad. Of course, we hope that our work will be some encouragement to those facing the daunting responsibilities of setting up and monitoring the cost and impacts of new health systems on health in, for example, America and Eastern Europe. Such investigators overseas will no doubt look back soon at our efforts as inadequate compared to the methods they will by then have evolved. In all this we wish them well. And I hope they enjoy colleagues to work with comparable to the ones I have had here over the last decades.

# INTRODUCTION

## The Health and Lifestyle Survey 1984/5 (HALS1)

The Health and Lifestyle Survey was carried out in 1984/5 on a nationwide sample of adults in England, Scotland and Wales, and funded by the Health Promotion Research Trust. It was conducted by a multidisciplinary team from the University of Cambridge School of Clinical Medicine, with the principal objectives of examining the relationships of lifestyle, behaviours and circumstances to the physical and mental health of a large representative sample of the British population. It was the largest cross sectional study of its kind, covering information obtained at interview, from physiological measurements and from psychological assessment on the complete age range of adults in Great Britain.

The preliminary findings of HALS1 are set out in a book entitled 'The Health and Lifestyle Survey' (1987). The very large database – of well over 1000 variables on each of the 9003 respondents – provided the potential for a great deal of research. The database was deposited at the ESRC data archive at the University of Essex from where it has been accessible to those wishing to carry out further analyses.

The many publications from the survey by both the survey team and secondary database users have provided considerable insight into the relationships between various measures of health, lifestyle and circumstances in the adult British population in 1984-5 and generated much interest in many quarters.

## Background to the 1991/2 Health and Lifestyle Survey (HALS2)

Both in Britain and elsewhere, health surveys of local and national populations have become more common in recent decades. In Britain, a particular impetus has been provided by the Government White Paper 'The Health of the Nation' (1992), and the requirement that Directors of Public Health should produce annual reports on the health of their populations. Regularly repeated national surveys, such as the General Household Survey in Britain, the NIH surveys in the United States, the CREDOC surveys in France, the 'Level of Living' surveys in Norway, and the surveys of the Danish National Institute of Social Medicine, have been conducted for many years.

The common pattern, however, is for surveys to be repeated on new samples of respondents. Longitudinal studies on the same individuals obviously have a greater potential for uncovering the relationship between lifestyles and health because changes in one dimension measured can be compared with changes in others. This has been shown by the pioneering Alameda County study in the United States, and the more recent National Health and Nutrition Examination Survey, also in the USA, as well as the studies of birth cohorts (such as the National Child Development Study and the National Survey of Health and Development) and of particular groups (such as the Whitehall Study of civil servants) in Britain.

When funding became available to the original team, again from the Health Promotion Research Trust, to carry out a further study, it seemed obvious that a similar survey would be invaluable. The first question was, should this be a repeat of the 1984-5 study on a random sample of the adult population, selected and studied in the same way as before, or should the original 'snapshot' survey be converted into a longitudinal study by following up the respondents who took part previously? Although administratively it might have been simpler to take another random sample, it seemed preferable to take the opportunity of carrying out a longitudinal survey which could provide more information about cause and effect, in this case focussing on health.

Attrition due to various factors – death, removal abroad or to areas too remote from survey points, refusals, illness, senility and not being traced – reduced the interviewed population size from 9003 in HALS1 to 5352 in HALS2.

HALS2 has focussed particularly on changes that have taken place in the seven years since the first survey. It offers the opportunity to determine to what extent 'health messages', especially those related to the prevention of diseases with an environmental component, such as heart disease, have been received and acted upon, changing lifestyles, in adults aged now from 25 to 99 and living in all parts of Great Britain. Social conditions have changed considerably since HALS1. Unemployment has grown, as has the divorce rate, and HALS2 offers the opportunity to investigate some of the health consequences of these changes. Some health issues have attained more prominence since the first survey, and targets for changes in diet, smoking habits, alcohol consumption and exercise in relation to health have been widely promoted.

HALS1 contributed to the debate on inequality in health by documenting social differences in the prevalence of physical and psychological ill health and in lifestyles and attitudes to health. Since then 'The Health Divide' (1987) and 'Income and Health' (1991) have shown that inequalities in health continue to exist. In HALS2, some attempt can also be made to identify the effect of change in individual circumstances upon physical and mental health.

## Content of the Follow-up Survey

The follow-up survey has been conducted in three parts, all taking place in the respondent's place of residence, as was the original survey. HALS1 only covered those living in their own homes, and therefore excluded many of the more frail and ill members of society, who were in hospitals, residential or nursing homes. In HALS2 all respondents who took part in the first survey were eligible for inclusion, regardless of their living accommodation. First, an interviewer visited the respondent and administered a questionnaire, the content of which covered the main lifestyle habits – diet, alcohol consumption, smoking and exercise – as well as self-reported health, attitudes to and beliefs about health, and demographic details. This was followed by a nurse carrying out simple physiological measurements and psychological tests and handing over a self-completion questionnaire concerned with personality and psychological health. This questionnaire was returned by post.

The design of all three sections has been to repeat, where feasible and appropriate, the questions and measurements of the first survey, and to include, in addition, questions relating to the respondent's experiences of change in the previous seven years. The interview questionnaire and the measurements form used in the survey are set out in Appendix C.

As the main object of HALS2 was to examine changes over the past seven years, this book concentrates on comparing the findings in the present survey with those on the same respondents in HALS1. A selection has been made of the data which seem most interesting or important, although as the survey questionnaires (Appendix C) show, there is much that has had to be excluded. The intention has been to provide a descriptive account of the changes in health and health-related behaviour in the survey populations in a form which is accessible to as wide a readership as possible. To this end, the information is presented principally in tabular form, without the use of statistics or complex technical or methodological detail. This provides the basis on which complex statistical analyses can be undertaken in the future.

## Future of the Database

As before, a complete data file with a comprehensive User's Manual (ESRC) will be deposited with the Data Archive of the Economic and Social Research Council at the University of Essex. A subset of the HALS1 dataset relating to those interviewed at HALS2 will also be deposited. Since HALS1 is 'flagged' with the National Health Service Register at the Office of Population Censuses and Surveys (OPCS) data giving the date and cause of death of respondents will be deposited in due course. Mortality can then be examined in relation to circumstances and lifestyle at the time of HALS1. Information from the Cancer Registry is also available on the site of cancer, for all notified cancer cases. It is hoped that these datasets will provide a resource for researchers in many fields, and in many locations.

The two Health and Lifestyle Surveys offer a unique opportunity to study the inter-relationships of changes in many aspects of health – reported and measured, physical and psychological – and lifestyles in a nationwide population of adults, from all walks of life and of all ages, all studied in their own place of residence.

**References**

Cox, B.D. et al. (1987), 'The Health and Lifestyle Survey', London: The Health Promotion Research Trust.

Quick, A. and Wilkinson, R.G. (1991), 'Income and Health', London: Socialist Health Association.

'The Health of the Nation: A strategy document for health in England', (1992), London: HMSO.

Whitehead, M. (1987), 'The Health Divide: inequalities in health in the 1980s', London: Health Education Council.

# Acknowledgements

We are happy to acknowledge the important role played by Lord Butterfield in the initiation of this survey.

We are indebted to those who were involved at various stages of the survey, to Professor N.E. Day for support and advice, to Ms Barbara White for her invaluable assistance with the data handling, and to Mrs Karen Halket and Mrs Enid Palmer, for secretarial assistance. Our thanks are due to Ms Patricia Prescott-Clarke and the other staff of SCPR who organized the smooth running of the survey, the data collection and preparation of the data file and the many interviewers and nurses who diligently carried out the fieldwork.

To the 5,352 respondents who so willingly and cheerfully spared the time to be interviewed and gave us such interesting accounts of their lifestyles we are especially grateful. Needless to say without them this Survey would have been impossible.

The Survey was generously supported by a grant from The Health Promotion Research Trust. We are grateful to the Trust for their encouragement and for facilitating the production of this report.

# THE

# SAMPLE

# SAMPLE STRUCTURE, DATA COLLECTION AND TRACING PROCEDURES

Brian D Cox and Margaret J Whichelow

## The HALS1 (1984/5) sample

The population for the 1984/5 survey was defined as individuals aged 18 years and over living in private households in England, Wales and Scotland.

Preliminary selection of addresses was made randomly from English, Welsh and Scottish Electoral Registers using a three-stage design. Within Standard Regions, parliamentary constituencies were allocated to one of three population density bands, and 198 constituencies were then selected with probability proportional to the size of the electorate. Two wards were selected from each, again with probability proportional to the electorate. In each household, one individual aged 18 or over was selected from all those resident, by application of a standard sampling technique. This procedure was necessary because Electoral Registers are not usually sufficiently up to date to provide a reliable list of individuals.

A total of 12254 addresses yielded interviews in their own homes with 9003 individuals, a response rate of 73.5%. A high proportion (82.4%) of those who were interviewed were also measured, and a high proportion (88.6%) of those who received a self-completion booklet returned it. The highest response rates were achieved in Scotland, Wales and the Northern Region of England, and the lowest in Greater London. Details of these response rates are shown in the first chapter of the report of HALS1 (Cox et al, 1987).

Because of inevitable losses from the sample at each stage (caused by death, illness and household movements as well as non-response), the three parts of the study necessarily produced samples of differing sizes so that overall response rates, related to the original sample, were reduced to 60.6% for the measured sample and 53.7% for the self-completion booklet.

The study population was compared to the 1981 Census, in order to demonstrate whether or not it could be assumed to represent accurately the population of England, Wales and Scotland in respect of major demographic variables. The HALS1 Survey had a slight excess of women, and some differences from the expected population among the youngest respondents and elderly women. This was likely to be due to differences in availability for interview. Other sources of bias were considered to be relatively small, and the HALS1 sample appeared to offer a good and representative sample of the population. The Survey population was also 'flagged' with the central National Health Service (NHS) Register at OPCS, Southport, Lancashire, so that the team was notified of deaths and sent copies of the death certificates. Further details of the sample and the sampling procedure can be found in the User's Manual to the HALS1 database, obtainable from the Economic and Social Research Council data archive at the University of Essex, Colchester.

## The HALS2 (1991/2) sample

Since the 1984/5 Survey was originally designed as a 'snapshot' survey, no attempt was made to stay in contact with the 9003 respondents, nor to keep track of their movements. The initial stages of the planning, in 1990-1, for the HALS2 follow-up survey involved exploring the most effective ways

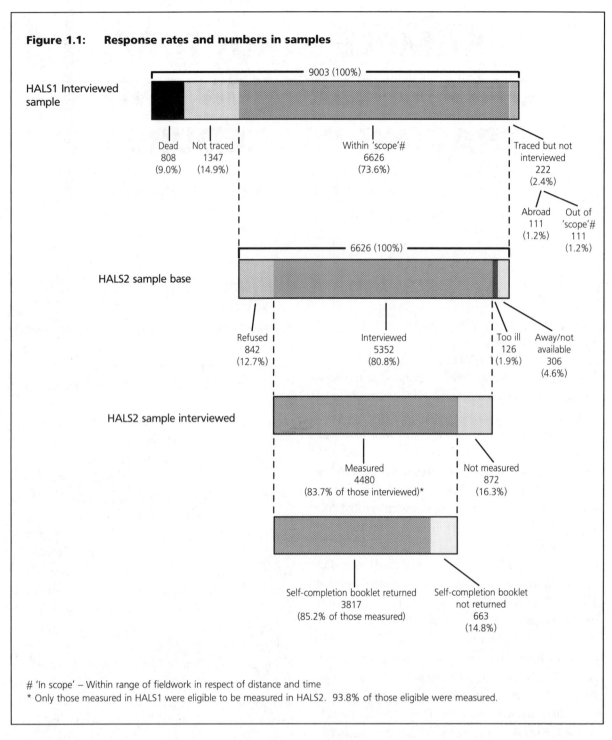

**Figure 1.1: Response rates and numbers in samples**

# 'In scope' – Within range of fieldwork in respect of distance and time
* Only those measured in HALS1 were eligible to be measured in HALS2. 93.8% of those eligible were measured.

of tracing the respondents. The stages of the tracing operations are covered in detail later in this chapter.

During the fieldwork a total of 6737 'good' addresses of living respondents (74.8% of the original 9003) were found within Great Britain, but due to household movements to areas too far away to be visited the total of 'within scope' addresses fell to 6626. These addresses yielded a total of 5352 interviews, a response rate of 80.8% (Figure 1.1). A

high proportion of these respondents were also measured (83.7%) and since only those who were measured in HALS1 were measured in HALS2 the response rate in those eligible was 93.8%. 85.2% of those measured returned the self-completion questionnaires concerned with personality and psychological health.

The success rates for interviews, for the respondents who were 'in scope', are shown in

Tables 1.1, 1.2 and 1.3 by 1984/5 age, socio-economic group and Standard Region respectively, together with the reasons for interviews not being obtained. A high proportion of those over eighty were not interviewed because they were too ill or infirm (15.3%).

Successful interviews were more likely to be obtained on the non-manual (Table 1.2) than the manual or 'other' respondents. Those in the manual groups were more likely to refuse to take part in HALS2 and also to be too ill to do so. There were regional differences in the success rate for interviews (Table 1.3), with Scotland having the highest and, as expected, London the lowest. Scotland also showed the lowest rate of refusals at 8.4% compared to an overall refusal rate of 12.7%. The highest proportion of respondents who were away from home at the time of interview was in London. In contrast, Wales had the lowest number of people away or otherwise not available, but the highest number of those who were too sick or infirm to take part.

By the very nature of the tracing procedures and the fact that the youngest of the HALS2 respondents were aged 25 at interview, the survey population cannot be considered to be representative of the adult population of Great Britain as were the HALS1 respondents. Tables 1.4 and 1.5 show the 1991 Census distribution by age and Standard Region for comparison with the HALS2 sample. The HALS2 sample is proportionately reduced in the two youngest age groups and in the oldest, and is increased in the middle age groups. The distribution of the HALS2 sample by region is similar to that of the 1991 census, with the exception of a reduced number in Greater London and a higher proportion in Scotland. Although the differences for most of the age groups and for Scotland and Greater London are significant, the percentage differences are small, so that adjustment can be made for comparison with a representative British population sample.

## Data collection

The data collection procedure was essentially the same for both the HALS1 and the HALS2 surveys.

Information was collected at two home visits. The first was carried out by an interviewer and lasted approximately one hour. At this visit information on self-reported health, health attitudes and beliefs, dietary habits, exercise, leisure, smoking habits and alcohol consumption was collected. Questions were also asked about the subject's home and family circumstances, employment, education and income. For HALS2, supplementary questions were asked about changes in personal circumstances, health and behaviours which had taken place in the seven years since HALS1, and a section on life events was included.

A second visit was made by a nurse who carried out the physiological measurements of height, weight, girth, hips, blood pressure, pulse rate, and respiratory function. In HALS1 environmental and exhaled carbon monoxide were also measured, but in HALS2 these were replaced by a sample taken for the measurement of salivary cotinine, a breakdown product of nicotine. At the same visit simple tests of cognitive function (reaction time, memory and reasoning) were also carried out. The instruments and methods used for these physiological and cognitive measures are discussed in Chapters 5, 6, 8 and 9 and Appendices A and B.

The nurse introduced the respondent to a self-completion questionnaire which assessed personality and psychiatric status, and was later returned by post. The schedules for the study, excluding those of personality and psychiatric status, which are under copyright, are reproduced at Appendix C.

The original sample selection for HALS1 was carried out by Social and Community Planning Research (SCPR), London, who also carried out the fieldwork for both the 1984/5 and 1991/2 studies. Interviewing was carried out in both surveys in three waves between autumn and summer in 1984/5 and 1991/2 respectively, with each region of the country represented in at least two waves, and most in all three, in order to ensure that different times of the year were represented in each area. This procedure ensured that in the majority of cases the respondents were also interviewed at the same time of year for both surveys. In addition a small 'mop up' wave was introduced in late summer 1992 in order to cover as many as possible of the respondents who had been found to have moved out of the survey areas, but were still resident in Great Britain.

In both surveys the interviewers provided potential respondents with an introductory letter explaining the purpose of the survey. At the close of each interview they introduced the second part of the study, the visit by the nurse, and, unless objections were made, the names of those who had been interviewed were passed to the nurse. In HALS2 the interviewer was asked to introduce the nurse's visit only to those respondents who had previously been measured by a nurse in HALS1. The nurse's visit, also accompanied by an explanatory letter, was made a week or so later. At the end of the visit the self-completion questionnaire booklet was given to the respondent together with a reply-paid envelope, and the method of completing it was explained.

To facilitate the smooth operation of the fieldwork, the Survey team kept in close contact with the nurses, who immediately reported any equipment failure. Replacement items for faulty equipment were dispatched at once, usually by overnight national carrier service. Upon completion of the interviews or measurements, the questionnaires and forms were sent to SCPR for checking and data entry, before being dispatched to Cambridge with the datafile. The survey team undertook the coding of the open-ended questions and logic checks of the datafile.

## Tracing procedures

Several techniques were investigated for tracing the individuals who took part in HALS1 in 1984/5. One of the most logical seemed to be to use the Family Health Service Authorities (FHSA) who keep a current register of patients on their lists and who might be expected to respond favourably to requests for assistance with health surveys.

Letters were sent to all the FHSAs in England, Scotland and Wales informing them of the first Health and Lifestyle Survey, and of the nature of the follow-up study, and enquiring whether they would assist the team in locating the respondents registered in their area. Replies were received from only half of the FHSAs and although a few of those who did reply agreed to release addresses, most offered only to pass on any letter that the team might wish to send. As it would therefore have been impossible to guarantee being able to locate more than a small proportion of the respondents through the FHSAs, this line of approach was abandoned.

### Tracing via the Electoral Register

The respondents had originally been selected from the Electoral Registers of two wards in constituencies representative of that area. Although boundary changes had occurred since 1984-5, on the whole these had been minor, making checking of the Electoral Registers feasible. For reasons of confidentiality the names and addresses of the respondents had been kept in a separate location from the data, with only serial numbers connecting the two. In order to preserve this confidentiality, new serial numbers were created for the names and addresses file when being used at Cambridge.

The Electoral Registers for the appropriate wards were examined in late 1990. Those known to be dead at the time of this operation (602) were excluded from the search, as were those where there was an incomplete name or address on the original contact sheets (40). As a result of this exercise 62.5% of respondents were identified as still being at their original address in 1990. In some cases (6.4%) there was a resident of the same surname at the listed address, but not the respondent. For 4.6% of addresses there was no record, which may have been because the dwelling was unoccupied, or had been demolished, or because the occupants wished to avoid registration for the Community Charge. In 26.5% of identified addresses there were no residents of the same surname present, indicating a household move. Table 1.6 shows the results of the Electoral Register searches by HALS1 age. In the 18-29 age group there was a major difference between the sexes in those cases where there was someone of the same surname listed but not the respondent. In this age group (where respondents had been likely to be living with their parents) more young men than women seem to have left home. Overall, the younger respondents were less likely to be at their original address. There were no great or consistent differences between socio-economic groups or the regions with respect to the results of these searches.

As previously indicated, notification of death had been received from OPCS for 602 subjects. However as there was often a delay in these notifications, it was probable that a number of the respondents who could not be traced were, in fact, dead.

### Tracing by mailshot

In an attempt to locate those respondents who could not be found on the Electoral Registers and who were not known to be dead, a letter was sent to the 3135 addresses where respondents were apparently no longer resident. This letter asked the present occupants to complete a form, giving information, if known, of the current address and telephone number of the respondent. A stamped addressed envelope was enclosed for reply. As a result of this operation a further 975 new addresses in Great Britain for the original respondents were obtained, and 138 respondents were confirmed as being at their original address, although not listed on the electoral roll. In a few instances this was because the respondents had changed their names, usually as result of marriage. Information was received that a further 68 respondents had died. 33 respondents had gone abroad and these were not followed up further. Where some of the new addresses appeared incomplete, and for respondents with unusual names, local telephone directories were checked: in this way the necessary details were found for another 55 respondents.

### Tracing by the Interviewers

In order to carry out the fieldwork of the HALS2 survey the interviewers were issued with lists of the last known address of each respondent. These comprised 'good' addresses, where the respondents had been traced via the Electoral Register or through the mailshot, and 'bad' addresses where the respondents appeared to have moved and had not been traced by letter or telephone directory. If a respondent was found to have moved from the issued address, the interviewer was instructed to explore every available avenue to find the new address, by contacting neighbours, local shops, the police and the post office, checking the local telephone directory and enquiring at the Local Authority Housing Department, if appropriate. By these means further new addresses were obtained.

## Outcome of Tracing Procedures

A summary of the results of the various methods of tracing are shown in Tables 1.7, 1.8 and 1.9. These tables include all those known to be dead, whether the information was from OPCS or found via the

mailshot or the interviewers. The lowest proportion of those who could be located was amongst the youngest age group, and almost half those who were identified as having gone abroad were in this group. The oldest respondents — over 70 years — were the easiest to trace, and, of course, the most likely to have died.

Examination of socio-economic characteristics (Table 1.8) showed that there was some difference between the groups in the proportions who were traced, with more non-manual than manual respondents being traced. There was also a higher number of deaths amongst the manual groups, and the non-manual respondents were more likely to have gone abroad. The 'other' group includes the armed forces, students and those who have never worked, which could explain the small proportion who could not be traced and the relatively high proportion who had gone abroad.

Regional variations (Table 1.9) were, in general, small, but Greater London had the highest proportion of respondents who could not be traced. In the first survey the lowest response rates were in Greater London, 64.2% compared to 73.5% overall. These problems in the capital are not unique to the Health and Lifestyle Survey (General Household Survey, 1990). In contrast, more respondents were traced in East Anglia, 91.6%, than in any other region. The highest proportion of deaths were in the North and the South West. Detailed analysis of the characteristics of those who had died or had moved between the two surveys are described in later chapters.

## Data Presentation

In the tables that follow sample numbers will not always be the same because of non-response to specific questions in either survey or where change is being demonstrated. The physiological measures and psychological data will always refer to smaller samples than the interview material.

The basic categories which are used to describe people — age grouping, social class, education, income and so on — may also differ slightly as appropriate to the topic. The wealth of detailed information permits many different forms of categorisation, and the principle has been to use the one most useful in any particular context.

Those categories, measures, scores, and variables

derived from a number of different items of information which are not entirely self-explanatory are defined in Appendix A.

For the reasons noted in the introduction, statistical tests of significance are not included in any Tables. The significance of any given distribution has, however, always been taken into account in the text, and if associations are clearly claimed they may be assumed to be statistically significant. The base numbers on which percentages are based are given in all Tables in italic type for those who wish to examine the data more closely, or consider further analyses.

The following conventions have been adopted:
φ: 0.9% or less in tables of percentages
0: zero count
(bracketed figure): number rather than percentage, in tables of percentages, where count or base number is small.

### References

Blaxter, M. (1987), 'Sample and data collection' in Cox, B D, et al, 'The Health and Lifestyle Survey', London: The Health Promotion Research Trust.

Smyth, M. and Browne, F. (1992), 'General Household Survey 1990', London: HMSO.

**Table 1.1**     **Fieldwork response rates in 1991/2 for respondents traced and 'in scope' as a percentage of the 1984/5 age group**

| | HALS1 (1984/5) age group | | | | | | | |
| | 18-29 | 30-39 | 40-49 | 50-59 | 60-69 | 70-79 | 80+ | ALL |
|---|---|---|---|---|---|---|---|---|
| Respondent interviewed | 82.1 | 83.9 | 81.5 | 81.3 | 77.3 | 75.1 | 63.3 | 80.8 |
| Respondent not interviewed: | | | | | | | | |
|    respondent away / not available | 8.0 | 4.6 | 5.0 | 3.5 | 2.2 | 1.5 | 3.1 | 4.6 |
|    refused or proxy refused | 9.7 | 11.1 | 13.0 | 13.5 | 15.9 | 15.4 | 18.4 | 12.7 |
|    too infirm or too ill | 0.2 | 0.3 | 0.4 | 1.7 | 4.7 | 8.0 | 15.3 | 1.9 |
| *Base = 100%* | *1276* | *1474* | *1252* | *1099* | *965* | *462* | *98* | *6626* |

**Table 1.2**     **Fieldwork response rates in 1991/2 for respondents traced and 'in scope' as a percentage of the 1984/5 socio-economic group**

| | HALS1 (1984/5) socio-economic group | | | | | | | |
| | Profes-sional | Managers & exec. | Other non-man. | Skilled manual | Semi-skilled | Unskilled manual | Others | All |
|---|---|---|---|---|---|---|---|---|
| Respondent interviewed | 84.8 | 82.7 | 82.8 | 80.3 | 78.0 | 75.4 | 74.5 | 80.8 |
| Respondent not interviewed: | | | | | | | | |
|    respondent away / not available | 5.0 | 3.9 | 4.3 | 4.4 | 5.6 | 5.0 | 6.9 | 4.6 |
|    refused or proxy refused | 8.8 | 11.9 | 11.5 | 13.3 | 13.8 | 15.8 | 16.7 | 12.7 |
|    too infirm or too ill | 1.5 | 1.4 | 1.4 | 2.0 | 2.6 | 3.8 | 2.0 | 1.9 |
| *Base = 100%* | *342* | *1194* | *1339* | *2257* | *1075* | *317* | *102* | *6626* |

**Table 1.3**     **Fieldwork response rates in 1991/2 for respondents traced and 'in scope' as a percentage of the standard region of residence in 1984/5**

| | HALS1 (1984/5) region of residence | | | | | | | | | | |
| | Scotland | Wales | North | North West | Yorks/ Humber | West Mids | East Mids | East Anglia | South West | South East | Greater London | All |
|---|---|---|---|---|---|---|---|---|---|---|---|---|
| Respondent interviewed | 85.7 | 80.3 | 81.1 | 81.6 | 79.8 | 77.4 | 80.0 | 82.1 | 80.5 | 82.3 | 76.6 | 80.8 |
| Respondent not interviewed: | | | | | | | | | | | | |
|    away / not available | 4.2 | 1.6 | 3.1 | 4.9 | 3.7 | 7.0 | 3.4 | 3.8 | 3.1 | 4.5 | 8.4 | 4.6 |
|    refused or proxy refused | 8.4 | 15.2 | 13.7 | 11.6 | 14.4 | 13.2 | 15.5 | 13.0 | 14.6 | 11.5 | 12.6 | 12.7 |
|    too infirm or too ill | 1.7 | 2.9 | 2.1 | 1.8 | 2.1 | 2.4 | 1.1 | 1.1 | 1.9 | 1.7 | 2.4 | 1.9 |
| *Base = 100%* | *663* | *376* | *387* | *817* | *619* | *615* | *534* | *262* | *522* | *1202* | *629* | *6626* |

**Table 1.4  Comparison of HALS2 Sample and Census 1991: age and sex**

| Age | Census | Inter-viewed | Meas-ured | Self-comple-tion | Census | Inter-viewed | Meas-ured | Self-comple-tion | Census | Inter-viewed | Meas-ured | Self-comple-tion |
|---|---|---|---|---|---|---|---|---|---|---|---|---|
| | Percentage of men | | | | Percentage of women | | | | Total percentage | | | |
| 25-29 | 12.3 | 9.3 | 8.8 | 8.2 | 11.4 | 7.2 | 6.5 | 5.4 | 11.8 | 8.1 | 7.5 | 6.6 |
| 30-39 | 21.8 | 16.0 | 15.5 | 14.2 | 19.8 | 18.4 | 19.1 | 19.1 | 20.7 | 17.4 | 17.5 | 17.0 |
| 40-49 | 21.1 | 23.1 | 23.6 | 22.9 | 19.1 | 24.0 | 25.7 | 26.1 | 20.0 | 23.6 | 24.8 | 24.7 |
| 50-59 | 16.7 | 18.0 | 18.3 | 19.1 | 15.1 | 18.4 | 19.1 | 18.8 | 15.8 | 18.2 | 18.7 | 18.9 |
| 60-69 | 15.1 | 17.2 | 17.7 | 18.5 | 15.1 | 15.2 | 15.0 | 15.9 | 15.1 | 16.1 | 16.2 | 17.0 |
| 70-79 | 9.5 | 11.8 | 11.9 | 13.1 | 12.2 | 11.6 | 10.4 | 11.2 | 10.9 | 11.7 | 11.1 | 12.0 |
| 80+ | 3.5 | 4.5 | 4.2 | 4.1 | 7.4 | 5.2 | 4.3 | 3.6 | 5.6 | 4.9 | 4.2 | 3.8 |
| All ages | 48.4 | 43.0 | 44.3 | 43.3 | 51.6 | 57.0 | 55.7 | 56.7 | | | | |
| Base = 100% | | 2300 | 1984 | 1652 | | 3052 | 2495 | 2165 | | 5352 | 4480 | 3817 |

**Table 1.5  Comparison of HALS2 Sample and Census 1991: standard region and sex**

| Standard Region | Census | Inter-viewed | Meas-ured | Self-comple-tion | Census | Inter-viewed | Meas-ured | Self-comple-tion | Census | Inter-viewed | Meas-ured | Self-comple-tion |
|---|---|---|---|---|---|---|---|---|---|---|---|---|
| | Percentage of males | | | | Percentage of females | | | | Total percentage | | | |
| Scotland | 9.0 | 10.8 | 10.8 | 10.7 | 9.2 | 10.4 | 9.8 | 9.7 | 9.1 | 10.6 | 10.3 | 10.2 |
| Wales | 5.2 | 5.9 | 5.8 | 6.1 | 5.2 | 5.4 | 5.7 | 5.5 | 5.2 | 5.6 | 5.7 | 5.7 |
| North | 5.5 | 5.0 | 5.0 | 5.0 | 5.5 | 6.6 | 6.7 | 6.7 | 5.5 | 5.9 | 5.9 | 5.9 |
| North West | 11.3 | 10.9 | 10.7 | 10.7 | 11.4 | 13.7 | 13.0 | 12.4 | 11.4 | 12.5 | 12.0 | 11.7 |
| Yorks/Humber | 8.8 | 9.6 | 9.6 | 9.0 | 8.8 | 9.0 | 9.0 | 8.6 | 8.8 | 9.3 | 9.3 | 8.8 |
| West Midlands | 9.5 | 8.7 | 8.4 | 8.9 | 9.3 | 9.1 | 8.8 | 8.8 | 9.4 | 8.9 | 8.6 | 8.9 |
| East Midlands | 7.3 | 8.5 | 8.8 | 9.1 | 7.1 | 7.7 | 7.9 | 8.1 | 7.2 | 8.0 | 8.3 | 8.5 |
| East Anglia | 3.7 | 3.6 | 3.9 | 4.2 | 3.7 | 4.3 | 4.6 | 5.0 | 3.7 | 4.0 | 4.3 | 4.6 |
| South West | 8.4 | 8.3 | 7.9 | 7.6 | 8.4 | 7.8 | 7.7 | 7.8 | 8.4 | 8.0 | 7.8 | 7.7 |
| South East | 19.3 | 19.5 | 19.9 | 20.4 | 19.1 | 17.5 | 18.4 | 19.1 | 19.2 | 18.4 | 19.0 | 19.6 |
| Gtr London | 12.1 | 9.3 | 9.0 | 8.5 | 12.3 | 8.5 | 8.5 | 8.3 | 12.2 | 8.9 | 8.7 | 8.4 |
| Base = 100% | | 2300 | 1984 | 1652 | | 3052 | 2495 | 2165 | | 5352 | 4480 | 3817 |

**Table 1.6** **Results of electoral register searches in 1990 for respondents as percentages of the 1984/5 age group – known dead excluded**

| | HALS1 (1984/5) age group | | | | | | | |
| --- | --- | --- | --- | --- | --- | --- | --- | --- |
| | 18-29 | 30-39 | 40-49 | 50-59 | 60-69 | 70-79 | 80+ | All |
| **Males** | | | | | | | | |
| Respondent listed at 1984/5 address | 34.7 | 57.4 | 72.6 | 75.4 | 75.4 | 81.4 | 64.4 | 61.3 |
| Respondent not listed at 1984/5 address: | | | | | | | | |
| same surname listed | 22.1 | 4.1 | 2.7 | 3.6 | 3.2 | 2.9 | 2.2 | 8.0 |
| surname not listed | 36.2 | 33.3 | 20.6 | 18.0 | 17.6 | 14.0 | 22.2 | 25.9 |
| address not listed on Electoral Register | 7.0 | 5.3 | 4.1 | 3.1 | 3.9 | 1.7 | 11.1 | 4.8 |
| *Base = 100%* | *885* | *760* | *631* | *556* | *467* | *242* | *45* | *3586* |
| **Females** | | | | | | | | |
| Respondent listed at 1984/5 address | 35.7 | 64.0 | 74.2 | 75.6 | 74.3 | 75.2 | 66.3 | 63.4 |
| Respondent not listed at 1984/85 address: | | | | | | | | |
| same surname listed | 15.1 | 2.9 | 2.2 | 1.7 | 2.1 | 2.7 | 2.1 | 5.2 |
| surname not listed | 42.3 | 29.8 | 19.9 | 19.8 | 18.6 | 19.0 | 24.2 | 27.0 |
| address not listed on Electoral Register | 6.9 | 3.4 | 3.7 | 2.9 | 5.1 | 3.0 | 7.4 | 4.5 |
| *Base = 100%* | *1085* | *1044* | *831* | *716* | *673* | *331* | *95* | *4775* |

**Table 1.7** **Summary of all tracing procedures in 1992 for HALS1 respondents as percentages of the 1984/5 age group**

| | HALS1 (1984/5) age group | | | | | | | |
| --- | --- | --- | --- | --- | --- | --- | --- | --- |
| | 18-29 | 30-39 | 40-49 | 50-59 | 60-69 | 70-79 | 80+ | All |
| Respondent located in great Britain | 66.7 | 81.6 | 84.4 | 83.2 | 76.3 | 57.2 | 38.7 | 74.8 |
| Respondent abroad | 2.5 | 1.0 | 1.0 | 1.0 | 0.8 | 0.7 | 0.0 | 1.2 |
| Respondent not traced | 30.0 | 15.9 | 11.9 | 7.9 | 6.9 | 3.9 | 5.9 | 14.5 |
| Respondent dead | 0.5 | 0.9 | 1.9 | 7.7 | 15.6 | 38.0 | 55.1 | 9.0 |
| Insufficient information for search | 0.4 | 0.6 | 0.7 | 0.2 | 0.5 | 0.1 | 0.4 | 0.4 |
| *Base = 100%* | *1990* | *1828* | *1497* | *1339* | *1280* | *813* | *256* | *9003* |

**Table 1.8**   **Summary of all tracing procedures in 1992 for HALS1 respondents as percentage of the 1984/5 socio-economic group**

| | HALS1 (1984/5) socio-economic group | | | | | | | |
| --- | --- | --- | --- | --- | --- | --- | --- | --- |
| | Profes-sional | Managers & exec. | Other non-man. | Skilled manual | Semi-skilled | Unskilled manual | Others | All |
| Respondent located in Great Britain | 77.1 | 78.2 | 74.2 | 75.8 | 73.0 | 72.9 | 52.5 | 74.8 |
| Respondent abroad | 2.7 | 1.3 | 1.5 | 0.7 | 1.1 | 0.2 | 7.4 | 1.2 |
| Respondent not traced | 14.0 | 12.7 | 17.3 | 12.5 | 14.9 | 14.4 | 32.2 | 14.5 |
| Respondent dead | 6.0 | 7.1 | 6.5 | 10.8 | 10.5 | 12.0 | 7.4 | 9.0 |
| Insufficient information for search | 0.2 | 0.6 | 0.5 | 0.3 | 0.5 | 0.5 | 0.5 | 0.4 |
| *Base = 100%* | *450* | *1563* | *1842* | *3012* | *1491* | *443* | *202* | *9003* |

**Table 1.9**   **Summary of all tracing procedures in 1992 for HALS1 respondents as percentages of the standard region of residence in 1984/5**

| | HALS1 (1984/5) region of residence | | | | | | | | | | | |
| --- | --- | --- | --- | --- | --- | --- | --- | --- | --- | --- | --- | --- |
| | Scotland | Wales | North | North West | Yorks/ Humber | West Mids | East Mids | East Anglia | South West | South East | Greater London | All |
| Respondent located in GB | 74.1 | 77.0 | 72.0 | 75.2 | 76.6 | 75.3 | 79.1 | 79.9 | 73.5 | 76.2 | 67.5 | 74.8 |
| Respondent abroad | 0.9 | 1.0 | 0.6 | 1.3 | 0.5 | 1.2 | 0.4 | 2.1 | 1.1 | 2.2 | 1.5 | 1.2 |
| Respondent not traced | 15.6 | 12.4 | 12.5 | 15.4 | 13.4 | 13.2 | 12.1 | 8.4 | 13.3 | 14.4 | 21.8 | 14.5 |
| Respondent dead | 9.4 | 9.0 | 14.2 | 7.4 | 9.4 | 10.0 | 8.3 | 8.1 | 11.4 | 6.6 | 9.1 | 9.0 |
| Insufficient information for search | 0.1 | 0.6 | 0.7 | 0.7 | 0.1 | 0.2 | 0.0 | 1.5 | 0.7 | 0.6 | 0.1 | 0.4 |
| *Base = 100%* | *925* | *501* | *542* | *1098* | *812* | *827* | *685* | *333* | *720* | *1615* | *945* | *9003* |

# DEMOGRAPHIC CHANGES | 2

Margaret J Whichelow, Virginia J Swain and Brian D Cox

The data presented in this chapter form a background to the findings presented in following chapters in this book, an overview and a preliminary report of HALS2. They also form a point of reference for those wishing to carry out further analysis. A limited selection of demographic variables are presented here, and others will be available on the dataset to be lodged with the ESRC Data Archive (see Chapter 1). The 5352 respondents who took part in both Surveys are considered sometimes compared at HALS1 and HALS2, and in other cases in relation to the full 9003 HALS1 sample. Unlike Chapter 1, where analysis was conducted on all those who could be traced in 1991/2, this chapter is concerned only with those who were re-interviewed in HALS2. Common to all who took part in HALS2 is that they are seven years older than at HALS1, but in all other respects there is potential for a variety of changes.

For marital status, household structure, employment status, socio-economic group and educational qualifications, the data are presented in seven year age groups with the results from the full HALS1 sample and the HALS2 sub-sample at HALS1 and HALS2. This enables the attrition rate between HALS1 and HALS2 for each demographic variable in each group to be assessed and the change over seven years of each group and each cohort to be examined. Further tables show the changes within each group between 1984/5 and 1991/2.

## Region of Residence

Table 2.1 shows the movement into and out of regions of the HALS2 sample. Those who moved were, of course, less likely to be traced. The greatest amount of movement into a region occurred in the South-West followed by the South-East. The South-East and Greater London also saw the largest movement of respondents away from the area.

## Marital Status

The marital status of the respondents in each age group is shown in Tables 2.2 and 2.3. The main losses between the HALS1 full sample and the HALS2 sub-sample at HALS1 have occurred in the youngest married and oldest married men and the single men aged 25-38 at HALS1. After 7 years at HALS2 the sample included a smaller proportion of single men and women, and slightly higher proportions of people who were widowed and divorced.

By 1991/2 many of the youngest respondents had become married, but for both men and women aged between 25 and 38 at HALS2, a smaller proportion were married than in the equivalent age group at HALS1. This was partly because of an increase in the proportion of divorced respondents in these age groups and partly because more respondents remained single. These trends have also been noted by the General Household Survey (Bridgwood and Savage, 1993). The increase in the proportion of widows between 60 and 73 and of widowers between 67 and 80 at HALS1 is less than would be expected for the seven year advance in age, so that the proportion of married respondents at these ages is higher. This may be associated with increasing life expectancy.

There has been considerable change over the seven year period, as would be expected (Table 2.4), with single people in the younger age groups getting married, and divorce or separation occurring for some respondents who were either single or married at HALS1, whilst widowhood is the predominant feature in the over-60s. These changes, the birth of children and adult children leaving the parental home, are reflected in changes in household structure.

## Household Structure

Table 2.5 to Table 2.8 show the distributions of household types in each seven year age band at HALS1 and HALS2 and the changes that have occurred between the groups. Those most likely to be lost from the original sample were men in the youngest group who were, in 1984/5, in households where there was a couple with dependent children, and both men and women who were living alone or with unrelated others. Respondents who were, at HALS1, living with relatives – mostly parents – were less likely to be lost from the sample. It was easier to trace these respondents, as the parents had usually not moved and knew where their offspring were living. There was less difference in the other age groups between the HALS1 full sample and the sub-sample at HALS1 (the respondents who were re-interviewed at HALS2). Overall, those who were living alone were less likely to be traced and re-interviewed. In the youngest two age groups at HALS2 there has been an increase in the proportion of households with a couple and dependent children, but it is less than would have been expected when the percentage is compared with the same age group in 1984/5. On the other hand the proportions of couples without children, and of those still living with relatives in the youngest age group are higher than for the same age group at HALS1. Over half of the men aged 18 to 38 and living alone in 1984/5 are now in a household with a partner compared with 43% of the equivalent women, but 8% of the women who were with a partner and dependent children at HALS1 are now lone parents. In the oldest age group more women than men have changed from living with a partner to living alone – 24% compared to 13% – most probably due to widowhood, or in some

cases because the partner has moved to a nursing home.

## Employment Status

Unemployed men and students of both sexes, tended to be lost disproportionately from the HALS1 sample (Tables 2.9 and 2.10). Those in employment were presumably more settled and easier to trace. More women of working age are in full time and part time employment at HALS2 than those of the same age at HALS1. Amongst the men, but not the women there is an increase in the proportion who have become permanently sick or disabled especially for those aged 60-66 at HALS2.

The changes in employment status (Table 2.11) show that the majority of the young men who were employed full time at HALS1 have remained so. Two-thirds of the younger men, who were unemployed at HALS1 are now in full time employment but only a quarter of the 39 to 59 group have become employed and another quarter have become permanently sick or disabled. Retirement accounts for the biggest changes in the elderly, and also for a high percentage of the changes in the middle aged, particularly for women. Most of the oldest group of men, who are now aged 67 and over, have become retired, but 14% reported working part time and 7% are still in full time occupation. For young women there has been more change, to part time employment and housekeeping, reflecting changes in their domestic situation with child rearing. In middle aged women the return to work, predominantly part time, is apparent.

## Education

The respondents were asked in both Surveys to identify the highest educational qualifications achieved. These should only have gone up between HALS1 and HALS2, and as only the youngest age group included an appreciable number of students, the main changes would be expected to occur among them.

Tables 2.12 and 2.13 show that attrition between HALS1 and HALS2 has occurred disproportionately in those over 46 at HALS1 who reported having no qualifications in 1984/5. A greater proportion of young respondents with professional qualifications or degrees at HALS1 were not interviewed at HALS2. There are smaller proportions of respondents reporting no qualifications in most cohorts, and always less than for the comparable HALS1 age group.

However, Table 2.14 shows that the distributions in Tables 2.12 and 2.13 mask considerable changes within groups. Whilst the majority of those with no qualifications and the highest qualifications (degrees) maintain that status in both surveys, there is greater change in the other groups towards claiming both more and fewer qualifications. These trends are even apparent in the oldest age group, where almost no change would have been expected. These findings raise doubt about the reliability of the questions. It is possible that asking respondents to identify their highest qualification may have caused confusion.

## Socio-economic group

The head of household's socio-economic group is reported; for men this is almost invariably their own socio-economic group, as it is for single, divorced and separated women. Married and widowed women are classified by their (former) husbands' occupation. Appendix A describes how socio-economic groups are defined. Elsewhere in this report socio-economic group usually refers to the HALS1 group, but in this chapter the HALS1 and HALS2 groups are compared.

Overall there was little difference between socio-economic groups in the proportions of the sample lost, amongst either men or women, between HALS1 and HALS2 (Tables 2.15 and 2.16), except for those in the armed forces at HALS1, and those unclassified, where proportionally more respondents were lost. However, some loss of the sample between HALS1 and HALS2 has occurred in some age groups, particularly in the 18-24 year old semi-skilled men and the 25-31 year old 'other' non-manual women. A higher proportion of respondents in the employer/ managers category were interviewed at HALS2 in the older age groups in both sexes. By HALS2, in those now aged 25 – 38, the proportions in the professional and employers/managers groups had risen to the levels for the equivalent HALS1 ages. For women, but not for men there is a fall in the proportion of skilled workers between the two Surveys, particularly

from age 53 at HALS2 onwards.

The change amongst individuals from HALS1 to HALS2 (Tables 2.18 and 2.19), show a considerable movement between groups, as has been found elsewhere (Goldblatt, 1988). With the change in the economy in Great Britain since 1984/5 a number of respondents of all ages may have changed their type of job in order to remain employed. Amongst the elderly women only 54% of those who declared their husbands (or more rarely, their own) occupation to be in the employer/managers group at HALS1 are in the same group in HALS2, compared to 92% for the elderly men. Indeed, for each age band and socio-economic group, women are less likely than men to report being in the same socio-economic group at both Surveys. As the same questions were used in both Surveys, some lack of clarity about their husband's occupation can be assumed.

## Summary

Some marked and unexpected changes have occurred between HALS1 and HALS2. There were smaller proportions of married respondents and couples with dependent children amongst the younger respondents at HALS1 than at comparable ages at HALS2. A higher proportion of women were in part-time, and more notably, full-time employment at HALS2, resulting in fewer housewives. Anomalies have occurred in the reporting of educational qualifications, at all ages, with some respondents apparently having lower qualifications at HALS2 than at HALS1. The oldest women revealed a higher level of change in socio-economic status between HALS1 and HALS2 than the men.

### References

Bridgwood, A and Savage, D. (1993), 'General Household Survey 1991', HMSO, London.

Goldblatt, P. (1988), 'Changes in social class between 1971 and 1981: could these affect mortality differences among men of working ages?' Population Trends, 51, 9-17.

**Table 2.1**   **Change in region of residence of HALS2 sample between HALS1 and HALS2 (males and females combined)**

| | Scotland | Wales | North | North West | Yorks/ Humber | West Midlands | East Midlands | East Anglia | South West | South East | Greater London |
|---|---|---|---|---|---|---|---|---|---|---|---|
| % of HALS1 in region at HALS2 | 99.8 | 99.7 | 99.7 | 100 | 99.8 | 99.4 | 99.3 | 99.5 | 99.0 | 98.4 | 97.5 |
| *Base = 100%* | *569* | *302* | *314* | *667* | *493* | *476* | *427* | *215* | *420* | *987* | *482* |
| **Numbers moved:-** | | | | | | | | | | | |
| into region | 0 | 0 | 1 | 1 | 4 | 2 | 5 | 1 | 13 | 11 | 5 |
| from region | 1 | 1 | 1 | 0 | 1 | 3 | 3 | 1 | 4 | 16 | 12 |

**Table 2.2**   **Age variations in marital status for males for the HALS1 full sample and HALS2 sub-sample at HALS1 and HALS2. Percentage of age group**

| Age at HALS1 | 18-24 | | 25-31 | | 32-38 | | 39-45 | | 46-52 | | 53-59 | | 60-66 | | 67-73 | | 74+ | | All | |
|---|---|---|---|---|---|---|---|---|---|---|---|---|---|---|---|---|---|---|---|---|
| **Age at HALS2** | | 25-31 | | 32-38 | | 39-45 | | 46-52 | | 53-59 | | 60-66 | | 67-73 | | 74-80 | | 81+ | | All |
| **Single** | | | | | | | | | | | | | | | | | | | | |
| HALS1 sample | 80 | | 32 | | 11 | | 6 | | 7 | | 7 | | 7 | | 5 | | 7 | | 21 | |
| HALS2 sub-sample | 83 | 45 | 29 | 16 | 8 | 6 | 5 | 5 | 6 | 6 | 6 | 5 | 6 | 5 | 3 | 3 | 8 | 8 | 18 | 11 |
| **Married** | | | | | | | | | | | | | | | | | | | | |
| HALS1 sample | 18 | | 63 | | 82 | | 86 | | 84 | | 86 | | 84 | | 78 | | 62 | | 70 | |
| HALS2 sub-sample | 15 | 50 | 67 | 71 | 86 | 85 | 90 | 88 | 87 | 86 | 88 | 83 | 87 | 82 | 82 | 72 | 58 | 33 | 75 | 76 |
| **Separated** | | | | | | | | | | | | | | | | | | | | |
| HALS1 sample | 1 | | 2 | | 3 | | 2 | | 3 | | 2 | | 2 | | 0 | | 1 | | 2 | |
| HALS2 sub-sample | 1 | 2 | 3 | 4 | 3 | 3 | 1 | 2 | 2 | 1 | 1 | (2) | (2) | (2) | 0 | (1) | 2 | 0 | 2 | 2 |
| **Divorced** | | | | | | | | | | | | | | | | | | | | |
| HALS1 sample | (3) | | 2 | | 4 | | 6 | | 5 | | 2 | | 2 | | 1 | | 1 | | 3 | |
| HALS2 sub-sample | (1) | 3 | 2 | 9 | 4 | 7 | 4 | 5 | 4 | 4 | 2 | 3 | 2 | 3 | 0 | 1 | 2 | 2 | 3 | 4 |
| **Widowed** | | | | | | | | | | | | | | | | | | | | |
| HALS1 sample | 0 | | 0 | | 0 | | (1) | | 1 | | 3 | | 5 | | 16 | | 29 | | 4 | |
| HALS2 sub-sample | 0 | 0 | 0 | 0 | 0 | 0 | 0 | 2 | 1 | 4 | 3 | 8 | 5 | 9 | 14 | 23 | 30 | 56 | 3 | 6 |
| *Base = 100%* | *534* | | *489* | | *573* | | *474* | | *419* | | *417* | | *412* | | *314* | | *273* | | *3905* | |
| | *288* | *288* | *238* | *238* | *382* | *382* | *323* | *323* | *279* | *279* | *278* | *278* | *259* | *259* | *147* | *147* | *87* | *87* | *2281* | *2281* |

**Table 2.3** **Age variations in marital status for females for the HALS1 full sample and HALS2 sub-sample at HALS1 and HALS2. Percentage of age group**

| | 18-24 | | 25-31 | | 32-38 | | 39-45 | | 46-52 | | 53-59 | | 60-66 | | 67-73 | | 74+ | | All | |
|---|---|---|---|---|---|---|---|---|---|---|---|---|---|---|---|---|---|---|---|---|
| **Age at HALS2** | | 25-31 | | 32-38 | | 39-45 | | 46-52 | | 53-59 | | 60-66 | | 67-73 | | 74-80 | | 81+ | | All |
| **Single** | | | | | | | | | | | | | | | | | | | | |
| HALS1 sample | 66 | | 15 | | 6 | | 3 | | 5 | | 6 | | 5 | | 7 | | 11 | | 14 | |
| HALS2 sub-sample | 65 | 30 | 12 | 8 | 6 | 5 | 2 | 2 | 5 | 5 | 5 | 5 | 6 | 6 | 7 | 7 | 11 | 11 | 12 | 8 |
| **Married** | | | | | | | | | | | | | | | | | | | | |
| HALS1 sample | 30 | | 76 | | 83 | | 85 | | 81 | | 79 | | 67 | | 50 | | 31 | | 67 | |
| HALS2 sub-sample | 33 | 59 | 81 | 77 | 85 | 82 | 87 | 84 | 81 | 77 | 79 | 68 | 68 | 55 | 51 | 33 | 34 | 19 | 72 | 69 |
| **Separated** | | | | | | | | | | | | | | | | | | | | |
| HALS1 sample | 2 | | 3 | | 3 | | 4 | | 2 | | 3 | | 2 | | 1 | | (1) | | 2 | |
| HALS2 sub-sample | 1 | 4 | 2 | 4 | 2 | 3 | 3 | 2 | 1 | 1 | 2 | 1 | 2 | (3) | 2 | 1 | 0 | 0 | 2 | 2 |
| **Divorced** | | | | | | | | | | | | | | | | | | | | |
| HALS1 sample | 2 | | 5 | | 6 | | 6 | | 8 | | 5 | | 3 | | 1 | | 1 | | 5 | |
| HALS2 sub-sample | 1 | 7 | 6 | 11 | 5 | 9 | 6 | 8 | 7 | 8 | 4 | 6 | 3 | 3 | 1 | 1 | (1) | 1 | 4 | 7 |
| **Widowed** | | | | | | | | | | | | | | | | | | | | |
| HALS1 sample | (1) | | (2) | | 1 | | 2 | | 5 | | 9 | | 23 | | 40 | | 57 | | 12 | |
| HALS2 sub-sample | 0 | 0 | 0 | (1) | 2 | 1 | 2 | 4 | 5 | 9 | 10 | 19 | 22 | 35 | 39 | 57 | 54 | 69 | 10 | 15 |
| *Base = 100%* | 626 | | 672 | | 766 | | 618 | | 576 | | 486 | | 553 | | 391 | | 410 | | 5098 | |
| | 308 | 308 | 392 | 392 | 544 | 544 | 431 | 431 | 390 | 390 | 315 | 315 | 326 | 326 | 190 | 190 | 143 | 143 | 3039 | 3039 |

**Table 2.4    Change in marital status between HALS1 and HALS2. Percentage of marital group at HALS1**

| HALS1 Age | 18-38 | | | | | 39-59 | | | | | 60+ | | | | |
|---|---|---|---|---|---|---|---|---|---|---|---|---|---|---|---|
| HALS1 | Sg | Mrd | Sep | Div | Wid | Sg | Mrd | Sep | Div | Wid | Sg | Mrd | Sep | Div | Wid |
| **HALS2 marital group** | | | | | | | | **Males** | | | | | | | |
| Single | 56 | – | 0 | 0 | – | 94 | – | – | – | – | 93 | – | – | – | – |
| Married | 39 | 93 | (7) | 40 | – | 4 | 95 | (4) | 23 | (1) | 4 | 86 | (1) | 0 | 7 |
| Separated | 3 | 3 | (3) | 0 | – | 0 | 1 | (2) | 0 | 0 | 0 | (3) | 0 | 0 | 0 |
| Divorced | 2 | 5 | (9) | 60 | – | 2 | (6) | (5) | 73 | 0 | 0 | (2) | 0 | (8) | 2 |
| Widowed | 0 | 0 | 0 | 0 | – | 0 | 3 | (2) | 3 | (11) | 4 | 12 | (3) | 0 | 92 |
| | | | | | | | | **Females** | | | | | | | |
| Single | 54 | (1) | – | – | – | 94 | – | – | – | – | 100 | – | – | – | – |
| Married | 40 | 90 | 23 | 42 | (4) | 4 | 91 | 15 | 16 | 7 | 0 | 73 | 0 | 0 | 1 |
| Separated | 3 | 4 | 8 | 0 | 0 | 0 | 1 | 27 | 0 | 0 | 0 | (1) | (4) | 0 | 0 |
| Divorced | 4 | 6 | 69 | 59 | 0 | 2 | 2 | 50 | 84 | 5 | 0 | (1) | (3) | (6) | 2 |
| Widowed | 0 | (3) | 0 | 0 | (4) | 0 | 6 | 8 | 0 | 88 | 0 | 27 | (3) | (6) | 97 |
| *Base =* | *339* | *530* | *19* | *20* | *0* | *49* | *776* | *13* | *30* | *12* | *27* | *395* | *4* | *8* | *59* |
| *100%* | *278* | *879* | *26* | *53* | *8* | *46* | *942* | *26* | *62* | *60* | *49* | *367* | *10* | *12* | *221* |

**Table 2.5    Age variations in household structure for males for the HALS1 full sample and HALS2 sub-sample at HALS1 and HALS2. Percentage of age group**

| Age at HALS1 | 18-24 | | 25-31 | | 32-38 | | 39-45 | | 46-52 | | 53-59 | | 60-66 | | 67-73 | | 74+ | | All | |
|---|---|---|---|---|---|---|---|---|---|---|---|---|---|---|---|---|---|---|---|---|
| Age at HALS2 | | 25-31 | | 32-38 | | 39-45 | | 46-52 | | 53-59 | | 60-66 | | 67-73 | | 74-80 | | 81+ | | All |
| **Couple with dependent children** | | | | | | | | | | | | | | | | | | | | |
| HALS1 sample | 17 | | 46 | | 71 | | 61 | | 28 | | 10 | | 2 | | (2) | | 0 | | 29 | |
| HALS2 sub-sample | 9 | 37 | 50 | 63 | 75 | 62 | 63 | 28 | 29 | 7 | 10 | 2 | 1 | 0 | (1) | (1) | 0 | 0 | 33 | 27 |
| **Couple with adult children** | | | | | | | | | | | | | | | | | | | | |
| HALS1 sample | 0 | | 0 | | 2 | | 13 | | 32 | | 31 | | 17 | | 5 | | 6 | | 11 | |
| HALS2 sub-sample | 0 | 0 | 0 | 2 | 2 | 14 | 15 | 37 | 33 | 29 | 33 | 21 | 18 | 8 | 7 | 5 | 6 | 1 | 13 | 15 |
| **Couple (with or without others)** | | | | | | | | | | | | | | | | | | | | |
| HALS1 sample | 11 | | 22 | | 11 | | 12 | | 24 | | 45 | | 65 | | 72 | | 56 | | 31 | |
| HALS2 sub-sample | 8 | 25 | 22 | 12 | 10 | 13 | 11 | 24 | 26 | 51 | 44 | 61 | 67 | 73 | 74 | 66 | 52 | 32 | 29 | 37 |
| **Lone parent with dependent children** | | | | | | | | | | | | | | | | | | | | |
| HALS1 sample | (4) | | (2) | | (5) | | 2 | | 1 | | 0 | | (1) | | (1) | | 0 | | (26) | |
| HALS2 sub-sample | 1 | (2) | 0 | 2 | (3) | 1 | 2 | (3) | 1 | (1) | 0 | 0 | (1) | 0 | (1) | 0 | 0 | 0 | (19) | (15) |
| **Lone parent with adult children** | | | | | | | | | | | | | | | | | | | | |
| HALS1 sample | 0 | | 0 | | 0 | | (4) | | 1 | | 1 | | 1 | | 2 | | 5 | | 1 | |
| HALS2 sub-sample | 0 | 0 | 0 | 0 | 0 | (3) | (1) | 3 | 2 | 3 | 1 | 3 | (2) | 2 | 2 | 2 | 2 | 9 | (17) | 2 |
| **One person** | | | | | | | | | | | | | | | | | | | | |
| HALS1 sample | 5 | | 12 | | 7 | | 7 | | 7 | | 8 | | 11 | | 17 | | 28 | | 10 | |
| HALS2 sub-sample | 1 | 10 | 9 | 8 | 5 | 6 | 4 | 5 | 5 | 6 | 7 | 11 | 9 | 14 | 12 | 21 | 35 | 49 | 7 | 11 |
| **One with relatives** | | | | | | | | | | | | | | | | | | | | |
| HALS1 sample | 66 | | 17 | | 7 | | 3 | | 5 | | 2 | | 3 | | 2 | | 5 | | 14 | |
| HALS2 sub-sample | 79 | 25 | 17 | 12 | 6 | 3 | 3 | 2 | 3 | 3 | 3 | 2 | 4 | 2 | 1 | 2 | 5 | 5 | 15 | 6 |
| **One with others** | | | | | | | | | | | | | | | | | | | | |
| HALS1 sample | 7 | | 4 | | 2 | | 2 | | 2 | | 2 | | 1 | | 1 | | (2) | | 3 | |
| HALS2 sub-sample | 2 | 3 | 3 | 2 | 2 | (3) | 2 | (2) | 1 | 1 | 2 | (1) | (2) | (2) | 1 | (3) | 0 | (5) | 2 | 1 |
| *Base = 100%* | 534 | | 489 | | 573 | | 474 | | 419 | | 417 | | 412 | | 314 | | 273 | | 3905 | |
| | 299 | 299 | 241 | 241 | 383 | 383 | 324 | 324 | 280 | 280 | 278 | 278 | 259 | 259 | 148 | 148 | 88 | 88 | 2300 | 2300 |

**Table 2.6** **Age variations in household structure for females for the HALS1 full sample and HALS2 sub-sample at HALS1 and HALS2. Percentage of age group**

| Age at HALS1 | 18-24 | | 25-31 | | 32-38 | | 39-45 | | 46-52 | | 53-59 | | 60-66 | | 67-73 | | 74+ | | All | |
|---|---|---|---|---|---|---|---|---|---|---|---|---|---|---|---|---|---|---|---|---|
| Age at HALS2 | | 25-31 | | 32-38 | | 39-45 | | 46-52 | | 53-59 | | 60-66 | | 67-73 | | 74-80 | | 81+ | | All |
| **Couple with dependent children** | | | | | | | | | | | | | | | | | | | | |
| HALS1 sample | 17 | | 59 | | 74 | | 58 | | 18 | | 3 | | (1) | | 0 | | 0 | | 30 | |
| HALS2 sub-sample | 19 | 48 | 63 | 68 | 76 | 51 | 59 | 19 | 20 | 2 | 3 | 0 | (1) | 0 | 0 | 0 | 0 | 0 | 35 | 26 |
| **Couple with adult children** | | | | | | | | | | | | | | | | | | | | |
| HALS1 sample | 0 | | (1) | | 3 | | 19 | | 35 | | 28 | | 9 | | 6 | | (3) | | 11 | |
| HALS2 sub-sample | 0 | 0 | 0 | 4 | 3 | 23 | 20 | 39 | 37 | 23 | 28 | 10 | 10 | 4 | 5 | 3 | (1) | (1) | 13 | 15 |
| **Couple (with or without others)** | | | | | | | | | | | | | | | | | | | | |
| HALS1 sample | 19 | | 19 | | 8 | | 9 | | 28 | | 48 | | 57 | | 44 | | 30 | | 27 | |
| HALS sub-sample | 17 | 21 | 19 | 10 | 8 | 11 | 8 | 27 | 23 | 54 | 48 | 59 | 57 | 51 | 45 | 30 | 33 | 18 | 25 | 30 |
| **Lone parent with dependent children** | | | | | | | | | | | | | | | | | | | | |
| HALS1 sample | 6 | | 9 | | 9 | | 6 | | 3 | | (3) | | 0 | | 0 | | 0 | | 4 | |
| HALS2 sub-sample | 6 | 9 | 9 | 13 | 7 | 5 | 5 | 2 | 3 | 0 | (1) | 0 | 0 | 0 | 0 | 0 | 0 | 0 | 4 | 4 |
| **Lone parent with adult children** | | | | | | | | | | | | | | | | | | | | |
| HALS1 sample | 0 | | (1) | | (4) | | 4 | | 5 | | 5 | | 6 | | 7 | | 9 | | 4 | |
| HALS2 sub-sample | 0 | 0 | 0 | (3) | (1) | 4 | 4 | 5 | 5 | 7 | 5 | 5 | 6 | 5 | 7 | 8 | 9 | 9 | 3 | 4 |
| **One person** | | | | | | | | | | | | | | | | | | | | |
| HALS1 sample | 4 | | 5 | | 3 | | 3 | | 8 | | 12 | | 25 | | 40 | | 54 | | 14 | |
| HALS2 sub-sample | 1 | 5 | 3 | 3 | 2 | 3 | 3 | 7 | 8 | 13 | 11 | 23 | 23 | 37 | 39 | 55 | 51 | 58 | 11 | 17 |
| **One with relatives** | | | | | | | | | | | | | | | | | | | | |
| HALS1 sample | 46 | | 6 | | 3 | | (5) | | 2 | | 4 | | 3 | | 2 | | 7 | | 8 | |
| HALS2 sub-sample | 55 | 13 | 5 | 2 | 3 | 3 | (3) | (4) | 2 | 1 | 3 | 4 | 3 | 3 | 3 | 2 | 6 | 4 | 8 | 3 |
| **One with others** | | | | | | | | | | | | | | | | | | | | |
| HALS1 sample | 8 | | 3 | | 1 | | (5) | | 1 | | (2) | | (4) | | 1 | | (2) | | 2 | |
| HALS2 sub-sample | 2 | 5 | 2 | (2) | 1 | (2) | (2) | 0 | 1 | (1) | (2) | (1) | (2) | (3) | (1) | (2) | (1) | 10 | 1 | 1 |
| *Base = 100%* | *626* | | *672* | | *766* | | *617* | | *576* | | *485* | | *553* | | *391* | | *410* | | *5096* | |
| | *311* | *311* | *394* | *394* | *545* | *545* | *431* | *431* | *391* | *391* | *315* | *314* | *327* | *326* | *191* | *190* | *146* | *143* | *3050* | *3046* |

**Table 2.7** **Change in household structure between HALS1 and HALS2 for males.
Percentage of HALS1 household group**

| | HALS1 household structure | | | | | | | |
|---|---|---|---|---|---|---|---|---|
| | Couple + dep. child | Couple + adult child | Couple ± others | Lone parent + dep. child | Lone parent + adult | One person | One + relative | One + others |
| **HALS2 household structure** | **HALS1 Age 18-38** | | | | | | | |
| Couple + dependent child | 77 | 0 | 63 | (1) | – | 31 | 23 | 30 |
| Couple + adult child | 12 | (3) | (1) | (1) | – | 0 | 0 | 5 |
| Couple ± others | 6 | (4) | 28 | 0 | – | 21 | 25 | 30 |
| Lone parent + dependent child | 1 | 0 | 0 | (1) | – | 0 | 1 | 5 |
| Lone parent + adult child | (1) | (1) | 0 | (1) | – | 0 | 0 | 0 |
| One person | 1 | 0 | 8 | 0 | – | 38 | 13 | 15 |
| One person + relative | 1 | 0 | 0 | (2) | – | 2 | 34 | 10 |
| One person + others | (3) | 0 | 0 | 0 | – | 7 | 3 | 5 |
| *Base = 100%* | *434* | *8* | *114* | *6* | *0* | *42* | *299* | *20* |
| | **HALS1 Age 39-59** | | | | | | | |
| Couple + dependent child | 32 | (2) | 2 | (1) | (1) | 0 | 0 | (4) |
| Couple + adult child | 50 | 36 | 4 | (2) | (1) | 0 | 4 | (2) |
| Couple ± others | 13 | 58 | 89 | 0 | (3) | 16 | 4 | (2) |
| Lone parent + dependent child | (1) | 0 | 0 | (2) | 0 | 0 | 0 | (1) |
| Lone parent + adult child | 3 | 2 | (2) | (4) | (2) | 2 | 0 | 0 |
| One person | 1 | 3 | 4 | (2) | (3) | 76 | 25 | (3) |
| One person + relative | (1) | 0 | (1) | 0 | 0 | 2 | 63 | (1) |
| One person + others | 0 | 0 | 0 | 0 | 0 | 4 | 4 | (3) |
| *Base = 100%* | *316* | *232* | *228* | *11* | *10* | *45* | *24* | *16* |
| | **HALS1 Age 60+** | | | | | | | |
| Couple + dependent child | (1) | 0 | 0 | 0 | 0 | 0 | 0 | 0 |
| Couple + adult child | (3) | 38 | (2) | 0 | 0 | 0 | 0 | 0 |
| Couple ± others | 0 | 46 | 85 | 0 | 0 | 9 | 0 | (1) |
| Lone parent + dependent child | 0 | 0 | 0 | 0 | 0 | 0 | 0 | 0 |
| Lone parent + adult child | 0 | 8 | (3) | (1) | (2) | 7 | 0 | 0 |
| One person | 0 | 6 | 13 | (1) | (4) | 76 | (5) | 0 |
| One person + relative | 0 | 0 | 0 | 0 | (1) | 1 | (10) | (1) |
| One person + others | 0 | 2 | (3) | 0 | 0 | 7 | 0 | (2) |
| *Base = 100%* | *4* | *63* | *329* | *2* | *7* | *71* | *15* | *4* |

**Table 2.8    Change in household structure between HALS1 and HALS2 for females. Percentage of HALS1 household group**

| | HALS1 household structure | | | | | | | |
| HALS2 household structure | Couple + dep. child | Couple + adult child | Couple ± others | Lone parent + dep. child | Lone parent + adult | One person | One + relative | One + others |
|---|---|---|---|---|---|---|---|---|
| | **HALS1 Age 18-38** | | | | | | | |
| Couple + dependent child | 70 | (1) | 55 | 31 | 0 | 14 | 29 | 25 |
| Couple + adult child | 17 | (5) | 1 | 4 | 0 | 0 | (1) | 10 |
| Couple ± others | 4 | (6) | 36 | 2 | (1) | 29 | 26 | 25 |
| Lone parent + dependent child | 6 | – | 5 | 46 | 0 | 0 | 3 | 15 |
| Lone parent + adult child | 2 | (1) | 0 | 9 | 0 | 0 | 0 | 5 |
| One person | (6) | (1) | (1) | 6 | 0 | 50 | 8 | 0 |
| One person + relative | 0 | 0 | (1) | 2 | 0 | 4 | 28 | 5 |
| One person + others | (1) | 0 | 1 | 0 | 0 | 4 | 5 | 15 |
| *Base = 100%* | *723* | *14* | *168* | *91* | *1* | *28* | *206* | *20* |
| | **HALS1 Age 39-59** | | | | | | | |
| Couple + dependent child | 25 | 0 | 0 | 10 | 0 | 0 | 0 | 0 |
| Couple + adult child | 52 | 29 | 4 | 10 | 2 | 0 | 0 | (1) |
| Couple ± others | 15 | 62 | 87 | 10 | 13 | 13 | 0 | (4) |
| Lone parent + dependent child | 2 | 0 | 0 | 0 | 0 | 0 | 0 | 0 |
| Lone parent + adult child | 5 | 4 | 0 | 55 | 32 | 3 | 10 | 0 |
| One person | 1 | 5 | 10 | 13 | 42 | 83 | 38 | (2) |
| One person + relative | 0 | 0 | (1) | 3 | 8 | 3 | 52 | 0 |
| One person + others | 0 | 0 | 0 | 0 | 4 | 0 | 0 | (1) |
| *Base = 100%* | *345* | *323* | *275* | *31* | *53* | *80* | *21* | *8* |
| | **HALS1 Age 60+** | | | | | | | |
| Couple + dependent child | 0 | 0 | 0 | – | 0 | 0 | 0 | 0 |
| Couple + adult child | 0 | 38 | (2) | – | 0 | 0 | 0 | (1) |
| Couple ± others | 0 | 36 | 72 | – | 2 | 1 | 0 | 0 |
| Lone parent + dependent child | 0 | 0 | 0 | – | 0 | 0 | 0 | 0 |
| Lone parent + adult child | (1) | 17 | (1) | – | 68 | 1 | 8 | 0 |
| One person | 0 | 7 | 24 | – | 25 | 93 | 29 | 0 |
| One person + relative | 0 | 2 | (2) | – | 0 | (1) | 63 | 0 |
| One person + others | 0 | 0 | 2 | – | 5 | 4 | 0 | (3) |
| *Base = 100%* | *1* | *42* | *320* | *0* | *44* | *224* | *24* | *4* |

**Table 2.9    Age variations in employment status for males for the HALS1 full sample and HALS2 sub-sample at HALS1 and HALS2. Percentage of age group**

| Age at HALS1 | 18-24 | | 25-31 | | 32-38 | | 39-45 | | 46-52 | | 53-59 | | 60-66 | | 67-73 | | 74+ | | All | |
| --- | --- | --- | --- | --- | --- | --- | --- | --- | --- | --- | --- | --- | --- | --- | --- | --- | --- | --- | --- | --- |
| Age at HALS2 | | 25-31 | | 32-38 | | 39-45 | | 46-52 | | 53-59 | | 60-66 | | 67-73 | | 74-80 | | 81+ | | All |
| **Full time** | | | | | | | | | | | | | | | | | | | | |
| HALS1 sample | 69 | | 84 | | 91 | | 90 | | 86 | | 71 | | 39 | | 3 | | 0 | | 65 | |
| HALS2 sub-sample | 73 | 86 | 87 | 90 | 92 | 90 | 92 | 88 | 88 | 68 | 74 | 33 | 40 | 3 | 4 | (1) | 0 | 0 | 71 | 67 |
| **Part time** | | | | | | | | | | | | | | | | | | | | |
| HALS1 sample | 4 | | (4) | | 1 | | (1) | | 1 | | 1 | | 4 | | 8 | | 3 | | 2 | |
| HALS2 sub-sample | 5 | 2 | 0 | 1 | (3) | 2 | (1) | 2 | 1 | 4 | 1 | 7 | 5 | 9 | 10 | 5 | 2 | 0 | 2 | 4 |
| **Unemployed** | | | | | | | | | | | | | | | | | | | | |
| HALS1 sample | 19 | | 14 | | 7 | | 8 | | 8 | | 11 | | 3 | | 0 | | 0 | | 9 | |
| HALS2 sub-sample | 16 | 10 | 11 | 5 | 6 | 4 | 6 | 5 | 7 | 6 | 10 | 4 | 4 | 0 | 0 | 0 | 0 | 0 | 8 | 4 |
| **Disabled/sick** | | | | | | | | | | | | | | | | | | | | |
| HALS1 sample | 0 | | 1 | | 1 | | 1 | | 3 | | 13 | | 8 | | 0 | | 0 | | 3 | |
| HALS2 sub-sample | 0 | 1 | 2 | 3 | (3) | 2 | 1 | 4 | 3 | 14 | 10 | 13 | 5 | 0 | 0 | 0 | 0 | 0 | 3 | 5 |
| **Retired** | | | | | | | | | | | | | | | | | | | | |
| HALS1 sample | 0 | | 0 | | 0 | | (2) | | (3) | | 5 | | 46 | | 89 | | 97 | | 19 | |
| HALS2 sub-sample | 0 | 0 | 0 | 0 | 0 | (1) | (1) | (3) | (2) | 8 | 5 | 44 | 46 | 88 | 85 | 95 | 98 | 100 | 15 | 26 |
| **Student** | | | | | | | | | | | | | | | | | | | | |
| HALS1 sample | 8 | | (2) | | (3) | | (1) | | 0 | | 0 | | 0 | | 0 | | 0 | | 1 | |
| HALS2 sub-sample | 6 | 1 | 0 | (2) | 0 | 0 | (1) | 0 | 0 | 0 | 0 | 0 | 0 | 0 | 0 | 0 | 0 | 0 | (19) | (5) |
| *Base = 100%* | 534 | | 489 | | 573 | | 474 | | 419 | | 417 | | 412 | | 314 | | 273 | | 3894 | |
| | 299 | 299 | 241 | 241 | 383 | 383 | 324 | 324 | 280 | 280 | 278 | 278 | 259 | 259 | 147 | 147 | 87 | 87 | 2298 | 2298 |

**Table 2.10**  **Age variations in employment status for females for the HALS1 full sample and HALS2 sub-sample at HALS1 and HALS2. Percentage of age group**

| | 18-24 | | 25-31 | | 32-38 | | 39-45 | | 46-52 | | 53-59 | | 60-66 | | 67-73 | | 74+ | | All | |
| --- | --- | --- | --- | --- | --- | --- | --- | --- | --- | --- | --- | --- | --- | --- | --- | --- | --- | --- | --- | --- |
| Age at HALS2 | | 25-31 | | 32-38 | | 39-45 | | 46-52 | | 53-59 | | 60-66 | | 67-73 | | 74-80 | | 81+ | | All |
| **Full time** | | | | | | | | | | | | | | | | | | | | |
| HALS1 sample | 58 | | 33 | | 28 | | 34 | | 34 | | 25 | | 5 | | 1 | | 0 | | 27 | |
| HALS2 sub-sample | 61 | 47 | 31 | 35 | 25 | 45 | 35 | 39 | 36 | 29 | 27 | 4 | 5 | (2) | 1 | 0 | 0 | 0 | 28 | 27 |
| **Part time** | | | | | | | | | | | | | | | | | | | | |
| HALS1 sample | 6 | | 18 | | 32 | | 37 | | 28 | | 25 | | 12 | | 5 | | 1 | | 20 | |
| HALS2 sub-sample | 6 | 22 | 20 | 37 | 36 | 35 | 39 | 38 | 28 | 29 | 28 | 13 | 14 | 5 | 8 | 2 | 2 | 0 | 24 | 24 |
| **Unemployed** | | | | | | | | | | | | | | | | | | | | |
| HALS1 sample | 8 | | 3 | | 2 | | 2 | | 2 | | 2 | | 0 | | 0 | | 0 | | 2 | |
| HALS2 sub-sample | 9 | 2 | 3 | 2 | 2 | 2 | 2 | (3) | 2 | 4 | 2 | (2) | 0 | 0 | 0 | 0 | 0 | 0 | 2 | 2 |
| **Disabled/sick** | | | | | | | | | | | | | | | | | | | | |
| HALS1 sample | (2) | | (2) | | (3) | | (5) | | 2 | | 5 | | 0 | | 0 | | 0 | | 1 | |
| HALS2 sub-sample | (1) | 1 | (1) | 1 | (2) | 2 | (4) | 3 | 2 | 6 | 4 | 0 | 0 | 0 | 0 | 0 | 0 | 0 | 1 | 3 |
| **Retired** | | | | | | | | | | | | | | | | | | | | |
| HALS1 sample | 0 | | 0 | | 0 | | (2) | | 1 | | 5 | | 83 | | 94 | | 99 | | 24 | |
| HAL52 sub-sample | 0 | 0 | 0 | 0 | 0 | (1) | (2) | 1 | 1 | 7 | 5 | 83 | 81 | 95 | 91 | 98 | 98 | 100 | 19 | 30 |
| **Student** | | | | | | | | | | | | | | | | | | | | |
| HALS1 sample | 8 | | (4) | | (4) | | (1) | | 0 | | 0 | | 0 | | 0 | | 0 | | 1 | |
| HALS2 sub-sample | 4 | 2 | 0 | 2 | (1) | 1 | (1) | (3) | 0 | 0 | 0 | 0 | 0 | 0 | 0 | 0 | 0 | 0 | (14) | (24) |
| **Housekeeping** | | | | | | | | | | | | | | | | | | | | |
| HALS1 sample | 20 | | 45 | | 38 | | 26 | | 32 | | 38 | | (1) | | 0 | | 0 | | 25 | |
| HALS2 sub-sample | 20 | 26 | 46 | 23 | 36 | 14 | 24 | 17 | 32 | 25 | 34 | 0 | (1) | 0 | 0 | 0 | 0 | 0 | 25 | 14 |
| *Base = 100%* | 626 | | 672 | | 766 | | 618 | | 576 | | 486 | | 553 | | 391 | | 410 | | 5097 | |
| | 311 | 311 | 393 | 393 | 545 | 545 | 432 | 432 | 391 | 391 | 315 | 315 | 326 | 326 | 190 | 190 | 143 | 143 | 3046 | 3046 |

*Age at HALS1*

**Table 2.11  Change in employment status between HALS1 and HALS2. Percentage of HALS1 employment group**

| HALS1 Age | 18-38 | | | | | | 39-59 | | | | | | | 60+ | | | | | |
|---|---|---|---|---|---|---|---|---|---|---|---|---|---|---|---|---|---|---|---|
| HALS1 employment status / HALS2 employment status | Full time | Part time | Unem-ployed | Dis-abled | Student | House-keeping | Full time | Part time | Unem-ployed | Dis-abled | Retired | Student | House-keeping | Full time | Part time | Unem-ployed | Dis-abled | Retired | House-keeping |
| **Males** | | | | | | | | | | | | | | | | | | | |
| Full time | 94 | (10) | 60 | (2) | (18) | (1) | 72 | (5) | 26 | 5 | 0 | (1) | (1) | 7 | 3 | 0 | 0 | 0 | 0 |
| Part time | 2 | 0 | 3 | 0 | 0 | (1) | 4 | (2) | 6 | 5 | 0 | 0 | 0 | 14 | 28 | (1) | 0 | 2 | 0 |
| Unemployed | 3 | (4) | 30 | 0 | 0 | 0 | 3 | 0 | 29 | 0 | 0 | 0 | 0 | 0 | 0 | 0 | 0 | 0 | 0 |
| Disabled/sick | 1 | (2) | 3 | (5) | 0 | 0 | 6 | 0 | 23 | 63 | (1) | 0 | 0 | 0 | 0 | 0 | (5) | 2 | 0 |
| Retired | (1) | 0 | 0 | 0 | 0 | 0 | 15 | (1) | 17 | 25 | (15) | 0 | 0 | 79 | 69 | (8) | (10) | 96 | (1) |
| Student | (3) | 0 | 2 | 0 | 0 | 0 | 0 | 0 | 0 | 0 | 0 | 0 | 0 | 0 | 0 | 0 | 0 | 0 | 0 |
| Housekeeping | (1) | (2) | 2 | 0 | 0 | (1) | 0 | 0 | 0 | 3 | 0 | 0 | (1) | 0 | 0 | 0 | 0 | 0 | 0 |
| **Females** | | | | | | | | | | | | | | | | | | | |
| Full time | 66 | 39 | 42 | (1) | (10) | 19 | 55 | 18 | 17 | 0 | 0 | 0 | 5 | (1) | 2 | – | 0 | 0 | 0 |
| Part time | 18 | 47 | 17 | 0 | (2) | 40 | 14 | 50 | 26 | 4 | 5 | 0 | 23 | (2) | 22 | – | 0 | (4) | 0 |
| Unemployed | 1 | 2 | 10 | 0 | 0 | 3 | 2 | 1 | 13 | 4 | 0 | 0 | (3) | 0 | 0 | – | 0 | 0 | 0 |
| Disabled/sick | (3) | (2) | 6 | (2) | 0 | 2 | 3 | 2 | 13 | 40 | 14 | 0 | 4 | 0 | 2 | – | (1) | 3 | 0 |
| Retired | (1) | 0 | 0 | 0 | 0 | 0 | 21 | 20 | 22 | 40 | 71 | 0 | 33 | (15) | 75 | – | (6) | 97 | 0 |
| Student | 2 | 1 | 0 | 0 | 0 | 2 | (1) | (1) | 0 | 0 | 0 | 0 | (1) | 0 | 0 | – | 0 | 0 | 0 |
| Housekeeping | 12 | 10 | 25 | (1) | (1) | 35 | 5 | 8 | 9 | 12 | 10 | (1) | 35 | 0 | 0 | – | 0 | 0 | (1) |
| *Base = 100%* | *780* | *18* | *97* | *7* | *18* | *3* | *749* | *8* | *66* | *40* | *16* | *1* | *2* | *110* | *29* | *9* | *15* | *329* | *1* |
| | *451* | *296* | *48* | *4* | *13* | *437* | *373* | *363* | *23* | *25* | *21* | *1* | *332* | *18* | *63* | *0* | *7* | *570* | *1* |

**Table 2.12**  **Age variations in highest educational qualification for men for the HALS1 full sample and HALS2 sub-sample at HALS1 and HALS2 (foreign qualifications excluded). Percentage of age group**

| Age at HALS1 | 18-24 | | 25-31 | | 32-38 | | 39-45 | | 46-52 | | 53-59 | | 60-66 | | 67-73 | | 74+ | | All | |
|---|---|---|---|---|---|---|---|---|---|---|---|---|---|---|---|---|---|---|---|---|---|
| Age at HALS2 | | 25-31 | | 32-38 | | 39-45 | | 46-52 | | 53-59 | | 60-66 | | 67-73 | | 74-80 | | 81+ | | All |
| **None** | | | | | | | | | | | | | | | | | | | | | |
| HALS1 sample | 17 | | 28 | | 33 | | 44 | | 53 | | 64 | | 62 | | 69 | | 80 | | 46 | |
| HALS2 sub-sample | 16 | 16 | 29 | 22 | 32 | 27 | 43 | 38 | 47 | 42 | 61 | 57 | 63 | 59 | 65 | 69 | 68 | 72 | 43 | 40 |
| **Work related** | | | | | | | | | | | | | | | | | | | | | |
| HALS1 sample | 4 | | 5 | | 6 | | 9 | | 7 | | 8 | | 7 | | 9 | | 4 | | 7 | |
| HALS2 sub-sample | 4 | 4 | 3 | 6 | 5 | 9 | 10 | 11 | 6 | 9 | 8 | 10 | 7 | 10 | 10 | 9 | 6 | 3 | 6 | 8 |
| **'O' level or equivalent** | | | | | | | | | | | | | | | | | | | | | |
| HALS1 sample | 47 | | 28 | | 18 | | 16 | | 11 | | 7 | | 8 | | 4 | | 3 | | 18 | |
| HALS2 sub-sample | 52 | 38 | 25 | 25 | 18 | 20 | 17 | 14 | 13 | 13 | 8 | 8 | 8 | 6 | 4 | 3 | 5 | 1 | 19 | 16 |
| **'A' level or equivalent** | | | | | | | | | | | | | | | | | | | | | |
| HALS1 sample | 27 | | 25 | | 22 | | 15 | | 15 | | 11 | | 9 | | 10 | | 5 | | 17 | |
| HALS2 sub-sample | 26 | 32 | 31 | 32 | 22 | 19 | 15 | 19 | 15 | 14 | 13 | 14 | 9 | 11 | 10 | 7 | 9 | 9 | 18 | 19 |
| **Professional qualifications** | | | | | | | | | | | | | | | | | | | | | |
| HALS1 sample | 2 | | 6 | | 10 | | 9 | | 9 | | 6 | | 11 | | 6 | | 4 | | 7 | |
| HALS2 sub-sample | 1 | 5 | 4 | 7 | 9 | 10 | 9 | 9 | 11 | 13 | 7 | 6 | 10 | 10 | 7 | 9 | 9 | 10 | 8 | 9 |
| **Degree** | | | | | | | | | | | | | | | | | | | | | |
| HALS1 sample | 4 | | 9 | | 12 | | 7 | | 6 | | 4 | | 3 | | 3 | | 3 | | 6 | |
| HALS2 sub-sample | 1 | 6 | 8 | 8 | 13 | 15 | 7 | 9 | 9 | 10 | 4 | 5 | 4 | 4 | 4 | 3 | 3 | 3 | 7 | 8 |
| *Base = 100%* | *532* | | *489* | | *570* | | *471* | | *418* | | *416* | | *410* | | *314* | | *273* | | *3893* | |
| | *298* | *299* | *241* | *238* | *383* | *381* | *321* | *323* | *280* | *279* | *278* | *277* | *258* | *257* | *148* | *147* | *88* | *87* | *2295* | *2288* |

**Table 2.13** Age variations in highest educational qualification for women for the HALS1 full sample and HALS2 sub-sample at HALS1 and HALS2 (foreign qualifications excluded). Percentage of age group

| | 18-24 | | 25-31 | | 32-38 | | 39-45 | | 46-52 | | 53-59 | | 60-66 | | 67-73 | | 74+ | | All | |
|---|---|---|---|---|---|---|---|---|---|---|---|---|---|---|---|---|---|---|---|---|
| **Age at HALS1** | 18-24 | | 25-31 | | 32-38 | | 39-45 | | 46-52 | | 53-59 | | 60-66 | | 67-73 | | 74+ | | All | |
| **Age at HALS2** | | 25-31 | | 32-38 | | 39-45 | | 46-52 | | 53-59 | | 60-66 | | 67-73 | | 74-80 | | 81+ | | All |
| **None** | | | | | | | | | | | | | | | | | | | | |
| HALS1 sample | 16 | | 33 | | 43 | | 49 | | 61 | | 67 | | 73 | | 79 | | 82 | | 53 | |
| HALS2 sub-sample | 15 | 14 | 35 | 35 | 44 | 39 | 46 | 41 | 56 | 53 | 64 | 65 | 67 | 68 | 76 | 81 | 81 | 80 | 50 | 48 |
| **Work related** | | | | | | | | | | | | | | | | | | | | |
| HALS1 sample | 2 | | 3 | | 4 | | 3 | | 2 | | 3 | | 3 | | 3 | | 4 | | 3 | |
| HALS2 sub-sample | 4 | 7 | 3 | 4 | 4 | 4 | 3 | 4 | 3 | 4 | 4 | 3 | 3 | 3 | 4 | 2 | 2 | 3 | 3 | 4 |
| **'O' level and equivalent** | | | | | | | | | | | | | | | | | | | | |
| HALS1 sample | 47 | | 27 | | 20 | | 17 | | 10 | | 9 | | 7 | | 4 | | 4 | | 18 | |
| HALS2 sub-sample | 50 | 43 | 26 | 23 | 21 | 22 | 18 | 17 | 11 | 10 | 10 | 7 | 9 | 9 | 4 | 2 | 4 | 5 | 18 | 17 |
| **'A' level and equivalent** | | | | | | | | | | | | | | | | | | | | |
| HALS1 sample | 28 | | 18 | | 17 | | 16 | | 11 | | 12 | | 9 | | 7 | | 5 | | 15 | |
| HALS2 sub-sample | 27 | 25 | 18 | 17 | 16 | 17 | 17 | 18 | 14 | 16 | 12 | 15 | 13 | 9 | 7 | 6 | 6 | 6 | 15 | 16 |
| **Professional qualifications** | | | | | | | | | | | | | | | | | | | | |
| HALS1 sample | 4 | | 10 | | 11 | | 10 | | 12 | | 7 | | 7 | | 6 | | 3 | | 8 | |
| HALS2 sub-sample | 4 | 9 | 13 | 13 | 11 | 13 | 11 | 13 | 14 | 13 | 7 | 8 | 9 | 10 | 8 | 10 | 6 | 5 | 10 | 11 |
| **Degree** | | | | | | | | | | | | | | | | | | | | |
| HALS1 sample | 2 | | 8 | | 5 | | 5 | | 3 | | 2 | | 1 | | (3) | | 1 | | 4 | |
| HALS2 sub-sample | 1 | 3 | 6 | 7 | 5 | 6 | 6 | 7 | 3 | 4 | 2 | 2 | (3) | 2 | (1) | (1) | 2 | 2 | 4 | 4 |
| *Base = 100%* | 622 | | 670 | | 763 | | 613 | | 571 | | 484 | | 552 | | 388 | | 407 | | 5070 | |
| | 310 | 309 | 392 | 393 | 543 | 542 | 429 | 430 | 387 | 388 | 315 | 315 | 327 | 324 | 191 | 190 | 145 | 142 | 3039 | 3033 |

**Table 2.14  Change between HALS1 and HALS2 in highest educational qualification reported. Percentage of HALS1 education group**

| HALS1 Age | 18-38 | | | | | | 39-59 | | | | | | 60+ | | | | | |
|---|---|---|---|---|---|---|---|---|---|---|---|---|---|---|---|---|---|---|
| **HALS1 education** | None | Work etc | 'O' Lev etc | 'A' lev etc | Profess-ional | Degree | None | Work etc | 'O' Lev etc | 'A' lev etc | Profess-ional | Degree | None | Work etc | 'O' Lev etc | 'A' lev etc | Profess-ional | Degree |
| **HALS2 education group** | | | | | | | | | | | | | | | | | | |
| **Males** | | | | | | | | | | | | | | | | | | |
| None | 72 | 18 | 5 | 2 | 6 | 0 | 80 | 9 | 4 | 0 | 0 | 0 | 89 | 51 | 27 | 11 | 2 | (1) |
| Work related | 10 | 18 | 6 | 3 | 4 | 0 | 9 | 31 | 6 | 4 | 2 | 0 | 5 | 27 | 10 | 9 | 18 | 0 |
| 'O'level etc | 10 | 28 | 60 | 18 | 6 | 0 | 6 | 14 | 41 | 13 | 6 | 0 | 2 | 5 | 23 | 13 | 2 | 0 |
| 'A'level etc | 6 | 26 | 24 | 63 | 4 | 3 | 3 | 9 | 21 | 73 | 6 | 2 | 3 | 11 | 23 | 59 | 2 | 0 |
| Professional | 2 | 10 | 3 | 9 | 52 | 7 | 1 | 11 | 8 | 2 | 68 | 2 | 1 | 3 | 17 | 9 | 64 | (6) |
| Degree | (1) | 0 | 2 | 4 | 26 | 87 | 0 | 3 | 0 | 2 | 17 | 97 | 0 | 3 | 0 | 0 | 11 | (12) |
| Base = 100% | 239 | 39 | 280 | 235 | 50 | 74 | 437 | 70 | 110 | 124 | 78 | 57 | 314 | 37 | 30 | 46 | 44 | 19 |
| **Females** | | | | | | | | | | | | | | | | | | |
| None | 82 | 8 | 4 | 0 | 0 | 0 | 88 | 31 | 10 | 10 | 3 | 2 | 94 | 51 | 46 | 23 | 4 | 0 |
| Work related | 3 | 25 | 4 | 2 | 0 | 0 | 4 | 21 | 3 | 6 | 2 | 2 | 1 | 27 | 5 | 7 | 0 | 0 |
| 'O'level etc | 9 | 32 | 62 | 23 | 4 | 0 | 3 | 13 | 58 | 11 | 4 | 0 | 3 | 23 | 27 | 15 | 4 | 0 |
| 'A'Level etc | 4 | 14 | 20 | 58 | 2 | 2 | 6 | 20 | 20 | 69 | 2 | 2 | 2 | 23 | 10 | 50 | 4 | 0 |
| Professional | 2 | 9 | 7 | 5 | 83 | 4 | 1 | 8 | 2 | 2 | 85 | 4 | (4) | (1) | 7 | 12 | 50 | 4 |
| Degree | 0 | 2 | (1) | 3 | 9 | 94 | 0 | 3 | 0 | 2 | 4 | 89 | 0 | (1) | 0 | 0 | (7) | (7) |
| Base = 100% | 418 | 44 | 369 | 236 | 119 | 53 | 614 | 39 | 147 | 161 | 121 | 45 | 476 | 18 | 41 | 62 | 51 | 7 |

**Table 2.15    Age variations in socio-economic group for males in the HALS1 full sample and the HALS2 sub-sample at HALS1 and HALS2. Percentage of age group**

| Age at HALS1 | 18-24 | | 25-31 | | 32-38 | | 39-45 | | 46-52 | | 53-59 | | 60-66 | | 67-73 | | 74+ | | All | |
| Age at HALS2 | | 25-31 | | 32-38 | | 39-45 | | 46-52 | | 53-59 | | 60-66 | | 67-73 | | 74-80 | | 81+ | | All |
|---|---|---|---|---|---|---|---|---|---|---|---|---|---|---|---|---|---|---|---|---|
| **Males** | | | | | | | | | | | | | | | | | | | | |
| **Professional** | | | | | | | | | | | | | | | | | | | | |
| HALS1 sample | 3 | | 5 | | 7 | | 6 | | 4 | | 5 | | 6 | | 5 | | 2 | | 5 | |
| HALS2 sub-sample | 2 | 4 | 4 | 5 | 8 | 8 | 7 | 8 | 5 | 6 | 5 | 5 | 6 | 7 | 4 | 4 | 2 | 2 | 5 | 6 |
| **Employers/managers** | | | | | | | | | | | | | | | | | | | | |
| HALS1 sample | 6 | | 14 | | 24 | | 28 | | 21 | | 16 | | 18 | | 18 | | 17 | | 18 | |
| HALS2 sub-sample | 5 | 12 | 14 | 25 | 24 | 28 | 28 | 28 | 21 | 21 | 18 | 16 | 18 | 17 | 22 | 21 | 22 | 22 | 19 | 22 |
| **Other non-manual** | | | | | | | | | | | | | | | | | | | | |
| HALS1 sample | 18 | | 23 | | 19 | | 14 | | 19 | | 16 | | 16 | | 14 | | 14 | | 18 | |
| HALS2 sub-sample | 21 | 27 | 23 | 17 | 20 | 19 | 14 | 13 | 22 | 18 | 18 | 18 | 17 | 17 | 13 | 12 | 14 | 14 | 19 | 18 |
| **Skilled manual** | | | | | | | | | | | | | | | | | | | | |
| HALS1 sample | 35 | | 36 | | 35 | | 36 | | 36 | | 37 | | 35 | | 38 | | 40 | | 36 | |
| HALS2 sub-sample | 40 | 36 | 41 | 35 | 34 | 33 | 37 | 37 | 34 | 38 | 35 | 34 | 35 | 33 | 37 | 39 | 38 | 38 | 36 | 35 |
| **Semi-skilled** | | | | | | | | | | | | | | | | | | | | |
| HALS1 sample | 22 | | 14 | | 13 | | 12 | | 15 | | 19 | | 19 | | 18 | | 18 | | 17 | |
| HALS2 sub-sample | 19 | 16 | 12 | 15 | 12 | 9 | 10 | 10 | 14 | 13 | 19 | 21 | 18 | 19 | 18 | 18 | 16 | 16 | 15 | 15 |
| **Unskilled** | | | | | | | | | | | | | | | | | | | | |
| HALS1 sample | 7 | | 6 | | 2 | | 4 | | 5 | | 6 | | 5 | | 7 | | 8 | | 5 | |
| HALS2 sub-sample | 6 | 4 | 5 | 3 | 2 | 3 | 5 | 4 | 4 | 4 | 5 | 5 | 5 | 6 | 6 | 7 | 8 | 8 | 5 | 4 |
| **Unclassified/never employed** | | | | | | | | | | | | | | | | | | | | |
| HALS1 sample | 9 | | 1 | | (1) | | 0 | | 0 | | 0 | | 0 | | 0 | | 0 | | 2 | |
| HALS2 sub-sample | 7 | (2) | 1 | (2) | 0 | 0 | 0 | 0 | 0 | 0 | 0 | 0 | 0 | 0 | 0 | 0 | 0 | 0 | 1 | (4) |
| **Armed forces** | | | | | | | | | | | | | | | | | | | | |
| HALS1 sample | (3) | | 1 | | 1 | | (1) | | (1) | | 0 | | (3) | | (1) | | (1) | | (21) | |
| HALS2 sub-sample | (2) | (1) | (1) | (1) | 0 | 0 | 0 | 0 | (1) | 0 | 0 | 0 | (2) | (2) | 0 | 0 | (1) | (1) | (7) | (5) |
| *Base = 100%* | *534* | | *489* | | *573* | | *474* | | *419* | | *417* | | *412* | | *314* | | *273* | | *3905* | |
| | *299* | *299* | *241* | *241* | *383* | *383* | *324* | *324* | *280* | *280* | *278* | *278* | *259* | *259* | *148* | *148* | *88* | *88* | *2300* | *2300* |

**Table 2.16** **Age variations in socio-economic group for females for the full HALS1 sample and the HALS2 sub-sample at HALS1 and HALS2. Percentage of age group**

| | 18-24 | | 25-31 | | 32-38 | | 39-45 | | 46-52 | | 53-59 | | 60-66 | | 67-73 | | 74+ | | All | |
|---|---|---|---|---|---|---|---|---|---|---|---|---|---|---|---|---|---|---|---|---|
| **Age at HALS1** | | | | | | | | | | | | | | | | | | | | |
| **Age at HALS2** | | 25-31 | | 32-38 | | 39-45 | | 46-52 | | 53-59 | | 60-66 | | 67-73 | | 74-80 | | 81+ | | All |
| *Females* | | | | | | | | | | | | | | | | | | | | |
| **Professional** | | | | | | | | | | | | | | | | | | | | |
| HALS1 sample | 2 | | 5 | | 7 | | 7 | | 6 | | 5 | | 5 | | 5 | | 4 | | 5 | |
| HALS sub-sample | 2 | 4 | 4 | 4 | 8 | 8 | 8 | 9 | 6 | 7 | 6 | 5 | 5 | 5 | 6 | 4 | 6 | 2 | 6 | 6 |
| **Employers/managers** | | | | | | | | | | | | | | | | | | | | |
| HALS1 sample | 6 | | 14 | | 19 | | 23 | | 27 | | 18 | | 17 | | 14 | | 16 | | 17 | |
| HALS2 sub-sample | 4 | 14 | 13 | 20 | 19 | 25 | 23 | 22 | 27 | 25 | 20 | 15 | 17 | 10 | 17 | 14 | 19 | 14 | 18 | 19 |
| **Other non-manual** | | | | | | | | | | | | | | | | | | | | |
| HALS1 sample | 39 | | 26 | | 23 | | 19 | | 17 | | 19 | | 19 | | 17 | | 19 | | 23 | |
| HALS2 sub-sample | 41 | 31 | 23 | 21 | 23 | 18 | 19 | 23 | 19 | 21 | 19 | 26 | 21 | 28 | 19 | 31 | 13 | 24 | 22 | 24 |
| **Skilled manual** | | | | | | | | | | | | | | | | | | | | |
| HALS1 sample | 21 | | 34 | | 33 | | 31 | | 31 | | 35 | | 33 | | 35 | | 35 | | 32 | |
| HALS2 sub-sample | 24 | 30 | 40 | 33 | 33 | 32 | 32 | 31 | 29 | 25 | 35 | 28 | 31 | 26 | 30 | 19 | 34 | 16 | 32 | 28 |
| **Semi-skilled** | | | | | | | | | | | | | | | | | | | | |
| HALS1 sample | 23 | | 16 | | 12 | | 15 | | 13 | | 16 | | 19 | | 21 | | 18 | | 17 | |
| HALS2 sub-sample | 25 | 18 | 15 | 18 | 13 | 13 | 13 | 11 | 13 | 15 | 14 | 17 | 21 | 21 | 20 | 23 | 22 | 35 | 16 | 17 |
| **Unskilled** | | | | | | | | | | | | | | | | | | | | |
| HALS1 sample | 3 | | 4 | | 3 | | 4 | | 5 | | 7 | | 6 | | 6 | | 5 | | 5 | |
| HALS2 sub-sample | 2 | 4 | 5 | 4 | 3 | 4 | 4 | 4 | 4 | 7 | 6 | 10 | 5 | 10 | 7 | 8 | 6 | 8 | 4 | 6 |
| **Unclassified/never employed** | | | | | | | | | | | | | | | | | | | | |
| HALS1 sample | 6 | | (3) | | (2) | | (3) | | (4) | | (2) | | 1 | | 2 | | 2 | | 1 | |
| HALS2 sub-sample | 4 | (2) | (1) | (1) | (1) | 0 | (1) | 0 | (2) | (1) | (1) | 0 | (2) | (2) | (1) | (1) | (2) | (2) | (22) | 9 |
| **Armed forces** | | | | | | | | | | | | | | | | | | | | |
| HALS1 sample | (5) | | 1 | | 1 | | (5) | | (2) | | (3) | | (4) | | (2) | | 1 | | (43) | |
| HALS2 sub-sample | (1) | (1) | (1) | 0 | (5) | 0 | (3) | (2) | (2) | 0 | (2) | 0 | (2) | (1) | (1) | (1) | (1) | 0 | (18) | 0 |
| *Base = 100%* | 621 | | 669 | | 764 | | 616 | | 576 | | 485 | | 553 | | 391 | | 410 | | 5085 | |
| | 309 | 309 | 392 | 392 | 545 | 545 | 430 | 430 | 391 | 391 | 314 | 314 | 327 | 327 | 191 | 191 | 146 | 146 | 3045 | 3045 |

**Table 2.17    Change in socio-economic group in males between HALS1 and HALS2.
Percentage of HALS1 socio-economic group**

| | HALS1 socio-economic group | | | | | | | |
|---|---|---|---|---|---|---|---|---|
| | Profsnl. | Emplyr./ manag. | Other non-manual | Skilled manual | Semi-skilled | Un-skilled | Unclass | Armed services |
| **HALS2 socio-economic group** | | | | **HALS1 Age 18-38** | | | | |
| Professional | 57 | 4 | 8 | 1 | (1) | 0 | 8 | 0 |
| Employers, managers | 23 | 71 | 21 | 11 | 11 | 3 | 0 | 0 |
| Other non-manual | 14 | 14 | 63 | 7 | 7 | 11 | 36 | 0 |
| Skilled manual | 7 | 11 | 5 | 70 | 25 | 21 | 12 | (1) |
| Semi-skilled manual | 0 | 0 | 4 | 10 | 53 | 11 | 24 | 0 |
| Unskilled | 0 | (1) | 0 | (3) | 3 | 55 | 4 | 0 |
| Unclassified or never employed | 0 | 0 | 0 | 0 | 0 | 0 | 16 | 0 |
| Armed services | 0 | 0 | 0 | 0 | 0 | 0 | 0 | (2) |
| *Base = 100%* | *44* | *141* | *195* | *347* | *130* | *38* | *25* | *3* |
| | | | | **HALS1 Age 39-59** | | | | |
| Professional | 78 | 4 | 6 | 2 | 0 | 0 | – | 0 |
| Employers, managers | 12 | 75 | 13 | 6 | 3 | 0 | – | 0 |
| Other non-manual | 8 | 9 | 72 | 2 | 2 | 0 | – | (1) |
| Skilled manual | 2 | 11 | 7 | 82 | 18 | 24 | – | 0 |
| Semi-skilled manual | 0 | 3 | 3 | 7 | 72 | 12 | – | 0 |
| Unskilled | 0 | 0 | 0 | 2 | 5 | 63 | – | 0 |
| Unclassified or never employed | 0 | 0 | 0 | 0 | 0 | 0 | – | 0 |
| Armed services | 0 | 0 | 0 | 0 | 0 | 0 | – | 0 |
| *Base = 100%* | *49* | *201* | *155* | *311* | *124* | *41* | *0* | *1* |
| | | | | **HALS1 Age 60+** | | | | |
| Professional | 96 | 2 | 1 | 0 | 1 | 0 | – | 0 |
| Employers, managers | 0 | 92 | 3 | 2 | 1 | 0 | – | 0 |
| Other non-manual | 4 | 2 | 90 | (1) | 1 | 0 | – | 0 |
| Skilled manual | 0 | 2 | 5 | 91 | 7 | 3 | – | 0 |
| Semi-skilled manual | 0 | 2 | 1 | 4 | 89 | 3 | – | 0 |
| Unskilled | 0 | 0 | 0 | 3 | 1 | 93 | – | 0 |
| Unclassified or never employed | 0 | 0 | 0 | 0 | 0 | 0 | – | 0 |
| Armed services | 0 | 0 | 0 | 0 | 0 | 0 | – | (3) |
| *Base = 100%* | *23* | *97* | *76* | *179* | *88* | *29* | *0* | *3* |

**Table 2.18** **Change in socio-economic group in females between HALS1 and HALS2.**
**Percentage of HALS1 socio-economic group**

| | HALS1 socio-economic group | | | | | | | |
| --- | --- | --- | --- | --- | --- | --- | --- | --- |
| | Profsnl. | Emplyr./ manag. | Other non-manual | Skilled manual | Semi-skilled | Un-skilled | Unclass | Armed services |
| **HALS2 socio-economic group** | | | | HALS1 Age 18-38 | | | | |
| Professional | 60 | 2 | 4 | 2 | 2 | 0 | 0 | 0 |
| Employers, managers | 18 | 62 | 21 | 13 | 9 | 2 | 0 | (2) |
| Other non-manual | 19 | 13 | 49 | 7 | 17 | 2 | (7) | (2) |
| Skilled manual | 3 | 17 | 16 | 61 | 23 | 24 | (2) | (2) |
| Semi-skilled manual | 0 | 6 | 7 | 14 | 44 | 31 | (1) | (1) |
| Unskilled | 0 | (1) | 2 | 3 | 6 | 41 | 0 | 0 |
| Unclassified or never employed | 0 | 0 | 0 | 0 | 0 | 0 | (3) | 0 |
| Armed services | 0 | 0 | (1) | 0 | 0 | 0 | 0 | 0 |
| *Base = 100%* | *63* | *164* | *342* | *407* | *208* | *42* | *13* | *7* |
| | | | | HALS1 Age 39-59 | | | | |
| Professional | 71 | 2 | 7 | 2 | 0 | 0 | 0 | 0 |
| Employers, managers | 12 | 62 | 11 | 8 | 5 | 0 | (2) | 0 |
| Other non-manual | 15 | 19 | 71 | 9 | 8 | 6 | 0 | (1) |
| Skilled manual | 1 | 10 | 5 | 67 | 16 | 15 | (1) | (2) |
| Semi-skilled manual | 1 | 5 | 6 | 9 | 61 | 17 | 0 | (2) |
| Unskilled | 0 | 2 | (1) | 6 | 9 | 62 | 0 | 0 |
| Unclassified or never employed | 0 | 0 | 0 | 0 | 0 | 0 | (1) | 0 |
| Armed services | 0 | 0 | 0 | 0 | 0 | 0 | 0 | (2) |
| *Base = 100%* | *76* | *268* | *213* | *362* | *152* | *53* | *4* | *7* |
| | | | | HALS1 Age 60+ | | | | |
| Professional | 66 | 0 | 2 | 0 | 0 | 0 | 0 | 0 |
| Employers, managers | 6 | 54 | 2 | 4 | 2 | 0 | 0 | (1) |
| Other non-manual | 23 | 25 | 80 | 13 | 13 | 6 | 0 | (1) |
| Skilled manual | 0 | 9 | 4 | 58 | 7 | 3 | 0 | 0 |
| Semi-skilled manual | 6 | 10 | 11 | 17 | 67 | 28 | 0 | 0 |
| Unskilled | 0 | 2 | (1) | 7 | 12 | 64 | 0 | (1) |
| Unclassified or never employed | 0 | 0 | 0 | 0 | 0 | 0 | (5) | 0 |
| Armed services | 0 | 0 | 0 | (1) | 0 | 0 | 0 | (1) |
| *Base = 100%* | *35* | *115* | *125* | *206* | *138* | *36* | *5* | *4* |

# PATTERNS OF MORTALITY | 3

## Mildred Blaxter and A Toby Prevost

Between the first and second Surveys, deaths of respondents were notified by the Office of Population Censuses and Surveys (OPCS). Thus it is possible, for the first time in a British all-age population sample, to relate mortality, over the limited time-span of 7 years, to the very wide range of characteristics recorded in 1984/5.

A small proportion of the sample (323 individuals) had unknown survival status at the time of the second Survey: they were neither reported as dead, nor traced for re-interview. Thus the original sample of 9003 is reduced, for the purpose of this chapter, to 8680, the number known to be either dead or alive in 1991/2.

There were 808 known deaths at the time of the second Survey: 687 reported by OPCS and an additional 121 found to have died, from information from relatives or householders, when the sample was being contacted in 1991. Of the OPCS-reported deaths, death certificates were not available in 20 cases, nor were they available for the additional 121. The number of deaths where cause of death is known is, therefore, reduced to 667.

The respondents entered the study at different times during the first rounds of fieldwork in 1984/5. This analysis is based, however, on exactly seven years for each respondent, from the date of the first interview in 1984/5 to the date when the second interview would have been held in 1991/2.

Mortality rates over the 7 years, by age in 1984/5 (Figure 3.1), were compared for England and Wales with the cumulative national OPCS rates for the relevant years. (Mortality rates for Scotland are published separately, and the numbers in the survey sample are too small for accurate rates by age for this Region separately.) Taking into account the age-distribution of the sample, expected deaths among men, excluding Scotland, should have totalled 388, and among women 358. Ascertained deaths in England and Wales were 366 and 354 respectively.

Among women, expected and observed deaths matched closely at almost all ages, though there was some shortfall in observed deaths at ages 18-44. Any rates for young women should be regarded with caution, because of the effect of this discrepancy combined with the very small numbers of deaths at these ages. For men, there was some excess of observed over expected deaths among the 18-44 age group, and fewer deaths than expected mainly among those aged 65-74 in 1984/5: 121 compared with an expected 135. In general, however, it appears that the rates presented here are a representative sample of mortality experience in the population between 1984/5 and 1991/2. Table 3.1 shows the cause of death for the 667 deaths with this information.

## Mortality by area of residence

Mortality rates are known to be higher in the north of the country than in the south. Figure 3.2 demonstrates that the northern excess was, as expected, primarily in middle age, though for men higher rates appeared in the North and West at every age up to the 75 + group. In old age, rates obviously converge. Overall, controlling for age distribution in 5-year bands up to 85 +, males in the North and West had 1.56 times the odds of dying during the 7 years, compared with males in the South and East.

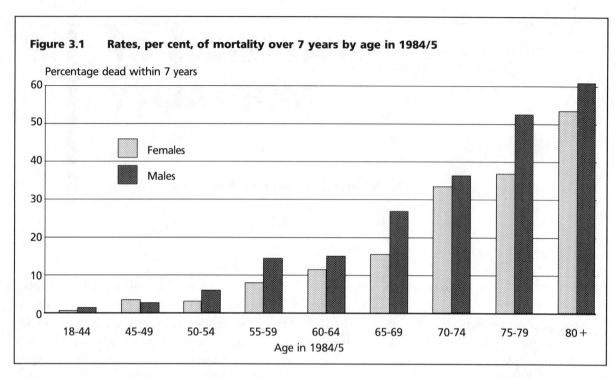

**Figure 3.1    Rates, per cent, of mortality over 7 years by age in 1984/5**

In the South and East, the mortality experience of the different Regions did not differ greatly. The North and West disadvantage was, however, primarily in the North Region and in Scotland and Wales for both men and women, and in the West Midlands for men. The North West Region's mortality was less, and similar to that of southern regions (Table 3.2).

## Mortality by social class

The report of the first Survey offered much evidence about class differences in illness experience. Figure 3.3 and Table 3.3 demonstrate the parallel trends in mortality. As usual, differences between non-manual and manual classes were greatest, especially for men, in late middle age. Table 3.3, distinguishing classes more precisely, shows the remarkably smooth gradients in all-age mortality which run through them, though patterns for specific age-groups may be more irregular. Table 3.4, considering the most numerous causes of death, shows that of the four major causes of mortality, it was very notably ischaemic heart disease (IHD) that accounted for the manual class disadvantage, especially at older ages. Under 65 (though numbers of deaths are often too small for reliable rates) each of the four disease categories contributed to class differences, with IHD prominent for men and cancers prominent for women. After age 65 rates of IHD and of lung

cancer were notably higher for both men and women in manual classes, but rates of other cancers were lower than those in non-manual classes.

The higher mortality rates in the North and West, compared with the South and East, which were demonstrated in Figure 3.2 are confounded by social class, since the North contains a higher proportion of manual classes. Table 3.5 considers rates for non-manual/manual social classes according to region of residence in 1984/5. For most age/sex groups, certainly over the age of 54, the class differences are apparent in both areas. In non-manual classes, however, the difference attributable to region was small or, at some ages, even reversed. Overall, the mortality rate was slightly higher in the South than in the North. Among manual classes, on the other hand, the mortality rate was consistently higher (up to 75+) in the North. The possibility that 'manual' occupations differ in the North and South must be considered: this does, however, support the general finding reported for the 1984/5 Survey, that the environment appeared to weigh more heavily on manual than on non-manual social classes.

## Mortality by marital status

Marital status is another characteristic which is considered in national mortality figures, showing that those who remain single after youth, and those who are separated, divorced or widowed, have a

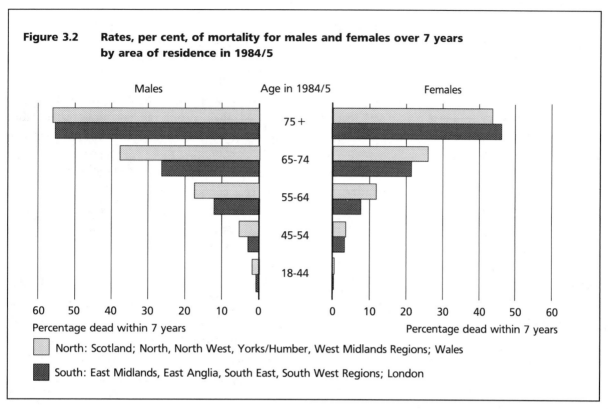

**Figure 3.2    Rates, per cent, of mortality for males and females over 7 years by area of residence in 1984/5**

North: Scotland; North, North West, Yorks/Humber, West Midlands Regions; Wales

South: East Midlands, East Anglia, South East, South West Regions; London

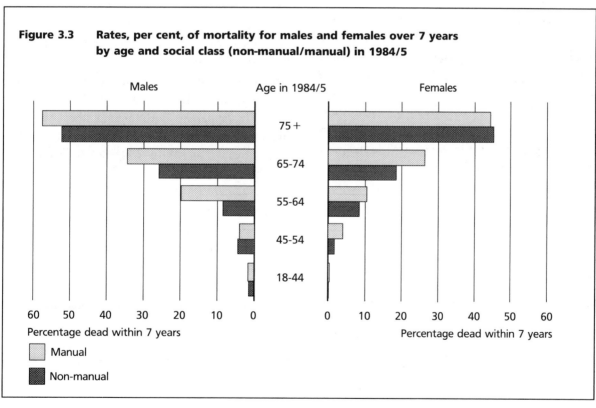

**Figure 3.3    Rates, per cent, of mortality for males and females over 7 years by age and social class (non-manual/manual) in 1984/5**

Manual

Non-manual

greater likelihood of death at earlier ages than the married. It was demonstrated clearly in the first Survey that married men (but not women) tended to be healthier, age for age, than those who were not married. These differences are confirmed by the mortality rates shown in Table 3.6. It must be noted that they are based on marital status in 1984/5, which in many cases will have changed. The rates must also be considered in relation to the 'normal' status at each age. For the youngest group, the 'not married' are predominantly single, and are on average younger within the group than the married. In the oldest group, the majority of the 'not married' are widowed, and are older on average. It is not surprising that, for both men and women, the 'not married' had higher death rates after the age of 65. Despite the weighting of age within the group, however, the married had lower mortality than the unmarried, among men but not women, at every age to 55. The different 'not married' categories have, for most age groups, both numbers of deaths and base numbers which are too small for reliable rates. Notable rates do, however, include a relatively very high rate of 2.3% for separated/divorced women aged 18-44 (on a base number of 176 individuals).

## Predictors of mortality

The most powerful predictor for the probability of earlier death is, of course, the existence of serious disease. All-age seven-year mortality rates for those who, in 1984/5, had 'limiting' chronic conditions were 21.3% for males and 19.6% for females, compared with 8.7% and 5.9% for those with no such disease.

Severe ill-health also affects the characteristics – life circumstances, behavioural patterns – which may be investigated as possible predictors. The analysis of the first Survey showed, however, that it was only those people who declared that they suffered from what was defined as limiting disease who differed, in behaviour and other characteristics, from those with no disease. It was also demonstrated that there was a considerable social class or educational bias in the replies to the question about 'any longstanding illness', but that this did not apply to limiting conditions.

For these reasons, Tables 3.7-3.11 focus on those who, in 1984/5, had no limiting disease: they present a preliminary analysis of possible predictors of earlier death without the complicating factor of the presence, at the date when predictor variables were established, of (known or declared) more serious ill health.

One of the strongest predictors was the reply to the question 'Would you say that for someone of your own age your health in general is excellent/ good/fair/poor?' This would not be surprising for those who were aware that they were suffering from serious disease, but as Table 3.7 shows, even among those without current limiting disease, mortality rates were higher at all ages, among men, for those who described their health as fair/poor, rather than excellent/good. For women this was true only after age 55. Among men, those who thought their health was fair/poor were almost twice as likely to die in the seven-year period as those who thought that it was excellent/good. It has to be concluded, as found in other studies (Berkham and Syme, 1979), that subjective knowledge of ill health, even in the absence of (known) disease, has validity.

Symptoms of general malaise (tiredness, worrying, stress, etc.) were also associated with the probability of mortality, though only among older people. An absence of malaise (low scores on the malaise scale used in the analysis of the 1984/5 survey) appeared to be protective in older age, when compared with average/high malaise scores (Table 3.8).

Scores on the General Health Questionnaire were also predictive (Table 3.9), particularly at older ages. The presence of physical ill health is, of course, strongly associated with higher GHQ scores, as the table indicates. The association with mortality is, however, apparent both among those without limiting disease at the time when the GHQ schedule was answered, and those who did have chronic ill health: indeed, it appears to be stronger, in late middle age, for those without disease than for those with.

Among the physiological measures made in 1984/5, Body Mass Index provided a clear association with mortality over the next 7 years. Those who had limiting disease at the time were more likely to be under- or overweight than those without disease: 10.6% of the female measured sample with disease were underweight, for instance, compared with 4.1% of those without disease; 64.1% of those with disease were overweight, compared with 26.9%. The age-distribution of those with and without disease was of course different, with the diseased being older. Underweight appeared to be a particular risk factor for men with disease (all-age odds ratio (OR) 2.5 (1.52, 4.10)), but – as far as can be shown with sometimes small numbers – deviation

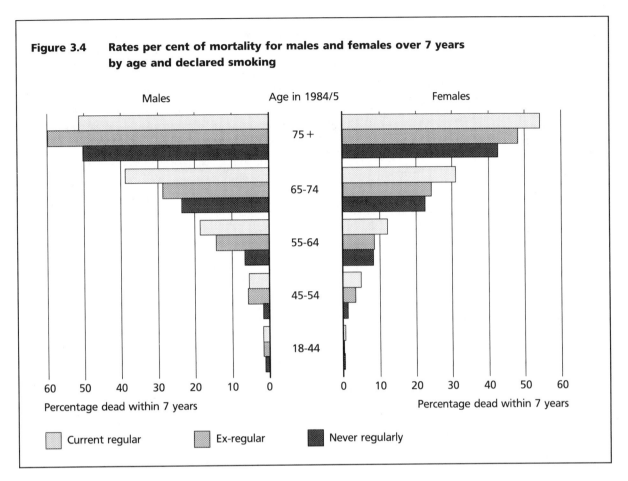

**Figure 3.4    Rates per cent of mortality for males and females over 7 years by age and declared smoking**

Males          Age in 1984/5          Females

75 +

65-74

55-64

45-54

18-44

60  50  40  30  20  10   0        0  10  20  30  40  50  60

Percentage dead within 7 years          Percentage dead within 7 years

Current regular      Ex-regular      Never regularly

from an 'acceptable' weight was not otherwise clearly associated with mortality for men or women already suffering serious ill health.

For those with no (known) disease at the time, on the other hand, both under- and overweight were predictive of mortality from the age of 60 for men and the age of 65 for women, though not at younger ages (Table 3.10). Underweight men 60+ had a particularly high risk, with OR 4.02 (1.93, 8.37), as did underweight women 65+ (but on small numbers).

Because of evidence from elsewhere (Syme, 1974) that 'usual' hours of sleep is predictive of ill health and even mortality, this was also tested in this sample. Here, it is similarly important to control for existing disease, since more or (particularly) less than an average range is a characteristic of ill health: 16.4% of those who declared a limiting disease said, in 1984/5, that they slept under 6 hours, compared with 7.6% of those without disease. Confining the analysis to those without disease (Table 3.11), to sleep less than the standard 6-8 hours was strongly predictive of mortality rates, especially among older men. To sleep for over 8 hours was also associated with

mortality rates, especially for older women, though to a lesser degree.

Among behavioural habits, smoking provides an example of a remarkably regular association with mortality for both men and women at all ages up to the very oldest (Figure 3.4). (Here, there is no reason to distinguish those with disease or without, since there is no confusion about the direction of assumed causation.)

Table 3.12 explores further the effect of giving up smoking, distinguishing those who, in 1984/5, were long-term ex-smokers and those who had given up within the previous 10 years. It must be emphasised that there is no information about smoking habits between 1984/5 and the time of death: while never-smokers and very long-term ex-smokers may have been unlikely to begin, many of the 'ex-smokers', if the period was short, may have become smokers again – in the first Survey many described frequent abortive attempts to stop. Even long-term ex-smokers, however, had poorer mortality rates than never-smokers, from middle-age in men but only after 65 for women.

## Summary

Some of the potential of this sample for the investigation of characteristics associated with mortality has been illustrated, though many possible factors remain to be investigated. Unemployment, and the nature of work, are obviously factors of interest, but deaths are too few at young ages for reliable analysis. Other variables which may prove to be important include, in particular, the effects of social support and social interaction, shown in many studies to have important independent effects (Welin et al. 1985, Orth-Gomer and Johnson, 1987), detailed aspects of diet, and various possible predictors among the physiological and psychological measurements which are available.

### References

Berkman, L.F. and Syme S.L. (1979), 'Social networks, host resistance and mortality: a nine-year follow-up study of Alameda County Residents', Am. J. Epidemiology, 109, 186-204.

Orth-Gomer, K., and Johnson, J.V. (1987), 'Social interaction and mortality: a six-year follow-up study of a random sample of the Swedish population', J. Chronic Disease, 40, 949-57.

Syme, S.L. (1974), 'Behavioural factors associated with the etiology of physical disease', Am. J. Public Health, 64, 1043-5.

Welin, L., Tibblin, G., Svardsudd, K., et al. (1985), 'Prospective study of social influences on mortality', Lancet 1, 915-18.

**Table 3.1    Rates/1000 of mortality over 7 years by cause of death (number of deaths in brackets)**

| Age in 1984/5 | Males | | | | Females | | | |
|---|---|---|---|---|---|---|---|---|
| | 18-44 | 45-64 | 65-74 | 75+ | 18-44 | 45-64 | 65-74 | 75+ |
| Neoplasm of lung etc ICD162 | – | 10.9 (13) | 32.0 (14) | 37.8 (8) | – | 7.2 (11) | 8.7 (5) | – (2) |
| Neoplasm of uterus, breast, cervix ICD 174-182 | – | – | – | – (3) | – | 3.9 (6) | 5.2 (7) | – (3) |
| Other neoplasm ICD140-161, 163-173, 183-239 | 3.1 (6) | 11.8 (14) | 66.2 (29) | 73.9 (17) | – (2) | 15.1 (23) | 22.6 (13) | 43.9 (16) |
| Diseases of respiratory system ICD 460-519 | – | 7.6 (9) | 32.0 (14) | 65.2 (15) | – (1) | – (3) | 17.4 (10) | 46.8 (16) |
| Ischaemic heart disease ICD 410-414 | 2.1 (4) | 32.8 (39) | 73.1 (32) | 152.2 (35) | – | 4.6 (7) | 53.9 (31) | 131.6 (45) |
| Other diseases of circulatory system ICD 390-409, 415-458 | – (1) | 8.4 (10) | 32.0 (14) | 104.3 (24) | – (1) | 9.2 (14) | 50.4 (29) | 99.4 (34) |
| Other causes | 3.7 (7) | 8.4 (10) | 25.1 (11) | 65.2 (15) | – (2) | 9.2 (14) | 24.3 (14) | 40.9 (14) |
| Cause unknown % of all deaths | (8) 31 | (20) 17 | (24) 17 | (14) 11 | (2) 18 | (21) 21 | (28) 20 | (24) 16 |
| *Base* | *1909* | *1188* | *438* | *230* | *2471* | *1527* | *575* | *342* |

ICD Chapters with numbers too small for useful rates included in 'other causes of death' above, include: diseases of nervous system, 8 deaths in total; endocrine etc. disorders (including diabetes), 14; mental disorders, 8; diseases of digestive system, 20; diseases of genito-urinary system, 8; accidents, poisoning and violence, 18.

**Table 3.2    Odds ratios for the greater probability of mortality over 7 years in the 'North and West' Regions, compared with the 'South and East'**

| | Males | | Females | |
|---|---|---|---|---|
| Overall Odds Ratios for N and W compared with S and E (95% confidence intervals in brackets) | 1.56 | (1.23, 1.98) | 1.24 | (0.98, 1.57) |
| Separate Regions: | | | | |
| Scotland | 1.56 | (1.03, 2.35) | 1.48 | (1.01, 2.19) |
| North | 2.77 | (1.74, 4.41) | 2.03 | (1.31, 3.12) |
| North West | 0.99 | (0.66, 1.48) | 0.84 | (0.56, 1.26) |
| Yorks/Humber | 1.48 | (0.97, 2.26) | 1.04 | (0.68, 1.58) |
| West Midlands | 1.92 | (1.27, 2.91) | 1.14 | (0.74, 1.74) |
| Wales | 1.54 | (0.88, 2.69) | 1.47 | (0.89, 2.44) |

**Table 3.3**  **Mortality, per cent, over 7 years by respondent's social class in 1984/5 (Sample sizes in brackets)**

| Age in 1984/5 | 18-44 | 45-54 | 55-64 | 65-74 | 75+ | All |
|---|---|---|---|---|---|---|
| | | | **Males** | | | |
| Professional and managerial | 0.8 | 4.8 | 8.8 | 21.5 | 58.7 | 7.8 |
| | (490) | (187) | (170) | (107) | (46) | (1000) |
| Other non-manual | 2.1 | 3.4 | 6.7 | 35.4 | 40.0 | 8.7 |
| | (243) | (58) | (75) | (48) | (25) | (449) |
| Skilled manual | 2.0 | 3.2 | 18.4 | 31.8 | 59.6 | 12.1 |
| | (713) | (219) | (206) | (157) | (99) | (1394) |
| Semi and unskilled manual | 0.5 | 5.6 | 20.1 | 37.9 | 54.2 | 14.1 |
| | (398) | (107) | (164) | (124) | (59) | (852) |
| | | | **Females** | | | |
| Professional and managerial | 0.1 | 1.4 | 6.5 | 15.9 | 44.4 | 5.3 |
| | (674) | (277) | (201) | (138) | (72) | (1362) |
| Other non-manual | 0.2 | 3.7 | 12.7 | 23.5 | 46.0 | 8.2 |
| | (440) | (81) | (102) | (68) | (63) | (754) |
| Skilled manual | 0.5 | 5.5 | 9.6 | 27.8 | 46.7 | 9.6 |
| | (781) | (256) | (261) | (198) | (122) | (1618) |
| Semi and unskilled manual | 0.8 | 1.9 | 11.9 | 25.2 | 40.5 | 9.1 |
| | (516) | (156) | (176) | (159) | (74) | (1081) |

**Table 3.4**   **Mortality, per thousand, over 7 years from selected causes, by non-manual/manual social class in 1984/5 (number of deaths in brackets)**

| Cause | Males | | Females | |
|---|---|---|---|---|
| | Non-manual | Manual | Non-manual | Manual |
| | Age 18-64 in 1984/5 | | | |
| Neoplasm of lung etc. | – | 5.5 | 2.3 | 3.3 |
| | (3) | (10) | (4) | (7) |
| Other neoplasms | 5.7 | 7.2 | 3.9 | 11.6 |
| | (7) | (13) | (7) | (25) |
| Ischaemic heart disease | 9.0 | 17.7 | – | – |
| | (11) | (32) | (3) | (4) |
| Other diseases of circulatory system | – | 4.4 | – | 5.6 |
| | (3) | (8) | (3) | (12) |
| *Base* | *1233* | *1807* | *1775* | *2146* |
| | Age 65+ in 1984/5 | | | |
| Neoplasm of lung etc. | 22.1 | 38.7 | – | 9.0 |
| | (5) | (17) | (2) | (5) |
| Other neoplasms | 75.2 | 66.1 | 46.9 | 39.8 |
| | (17) | (29) | (16) | (22) |
| Ischaemic heart disease | 79.6 | 111.6 | 58.7 | 95.8 |
| | (18) | (49) | (20) | (53) |
| Other diseases of circulatory system | 57.5 | 56.9 | 64.5 | 68.7 |
| | (13) | (25) | (22) | (38) |
| *Base* | *226* | *439* | *341* | *553* |

**Table 3.5**  **Mortality, per cent, over 7 years, by social class and region of residence in 1984/5 (Sample sizes in brackets)**

| Age in 1984/5 | | 18-44 | 45-54 | 55-64 | 65-74 | 75+ | All |
|---|---|---|---|---|---|---|---|
| | | | | **Males** | | | |
| Non-manual | North | 1.8 (333) | 4.3 (117) | 11.9 (84) | 26.3 (57) | 46.7 (30) | 8.1 (621) |
| | South | 0.8 (400) | 4.7 (128) | 6.2 (161) | 25.5 (98) | 56.7 (41) | 8.1 (828) |
| Manual | North | 1.9 (646) | 5.9 (188) | 20.2 (203) | 42.6 (141) | 59.3 (86) | 13.8 (1264) |
| | South | 0.9 (465) | (2) (138) | 18.0 (167) | 26.4 (140) | 55.6 (72) | 11.5 (982) |
| | | | | **Females** | | | |
| Non-manual | North | (2) (526) | (2) (177) | 8.3 (133) | 19.8 (91) | 50.9 (53) | 6.1 (980) |
| | South | 0.0 (588) | 2.8 (181) | 8.8 (170) | 17.4 (115) | 41.5 (82) | 6.5 (1136) |
| Manual | North | 0.8 (760) | 4.6 (241) | 13.2 (272) | 28.4 (222) | 39.6 (106) | 9.9 (1601) |
| | South | (2) (537) | 3.5 (171) | 6.1 (165) | 23.7 (135) | 50.0 (90) | 8.7 (1098) |

Odds Ratios of North compared with South, controlling for age in ten 5-year bands (to 85 +): Non-manual males: 1.19 not significant, females: 1.19 not significant; Manual males: 1.58 (1.17, 2.12), females: 1.21 not significant. 'North' and 'South': See Figure. 3.2.

**Table 3.6**  **Mortality, per cent, over 7 years by marital status in 1984/5**

| Age in 1984/5 | **Males** | | | | **Females** | | | |
|---|---|---|---|---|---|---|---|---|
| | 18-44 | 45-54 | 55-64 | 65+ | 18-44 | 45-54 | 55-64 | 65+ |
| Married/partnered | 1.1 (1236) | 3.9 (490) | 13.6 (530) | 38.7 (486) | 0.4 (1793) | 3.2 (625) | 9.0 (544) | 25.8 (399) |
| Single, separated, divorced, widowed | 1.8 (672) | 6.2 (81) | 21.8 (87) | 42.9 (182) | 0.6 (678) | 3.3 (151) | 12.1 (207) | 36.3 (518) |

**Table 3.7**  **Mortality, per cent, over 7 years, according to own assessment of health as excellent/good or fair/poor in 1984/5 for those without chronic disease at that time (Sample sizes in brackets)**

| Age in 1984/5 | 18-44 | 45-54 | 55-64 | 65-74 | 75+ | All |
|---|---|---|---|---|---|---|
| | | | **Males** | | | |
| Excellent/good | 1.1 | 4.0 | 11.2 | 21.9 | 48.5 | 7.7 |
| | (1330) | (377) | (348) | (242) | (136) | (2433) |
| Fair/poor | 1.7 | 4.5 | 15.8 | 50.0 | 58.8 | 12.0 |
| | (403) | (88) | (95) | (74) | (34) | (694) |
| | | | **Females** | | | |
| Excellent/good | 0.4 | 2.8 | 5.9 | 16.4 | 35.2 | 4.9 |
| | (1782) | (500) | (442) | (304) | (165) | (3193) |
| Fair/poor | 0.2 | 2.0 | 16.3 | 28.9 | 49.2 | 9.3 |
| | (456) | (147) | (123) | (90) | (65) | (881) |

Odds ratios of fair/poor compared with excellent/good, controlling for age in ten 5-year bands (to 85+): Males: OR 2.00 (1.45, 2.75); Females: OR age 18-59, not significant; age 60+, 2.39 (1.69, 3.38).

**Table 3.8**  **Mortality, per cent, over 7 years in relation to malaise symptoms in 1984/5 for those without chronic disease at that time (Sample sizes in brackets)**

| Age in 1984/5 | 18-54 | 55-64 | 65-74 | 75+ |
|---|---|---|---|---|
| | | **Males** | | |
| Without malaise symptoms | 2.0 | 12.6 | 21.3 | 46.4 |
| | (933) | (253) | (197) | (97) |
| With malaise symptoms | 1.7 | 12.0 | 40.2 | 55.4 |
| | (1269) | (191) | (122) | (74) |
| | | **Females** | | |
| Without malaise symptoms | 1.0 | 6.8 | 16.6 | 31.7 |
| | (894) | (207) | (169) | (104) |
| With malaise symptoms | 0.8 | 8.9 | 21.2 | 46.2 |
| | (2001) | (361) | (226) | (130) |

**Table 3.9** **Mortality, per cent, over 7 years by scores on General Health Questionnaire in 1984/5 (Sample sizes in brackets)**

| Age in 1984/5 | 18-44 | 45-54 | 55-64 | 65-74 | 75+ | All |
|---|---|---|---|---|---|---|
| | | | Without chronic disease in 1984/5 | | | |
| **Males** | | | | | | |
| GHQ score < 5 | 1.0 | 4.2 | 9.7 | 21.5 | 44.4 | 6.9 |
| | (935) | (260) | (267) | (195) | (72) | (1729) |
| GHQ score 5+ | 2.7 | 3.8 | 9.7 | 40.0 | 60.0 | 10.7 |
| | (298) | (79) | (62) | (35) | (40) | (514) |
| **Females** | | | | | | |
| GHQ score < 5 | 0.3 | 2.8 | 6.7 | 14.3 | 26.6 | 3.8 |
| | (1142) | (327) | (282) | (168) | (79) | (1998) |
| GHQ score 5+ | 0.6 | 2.8 | 9.7 | 17.2 | 54.1 | 5.6 |
| | (503) | (145) | (93) | (64) | (37) | (842) |
| | | | With chronic disease in 1984/5 | | | |
| **Males** | | | | | | |
| GHQ score < 5 | (1) | (2) | 16.7 | 31.1 | 64.7 | 16.0 |
| | (71) | (45) | (78) | (45) | (17) | (256) |
| GHQ score 5+ | (1) | (2) | 25.9 | 46.2 | 66.7 | 22.9 |
| | (56) | (33) | (58) | (39) | (15) | (201) |
| **Females** | | | | | | |
| GHQ score < 5 | (1) | (1) | 13.0 | 29.7 | 46.7 | 13.7 |
| | (81) | (40) | (77) | (64) | (15) | (277) |
| GHQ score 5+ | (1) | 9.6 | 18.6 | 36.0 | 56.7 | 18.8 |
| | (86) | (52) | (59) | (50) | (30) | (277) |

Odds ratios of 5+ compared with < 5, controlling for age in ten 5-year bands (to 85+): Without chronic disease: males 1.74 (1.18, 2.58), females 1.67 (1.10, 2.53); with chronic disease: males 1.62 (0.95, 2.79), females 1.52 (0.91, 2.54).

**Table 3.10** **Mortality, per cent, over 7 years according to Body Mass Index (underweight, acceptable weight, overweight) in 1984/5 for those without chronic disease at that time (Sample sizes in brackets)**

| Age in 1984/5 | Males | | | Females | | |
|---|---|---|---|---|---|---|
| | 18-44 | 45-64 | 65+ | 18-44 | 45-64 | 65+ |
| Underweight | 0.0 | 20.0 | 68.0 | 0.0 | (1) | 60.0 |
| | (138) | (30) | (25) | (92) | (25) | (20) |
| Acceptable weight | 1.5 | 4.4 | 30.9 | 0.6 | 5.3 | 22.5 |
| | (843) | (293) | (178) | (1087) | (396) | (151) |
| Overweight | 1.0 | 8.0 | 32.3 | (1) | 4.2 | 24.2 |
| | (511) | (440) | (189) | (628) | (542) | (256) |

Odds ratios of underweight compared with acceptable, controlling for age in ten 5-year bands (to 85+): males: 2.72 (1.49, 4.98), females: 2.43 (1.11, 5.32).

**Table 3.11** **Mortality, per cent, over 7 years by declared 'usual' hours of sleep in 1984/5, for those without limiting disease at that time (Sample sizes in brackets)**

| Age in 1984/5 | 18-44 | 45-64 | 65+ | All |
|---|---|---|---|---|
| Hours of sleep | Males | | | |
| < 6 | 2.8 | 6.8 | 43.9 | 13.8 |
| | (109) | (74) | (57) | (240) |
| 6 – 8 | 1.1 | 7.8 | 33.2 | 7.2 |
| | (1160) | (650) | (253) | (2063) |
| 8+ | 1.3 | 9.2 | 37.8 | 11.0 |
| | (462) | (185) | (180) | (827) |
| | Females | | | |
| < 6 | 1.0 | 6.8 | 26.3 | 11.5 |
| | (104) | (133) | (118) | (355) |
| 6 – 8 | 0.2 | 4.7 | 24.1 | 4.9 |
| | (1369) | (779) | (340) | (2488) |
| 8+ | 0.5 | 5.6 | 32.7 | 6.0 |
| | (771) | (306) | (165) | (1242) |

**Table 3.12** **Mortality, per cent, over 7 years of those who described themselves as non-smokers or ex-smokers in 1984/5 (Sample sizes in brackets)**

| Age in 1984/5 | Males | | | Females | | |
|---|---|---|---|---|---|---|
| | 18-44 | 45-64 | 65+ | 18-44 | 45-64 | 65+ |
| Smoking in 1984/5 | | | | | | |
| Never smoked | 1.0 | 3.2 | 31.7 | 3.4 | 4.7 | 29.8 |
| | (743) | (249) | (101) | (1170) | (639) | (523) |
| Ex-smokers for over 10 years | (1) | 9.6 | 38.8 | 0.0 | 4.4 | 32.6 |
| | (83) | (218) | (188) | (116) | (158) | (132) |
| Ex-smokers for up to 10 years | 1.4 | 11.8 | 42.4 | 3.3 | 8.3 | 35.2 |
| | (278) | (212) | (139) | (304) | (169) | (88) |

# PHYSICAL
# HEALTH

# CHANGES IN SELF-REPORTED HEALTH | 4

**Virginia J Swain**

The validity and usefulness of self-reported data on health to epidemiologists, clinicians and others within the fields of medicine and health research is perhaps more widely accepted now than it was at the time of HALS1; nonetheless it is still a subject open to discussion and examination. Halabi et al. (1992) found, for example, that the reporting of well-defined chronic conditions, such as heart disease, was in close agreement with reports from proxy informants. Questions may also arise about the interpretation placed on the changing views of any given population under investigation. As the General Household Survey (1992) (GHS) for 1991 points out, when collecting information on people's subjective assessments of their own health, 'changes over time may reflect changes in people's expectations of their health as well as in the prevalence...of sickness'. Whether or not self-evaluation or changes in personal assessment of health are regarded as a reliable means of assessing 'objective' health or prevalence of morbidity, in Chapter 3 it is shown that self-evaluation of health is a predictor of mortality (even when disease is controlled for). Self-assessment and changes over time in views and attitudes are an important part of the multi-dimensional experience of health and ill-health.

Two trends are to be expected in the reporting of illness and disease when a population is re-interviewed after a 7 year interval. The first is that such reporting will largely follow an upward trend, and the second is that greater numbers of those suffering from more severe or chronic illness will be unavailable at the time of the second Survey. In the present work the latter potential problem has been overcome to some extent by including some tables divided into 7 year age groups, with the full HALS1 sample percentages included. This enables the reader to see the attrition rate in any particular group and then to compare people of the same age at two points in time or to follow the same group 7 years on in their life.

## Self Assessed Health Status

The question asking respondents in HALS2 whether they assessed their health as 'excellent', 'good', 'fair' or 'poor' was in the same format as in HALS1, asking people to judge their health status 'compared with someone of your age'.

The first Table (4.1) shows how the HALS population has changed in their assessment of their health, using the complete HALS1 sample, to see if certain groups have been disproportionately lost in the follow-up Survey. In fact, apart from a higher attrition rate with the youngest, male, age group it is not until the older age groups that wider gaps between HALS1 and HALS2 occur in both men and women who reported fair or poor health in 1984/5. More women up to age 66 are reporting excellent health in HALS2 both compared to the same age group seven years ago and their own group as it was in 1984/5. For men and women, at all ages, the reporting of fair or poor health has remained quite stable in most groups and has even fallen in some.

Differences in self-evaluated health, identified at HALS1 (Cox et al. 1987), are still apparent between socio-economic groups. (Table 4.2 – Table 4.4). Using HALS1 classifications, women in the non-manual socio-economic group are much more likely to report improved health status than are those in the manual group, wide differences being evident at all ages (Table 4.2). There is a similar trend for men after the age of 39, the biggest gap occurring between the groups after 60 years of age. However, for the men between 18 and 38 in the manual group there is an interesting anomaly: 64% reported that their health had changed from fair or poor to excellent or good compared with 55% in the non-manual group. Table 4.3 shows that men and women in the non-manual group who reported excellent or good health at HALS1, were much more likely to report the same 7 years on compared with their counterparts in the manual group. Only approximately 10% of those between 18 and 59 years of age reported a deterioration in their health status, whereas in the manual groups both sexes reported a greater decline of health at an earlier age. When the non-manual and manual groups are further divided in Table 4.4 the youngest men in the semi-skilled manual group at HALS1 have improved the most.

The standard Regions have been grouped into 'North': Scotland; Wales; North; North West; Yorks/ Humber; West Midlands and 'South': East Midlands; East Anglia; South East; South West; London. Table 4.5, shows a similar trend to that found in HALS1. In 1984/5 more people (except women in the oldest age group), in the North reported their health as only fair or poor and this pattern has been repeated in 1991/2; indeed the gap widens as age advances for all but the youngest group of men. The 'improvement' in health already referred to in young males in the manual social class is also evident at a regional level. Only 19% of 18-38 year old men in both North and South regions are now reporting fair or poor health compared with 28% in the North and 24% in the South at HALS1.

In the follow-up Survey respondents were asked 'do you think compared to 7 years ago your health is generally . . . better, worse or about the same?' Those who replied 'better' or 'worse', were asked if it was a bit or a lot better/worse. Table 4.6 shows the same pattern as before with an 'improvement' in health being reported by more young men in the manual social class than by their non-manual counterparts. After the age of 39 the more usual differences between the social classes are apparent. Men and women in the non-manual group and in the middle age group are more likely to report no change; men and women in the manual group are much more likely to say their health has deteriorated. This evens out slightly in the oldest group as more men in manual occupations, (but not women), assess their health as 'the same'. Nonetheless, men in the non-manual group, over 60, are still twice as likely to report better health than men in the manual class. For the oldest group of women, although differences between social class groups were small for reporting health as 'the same', more women in the non-manual group report better health whereas more women within the manual class report a decline in health.

Table 4.7 illustrates how people assessed improvement or deterioration of their health, according to their disease status at HALS1 and HALS2. As one might expect, women (and men under 60) who reported the presence of disease in 1984/5 but not in 1991/2, were most likely to describe their health as 'a lot better'. But, men and women in this group and between the ages of 38 and 59 were also more likely to describe their health as worse than those without disease at both Surveys. In the women over 60, 27% reported their health as a 'bit worse'; a figure very close to both the women who reported disease at both Surveys and also to those who reported disease at HALS2 for the first time. In the middle age group more men and women who have developed disease since HALS1 reported their health as slightly worse; in the oldest group the percentage was about equal to those who had disease on both occasions. The middle and older age group of people who reported disease at both Surveys show more deterioration than any other group. The greater degree of change, either identifying their health as better or worse, by respondents who declared chronic illness in 1984/5 but not in 1991/2, could be due to several factors. Reported improvement of health may be explained by remission from disease; 'coming to terms' with long-standing illness, or more improved and effective treatments being used for certain conditions. Those who report a deterioration in health may or may not be 'free' of chronic illness but may be perceiving their health differently because of other influences such as ageing. Further, more detailed, analysis is needed to examine the types of illness and level of disability which may be associated with different patterns of reporting.

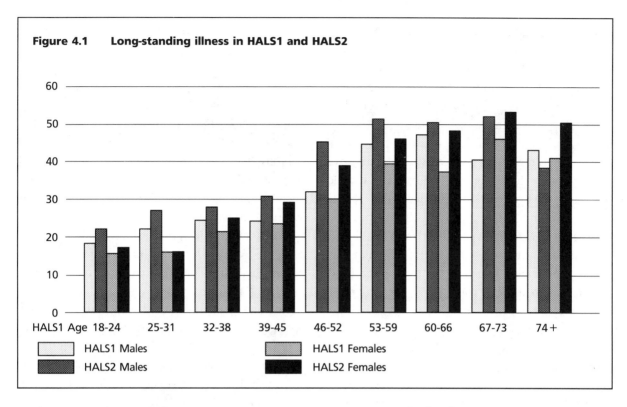

**Figure 4.1    Long-standing illness in HALS1 and HALS2**

## Disease and Disability

Although no changes were made to the open format question asking about current long-standing illness, disability or infirmity, slight modifications were made to the check-list of conditions 'ever suffered from' so that greater detail could be gained about different types of heart problems. Also, for the first time, respondents were asked if they had ever suffered from Myalgic Encephalomyelitis (ME) or Post-Viral Fatigue Syndrome. Information about the prevalence of ME is still scarce: Table 4.8 gives a breakdown of reported ME by sex, three broad age groups, social class and region. ME appears to be more common in women, at 2% compared to 1% for men overall. The percentage of women reporting ME was highest for those who live in the North or who are in non-manual occupational groups.

Figure 4.1 shows that the general trend of reported long-standing illness between HALS1 and HALS2 was slightly raised, although women who, at HALS2, were aged between 32 and 38 or 46 and 66 and men between 46 and 52 were less likely to report long-standing illness in HALS2 than respondents of the same age at HALS1. The GHS 1991 reports a fall in long-standing illness at all age groups between 1990 and 1991 after a steady increase during the

1980s. As with the first Survey, HALS2 showed slightly lower rates of long-standing illness and limiting long-standing illness than the GHS but finds similar differences between socio-economic groups. There have been quite a number of changes occurring during the 7 years for those who declared some degree of disease and disability in 1984/5, as shown in Table 4.9. Nearly a quarter of all men and almost a third of all women between 18 and 38 who reported having disease with moderate or severe handicap at HALS1 now report no chronic disease. Later analysis will examine these groups to see if they or their originally declared conditions differ in any way from other groups or illnesses.

The first Health and Lifestyle Report showed how respondents in the unemployed and manual groups in later years declared higher rates of chronic disease. Table 4.10 has been included to examine the changes in employment status of men who were aged 18-57 at HALS1 depending on their declared disease status at both Surveys. Although it is acknowledged that men at the oldest end of the age spectrum are more likely to be represented in the groups reporting long-standing illness, the overall employment 'snapshots' of three groups of working men at two points in time can still be examined. Of those who did not declare disease at either Survey, 93% were in employment when interviewed in 1984/5 and 1991/2 compared with only 79% of those who reported disease on both occasions and 76% who reported developing disease since 1984. The greatest changes have occurred to those who were unemployed in 1984/5. 62% of the 'healthy' men and 53% of those who declared chronic disease at both Surveys have moved into employment whereas only 28% of those who declared chronic disease for the first time at HALS2 have done so.

Some of the more prominent changes in the prevalence of diseases 'ever suffered from' are shown in Table 4.11 for men and women. Migraine has increased noticeably among the younger women and among men in the 25-31 and 60-66 age groups at HALS2. Heart problems have risen from 6.3% to 12.4% in men and from 5.4% to 9.7% in women. This increase is not only in the older groups but also occurs in the youngest group of men and in middle years for both sexes. The prevalence of asthma is known to be on the increase for adults as well as children (Alderson, 1987), as are other respiratory problems. The second Survey shows a marked increase in declared asthma, but not other respiratory problems, from 6.6% to 9.1% in men and from 5.1% to 8.6% in women, with a rise in reporting for both younger and older age groups. This has also been confirmed by higher rates of reported medication by the respondents when visited by the nurse (see Chapters 5 and 7). Diabetes also appears to be following an upward trend in the older groups. Among women between 60-66 at HALS2, 4.1% report having suffered from diabetes compared to only 1.8% of women aged 60-66 at HALS1. Similarly in men aged between 67 and 73 at HALS2, 7.3% reported diabetes at HALS2 compared with only 3.9% 7 years ago. The percentage of respondents declaring they had suffered with high blood-pressure at some time has risen during the 7 year period, despite the findings in the measured sample which show an overall decrease in median blood-pressure (see Chapter 5).

Although respondents were asked to identify, from a list, conditions or illnesses experienced at any time during their life, inconsistencies in reporting between HALS1 and HALS2 have occurred. Many illnesses which were reported as 'treated' or 'not-treated' at HALS1 were not reported at the second

Survey. For example, over a third of respondents who reported at HALS1 having had treatment for epilepsy at sometime in the past (n = 74), reported never having suffered from the condition at HALS2. Similarly – and more notably – 66% of those reporting, at HALS1, that they had suffered with, but not been treated for 'severe depression or other nervous illness' (n = 165) and 41% of those who had been treated (n = 756), when re-interviewed in 1991/2, stated that they had never been sufferers. It is not surprising to find such anomalies in reporting of this type of condition because despite campaigns both to promote knowledge and understanding about epilepsy and the widespread nature of mental illness in society, for many people there is still a sense of stigma and shame associated with such conditions. As expected, people were less likely to change in their reporting of any condition if it had been treated and were less likely to under-report an ailment such as asthma than say 'other chest problems'. However, even quite serious illnesses or events were not mentioned by some individuals and this will be investigated further at a later date.

It should be noted that in several instances the 'all' respondents values for the HALS2 sub-sample at HALS1 are slightly different from that for the HALS1 full sample. These differences when they occur are mostly due to the fact that the diseases or conditions being examined are contributors in terms of mortality to the attrition of the population in the older age groups. For example, this applies to heart and respiratory problems, but not apparently to asthma.

It must also be remembered that the HALS1 sample was selected from a population which had suffered some attrition from these very same diseases or conditions in the older age groups. With increasing age the HALS1 sample was sampling from a 'survivor' population. In almost all instances the HALS2 sub-sample is representative of the full HALS1 sample at the younger age groups when age standardised.

## Illness and Malaise

The same standard measure used at HALS1 for assessing illness and malaise has been used for the follow-up study. A check-list asked about symptoms experienced during the last month, and the illness and malaise scores are arrived at by adding together the number of symptoms reported (see Appendix A). Although respondents are only being asked about their recent experiences the score may have implications for more long-term self-evaluation of health. This information can be used to understand changing patterns in the types of symptoms declared by individuals and also to study possible relationships between the change in frequency of reporting particular symptoms and behavioural or social aspects of people's lives.

Table 4.12 shows examples of some symptoms which have been reported more or less frequently by respondents in the second Survey. Most people were interviewed at the same time of year on both occasions yet there has been a notable drop in the numbers of both men and women reporting having suffered with colds or flu during the last month before interview in 1991/2 compared with 1984/5. An overall increase in constipation has been reported by men, though not by women. For men the age groups most affected are between 32 and 45 and 53 and 59 at HALS2: there is a doubling of reported incidence compared with both the same group when they were seven years younger and the same age group in 1984/5. This may be associated with changing dietary habits identified in Chapter 11 and particularly in an apparent reduction in dietary fibre intake. Hay fever shows a consistent rise in both sexes over many age groups as does reporting of painful joints, even among the younger males. Although there has been no overall rise in reporting of headaches by women, the figures for younger women have gone up; a decrease after the age of 52 at HALS1 and HALS2 could be due to a post-menopausal effect. It should be noted that illness reporting is not necessarily expected to rise regularly with age, indeed, some symptoms are reported less as people get older.

Table 4.13 uses the additive score of illness to show the movement between 'low', 'average' and 'high' reporting of symptoms. The percentage of respondents reporting low rates of illness at HALS1 and HALS2 stays about the same in all age groups. However, men and women in the two oldest age groups who scored 'high' at the first Survey are much more likely to stay high scorers compared with their younger counterparts.

Analysis from the first Survey (Blaxter, 1990) demonstrated the beneficial effects of having a partner on psycho-social health (measured by malaise score) and perceived illness. Table 4.14 illustrates changes in illness and malaise scores for the 18-29 age group at HALS1 depending on whether the respondents were single at both times or whether they have subsequently become married. Men who were single on both occasions were slightly more likely to report low illness at HALS1 and HALS2 or to move to 'low' from 'average' and 'high'. Single women were more likely to stay 'low' but were also more likely to stay as average or high scorers at HALS1 and HALS2. In both cases the differences were not great, and much larger differences were evident when malaise scores were used. Here an apparent beneficial effect of having a partner is evident for men and women. Those who have become married are much more likely to declare low rates at both times or to move into the low category at HALS2. Of the married women who reported average or high malaise at the first Survey, 32% dropped to 'low' as compared with only 10% of those who remained single. However, a slightly more complex picture emerges when differences are examined between those who were married at both Surveys and those who now report being separated, divorced or widowed. When expected rates of illness or malaise (Table 4.15 – Table 4.18) for those who have remained married are applied to those who have become separated/divorced or widowed, the actual observed rates of those who are no longer married can be compared with those who are married. With this method, separated/divorced and widowed men appear to do less well than their married counterparts both for illness and malaise scores: older men who have become separated or divorced since HALS1 (Table 4.15a and Table 4.16a), reported more illness symptoms and the younger men reported higher levels of malaise. Although the numbers are small, widowed men experience more illness and considerably more malaise symptoms than those who are still married. Separated/divorced and widowed women, however, although reporting higher levels of malaise, have actual observed rates of illness symptoms which are lower than might be expected when using the transition rates for their married counterparts.

## Summary

The Survey has revealed many fascinating and important areas of changing perception and evaluation of health among the respondents who took part in the follow-up HALS study and has confirmed the increasing prevalence in particular diseases and conditions identified by other commentators. It is evident that social class and regional differences in reported health status still persist, yet certain groups, in particular men in the young manual occupations are viewing their health more positively. It has only been possible to illustrate a few of the changes in this Chapter, and further analysis will be necessary to examine some of the important changes in more detail, for example, the changing context within which individuals report disease and disability and the interaction between social roles such as employment, marital and parental status and reported health. It is evident that people's perception of their state of health, is associated with their environment and social relationships. Social contacts and their association with health status are examined in Chapter 15.

### References

Alderson M. (1987), 'Trends in morbidity and mortality from asthma', Population Trends, 49, 18-23.

Blaxter M. (1990), 'Health and Lifestyles', London/New York: Routledge, pp96-102.

Bridgwood A, and Savage D. (1992), 'General Household Survey 1991'. Office of Population Censuses and Surveys, London: HMSO.

Cox BD. et al. (1987), 'Health and Lifestyle Survey', London: Health Promotion Research Trust, pp5-15.

Halabi S, Zuray KH, Awaida R, Darwish M, and Saab B. (1992), 'Reliability and Validity of Self and Proxy Reporting of Morbidity Data: A Case Study from Beirut, Lebanon'. International Journal of Epidemiology, 21, 607-612

**Table 4.1**  **Self-assessed health compared to others of same age including complete HALS1 sample and HALS2 sub-sample at HALS1 and HALS2. Percentage of age group**

| | 18-24 | | 25-31 | | 32-38 | | 39-45 | | 46-52 | | 53-59 | | 60-66 | | 67-73 | | 74+ | | All | |
| HALS2 age | | 25-31 | | 32-38 | | 39-45 | | 46-52 | | 53-59 | | 60-66 | | 67-73 | | 74-80 | | 81+ | | All |
|---|---|---|---|---|---|---|---|---|---|---|---|---|---|---|---|---|---|---|---|---|---|
| **Self-assessed health — Males** | | | | | | | | | | | | | | | | | | | | | |
| **Excellent** | | | | | | | | | | | | | | | | | | | | | |
| HALS1 sample | 15 | | 21 | | 24 | | 24 | | 25 | | 20 | | 23 | | 20 | | 26 | | 22 | |
| HALS2 sub-sample | 15 | 20 | 17 | 19 | 26 | 23 | 25 | 26 | 25 | 22 | 21 | 21 | 23 | 18 | 24 | 26 | 30 | 21 | 22 | 22 |
| **Good** | | | | | | | | | | | | | | | | | | | | | |
| HALS1 sample | 55 | | 53 | | 53 | | 54 | | 48 | | 47 | | 45 | | 45 | | 42 | | 50 | |
| HALS2 sub-sample | 60 | 59 | 52 | 59 | 50 | 60 | 53 | 53 | 49 | 49 | 50 | 43 | 49 | 50 | 51 | 41 | 49 | 34 | 52 | 52 |
| **Fair** | | | | | | | | | | | | | | | | | | | | | |
| HALS1 sample | 27 | | 24 | | 21 | | 19 | | 22 | | 23 | | 24 | | 28 | | 24 | | 23 | |
| HALS2 sub-sample | 24 | 19 | 27 | 19 | 22 | 15 | 20 | 19 | 23 | 22 | 20 | 27 | 22 | 24 | 20 | 25 | 21 | 31 | 22 | 21 |
| **Poor** | | | | | | | | | | | | | | | | | | | | | |
| HALS1 sample | 4 | | 2 | | 2 | | 3 | | 6 | | 11 | | 7 | | 8 | | 7 | | 5 | |
| HALS2 sub-sample | 1 | 2 | 4 | 3 | 1 | 2 | 2 | 3 | 4 | 8 | 9 | 10 | 7 | 8 | 5 | 9 | 1 | 15 | 4 | 6 |
| *Base = 100%* | *534* | | *489* | | *572* | | *473* | | *417* | | *416* | | *410* | | *312* | | *271* | | *3894* | |
| | *299* | *298* | *241* | *241* | *383* | *383* | *324* | *324* | *278* | *280* | *278* | *278* | *258* | *258* | *147* | *148* | *88* | *88* | *2296* | *2298* |
| **Self-assessed health — Females** | | | | | | | | | | | | | | | | | | | | | |
| **Excellent** | | | | | | | | | | | | | | | | | | | | | |
| HALS1 sample | 17 | | 20 | | 22 | | 23 | | 23 | | 17 | | 18 | | 18 | | 18 | | 20 | |
| HALS2 sub-sample | 18 | 26 | 19 | 24 | 22 | 29 | 23 | 24 | 24 | 24 | 19 | 21 | 19 | 17 | 20 | 13 | 26 | 15 | 21 | 23 |
| **Good** | | | | | | | | | | | | | | | | | | | | | |
| HALS1 sample | 51 | | 57 | | 58 | | 55 | | 49 | | 47 | | 50 | | 46 | | 43 | | 52 | |
| HALS2 sub-sample | 49 | 52 | 59 | 58 | 58 | 53 | 55 | 55 | 50 | 49 | 46 | 45 | 54 | 54 | 49 | 52 | 46 | 49 | 53 | 52 |
| **Fair** | | | | | | | | | | | | | | | | | | | | | |
| HALS1 sample | 28 | | 20 | | 17 | | 18 | | 23 | | 25 | | 26 | | 27 | | 28 | | 23 | |
| HALS2 sub-sample | 28 | 19 | 19 | 15 | 18 | 15 | 18 | 17 | 21 | 22 | 26 | 26 | 24 | 22 | 25 | 27 | 21 | 27 | 22 | 20 |
| **Poor** | | | | | | | | | | | | | | | | | | | | | |
| HALS1 sample | 4 | | 3 | | 3 | | 4 | | 6 | | 10 | | 6 | | 10 | | 11 | | 6 | |
| HALS2 sub-sample | 5 | 3 | 3 | 3 | 2 | 4 | 4 | 4 | 6 | 6 | 9 | 7 | 3 | 7 | 5 | 8 | 6 | 8 | 5 | 5 |
| *Base = 100%* | *625* | | *669* | | *763* | | *614* | | *574* | | *485* | | *550* | | *391* | | *406* | | *5077* | |
| | *311* | *310* | *392* | *394* | *544* | *544* | *430* | *431* | *389* | *390* | *315* | *314* | *325* | *326* | *191* | *189* | *145* | *143* | *3042* | *3041* |

**Table 4.2    Self-assessed health in HALS2 of those reporting 'fair' or 'poor' health in HALS1 by socio-economic group (S.E.G.) at HALS1. Percentage of socio-economic group**

| HALS1 age | 18-38 | | 39-59 | | 60+ | |
|---|---|---|---|---|---|---|
| S.E.G. | Non-manual | Manual | Non-manual | Manual | Non-manual | Manual |
| **Self-assessed health at HALS2** | | | **Males** | | | |
| Excellent/good | 55 | 64 | 46 | 35 | 50 | 36 |
| Fair/poor | 45 | 36 | 54 | 65 | 50 | 64 |
| *Base = 100%* | *80* | *155* | *72* | *155* | *36* | *92* |
| | | | **Females** | | | |
| Excellent/good | 69 | 51 | 53 | 38 | 46 | 39 |
| Fair/poor | 31 | 49 | 47 | 62 | 54 | 61 |
| *Base = 100%* | *121* | *170* | *104* | *197* | *67* | *111* |

**Table 4.3    Self assessed health in HALS2 of those reporting 'excellent' or 'good' health in HALS1 by socio-economic group (S.E.G.) at HALS1. Percentage of socio-economic group**

| HALS1 age | 18-38 | | 39-59 | | 60+ | |
|---|---|---|---|---|---|---|
| S.E.G. | Non-manual | Manual | Non-manual | Manual | Non-manual | Manual |
| **Self-assessed health at HALS2** | | | **Males** | | | |
| Excellent/good | 89 | 86 | 89 | 75 | 77 | 73 |
| Fair/poor | 11 | 14 | 11 | 25 | 23 | 27 |
| *Base = 100%* | *312* | *359* | *331* | *321* | *159* | *202* |
| | | | **Females** | | | |
| Excellent/good | 90 | 86 | 87 | 80 | 85 | 73 |
| Fair/poor | 10 | 14 | 13 | 20 | 15 | 28 |
| *Base = 100%* | *453* | *485* | *453* | *364* | *206* | *262* |

**Table 4.4** **Percentage reporting 'fair' or 'poor' health at HALS1 and HALS2 by head of household's socio-economic group at HALS1 (HALS1 S.E.G.)**

| | Males | | | | | | | | |
|---|---|---|---|---|---|---|---|---|---|
| HALS1 age | 18-38 | | 39-59 | | 60+ | | 18-38 | 39-59 | 60+ |
| HALS | 1 | 2 | 1 | 2 | 1 | 2 | | | |
| HALS1 S.E.G. | | | | | | | | Base = 100% | |
| Professional | 16 | 21 | 12 | 10 | 13 | 4 | 44 | 49 | 23 |
| Managers\executives | 24 | 16 | 18 | 16 | 22 | 32 | 141 | 200 | 97 |
| Other non-manual | 18 | 18 | 20 | 25 | 16 | 29 | 194 | 154 | 75 |
| Skilled manual | 27 | 22 | 30 | 34 | 31 | 38 | 347 | 311 | 179 |
| Semi-skilled manual | 33 | 10 | 38 | 44 | 35 | 40 | 130 | 124 | 87 |
| Unskilled manual | 44 | 45 | 34 | 49 | 21 | 39 | 38 | 41 | 28 |
| | **Females** | | | | | | | | |
| Professional | 18 | 8 | 16 | 9 | 15 | 12 | 63 | 76 | 34 |
| Managers\executives | 15 | 12 | 16 | 18 | 26 | 20 | 165 | 267 | 115 |
| Other non-manual | 25 | 17 | 23 | 24 | 26 | 32 | 341 | 214 | 124 |
| Skilled manual | 22 | 21 | 31 | 31 | 29 | 38 | 406 | 358 | 202 |
| Semi-skilled manual | 31 | 25 | 38 | 37 | 35 | 39 | 207 | 150 | 135 |
| Unskilled manual | 41 | 38 | 53 | 51 | 14 | 28 | 42 | 53 | 36 |

**Table 4.5** **Regional changes in reporting health as 'fair' or 'poor' from HALS1 to HALS2. Percentage of age group in region**

| | Males | | | | | | | | |
|---|---|---|---|---|---|---|---|---|---|
| HALS1 age | 18-38 | | 39-59 | | 60+ | | | | |
| HALS | 1 | 2 | 1 | 2 | 1 | 2 | | Base = 100% | |
| North | 28 | 19 | 28 | 36 | 27 | 38 | 517 | 439 | 213 |
| South | 24 | 19 | 23 | 23 | 25 | 33 | 406 | 441 | 280 |
| Regional difference | +4 | 0 | +5 | +13 | +2 | +5 | | | |
| | **Females** | | | | | | | | |
| North | 26 | 22 | 30 | 31 | 28 | 37 | 668 | 623 | 352 |
| South | 22 | 16 | 23 | 21 | 29 | 27 | 579 | 511 | 309 |
| Regional difference | +4 | +6 | +7 | +10 | − 1 | +10 | | | |

**Table 4.6**    **Self-reported health at HALS2 compared to seven years ago by social class in 1984/5. Percentage of social class group**

| HALS1 age | 18-38 | | 39-59 | | 60+ | |
|---|---|---|---|---|---|---|
| | **Non-manual** | **Manual** | **Non-manual** | **Manual** | **Non-manual** | **Manual** |
| **Change in reported health** | | | **Males** | | | |
| Better | 16 | 23 | 18 | 16 | 14 | 7 |
| Same | 67 | 64 | 63 | 57 | 54 | 62 |
| Worse | 17 | 14 | 19 | 27 | 32 | 31 |
| *Base = 100%* | *400* | *550* | *363* | *470* | *195* | *296* |
| | | | **Females** | | | |
| Better | 24 | 22 | 19 | 19 | 14 | 10 |
| Same | 62 | 64 | 65 | 55 | 53 | 51 |
| Worse | 14 | 15 | 16 | 27 | 33 | 39 |
| *Base = 100%* | *578* | *718* | *504* | *558* | *268* | *378* |

**Table 4.7**  **Self-reported health at HALS2 compared to seven years ago by disease status in 1984/5 and 1991/2. Percentage of disease groups**

| | Reported health | | | | | | | | | | |
|---|---|---|---|---|---|---|---|---|---|---|---|
| | 'Lot' better | | 'Bit' better | | Same | | 'Bit' worse | | 'Lot' worse | | Base = 100% | |
| | Males | Females | Males | Females | Males | Females | Males | Females | Males | Females | Males | Females |
| **Disease status HALS1 & HALS2** | | | | | | | | | | | | |
| **HALS1 Age 18-38** | | | | | | | | | | | | |
| No disease HALS1/2 | 8 | 11 | 11 | 10 | 68 | 68 | 11 | 10 | 2 | 1 | 603 | 894 |
| No disease HALS1/ disease HALS2 | 6 | 9 | 13 | 12 | 54 | 50 | 20 | 16 | 7 | 13 | 117 | 121 |
| Disease HALS1/2 | 10 | 11 | 14 | 14 | 53 | 50 | 17 | 16 | 6 | 10 | 120 | 133 |
| Disease HALS1/ no disease HALS2 | 16 | 25 | 6 | 14 | 68 | 52 | 9 | 7 | 0 | 1 | 81 | 97 |
| **HALS1 Age 39-59** | | | | | | | | | | | | |
| No disease HALS1/2 | 8 | 11 | 7 | 6 | 71 | 70 | 12 | 11 | 2 | 2 | 430 | 604 |
| No disease HALS1/ disease HALS2 | 9 | 10 | 8 | 8 | 49 | 42 | 21 | 25 | 12 | 15 | 158 | 189 |
| Disease HALS1/2 | 9 | 11 | 9 | 8 | 46 | 50 | 17 | 15 | 19 | 15 | 208 | 232 |
| Disease HALS1/ no disease HALS2 | 10 | 16 | 10 | 9 | 60 | 58 | 17 | 13 | 4 | 4 | 82 | 108 |
| **HALS1 Age 60+** | | | | | | | | | | | | |
| No disease HALS1/2 | 4 | 5 | 5 | 5 | 72 | 68 | 15 | 17 | 5 | 5 | 199 | 250 |
| No disease HALS1/ disease HALS2 | 4 | 4 | 5 | 6 | 53 | 42 | 23 | 29 | 15 | 19 | 75 | 138 |
| Disease HALS1/2 | 4 | 8 | 7 | 8 | 43 | 34 | 23 | 30 | 23 | 20 | 167 | 184 |
| Disease HALS1/ no disease HALS2 | 2 | 8 | 11 | 4 | 66 | 55 | 13 | 27 | 8 | 6 | 53 | 78 |

**Table 4.8** **Number and percentage of respondents reporting having suffered from ME/Post Viral Fatigue Syndrome at HALS2. Percentage of age, region and social class (RGSC)**

| HALS2 age | 25-45 | 46-66 | 67+ | Total |
|---|---|---|---|---|
| | | Males | | |
| Number | 9 | 12 | 2 | 23 |
| Percentage | 1.0 | 1.4 | 0.4 | 1.0 |
| *Base = 100%* | *918* | *875* | *491* | *2284* |
| | | Females | | |
| Number | 28 | 25 | 9 | 62 |
| Percentage | 2.3 | 2.2 | 1.4 | 2.0 |
| *Base = 100%* | *1241* | *1132* | *655* | *3028* |

| Region | North | South | Total |
|---|---|---|---|
| | | Males | |
| Number | 11 | 12 | 23 |
| Percentage | 0.9 | 1.1 | 1.0 |
| *Base = 100%* | *1164* | *1120* | *2284* |
| | | Females | |
| Number | 37 | 25 | 62 |
| Percentage | 2.3 | 1.8 | 2.0 |
| *Base = 100%* | *1637* | *1391* | *3028* |

| RGSC | Non-manual | Manual | Total |
|---|---|---|---|
| | | Males | |
| Number | 9 | 14 | 23 |
| Percentage | 0.9 | 1.1 | 1.0 |
| *Base = 100%* | *957* | *1309* | *2266* |
| | | Females | |
| Number | 37 | 25 | 62 |
| Percentage | 2.7 | 1.5 | 2.0 |
| *Base = 100%* | *1349* | *1646* | *2995* |

**Table 4.9** **Percentage of HALS1 disease and disability group compared with disease and disability status at HALS2 for three age groups**

| HALS1 | No chronic disease | | Non-limiting disease | | Disease – mild handicap | | Disease – moderate severe handicap | |
|---|---|---|---|---|---|---|---|---|
| **HALS1 Age 18-38** | **Males** | **Females** | **Males** | **Females** | **Males** | **Females** | **Males** | **Females** |
| No chronic disease | 84 | 88 | 47 | 49 | 44 | 47 | 23 | 30 |
| Non-limiting disease | 9 | 6 | 40 | 31 | 22 | 14 | 25 | 21 |
| Disease – mild handicap | 3 | 2 | 2 | 9 | 4 | 11 | 8 | 7 |
| Disease – moderate/ severe handicap | 5 | 4 | 11 | 11 | 30 | 28 | 44 | 43 |
| *Base = 100%* | *718* | *1009* | *123* | *117* | *27* | *36* | *52* | *77* |
| | | | | | | | | |
| **HALS1 Age 39-59** | | | | | | | | |
| No chronic disease | 74 | 77 | 37 | 40 | 47 | 38 | 13 | 19 |
| Non-limiting disease | 13 | 13 | 36 | 37 | 23 | 24 | 12 | 16 |
| Disease – mild handicap | 2 | 2 | 6 | 7 | 0 | 12 | 3 | 4 |
| Disease – moderate/ severe handicap | 11 | 9 | 21 | 17 | 30 | 26 | 72 | 62 |
| *Base = 100%* | *574* | *769* | *140* | *164* | *30* | *42* | *123* | *138* |
| | | | | | | | | |
| **HALS1 Age 60+** | | | | | | | | |
| No chronic disease | 75 | 66 | 36 | 39 | 15 | 24 | 13 | 22 |
| Non-limiting disease | 11 | 18 | 36 | 31 | 35 | 24 | 17 | 13 |
| Disease – mild handicap | 1 | 1 | 2 | 3 | 5 | 14 | 2 | 5 |
| Disease – moderate/ severe handicap | 13 | 15 | 26 | 28 | 45 | 38 | 67 | 60 |
| *Base = 100%* | *260* | *361* | *102* | *110* | *20* | *21* | *98* | *136* |

**Table 4.10**  **Current employment status of men aged 18-57 at HALS1 reporting presence or absence of disease. Percentage of employment groups**

| HALS1 | With chronic disease 1984/5 and 1991/2 | | |
| --- | --- | --- | --- |
| | Employed | Unemployed | Permanently sick |
| **HALS2** | | | |
| Employed | 79 | 53 | 13 |
| Unemployed | 3 | 25 | 0 |
| Permanently sick | 12 | 19 | 77 |
| Retired | 6 | 3 | 10 |
| *Base = 100%* | *228* | *32* | *31* |

| | Without chronic disease 1984/5 and 1991/2 | | |
| --- | --- | --- | --- |
| Employed | 93 | 62 | 0 |
| Unemployed | 3 | 36 | 0 |
| Permanently sick | 1 | 0 | (1) |
| Retired | 4 | 3 | 0 |
| *Base = 100%* | *899* | *76* | *1* |

| | Developed chronic disease since 1984/5 | | |
| --- | --- | --- | --- |
| Employed | 76 | 28 | 0 |
| Unemployed | 6 | 24 | 0 |
| Permanently sick | 10 | 41 | (1) |
| Retired | 7 | 12 | 0 |
| *Base = 100%* | *212* | *29* | *1* |

**Table 4.11a    Selected diseases or conditions 'ever suffered from': differences between HALS1 and HALS2. Percentage of age group**

Males

| HALS1 age | 18-24 | | 25-31 | | 32-38 | | 39-45 | | 46-52 | | 53-59 | | 60-66 | | 67-73 | | 74+ | | All | |
|---|---|---|---|---|---|---|---|---|---|---|---|---|---|---|---|---|---|---|---|---|
| HALS2 age | | 25-31 | | 32-38 | | 39-45 | | 46-52 | | 53-59 | | 60-66 | | 67-73 | | 74-80 | | 81+ | | All |
| **Respiratory problems** | | | | | | | | | | | | | | | | | | | | |
| HALS1 sample | 25.1 | | 22.7 | | 25.5 | | 27.4 | | 28.6 | | 30.7 | | 35.4 | | 37.3 | | 41.4 | | 29.3 | |
| HALS2 sub-sample | 24.1 | 25.1 | 26.6 | 27.4 | 28.2 | 29.5 | 27.5 | 30.2 | 31.1 | 33.2 | 30.1 | 30.6 | 32.1 | 37.1 | 31.1 | 37.8 | 36.4 | 42.0 | 28.9 | 32.3 |
| **Asthma** | | | | | | | | | | | | | | | | | | | | |
| HALS1 sample | 10.5 | | 7.8 | | 6.8 | | 6.1 | | 6.2 | | 4.1 | | 5.3 | | 3.8 | | 5.5 | | 6.5 | |
| HALS2 sub-sample | 9.7 | 12.7 | 7.5 | 9.2 | 8.4 | 9.4 | 6.2 | 6.2 | 6.4 | 8.6 | 3.6 | 9.7 | 5.4 | 9.3 | 4.0 | 8.1 | 4.6 | 8.1 | 6.6 | 9.1 |
| **Bronchitis** | | | | | | | | | | | | | | | | | | | | |
| HALS1 sample | 4.9 | | 7.2 | | 6.8 | | 9.5 | | 8.4 | | 14.2 | | 16.5 | | 18.2 | | 23.4 | | 11.0 | |
| HALS2 sub-sample | 5.4 | 5.0 | 10.0 | 9.6 | 7.3 | 7.3 | 8.6 | 9.3 | 9.6 | 10.4 | 13.3 | 18.0 | 16.6 | 16.2 | 15.5 | 16.9 | 18.2 | 24.1 | 10.5 | 11.4 |
| **Other chest problems** | | | | | | | | | | | | | | | | | | | | |
| HALS1 sample | 13.3 | | 13.5 | | 16.8 | | 17.5 | | 19.3 | | 18.2 | | 21.6 | | 22.0 | | 21.6 | | 17.7 | |
| HALS2 sub-sample | 12.7 | 12.4 | 15.4 | 15.0 | 17.5 | 18.3 | 17.6 | 21.6 | 21.1 | 22.9 | 16.9 | 22.7 | 18.2 | 22.4 | 18.2 | 23.7 | 18.2 | 19.5 | 17.2 | 19.6 |
| **Diabetes** | | | | | | | | | | | | | | | | | | | | |
| HALS1 sample | 1.3 | | 0.4 | | 0.2 | | 1.1 | | 2.4 | | 4.8 | | 3.9 | | 3.5 | | 5.1 | | 2.2 | |
| HALS2 sub-sample | 1.3 | 2.0 | 0.4 | 0.8 | 0.3 | 0.8 | 1.5 | 2.1 | 2.9 | 4.7 | 3.2 | 6.1 | 3.9 | 7.3 | 4.1 | 8.8 | 3.4 | 8.1 | 2.0 | 3.8 |
| **High blood pressure** | | | | | | | | | | | | | | | | | | | | |
| HALS1 sample | 1.6 | | 3.6 | | 5.4 | | 7.5 | | 9.7 | | 20.8 | | 23.5 | | 22.9 | | 18.6 | | 11.3 | |
| HALS2 sub-sample | 0.3 | 5.0 | 4.1 | 7.9 | 5.4 | 12.2 | 5.8 | 15.1 | 10.7 | 20.0 | 20.1 | 33.5 | 22.7 | 31.5 | 19.5 | 26.3 | 12.5 | 22.0 | 10.2 | 18.2 |
| **Migraine** | | | | | | | | | | | | | | | | | | | | |
| HALS1 sample | 17.0 | | 11.4 | | 15.8 | | 17.9 | | 13.8 | | 14.8 | | 13.1 | | 7.6 | | 7.3 | | 13.8 | |
| HALS2 sub-sample | 14.3 | 20.7 | 12.8 | 13.3 | 15.1 | 14.6 | 15.4 | 20.4 | 15.0 | 16.4 | 14.3 | 15.4 | 13.9 | 12.7 | 7.4 | 7.4 | 6.8 | 12.6 | 13.7 | 15.6 |
| **Heart problems** | | | | | | | | | | | | | | | | | | | | |
| HALS1 sample | 1.3 | | 1.2 | | 2.2 | | 2.7 | | 6.4 | | 13.1 | | 17.4 | | 23.5 | | 19.4 | | 8.1 | |
| HALS2 sub-sample | 1.0 | 2.6 | 2.0 | 2.5 | 1.5 | 4.1 | 2.1 | 6.1 | 5.7 | 12.8 | 11.5 | 24.1 | 13.9 | 26.2 | 19.5 | 29.7 | 14.7 | 25.2 | 6.3 | 12.4 |
| *Base = 100%* | 534 | | 489 | | 573 | | 474 | | 419 | | 417 | | 412 | | 314 | | 273 | | 3905 | |
| | *299* | *299* | *241* | *241* | *383* | *382* | *324* | *324* | *280* | *279* | *278* | *278* | *259* | *259* | *148* | *148* | *88* | *87* | *2300* | *2297* |

**Table 4.11b Selected diseases or conditions 'ever suffered from': differences between HALS1 and HALS2. Percentage of age group**

Females

| | 18-24 | 25-31 | 32-38 | 39-45 | 46-52 | 53-59 | 60-66 | 67-73 | 74+ | All |
|---|---|---|---|---|---|---|---|---|---|---|
| HALS1 age | 18-24 | 25-31 | 32-38 | 39-45 | 46-52 | 53-59 | 60-66 | 67-73 | 74+ | All |
| HALS2 age | 25-31 | 32-38 | 39-45 | 46-52 | 53-59 | 60-66 | 67-73 | 74-80 | 81+ | All |

**Respiratory problems**

| | | | | | | | | | | |
|---|---|---|---|---|---|---|---|---|---|---|
| HALS1 sample | 21.2 | 18.9 | 22.7 | 25.2 | 26.6 | 34.2 | 35.1 | 30.4 | 34.6 | 26.8 |
| HALS2 sub-sample | 19.0 28.6 | 19.0 22.3 | 22.7 26.2 | 27.1 30.1 | 26.3 32.0 | 33.7 37.8 | 31.5 34.9 | 28.3 32.5 | 33.6 33.6 | 25.9 30.1 |

**Asthma**

| | | | | | | | | | | |
|---|---|---|---|---|---|---|---|---|---|---|
| HALS1 sample | 6.6 | 4.5 | 5.4 | 4.4 | 4.9 | 6.6 | 3.3 | 6.4 | 4.2 | 5.0 |
| HALS2 sub-sample | 6.8 12.9 | 4.3 7.6 | 5.0 7.2 | 4.2 8.6 | 5.1 8.2 | 6.7 9.6 | 3.4 6.2 | 6.3 10.5 | 4.8 9.2 | 5.1 8.6 |

**Bronchitis**

| | | | | | | | | | | |
|---|---|---|---|---|---|---|---|---|---|---|
| HALS1 sample | 5.9 | 5.8 | 6.7 | 9.2 | 11.5 | 14.6 | 15.2 | 18.2 | 20.5 | 11.0 |
| HALS2 sub-sample | 3.5 4.2 | 5.8 6.4 | 6.4 7.7 | 9.5 12.0 | 11.0 14.8 | 14.0 16.6 | 14.7 17.7 | 16.8 11.0 | 21.2 21.7 | 10.1 11.5 |

**Other chest problems**

| | | | | | | | | | | |
|---|---|---|---|---|---|---|---|---|---|---|
| HALS1 sample | 12.1 | 11.5 | 15.3 | 17.0 | 16.0 | 20.8 | 23.5 | 16.6 | 17.8 | 16.4 |
| HALS2 sub-sample | 11.6 16.7 | 12.2 14.0 | 15.6 16.8 | 18.1 18.1 | 16.1 19.7 | 20.0 22.4 | 19.9 20.4 | 14.7 20.1 | 17.1 19.9 | 16.1 18.3 |

**Diabetes**

| | | | | | | | | | | |
|---|---|---|---|---|---|---|---|---|---|---|
| HALS1 sample | 0.8 | 0.6 | 0.7 | 1.5 | 1.2 | 2.5 | 1.8 | 4.4 | 3.4 | 1.6 |
| HALS2 sub-sample | 1.0 1.9 | 0.5 0.5 | 0.9 0.9 | 2.1 3.0 | 1.3 2.0 | 2.5 4.1 | 1.5 3.7 | 1.1 5.3 | 2.1 5.6 | 1.4 2.5 |

**High blood pressure**

| | | | | | | | | | | |
|---|---|---|---|---|---|---|---|---|---|---|
| HALS1 sample | 8.9 | 16.6 | 15.8 | 14.8 | 16.6 | 24.4 | 21.8 | 25.5 | 30.0 | 18.4 |
| HALS2 sub-sample | 9.0 13.5 | 18.2 15.2 | 15.7 17.3 | 14.8 17.8 | 18.1 27.7 | 23.8 32.0 | 19.2 30.7 | 27.7 41.1 | 27.4 32.1 | 18.0 23.2 |

**Migraine**

| | | | | | | | | | | |
|---|---|---|---|---|---|---|---|---|---|---|
| HALS1 sample | 21.5 | 24.2 | 25.8 | 27.0 | 30.7 | 28.6 | 23.1 | 22.5 | 18.7 | 24.9 |
| HALS2 sub-sample | 21.5 28.0 | 23.1 33.7 | 25.5 28.6 | 28.0 30.3 | 30.9 30.1 | 28.8 28.5 | 22.9 21.5 | 20.9 20.7 | 21.9 20.9 | 25.4 28.0 |

**Heart problems**

| | | | | | | | | | | |
|---|---|---|---|---|---|---|---|---|---|---|
| HALS1 sample | 1.4 | 1.6 | 3.1 | 3.5 | 5.3 | 8.8 | 9.9 | 16.3 | 20.9 | 6.7 |
| HALS2 sub-sample | 0.6 1.2 | 1.0 2.0 | 3.6 5.6 | 3.7 5.3 | 5.3 12.2 | 7.6 14.6 | 7.0 16.9 | 14.1 22.1 | 19.1 25.1 | 5.4 9.6 |

| | | | | | | | | | | |
|---|---|---|---|---|---|---|---|---|---|---|
| *Base = 100%* | *626* | *672* | *766* | *618* | *576* | *486* | *553* | *391* | *410* | *5098* |
| | *311 311* | *394 394* | *545 544* | *432 432* | *391 391* | *315 314* | *327 325* | *191 190* | *146 142* | *3052 3043* |

**Table 4.12a   Change in prevalence reported 'during the past month' of selected symptoms by HALS1 and HALS2 age. Percentage of age group**

**Males**

| | 18-24 / 25-31 | 25-31 / 32-38 | 32-38 / 39-45 | 39-45 / 46-52 | 46-52 / 53-59 | 53-59 / 60-66 | 60-66 / 67-73 | 67-73 / 74-80 | 74+ / 81+ | Total / Total |
|---|---|---|---|---|---|---|---|---|---|---|
| **Constipation** | | | | | | | | | | |
| HALS1 sample | 3.0 | 2.4 | 2.6 | 2.7 | 3.1 | 3.8 | 8.2 | 10.5 | 11.7 | 4.7 |
| HALS2 sub-sample | 2.0 2.3 | 2.9 4.9 | 2.0 4.7 | 2.7 3.0 | 3.9 6.7 | 3.2 7.1 | 7.3 7.7 | 8.1 14.8 | 4.5 20.4 | 3.7 6.3 |
| **Hay fever** | | | | | | | | | | |
| HALS1 sample | 5.2 | 4.0 | 4.8 | 2.7 | 1.9 | 1.6 | 2.4 | 3.1 | 2.2 | 3.3 |
| HALS2 sub-sample | 4.6 8.3 | 3.3 4.5 | 4.7 4.9 | 3.7 5.2 | 1.0 5.0 | 2.1 7.5 | 3.0 5.4 | 2.0 3.3 | 3.4 3.4 | 3.2 5.6 |
| **Eye trouble** | | | | | | | | | | |
| HALS1 sample | 9.5 | 9.2 | 7.8 | 11.1 | 14.8 | 11.7 | 12.3 | 15.9 | 23.0 | 12.0 |
| HALS2 sub-sample | 8.7 7.3 | 9.9 10.3 | 8.8 12.7 | 9.8 20.3 | 13.5 17.8 | 8.9 17.2 | 10.4 20.4 | 15.5 24.3 | 20.4 31.8 | 10.7 16.3 |
| **Colds/flu** | | | | | | | | | | |
| HALS1 sample | 39.7 | 35.1 | 37.1 | 32.0 | 25.0 | 30.9 | 29.1 | 26.4 | 26.3 | 32.2 |
| HALS2 sub-sample | 42.1 37.1 | 37.3 28.2 | 37.0 25.3 | 30.8 23.1 | 23.9 26.4 | 30.5 26.6 | 28.5 22.3 | 29.7 18.2 | 27.2 25.0 | 32.7 26.3 |
| **Painful joints** | | | | | | | | | | |
| HALS1 sample | 8.2 | 10.6 | 13.0 | 17.3 | 21.9 | 28.3 | 31.0 | 30.5 | 34.4 | 20.0 |
| HALS2 sub-sample | 6.3 17.0 | 11.6 16.1 | 13.0 18.5 | 17.2 23.7 | 22.5 29.2 | 28.4 35.2 | 32.4 33.9 | 30.4 35.8 | 34.0 38.6 | 19.7 25.7 |
| *Base = 100%* | 534 | 489 | 573 | 474 | 419 | 417 | 412 | 314 | 273 | 3905 |
| | 299 299 | 241 241 | 383 383 | 324 324 | 280 280 | 278 278 | 259 259 | 148 148 | 88 88 | 2300 2300 |

**Table 4.12b   Change in prevalence reported 'during the past month' of selected symptoms by HALS1 and HALS2 age. Percentage of age group**

| | Females | | | | | | | | | |
|---|---|---|---|---|---|---|---|---|---|---|
| **HALS1 age** | 18-24 | 25-31 | 32-38 | 39-45 | 46-52 | 53-59 | 60-66 | 67-73 | 74+ | Total |
| **HALS2 age** | 25-31 | 32-38 | 39-45 | 46-52 | 53-59 | 60-66 | 67-73 | 74-80 | 81+ | Total |
| **Headaches** | | | | | | | | | | |
| HALS1 sample | 39.7 | 38.1 | 37.9 | 38.0 | 37.1 | 33.9 | 23.3 | 26.8 | 20.7 | 33.9 |
| HALS2 sub-sample | 37.3 42.7 | 38.5 43.6 | 37.6 36.7 | 36.1 38.4 | 37.0 33.5 | 32.3 24.7 | 23.2 22.0 | 25.6 19.3 | 19.8 17.1 | 33.7 33.2 |
| **Hay fever** | | | | | | | | | | |
| HALS1 sample | 7.0 | 2.6 | 4.1 | 5.3 | 5.3 | 3.9 | 3.8 | 4.0 | 4.1 | 4.5 |
| HALS2 sub-sample | 7.0 6.1 | 2.5 7.1 | 4.7 7.3 | 5.7 8.8 | 4.8 7.9 | 4.4 8.8 | 3.9 6.1 | 4.1 7.3 | 4.7 5.4 | 4.7 7.4 |
| **Colds/flu** | | | | | | | | | | |
| HALS1 sample | 43.9 | 38.2 | 34.0 | 26.3 | 33.5 | 28.8 | 29.2 | 27.3 | 23.1 | 32.4 |
| HALS2 sub-sample | 45.0 34.4 | 39.8 29.7 | 33.7 22.9 | 23.6 24.7 | 30.9 29.4 | 28.2 26.0 | 26.6 23.2 | 27.2 20.9 | 28.0 16.4 | 31.8 25.9 |
| **Painful joints** | | | | | | | | | | |
| HALS1 sample | 6.2 | 7.2 | 12.5 | 18.4 | 28.1 | 37.8 | 37.6 | 43.9 | 47.5 | 23.9 |
| HALS2 sub-sample | 5.7 8.3 | 6.6 11.9 | 13.2 22.7 | 18.2 29.8 | 27.6 43.4 | 38.1 46.6 | 37.0 46.6 | 46.6 53.9 | 41.1 52.7 | 22.7 31.9 |
| **Periods/menopause** | | | | | | | | | | |
| HALS1 sample | 17.8 | 16.9 | 20.5 | 23.9 | 20.8 | 7.6 | – | – | – | 17.9 |
| HALS2 sub-sample | 19.9 18.6 | 20.8 18.5 | 21.2 25.1 | 23.1 31.7 | 22.5 14.0 | 8.2 – | – – | – – | – – | 19.4 21.7 |
| *Base = 100%* | 626 | 672 | 766 | 618 | 576 | 486 | 553 | 391 | 410 | 5098 |
| | 311 311 | 394 394 | 545 545 | 432 432 | 391 391 | 315 315 | 327 327 | 191 191 | 146 146 | 3052 3052 |

**Table 4.13 Illness Scores: comparison of HALS1 and HALS2. Percentage of age group**

| | Males | | | | | | | | | | | |
|---|---|---|---|---|---|---|---|---|---|---|---|---|
| HALS1 age | | 18-38 | | | | 39-59 | | | | 60+ | | |
| HALS1 score | Low | Ave. | High | Total | Low | Ave. | High | Total | Low | Ave. | High | Total |
| **HALS2 score** | | | | | | | | | | | | |
| Low | 61 | 46 | 26 | 52 | 56 | 39 | 16 | 43 | 59 | 36 | 10 | 40 |
| Average | 30 | 36 | 42 | 33 | 32 | 36 | 32 | 34 | 28 | 35 | 36 | 32 |
| High | 9 | 19 | 32 | 15 | 11 | 25 | 52 | 23 | 13 | 29 | 54 | 28 |
| Total | 54 | 34 | 12 | | 48 | 36 | 16 | | 42 | 35 | 22 | |
| **Females** | | | | | | | | | | | | |
| Low | 53 | 33 | 23 | 39 | 49 | 31 | 12 | 32 | 54 | 22 | 8 | 27 |
| Average | 33 | 41 | 34 | 36 | 37 | 39 | 22 | 34 | 29 | 41 | 23 | 31 |
| High | 14 | 26 | 43 | 25 | 14 | 30 | 66 | 35 | 17 | 36 | 69 | 41 |
| Total | 41 | 37 | 22 | | 35 | 36 | 29 | | 31 | 36 | 33 | |
| *Base = 100%* | *497* | *313* | *111* | *921* | *420* | *317* | *145* | *882* | *209* | *175* | *111* | *495* |
| | *513* | *462* | *275* | *1250* | *394* | *411* | *333* | *1138* | *204* | *237* | *223* | *664* |

**Table 4.14**   **Changes in illness and malaise scores between HALS1 and HALS2 by marital status in 1984/5 and 1991/2. Percentages of age group 18-29 at HALS1**

| Marital status HALS1/2 | Single-Single | | Single-Married | |
|---|---|---|---|---|
| | Males | Females | Males | Females |
| **Illness at HALS2** | **Reported low illness in 1984/5** | | | |
| Low | 65 | 55 | 57 | 49 |
| Average/high | 36 | 45 | 43 | 51 |
| *Base = 100%* | *93* | *40* | *68* | *51* |
| | **Reported average/high illness 1984/5** | | | |
| Low | 37 | 23 | 31 | 34 |
| Average/high | 63 | 77 | 69 | 66 |
| *Base = 100%* | *68* | *74* | *55* | *55* |
| **Malaise at HALS2** | **Reported low malaise 1984/5** | | | |
| Low | 44 | 44 | 59 | 57 |
| Average/high | 56 | 56 | 41 | 43 |
| *Base = 100%* | *50* | *32* | *49* | *28* |
| | **Reported average/high malaise 1984/5** | | | |
| Low | 20 | 10 | 41 | 32 |
| Average/high | 80 | 90 | 60 | 68 |
| *Base = 100%* | *111* | *82* | *74* | *78* |

**Table 4.15a    Distribution of illness categories for those who were married at HALS1 and separated or divorced at HALS2, as percentage of age group**

| Illness | HALS1 age 18-34, N=29 | | | HALS1 age 35-64, N=28 | | |
| | HALS 1 | HALS 2 | | HALS 1 | HALS 2 | |
| | | Actual | Expected* | | Actual | Expected* |
| **Males** | | | | | | |
| Low | 65.5 | 51.7 | 54.6 | 32.1 | 32.1 | 41.9 |
| Average | 31.0 | 34.5 | 33.7 | 42.9 | 42.9 | 33.7 |
| High | 3.4 | 13.8 | 11.5 | 25.0 | 25.0 | 24.4 |
| **Females** | | | | | | |
| Low | 38.7 | 43.5 | 40.1 | 30.0 | 46.0 | 31.7 |
| Average | 43.5 | 38.7 | 37.6 | 48.0 | 20.0 | 36.8 |
| High | 17.7 | 17.7 | 22.3 | 22.0 | 34.0 | 31.5 |

* The 'expected' percentage is that which would occur if the separated/divorced group had experienced the same illness transition rates as the married group (Table 4.15b).

**Table 4.15b    Illness transition rate data from which 'expected' is calculated**

| HALS1 Illness | HALS1 age 18-34 | | | HALS1 age 35-64 | | |
| | Married at both surveys | | | Married at both surveys | | |
| | Low | Average | High | Low | Average | High |
| **Males** | | | | | | |
| HALS2 Illness | | | | | | |
| Low | 58.2 | 50.0 | 28.1 | 59.1 | 42.6 | 18.8 |
| Average | 33.3 | 34.0 | 37.5 | 31.0 | 36.0 | 33.0 |
| High | 8.5 | 16.0 | 34.4 | 9.8 | 21.4 | 48.2 |
| *Base = 100%* | *165* | *100* | *32* | *506* | *364* | *227* |
| **Females** | | | | | | |
| Low | 53.3 | 33.2 | 28.4 | 49.9 | 28.5 | 14.0 |
| Average | 34.9 | 41.1 | 34.9 | 35.4 | 43.3 | 24.4 |
| High | 11.8 | 25.7 | 36.7 | 14.7 | 28.2 | 48.4 |
| *Base = 100%* | *212* | *195* | *117* | *477* | *439* | *349* |

**Table 4.16a    Distribution of malaise categories for those who were married at HALS1 and separated or divorced at HALS2, as percentage of age group**

| | HALS1 age 18-34, N=29 | | | HALS1 age 35-64, N=28 | | |
|---|---|---|---|---|---|---|
| | HALS1 | HALS2 | | HALS1 | HALS2 | |
| **Males** | | | | | | |
| Malaise | | Actual | Expected* | | Actual | Expected* |
| Low | 37.9 | 27.6 | 39.1 | 25.0 | 25.0 | 45.5 |
| Average | 37.9 | 31.0 | 38.5 | 57.1 | 53.6 | 37.4 |
| High | 24.1 | 41.4 | 22.3 | 17.9 | 21.4 | 17.0 |
| **Females** | | | | | | |
| Low | 21.0 | 21.0 | 32.3 | 24.0 | 22.0 | 31.0 |
| Average | 30.6 | 40.3 | 33.9 | 34.0 | 38.0 | 34.5 |
| High | 48.4 | 38.7 | 33.8 | 42.0 | 40.0 | 34.5 |

\* The 'expected' percentage is that which would occur if the separated/divorced group had experienced the same malaise transition rates as the married group (Tables 4.16b).

**Table 4.16b    Malaise transition rate data from which 'expected' is calculated, as percentage of age group**

| | HALS1 aged 18-34 Married at both surveys | | | HALS1 aged 35-64 Married at both surveys | | |
|---|---|---|---|---|---|---|
| **Males** | | | | | | |
| HALS1 Malaise | Low | Average | High | Low | Average | High |
| **HALS2 Malaise** | | | | | | |
| Low | 64.3 | 34.5 | 6.9 | 72.0 | 41.9 | 20.3 |
| Average | 31.0 | 44.2 | 41.4 | 20.2 | 45.6 | 35.5 |
| High | 4.8 | 21.2 | 51.7 | 7.8 | 12.5 | 44.2 |
| *Base = 100%* | *126* | *113* | *58* | *525* | *375* | *197* |
| **Females** | | | | | | |
| Low | 59.5 | 31.9 | 20.8 | 62.1 | 33.8 | 10.9 |
| Average | 31.1 | 40.7 | 30.8 | 27.2 | 45.1 | 30.1 |
| High | 9.5 | 27.3 | 48.4 | 10.7 | 21.1 | 58.9 |
| *Base = 100%* | *148* | *216* | *159* | *449* | *441* | *275* |

**Table 4.17a    Distribution of illness categories for those who were married at HALS1 and widowed at HALS2. Percentage of age group**

| | HALS1 age 50-64, N=24 | | | HALS1 age 65-79, N=30 | | |
|---|---|---|---|---|---|---|
| | HALS1 | HALS2 | | HALS1 | HALS2 | |
| | | | **Males** | | | |
| Illness | | Actual | Expected* | | Actual | Expected* |
| Low | 41.7 | 29.2 | 36.4 | 46.7 | 33.3 | 38.4 |
| Average | 25.0 | 37.5 | 32.5 | 36.7 | 26.7 | 33.4 |
| High | 33.3 | 33.3 | 31.2 | 16.7 | 40.0 | 28.2 |
| | | | **Females** | | | |
| Low | 31.4 | 37.1 | 32.6 | 30.6 | 29.0 | 24.1 |
| Average | 40.0 | 22.9 | 33.2 | 35.5 | 25.8 | 30.1 |
| High | 28.6 | 40.0 | 34.3 | 33.9 | 45.2 | 45.8 |

* The 'expected' percentage is that which would occur if the widowed group had experienced the same illness transition rates as the married group (Table 4.17b).

**Table 4.17b    Illness transition rate data from which 'expected' is calculated. Percentage of age group**

| | HALS1 age 50-64 | | | HALS1 age 65-79 | | |
|---|---|---|---|---|---|---|
| | Married at both surveys | | | Married at both surveys | | |
| HALS1 Illness | Low | Average | High | Low | Average | High |
| HALS2 Illness | | | **Males** | | | |
| Low | 56.3 | 33.9 | 13.3 | 55.3 | 40.4 | 15.0 |
| Average | 29.7 | 38.9 | 31.1 | 38.2 | 28.1 | 35.0 |
| High | 14.0 | 27.2 | 55.6 | 6.6 | 31.6 | 50.0 |
| *Base = 100%* | *222* | *180* | *90* | *76* | *57* | *40* |
| | | | **Females** | | | |
| Low | 55.3 | 28.0 | 13.9 | 55.2 | 15.7 | 4.7 |
| Average | 29.2 | 43.3 | 23.5 | 20.7 | 47.1 | 20.9 |
| High | 15.5 | 28.7 | 62.7 | 24.1 | 37.3 | 74.4 |
| *Base = 100%* | *161* | *164* | *166* | *29* | *51* | *43* |

**Table 4.18a    Distribution of malaise categories for those who were married at HALS1 and widowed at HALS2. Percentage of age group**

| | HALS1 age 50-64, N=24 | | | HALS1 age 65-79, N=30 | | |
| | HALS1 | HALS2 | | HALS1 | HALS2 | |
| Malaise | | Actual | Expected* | | Actual | Expected* |
| | | | | **Males** | | |
| Low | 58.3 | 8.3 | 62.5 | 73.3 | 30.0 | 61.7 |
| Average | 33.3 | 41.7 | 27.0 | 16.7 | 26.7 | 22.8 |
| High | 8.3 | 50.0 | 10.5 | 10.0 | 43.3 | 15.5 |
| | | | | **Females** | | |
| Low | 25.7 | 20.0 | 37.5 | 37.1 | 22.6 | 38.4 |
| Average | 45.7 | 28.6 | 34.6 | 32.3 | 32.3 | 32.2 |
| High | 28.6 | 51.4 | 27.9 | 30.6 | 45.2 | 29.5 |

* The 'expected' percentage is that which would occur if the widowed group had experienced the same malaise transition rates as the married group (Table 4.18b).

**Table 4.18b    Malaise transition rate data from which 'expected' is calculated. Percentage of age group**

| | HALS1 age 50-64 | | | HALS1 age 65-79 | | |
| | Married at both surveys | | | Married at both surveys | | |
| HALS1 Malaise | Low | Average | High | Low | Average | High |
| HALS2 Malaise | | | **Males** | | | |
| Low | 78.8 | 44.1 | 22.2 | 72.4 | 47.6 | 6.7 |
| Average | 16.8 | 43.4 | 33.3 | 16.4 | 40.5 | 40.0 |
| High | 4.4 | 12.6 | 44.4 | 11.2 | 11.9 | 53.3 |
| *Base = 100%* | *250* | *143* | *99* | *116* | *42* | *15* |
| | | | **Females** | | | |
| Low | 65.9 | 38.8 | 10.0 | 58.3 | 37.9 | 14.7 |
| Average | 25.0 | 43.6 | 28.7 | 30.0 | 34.5 | 32.4 |
| High | 9.1 | 17.6 | 61.3 | 11.7 | 27.6 | 52.9 |
| *Base = 100%* | *176* | *165* | *150* | *60* | *29* | *34* |

# TRENDS IN BLOOD PRESSURE AND RESPIRATORY FUNCTION | 5

Brian D Cox

## BLOOD PRESSURE

In industrialised western populations blood pressure tends to rise with age (Epstein, 1983). This may be partly a reflection of lifestyle in these countries, as several studies have shown that in less industrialised countries ageing is not normally associated with an increase in blood pressure (Marmot, 1984). However, it has also been shown that genetic factors exert an influence on the development of hypertension (Cruz-Coke et al. 1973). More recently, evidence has been emerging regarding the possible influence of neonatal and very early development factors such as low birth weight and growth in the first year, as well as subsequent life environmental factors, as components in the later development of hypertension (Barker, 1991). There is still considerable debate about the factors affecting the association of rise in blood pressure with age: many studies are underway to evaluate the effect of modifying environmental and lifestyle factors on the steep rise in the prevalence of hypertension with age found in Western industrialised societies. It is hoped that the conversion of the HALS Survey from a cross-sectional to a longitudinal study may help to clarify the relationship between these factors and the development of hypertension.

The importance of research on levels of blood pressure lies in the fact that their chronic elevation above generally accepted norms (WHO Criteria) is associated with an increase in cardiovascular morbidity and mortality in both sexes, irrespective of geographical areas and ethnic origin (WHO, 1978; Lew, 1973).

## Methods

The procedures and the instrumentation used in the HALS2 1991/2 survey were identical to those used in the original HALS1 1984/5 study (Cox et al. 1987). The Datascope 'Accutorr' was used to measure blood pressures. This equipment, normally used for monitoring blood pressure in the clinical environment, was chosen after evaluation with intra-arterial catheterisation and comparison with the other machines available commercially. It was set to inflate and deflate the cuff automatically at one-minute intervals. The systolic, diastolic, and mean arterial pressures and heart rate were determined by oscillometry and the values displayed digitally to eliminate the type of observer bias which occurs with different operators using stethoscopes. The mean arterial pressure (a measurement only made possible with the advent of automated machines) is an integrated estimation of the mean pressure within the arterial system during the pulsatile cycle. The equipment was calibrated by reference to a mercury manometer (See Appendix B). In order to reduce stress which might have had an effect on blood pressure, these measurements were carried out near the end of the nurse's visit (by which time the respondent was expected to be relaxed), with the respondent seated in an upright chair and the right forearm supported in a resting position.

The clinical classification of blood pressure values requires at least three measures to be taken on two separate occasions. On both occasions in the HALS Surveys four blood pressure measurements were made on only a single occasion. However, several studies (WHO, 1978) have shown that the single estimate is predictive.

## Blood pressure values

Tables 5.1 and 5.2 show the systolic, diastolic and mean arterial blood pressure levels by seven-year age bands in the HALS1 and HALS2 sample populations. The data are presented as means of the whole HALS1 measured population, the means of the HALS2 sample (which is a sub-set of the HALS1 population) at both sampling times (1984/5 and 1991/2). The HALS1 population was regarded as being representative of the British population in comparison to the 1981 Census (Cox et al, 1987). The HALS2 sample, although not as representative of the 1991 Census as would have been wished, showing principally an imbalance of age distribution (see Chapter 1), nevertheless can in some respects be seen to be an indicator of population trends. The presentation in these tables of the mean values of both the whole HALS1 population and those of the group of them who were seen exactly seven years later at HALS2 enables an assessment to be made of how representative of the whole HALS1 sample is the HALS2 sub-set. The use of seven year age bands also enables a comparison to be made of the HALS2 1991/2 results with the values obtained for the next older age group at HALS1.

As far as blood pressure is concerned there is no discernible significant difference between the values obtained for the HALS1 group as a whole and the HALS2 sub-set at 1984/5, an unexpected finding. Mortality is a major reason for attrition in the older age groups of the original sample, and it might be anticipated that high blood pressure would be a significant contributor to their mortality. In those measured in HALS2 (the survivors) the mean blood pressure at HALS1 would be expected to be lower than in those not seen in HALS2 (which include a large number of respondents who will have died).

As previously reported (Cox et al. 1987) the blood pressure values obtained from the HALS1 population tended to rise with age, as was also described for the UK population by Miall and Lovell (1967). However, the mean rise in blood pressures over seven years in the HALS2 subjects in the younger age groups is consistently lower than would

have been expected to occur in comparison to that seen in the same age group at HALS1. This is despite a mean increase in body mass index which is higher than expected (see Chapter 6, Tables 6.3, 6.4). Also shown in these tables are the percentages in each age group who were currently being treated with drugs with anti-hypertensive effects. These include both those being actively treated for hypertension, and those for whom there was no previous report of hypertension but who were on medications with blood-pressure lowering effects. Overall, there has been an increase in subjects of all ages taking these drugs. In the older age groups the high proportions of respondents on them may have caused some lowering of the mean blood pressure. It may also be that the major changes seen in dietary patterns (Chapter 11) have had an influence on blood pressure levels.

For many of the following tables the blood pressure levels obtained have been categorised for ease of interpretation. The categories are those used by WHO (1978). All those being treated for high blood pressure by medication are categorised as treated hypertensives. In addition, as previously indicated, there was a small group who did not report to either the interviewer or nurse that they were hypertensive and who had normal blood pressure levels, but who were being treated with drugs with anti- hypertensive effects. The five categories are:-

1 Normotensive – normal blood pressure levels (≤140/90 mmHg).
2 Borderline – borderline blood pressure levels (between 141/91 and 159/94 mmHg).
3 Untreated hypertensive – hypertensive blood pressure levels but no medication (≥160/95mmHg).
4 Treated hypertensives – actively being treated for high blood pressure with drugs but with various levels of measured blood pressure.
5 Normotensive by measurement but being treated with drugs with blood pressure lowering effects – no self reported past history of high blood pressure (≤140/90mmHg).

The distribution of these groups in the HALS2 sample with age, as well as the changes that have occurred in each age group from HALS1 to HALS2 is shown in Table 5.3. As before there is a clear difference in the pattern of distribution of blood pressure categories between men and women, with a greater proportion of untreated hypertensives in the men in the younger age groups. In this table the notable feature is the proportion of each age group which is normotensive at HALS2 compared to the proportion who were normotensive at the same age in HALS1. As noted in the mean blood pressure tables, in the younger age groups more respondents remained normotensive than might have been expected from the proportions at that age in HALS1. In those respondents aged 60-66 at HALS2 the converse is generally true.

The proportion of respondents who did not report high blood pressure in the questionnaire or to the nurses but were on drugs with blood pressure lowering effects has greatly increased from HALS1 to HALS2. For example, in the younger age groups these were often ß-blockers (for migraine), in the older subjects, diuretics.

Table 5.4 shows how individuals have changed blood pressure categories in the seven years between the HALS1 and HALS2 measurements. 83.8% of the men and 87.0% of the women have remained normotensive. 35.1% of the men and 43.0% of the women who were measured hypertensive at HALS1 but were then untreated are now being treated with anti-hypertensive drugs. Of those treated hypertensives at HALS1 about 12% were no longer on drug therapy at HALS2 and approximately 6% of each sex measured normotensive.

Since losing weight is one of the measures often recommended for treating hypertension the mean percentage changes in Body Mass Index (BMI) relative to the change in blood pressure categories demonstrated in Table 5.4 is shown in Table 5.5. In those men and women who were normotensive at HALS1 there has been an increase in BMI in all HALS2 categories, averaging out at 4.2% and 5.8% for men and women respectively. This contrasts with the changes seen in all the other groups by their HALS1 categories where in all cases the average increase in BMI has been less than half that of the HALS1 normotensives and in some groups there has been a reduction in mean BMI. Thus it does appear that those previously diagnosed as having some degree of hypertension have made some attempt to control their weight.

To enable the distribution of blood pressure categories to be compared in subjects in similar age groups at both surveys, the proportions of respondents in each category by age at survey are shown in Table 5.6. As shown in earlier tables, the principal differences in the proportions of normotensives between HALS1 and HALS2 are in the youngest age group. Comparison of the ratio of untreated to treated hypertensives from HALS1 to HALS2 shows a great change. Table 5.7 shows the proportions of untreated to treated hypertensives by age at survey. A much greater proportion of the hypertensives were being treated at HALS2, especially in the older age groups, a possible result of the current policies of monitoring health. However, as the respondents found to be hypertensive but untreated at measurement in HALS1 were advised to visit their GP, they would now be more likely to be treated: this does not apply to those respondents who were normotensive or just borderline at HALS1 measurement, who were not given this advice. In these groups the similar increase in the proportions treated at HALS2 cannot be attributable to this factor. Many of the nurses' comments on the measurement proforma referred to routine check-ups at the respondent's GP clinics, even where results found at HALS2 were normal.

## High blood pressure: effectiveness of therapy

In HALS1 the proportion of those being treated with anti-hypertensive drugs whose blood pressure was in the normotensive range was less than those whose blood pressure at measurement was in the borderline or hypertensive range. Of the hypertensives, aged 40 and over at survey, who were receiving drug therapy (6.2% of men and 6.9% of women) only 42% of treated men were normotensive. Over 20% remained overtly hypertensive. The situation was much improved in HALS2 with 55% of the men and 60% of the women being normotensive at measurement and the proportion remaining hypertensive by measurement being 19% and 14% respectively (Table 5.8). Although there is an overall improvement, as seen in HALS1, drug therapy appears to be more effective in younger than in older women.

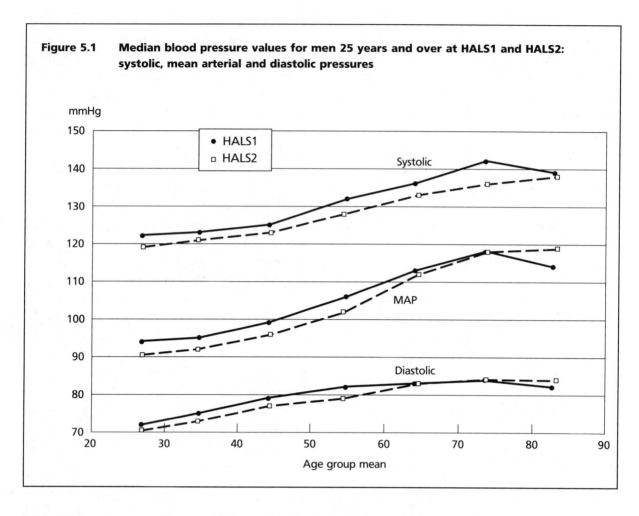

**Figure 5.1    Median blood pressure values for men 25 years and over at HALS1 and HALS2: systolic, mean arterial and diastolic pressures**

Compliance with the prescribed medication was impossible to assess, and this may indeed have been a factor since many of the drugs prescribed for hypertension have side effects such as depression (MRC, 1983) whilst hypertension itself is often asymptomatic.

## Median blood pressures

Since, especially in the older age groups, there were increasing numbers of treated hypertensives, a population mean value for blood pressure would be affected by those hypertensives who were being successfully treated and the true mean value cannot be ascertained. However, a valid median value can be obtained if the treated hypertensives are assumed to have values which are in the hypertensive range and if the median value so derived does not rise above the value at which treatment for hypertension would be instigated. The median values for systolic, diastolic and mean arterial pressure rose steadily with age in the HALS1 population and the rate of rise increased

in post menopausal women. The median values for HALS1 and HALS2 systolic, diastolic and mean arterial pressure for men and and women age 25 and over at survey are shown in Figure 5.1 and Figure 5.2. Bearing in mind the lower mean pressures for the younger ages demonstrated in Tables 5.1 and 5.2, the median values for HALS2 also show lower values than in HALS1, reducing the likelihood that the higher percentage of treated hypertensives would be the sole contributor to the lower mean blood pressures seen in the HALS2 sample.

## Blood pressure and body mass index

Obesity is known to be associated with high blood pressure (Tobian, 1978), and in a large number of cross-sectional studies it has been shown that blood pressure and body weight levels are correlated, not only in older adults but also in younger age groups (Wadsworth et al. 1985).

Body mass index (BMI), calculated from height and weight (see Appendix A), is one of the most

**Figure 5.2    Median blood pressure values for women 25 years and over at HALS1 and HALS2: systolic, mean arterial and diastolic pressures**

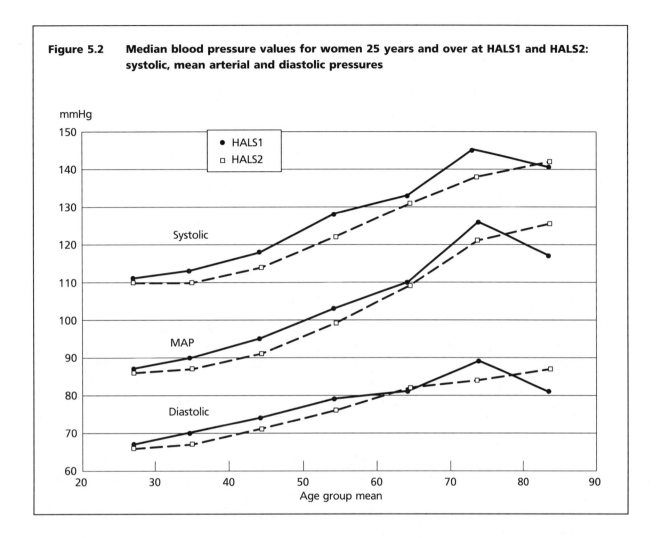

commonly used measures of obesity, and as with blood pressure there is a continuous distribution of values within a population (see Chapter 6). For simplicity, the BMI values were divided into the four categories – underweight, normal weight, over-weight and obese – following the Royal College of Physicians criteria (1983).

Table 5.9 shows the percentage of each BMI category who were normotensive in HALS1 and HALS2 by age at survey. Although the mean values of BMI for the acceptable, overweight and obese categories at HALS1 and HALS2 in these age bands are not shown, they are not significantly different. As was shown in HALS1, elevated blood pressures were strongly associated with obesity. Women who were not overweight were less likely to suffer from hypertension than men who were not overweight. With increasing adiposity the differences between the sexes in respect of hypertension were less marked. The overweight were more likely to have been diagnosed and treated for high blood pressure than

those who were in the acceptable weight groups.

In HALS2 the percentage in the middle aged group (40-59 years) who were normotensive was greater than in HALS1 in all BMI categories, and in both sexes. This also applied to the acceptable weight category in the next age group (60-79 years) but not to the overweight and obese or the older age group (80+ years).

## Blood pressure and socio-economic group: non-manual and manual

Several studies have indicated differences in the prevalence of hypertension between social groups, whichever form of classification is used (Rose and Marmot, 1981). Table 5.10 shows the blood pressure categories by age at Survey and by household socio-economic group. In the middle aged men and women (40-59 years) in the non-manual and manual socio-economic groups there there were no great differences between the patterns of blood pressure categories in either surveys. However, the previously reported pattern of more normotensives in the HALS2 sample aged 40-59 applied equally to both socio-economic groups. In the over 60s there were no major differences between the proportion of normotensives in HALS1 and HALS2, but a difference between the socio-economic groups had emerged, whereby there were fewer normotensives in the manual group in both surveys, especially in the men. The hypertensives in both socio-economic groups and both sexes were more likely to be treated in HALS2 than in HALS1 but there were no differences between the socio-economic groups.

## Blood pressure and smoking

The association of smoking with cardiovascular disease is well known (Royal College of Physicians, 1977) but the contribution of smoking to hypertension has not yet been fully evaluated. Several studies (Savdie, Grosslight and Adena, 1984; Seltzer, 1974; Kesteloot and Van Houte, 1974) suggest that smokers may have a lower incidence of hypertension than non-smokers and this was provisionally confirmed in the HALS1 report (Cox et al. 1987) where the age-standardised distribution of simple blood pressure categories and smoking habits demonstrated a slight negative association between blood pressure and smoking. However, as was stated in the HALS1 report, the non-smoking group contained a greater proportion of overweight and obese subjects compared to the regular smokers (Chapter 6). In further detailed analysis of the HALS1 data (Cox, unpublished), taking into account BMI, the negative association between high blood pressure and smoking in men virtually disappeared, but remained in women.

## Regional distribution

As has previously been reported (Cox et al. 1987; Shaper et al. 1981) there are regional differences in the prevalence of hypertension. The reduction in the sample size from HALS1 to HALS2 has meant that meaningful simple analysis cannot be carried out by Standard Region as in HALS1, so a dichotomised variable, North/South, has been used where the Standard Regions Scotland, North, North West, Yorks/Humber, Wales and West Midlands are combined as the 'North' and the East Midlands, East Anglia, South West, South East, and Greater London are combined as the 'South'.

Both by age group, and by sex, and in both surveys, there is a higher proportion of normotensives in the South than in the North (Table 5.11), an observation which may reflect the higher mean Body Mass Index seen in the North (Chapter 6). There is a higher proportion of normotensives in the middle aged group (40-59 years) in the South at both surveys. There were no marked or consistent differences in the likelihood of being treated for hypertension between the North and South.

## Pulse rate

In HALS1 a relationship between adiposity and pulse rate was demonstrated, and since the original report (Cox et al. 1987) the relationship between adiposity, smoking behaviour and pulse rate has been investigated (Cox and Whichelow, 1990). Table 5-12 shows the mean pulse rate of the HALS2 measured sample (excluding those on pulse rate modifying medication) by BMI and smoking category. There is a significant trend in that, with increasing adiposity, the mean pulse rate rises, and this is coupled with a further tonic effect for the regular smokers such that the mean pulse rate of obese men who are regular smokers is 74.6 ($\pm 0.45$ S.E.M.) beats per minute (bpm) and that of non-smoking men of acceptable weight is 65.0 ($\pm 0.65$ S.E.M.) bpm. For the women the figures are 73.7 ($\pm 0.90$ S.E.M.) and 68.7 ($\pm 0.44$ S.E.M.) bpm respectively.

Ex-smokers are a heterogeneous group in that some respondents will have given up many years ago, and some only recently. Analysis of the pulse rates of ex-smokers (Cox and Whichelow, 1990) has shown that in the first year following cessation of smoking the mean pulse rate is significantly lower than that of the non-smokers, but then rises.

# RESPIRATORY FUNCTION

Respiratory function is a composite of the purely mechanical process of breathing and the ability of the heart and the blood to transport oxygen to the tissues and carbon dioxide back to the lungs. The aspect measured in this Survey by a pocket spirometer is, of course, only the mechanical aspect of respiratory function. The device was an electronic pocket spirometer (Micro Medical Instruments Ltd.) and was selected after assessment against standard physiological laboratory displacement spirometers to be the most appropriate for this Survey in respect of portability and elimination of operator error (Appendix B).

Good respiratory function is essential to the maintenance of health, and recent studies in Baltimore (Beaty et al. 1985) have indicated that it appeared to be the most significant predictor of survival over a 24-year period for a group of subjects who were assessed at intervals for various measures, such as blood pressure, cholesterol, etc. Even when age and smoking habits were taken into consideration, the relationship of the observed forced expiratory volume in 1 second (FEV1) to its predicted value for that individual was significantly associated with mortality from all causes.

One of the goals of respiratory or lung function testing is to determine whether or not an individual is 'normal'. The term normal has many meanings in this context and can be used to indicate whether or not measured indices obtained from a subject have values which would be expected from an individual with the subject's characteristics in respect of age, height and sex. The equations derived for the estimation of normal values are obtained from the results of a large number of individuals who appear to be free of disease. Unfortunately, unlike blood pressures, there is no consensus as to normal values for groups of individuals. Many studies have been carried out on small populations, from different ethnic groups, and each centre seems to apply its own criteria for assessing pulmonary function.

More than fifty small surveys have examined 'normality' of respiratory function amongst their respective populations, and each has evolved multiple regression equations as a means of assessing 'normality'. These equations take into account stature and age in their derivation, weight being only weakly correlated with lung function. Lung size is positively correlated to a greater extent with stature than with any other body measurement and thus stature is the reference variable of choice for most purposes. The development of respiratory function reaches a maximum in the early 20s, and thereafter declines with age in a nearly linear fashion relative to stature. This enables multiple linear regression equations to be derived, for Forced Expiratory Volume in 1 second (FEV1), Forced Vital Capacity (FVC) and Peak Expiratory Flow (PEF) which are applicable, by taking account of stature and age, to males and females. Using these multiple linear regression models, subjects aged 18-25 appear to have poorer lung function than would be expected.

In HALS1 the regression equations of Knudson et al. (1976) were used for comparative assessment of lung function. These equations were derived from a population of white men and women aged 20-90, who had no evidence of respiratory disease, and were lifetime non-smokers. Another advantage in using these reference values at that time was that the equations were derived from a single population. Many of the regression equations often used are based on separate studies with different indices for men and women, and may include subjects with a history of smoking.

A publication by Schoenberg et al. (1978) examines the growth and decay of pulmonary function in a group of healthy blacks and whites in the USA, and is probably the most definitive study in this field. Unfortunately, the number of factors taken into consideration to derive their regression equations is more than it was practicable to measure in the HALS Surveys. However, the measurements of FEV1 and height obtained in HALS1 corresponded very closely to those obtained by Schoenberg et al. and Strachan et al. (1991) have published polynomial regression equations for lung function measures from over 1500 of the HALS1 subjects who were lifelong non-smokers with no history of respiratory disease: these are used in this study.

## Method

One problem in assessing lung function is that it requires the active co-operation of the respondent to a greater degree than the measurements of either weight or blood pressure. The respondent has to be instructed correctly, and then monitored by the nurse to ensure that the sequence of procedures is carried out according to the guidelines set down. Although in the majority of instances the procedure was carried out satisfactorily there were some instances where the respondent did not or could not follow the instructions, and in some cases satisfactory readings were not obtained because of language difficulties, as with some of the ethnic minorities, or because of problems with comprehension.

The respondent was instructed to take a deep breath, and then blow into the spirometer as hard and as fast and for as long as he or she could. Three measurements of lung function were then recorded by the spirometer: 1. FEV1 (Forced Expiratory Volume in 1 second) which is the volume of air in litres expelled in the first second, 2. PEF (Peak Expiratory Flow) which is the fastest rate of exhalation in litres per minute recorded during the measurements and 3. FVC (Forced Vital Capacity) which is the total amount of air in litres exhaled. This is a reflection of functional lung capacity.

All three measures of lung function depend on lung capacity, which is smaller in women than in men, and is related to stature, as mentioned, and ethnic origin. Black/African races have relatively smaller lungs than Caucasians (Schoenberg et al. 1978). The respiratory values for non- whites have been omitted from this report as the numbers are small, and the commonly used predicted values for lung function are not applicable for non-whites.

Of the three parameters, forced expiratory volume in one second (FEV1), forced vital capacity (FVC), and peak expiratory flow (PEF), only FEV1 results are reported here as it is the index least likely to have been affected by the respondent's inappropriate use of the spirometer.

## Respiratory function and age

Respiratory function declines with age, and the predicted values take this into account, so that useful comparisons of the observed values to the predicted values can be made and categories of assessed performance applied. Tables 5.13a and 5.13b show for men and women, by seven-year age bands, the mean FEV1, the mean of the predicted value for FEV1 (using the polynomial regression equations of Strachan et al. (1989)) and the percentage of each

group being treated for respiratory problems with broncho-dilators or steroidal anti-asthmatic preparations.

As for blood pressure the data are presented as means of the whole HALS1 measured population and of the HALS2 sample (which is a sub-sample of the HALS1 population) at both sampling times. For the rationale of this form of presentation see under 'Blood pressure values', earlier in this chapter. As previously stated, the presentation in these tables of the mean values of both the whole HALS1 population and those of the group who were seen exactly seven years later at HALS2 as well as at HALS1, enables an assessment to be made of how representative of the whole HALS1 sample is the HALS2 sub-set. The use of seven-year age bands also enables a comparison to be made of the HALS2 1991/2 results with the values obtained for the next older age group at HALS1.

The mean FEV1 can be seen to decline with increasing age in both men and women; the values obtained for the HALS2 sub-sample in 1984/5 are very similar to the whole HALS1 measured group at each age group under 52 years for men and under 59 years for women. The values obtained in 1991/2 for the first three age bands also correspond very closely with those seen in 1984/5 for the same age bands. This suggests that in these younger respondents the HALS2 sample is not only a representative sub-sample of the HALS1 population but that overall the decline in lung function is as might be expected for a seven year increase in age.

In the older age groups, especially in those over 60, there is a difference which is statistically significant in the values for FEV1 obtained for the HALS2 sub-sample compared to the whole HALS1 population, reflecting in some part the high death rate amongst those with poor respiratory function at HALS1 (Chapter 3). However, the HALS2 sub-sample values in 1991/2 are not statistically different from those of the same age band sub-sample values in 1984/5.

These trends are confirmed when the observed value is compared to the theoretical predicted value, where also there is a steady decline with age, which is partly the result of the increase in respiratory problems of the population as a whole with age and is also associated with the long-term effects of smoking on lung function.

What has changed dramatically over the seven years between HALS1 and HALS2 is the great increase in the use of broncho-dilators or anti-asthmatic medications by the measured sample which is associated with the increase in reported respiratory problems and asthma in Chapter 4.

In the youngest seven-year age band (aged 25-31 in HALS2) in both men and women the percentage using these medications greatly increased, from 2.7% to 5.8% in the men and from 3.9% to 5.4% in the women. In the next three age bands (aged 32-52 in HALS2) there have been no major changes in the use of these medications but the reported use in those aged 60-80 in HALS2 has doubled amongst both men and women. Overall, the change in usage by the measured HALS2 population has increased from 2.9% to 5.4% for the 1792 men and from 2.0% to 4.1% for the 2198 women reported in these tables. Some increase might have been expected as the sample aged by seven years but the order of magnitude is far greater than predicted. This change may reflect changes in prescribing and diagnostic patterns but may also reflect increasing prevalence of asthma and respiratory problems.

For simplicity of interpretation the respondents have been grouped into four categories, based on their performance in relation to predicted values. The first category 'Excellent' includes those whose performance with the spirometer was equal to or in excess of predicted values for a healthy person of their age, sex and height. The second category 'Good' comprises those whose measurements were up to 2.0 standard deviations below the predicted values. In the third category 'Fair to Poor' are those whose performance was between 2.0 and 4.0 standard deviations below the predicted values. Those respondents whose performance fell more than 4.0 standard deviations below the predicted values were included in the fourth category 'Very Poor' and were regarded as having grossly impaired respiratory function. In this category are those who were unable to undertake the measurements because of chronic respiratory problems. Respondents with transient acute respiratory problems, such as colds or flu, were excluded from the analysis.

Table 5.14 demonstrates the distribution in these categories at HALS1 (1984/5) and then at HALS2 (1991/2) by three age groups and with the proportion being treated with respiratory medication in each category. In both men and women there were no significant changes in the distribution of subjects by respiratory function category between HALS1 and HALS2. However an increase in the proportion on medication can be seen in each category, with the most dramatic changes occurring in the older age groups and in those with the poorest lung function. It might have been expected that the increase in the use of medication for respiratory problems would have resulted in an overall improvement in performance at measurement, but this does not seem to have occurred.

## Respiratory function and smoking

It has previously been reported (Higgins et al. 1971: Cox et al. 1987) that the respiratory function of smokers is poorer than that of non-smokers, even when there is no history of respiratory problems. In HALS1 the poorer respiratory function of regular smokers could clearly be seen even in young age groups. Respiratory function as a percentage of the predicted value and by smoking category at survey, of those subjects aged between 25 and 75 at HALS1 is shown in Table 5.15. The mean ages of those in each of the smoking categories at HALS1, 45.1 for non-smokers, 49.0 for ex-smokers, 45.1 for light regular smokers (1-15 cigarettes a day) and 43.8 for heavy regular smokers (16 or more cigarettes a day), were not very different. Although having the lowest mean age, the heavy regular smokers had the poorest lung function at approximately 88% of the predicted value. The ex- smoking men had poorer lung function values than the ex-smoking women, but this may reflect the fact that ex-smoking men were more likely to have been heavy regular smokers than were the women. It may be noted that the base numbers of the smoking categories change from HALS1 to HALS2, which reflects the change in smoking behaviour that has occurred in the seven years between the surveys (Chapter 12).

There is a complex pattern of changes which could and, in some instances, have occurred during the seven years between the two surveys. Table 5.16 shows the changes that have occurred in the mean of predicted values for FEV1 between HALS1 and HALS2 in relation to change or lack of change in the major smoking categories. In those subjects who

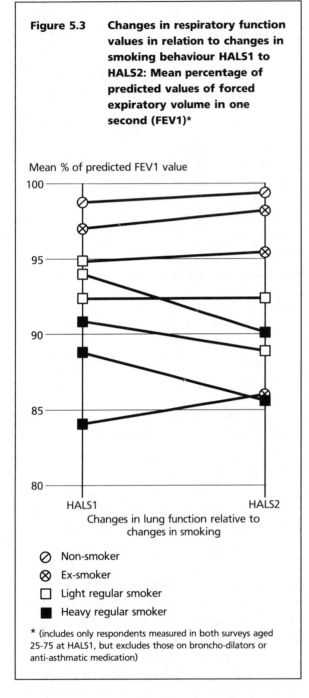

**Figure 5.3** **Changes in respiratory function values in relation to changes in smoking behaviour HALS1 to HALS2: Mean percentage of predicted values of forced expiratory volume in one second (FEV1)\***

Mean % of predicted FEV1 value

Changes in lung function relative to changes in smoking

⊘ Non-smoker
⊗ Ex-smoker
□ Light regular smoker
■ Heavy regular smoker

\* (includes only respondents measured in both surveys aged 25-75 at HALS1, but excludes those on broncho-dilators or anti-asthmatic medication)

improvement of lung function. These changes are graphically demonstrated in Figure 5.3.

## Respiratory function and socio-economic groups

In HALS1 (Cox et al. 1987) it was demonstrated that respiratory function varied with socio-economic group in both sexes. Because smoking patterns differ markedly between socio-economic groups with manual groups being more likely to be smokers (Chapter 12), analyses that take both factors into consideration are needed to demonstrate the differences between the performance of lung function measures that could be related to social group rather than just smoking behaviour. Table 5.17 shows the distribution of respondents by respiratory function categories, smoking behaviour and non-manual/manual household socio-economic group and by two age groups in those respondents who have not changed smoking behaviour HALS1 to HALS2. Taking the proportions of respondents with 'Excellent' respiratory function there is no marked difference between the non-manual and manual groups in the younger age group (aged 18-38 at HALS1), but the effect of current smoking behaviour can clearly be seen in the light and heavy regular smoking categories in both socio-economic groups.

In the older age group (aged 39-59 at HALS1) the manual groups show markedly poorer values in all but the heavy regular smoking groups. Figure 5.4 demonstrates the trends in lung function values seen in the HALS2 respondents in the non-manual and manual socio-economic groups who did not change their smoking behaviour from HALS1 to HALS2, and Figure 5.5 shows the trends in the non-manual and manual groups that were found in those respondents who were ex-smokers at HALS2 whatever their HALS1 smoking category. It does appear that ceasing smoking tends to lead to an improvement in measured FEV1. Those who were heavy smokers at HALS1 and were ex-smokers at HALS2 had the lowest mean lung function values at HALS1, suggesting that the development of respiratory problems led to the cessation of smoking activity. Investigation of the relationship between diet and lung function in the HALS1 sample led to the finding that good lung function is related to the frequent consumption of fresh fruit or fruit juice in non-

were non-smokers or ex-smokers in both surveys there has been a slight improvement in the mean percentage of predicted FEV1. In those continuing as light regular smokers there has been no change, but the overall values are lower than for the non-smokers or long-term ex-smokers. In those who were heavy regular smokers at both surveys there was a significant deterioration in lung function between HALS1 and HALS2. In subjects who were either light or heavy regular smokers at HALS1 and who were ex-smokers by HALS2 there appeared to be an

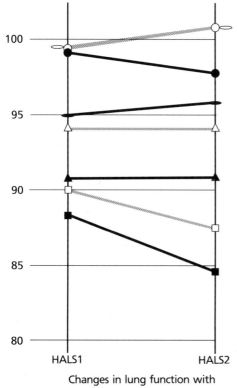

**Figure 5.4** **Changes in respiratory function values HALS1 to HALS2 by socio-economic group (non-manual and manual) where there were no changes in smoking behaviour: Mean percentage of predicted values of forced expiratory volume in one second (FEV1)***

Mean % of predicted FEV1 value

HALS1    HALS2

Changes in lung function with
no change in smoking category

○  Non-smoker, non-manual
●  Non-smoker, manual
◦  Ex-smoker, non-manual
━  Ex-smoker, manual
△  Light regular smoker, non-manual
▲  Light regular smoker, manual
□  Heavy regular smoker, non-manual
■  Heavy regular smoker, manual

* (includes only respondents measured in both surveys aged
25-75 at HALS1, but excludes those on broncho-dilators or anti-
asthmatic medication)

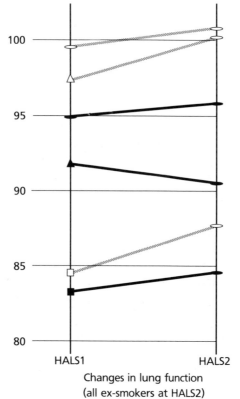

**Figure 5.5** **Changes in respiratory function values HALS1 to HALS2 by socio-economic group (non-manual and manual) and by various smoking categories at HALS1 but where all respondents were ex-smokers at HALS2: Mean percentage of predicted values of forced expiratory volume in one second (FEV1)***

Mean % of predicted FEV1 value

HALS1    HALS2

Changes in lung function
(all ex-smokers at HALS2)

◦  Ex-smoker, non-manual
━  Ex-smoker, manual
△  Light regular smoker, non-manual
▲  Light regular smoker, manual
□  Heavy regular smoker, non-manual
■  Heavy regular smoker, manual

* (includes only respondents measured in both surveys aged
25-75 at HALS1, but excludes those on broncho-dilators or anti-
asthmatic medication)

smokers and smokers (Cox and Whichelow, 1990; Strachan et al. 1991). Since the frequency of fruit consumption is also related to social group (Whichelow et al. 1988), the differences seen in lung function between socio-economic groups, independent of smoking behaviour, may be related in some part to different dietary patterns.

## Summary

Both mean and median blood pressure have risen less by HALS2 than would have been expected for the seven-year increase in age, and the increase in obesity. The proportion of treated to untreated hypertensives has risen considerably at HALS2, possibly reflecting an increased surveillance of the population. Treatments also appear to be more effective in that a higher proportion of respondents on medication have normal blood pressure levels at HALS2 than at HALS1.

Respiratory function values have changed as predicted by the increase in age but the proportion of respondents on broncho-dilators or anti-asthmatic preparations has risen considerably. Smoking has affected the rate of change in lung function more than has any other factor, that of heavy cigarette smokers having deteriorated faster than would be expected for the increase in age. In those who are now ex-smokers but who were heavy smokers at HALS1, there is some evidence of a recovery of lung function towards normal values.

## References

Barker, D.J.P. (1991), 'The foetal and infant origins of inequalities in health in Britain', Journal of Public Health Medicine, 13, 64-68.

Beaty, T.H., et al. (1985), 'Effects of pulmonary function on mortality', Journal of Chronic Disease, 38, 703-710.

Cox, B.D. et al. 1987), 'The Health and Lifestyle Survey, Preliminary report of a nationwide survey of the physical and mental health, attitudes and lifestyle of a random sample of 9,003 British adults', Health Promotion Research Trust, London.

Cox, B.D. and Whichelow, M.J. (1990), 'Body Mass Index, Waist/Hip ratio and pulse rate in non-smokers, smokers and ex-smokers relative to time of quitting', International Journal of Obesity, 14, S2.IP 69.

Cruz-Coke, R. Donaso, H. and Barrera, R.(1973), 'Genetic ecology of hypertension', Clinical Science, 45, 55s-56s.

Epstein, F. (1983), 'The Epidemiology of Essential Hypertension' in Robertson J.I.S. (ed) Handbook of Hypertension Vol.1 Clinical Aspects of Essential Hypertension, Elsevier, Oxford.

Higgins, I.T.T. et al. 1971), 'Smoking and chronic respiratory disease; findings in surveys carried out in 1957 and 1966 in Staveley in Derbyshire, England', Chest, 59, 345-351.

Kesteloot, H., and Van Houte, O. (1974), 'An epidemiological survey of arterial blood pressure in a large male population group', American Journal of Epidemiology, 99, 14-29.

Knudson, R.J., Slatin, R.C., Lebowitz, M.D. and Burrows, B. (1976), 'The maximal expiratory flow-volume curve. Normal standards, variability and effects of age', American Review of Respiratory Disease, 113, 587-600.

Lew, E. (1973), 'High blood pressure. Other risk factors and longevity: The insurance viewpoint', American Journal of Medicine, 55, 281-294.

Marmot, M. (1984), 'Geography of Blood Pressure and Hypertension', British Medical Bulletin, 40, 380-386.

Medical Research Council. (1985), 'MRC trial of treatment of mild hypertension: principal results', British Medical Journal, 291, 97-104.

Miall, W.E. and Lovell, H.G. (1967), 'Relation between change in blood pressure and age', British Medical Journal, 2, 660-664.

Rose, G. and Marmot, M.G. (1981), 'Social Class and Coronary Heart Disease', British Heart Journal, 45, 13-19.

Royal College of Physicians. (1983), 'Obesity Report', Journal of the Royal College of Physicians, 17, 5-65.

Royal College of Physicians. (1977), 'Third Report: Smoking or Health', Pitman Medical, London.

Savdie, E., Grosslight, G.M. and Adena, M.A. (1984), 'Relation of alcohol and cigarette consumption to blood pressure and serum creatinine levels', Journal of Chronic Disease, 37, 617-623.

Schoenberg, J.B., Beck, G.J. and Bouhuys A. (1978), 'Growth and decay of pulmonary function in healthy blacks and whites', Respiration Physiology, 33, 367-393.

Seltzer, C.C. (1974), 'Effect of smoking on blood pressure', American Heart Journal, 87, 558-564.

Shaper, A.G., et al. (1981), 'British Regional Heart Study: cardiovascular risk factors in middle aged men in 24 towns', British Medical Journal, 283, 179-186.

Strachan, D.P., Cox, B.D., Erzinclioglu, S.W., Walters, D.E. and Whichelow, M.J. (1991), 'Ventilatory function and winter fresh fruit consumption in a random sample of British adults', Thorax, 46, 624-629.

Tobian, L. (1978), 'Hypertension and obesity', New England Journal of Medicine, 298, 46-68.

Wadsworth, M.E.J., Cripps, H.A., Midwinter, R.E. and Colley, J.R.T.,(1985), 'Blood pressure in a national birth cohort at the age of 36 related to social and familial factors, smoking and body mass', British Medical Journal, 291, 1534-1538.

Whichelow, M.J., Erzinclioglu, S.W. and Cox, B.D. (1991), 'A comparison of the diets of non-smokers and smokers', British Journal of Addiction, 86, 71-81.

WHO (1978), Arterial Hypertension, World Health Organisation, Geneva.

**Table 5.1** Changes in systolic, mean arterial (M.A.P.) and diastolic blood pressure means in males (including those treated with anti-hypertensive drugs) analysed by age: HALS1 full sample in comparison to HALS2 sub-sample in 1984/5 and 1991/2 (Mean and ± standard error of the mean (S.E.M.))

| | Age | | | | | | | | | | | | | | | | | |
|---|---|---|---|---|---|---|---|---|---|---|---|---|---|---|---|---|---|---|
| **HALS1** | 18-24 | 25-31 | | 32-38 | | 39-45 | | 46-52 | | 53-59 | | 60-66 | | 67-73 | | >73 | | |
| **HALS2** | | | 25-31 | | 32-38 | | 39-45 | | 46-52 | | 53-59 | | 60-66 | | 67-73 | | 74-80 | >80 |
| **Systolic mean (mmHg.)** | | | | | | | | | | | | | | | | | | |
| HALS1 sample | 121.3 ±0.6 | 122.3 ±0.6 | | 124.2 ±0.6 | | 126.0 ±0.7 | | 129.6 ±0.8 | | 134.0 ±0.9 | | 137.3 ±1.0 | | 139.5 ±1.2 | | 140.2 ±1.5 | | |
| HALS2 sub-sample | 121.8 ±0.8 | 120.2 ±0.7 | 122.0 ±0.8 | 122.1 ±0.9 | 123.8 ±0.7 | 123.6 ±0.7 | 125.9 ±0.8 | 126.9 ±0.9 | 128.9 ±0.9 | 129.6 ±1.0 | 134.0 ±1.1 | 133.9 ±1.0 | 138.0 ±1.7 | 134.9 ±1.2 | 139.2 ±1.7 | 137.5 ±1.6 | 139.7 ±2.7 | 133.4 ±2.7 |
| **M.A.P. mean (mmHg.)** | | | | | | | | | | | | | | | | | | |
| HALS1 sample | 92.0 ±0.5 | 93.7 ±0.5 | | 96.6 ±0.5 | | 99.2 ±0.6 | | 103.2 ±0.7 | | 107.7 ±0.8 | | 110.9 ±0.9 | | 113.7 ±1.1 | | 113.4 ±1.3 | | |
| HALS2 sub-sample | 91.9 ±0.7 | 90.9 ±0.7 | 93.7 ±0.7 | 93.3 ±0.8 | 96.6 ±0.6 | 96.1 ±0.6 | 99.2 ±0.7 | 99.7 ±0.8 | 102.8 ±0.8 | 103.2 ±1.0 | 107.6 ±1.0 | 107.1 ±0.9 | 111.4 ±1.2 | 108.5 ±1.1 | 113.1 ±1.5 | 109.7 ±1.5 | 113.8 ±2.3 | 106.6 ±2.2 |
| **Diastolic mean (mmHg.)** | | | | | | | | | | | | | | | | | | |
| HALS1 sample | 70.6 ±0.4 | 73.3 ±0.4 | | 76.6 ±0.5 | | 78.8 ±0.5 | | 80.8 ±0.5 | | 82.7 ±0.6 | | 82.0 ±0.7 | | 81.7 ±0.8 | | 79.6 ±0.9 | | |
| HALS2 sub-sample | 70.7 ±0.6 | 71.7 ±0.7 | 73.4 ±0.7 | 74.7 ±0.7 | 76.1 ±0.5 | 77.1 ±0.5 | 78.3 ±0.6 | 78.3 ±0.6 | 80.2 ±0.6 | 79.4 ±0.7 | 82.8 ±0.7 | 79.9 ±0.6 | 82.5 ±0.8 | 77.6 ±0.7 | 81.5 ±1.0 | 77.8 ±1.0 | 79.7 ±1.7 | 74.2 ±1.6 |
| **Proportion on drugs with anti-hypertensive effects** | | | | | | | | | | | | | | | | | | |
| HALS1 sample | 1% | – | | 1% | | 1% | | 6% | | 15% | | 18% | | 23% | | 23% | | |
| HALS2 sub-sample | 1% | (1) | 1% | 1% | 4% | 5% | 7% | 15% | 15% | 27% | 16% | 34% | 18% | 35% | 11% | 35% | | |
| **Base = 100%** | | | | | | | | | | | | | | | | | | |
| HALS1 | 442 | 413 | | 510 | | 412 | | 357 | | 358 | | 339 | | 259 | | 211 | | |
| HALS2 | 240 | | 203 | | 339 | | 280 | | 241 | | 250 | | 219 | | 127 | | 71 |

**Table 5.2  Changes in systolic, mean arterial (M.A.P.) and diastolic blood pressure means in females (including those treated with anti-hypertensive drugs) analysed by age: HALS1 full sample in comparison to HALS2 sub-sample in 1984/5 and 1991/2 (Mean and ± standard error of the mean (S.E.M.)**

(In each column the first age band refers to HALS1, the second to the HALS2 sub-sample.)

| | 18-24 / 25-31 | 25-31 / 32-38 | 32-38 / 39-45 | 39-45 / 46-52 | 46-52 / 53-59 | 53-59 / 60-66 | 60-66 / 67-73 | 67-73 / 74-80 | >73 / >80 |
|---|---|---|---|---|---|---|---|---|---|
| **Systolic mean (mmHg.)** | | | | | | | | | |
| HALS1 sample | 111.6 ±0.5 | 112.0 ±0.6 | 114.9 ±0.5 | 117.2 ±0.6 | 124.0 ±0.7 | 129.9 ±0.9 | 133.9 ±0.9 | 143.6 ±1.4 | 144.2 ±1.4 |
| HALS2 sub-sample | 112.5 ±0.7 | 110.2 ±0.7 | 112.3 ±0.6 | 114.7 ±0.5 | 116.9 ±0.7 | 123.7 ±0.9 | 124.9 ±1.1 | 130.3 ±1.1 | 129.2 ±1.2 |
| **M.A.P. mean (mmHg.)** | | | | | | | | | |
| HALS1 sample | 86.2 ±0.4 | 87.6 ±0.4 | 91.2 ±0.4 | 93.4 ±0.6 | 99.2 ±0.7 | 104.5 ±0.8 | 107.8 ±0.8 | 115.7 ±1.1 | 115.0 ±1.3 |
| HALS2 sub-sample | 86.6 ±0.6 | 85.5 ±0.6 | 87.7 ±0.6 | 91.2 ±0.5 | 93.4 ±0.7 | 98.9 ±0.8 | 99.4 ±1.0 | 105.3 ±0.9 | 102.8 ±1.0 |
| **Diastolic mean (mmHg.)** | | | | | | | | | |
| HALS1 sample | 65.8 ±0.4 | 67.5 ±0.4 | 70.5 ±0.4 | 72.4 ±0.5 | 76.5 ±0.5 | 78.8 ±0.6 | 79.7 ±0.6 | 83.2 ±0.8 | 81.0 ±0.8 |
| HALS2 sub-sample | 66.6 ±0.6 | 66.2 ±0.6 | 67.8 ±0.5 | 70.3 ±0.4 | 70.5 ±0.4 | 72.2 ±0.6 | 72.2 ±0.5 | 75.2 ±0.8 | 76.3 ±0.8 |
| **Proportion on drugs with anti-hypertensive effects** | | | | | | | | | |
| HALS1 sample | (1) | (2) | % | 3% | 9% | 14% | 17% | 20% | 30% |
| HALS2 sub-smaple | (1) | (2) | 2% | 5% | 11% | 18% | 29% | 33% | 44% |
| **Base** | | | | | | | | | |
| HALS1 sample | 480 | 566 | 683 | 532 | 467 | 387 | 415 | 281 | 271 |
| HALS2 | 223 | 337 | 481 | 373 | 322 | 243 | 252 | 136 | 91 |

**Table 5.3   Changes in blood pressure categories from HALS1 to HALS2 analysed by age: percentage of age group**

| HALS1 age (HALS2 age) | 18-24 (25-31) | | 25-31 (32-38) | | 32-38 (39-45) | | 39-45 (46-52) | | 46-52 (53-59) | | 53-59 (60-66) | | 60-66 (67-73) | | 67-73 (74-80) | | >73 (>80) | |
|---|---|---|---|---|---|---|---|---|---|---|---|---|---|---|---|---|---|---|
| HALS | 1 | 2 | 1 | 2 | 1 | 2 | 1 | 2 | 1 | 2 | 1 | 2 | 1 | 2 | 1 | 2 | 1 | 2 |
| **Percentage** | | | | | | | | | | | | | | | | | | |
| **Males** | | | | | | | | | | | | | | | | | | |
| Normotensive (≤140/90 mmHg.) | 91 | 95 | 91 | 90 | 88 | 84 | 83 | 76 | 73 | 65 | 56 | 52 | 53 | 44 | 46 | 37 | 52 | 35 |
| Borderline (141/91 to 159/94 mmHg.) | 6 | 3 | 6 | 5 | 7 | 8 | 9 | 12 | 13 | 12 | 16 | 15 | 17 | 16 | 21 | 19 | 21 | 16 |
| Untreated hypertensive (≥160/95 mmHg.) | 1 | 2 | 3 | 3 | 4 | 4 | 7 | 6 | 7 | 7 | 14 | 6 | 14 | 6 | 15 | 9 | 16 | 14 |
| Treated Hypertensive | (2) | (1) | – | 1 | (2) | 4 | 1 | 5 | 5 | 12 | 12 | 23 | 16 | 29 | 14 | 25 | 10 | 18 |
| Normotensive but on drugs with anti-hypertensive effects (≤140/90 mmHg.) | (2) | – | – | – | – | – | (2) | (1) | 1 | 5 | 3 | 4 | (1) | 5 | 4 | 10 | 1 | 17 |
| *Base = 100%* | *240* | | *203* | | *339* | | *280* | | *242* | | *250* | | *219* | | *127* | | *71* | |
| **Females** | | | | | | | | | | | | | | | | | | |
| Normotensive (≤140/90 mmHg.) | 98 | 99 | 97 | 97 | 96 | 91 | 90 | 82 | 79 | 69 | 63 | 55 | 60 | 44 | 35 | 30 | 36 | 24 |
| Borderline (141/91 to 159/94 mmHg.) | 1 | (1) | 2 | (1) | 3 | 3 | 5 | 4 | 8 | 9 | 15 | 11 | 16 | 17 | 25 | 18 | 18 | 15 |
| Untreated hypertensive (≥160/95 mmHg.) | – | (1) | (1) | 1 | (3) | 1 | 2 | 2 | 4 | 5 | 9 | 5 | 10 | 6 | 17 | 8 | 22 | 13 |
| Treated Hypertensive | (1) | – | (2) | (2) | (1) | 3 | 2 | 7 | 9 | 16 | 12 | 24 | 12 | 27 | 19 | 35 | 20 | 30 |
| Normotensive but on drugs with anti-hypertensive effects (≤140/90 mmHg.) | – | – | – | 1 | (1) | 2 | (3) | 5 | (2) | 2 | 1 | 5 | 2 | 6 | 4 | 9 | 3 | 18 |
| *Base = 100%* | *223* | | *337* | | *482* | | *373* | | *322* | | *243* | | *252* | | *136* | | *91* | |

**Table 5.4**    **Seven-year changes in respondents' blood pressure categories: HALS2 blood pressure categories at measurement as a percentage of HALS1 categories**

| | Blood pressure category HALS1 (1984/5) | | | | | | | | | |
|---|---|---|---|---|---|---|---|---|---|---|
| | Normotensive (⩽140/90 mmHg.) | | Borderline (141/91 to 159/94 mmHg.) | | Untreated hypertensive (⩾160/95 mmHg.) | | Treated hypertensive (on medication) | | Normotensive but on drugs with anti-hypertensive effects (⩽140/90 mmHg.) | |
| | Males | Females | Males | Females | Males | Females | Males | Females | Males | Females |
| **Blood pressure category HALS2 (1991/2)** | | | | | | | | | | |
| Normotensive (⩽140/90 mmHg.) | 83.8 | 87.0 | 41.0 | 34.4 | 21.4 | 11.4 | 5.6 | 6.2 | (8) | (7) |
| Borderline (141/91 to 159/94 mmHg.) | 8.4 | 4.7 | 26.4 | 21.0 | 18.8 | 24.6 | 4.6 | 2.7 | (2) | – |
| Untreated hypertensive (⩾160/95 mmHg.) | 2.7 | 1.6 | 13.2 | 11.8 | 21.4 | 18.4 | (1) | 4.1 | – | – |
| Treated hypertensive (on medication) | 2.9 | 3.2 | 13.7 | 25.1 | 35.1 | 43.0 | 88.9 | 87.0 | (2) | (6) |
| Normotensive but on drugs with anti- hypertensive effects (⩽140/90 mmHg.) | 2.2 | 3.4 | 5.7 | 7.7 | 3.2 | 2.6 | – | – | (9) | (9) |
| *Base = 100%* | *1461* | *1981* | *227* | *195* | *154* | *114* | *108* | *146* | *21* | *22* |

**Table 5.5** **Mean percentage changes in Body Mass Index values over seven years in relation to changes in blood pressure categories**

| | Blood pressure category HALS1 (1984/5) | | | | | | | |
| | Normotensive (⩽140/90 mmHg.) | | Borderline (141/91 to 159/94 mmHg.) | | Untreated hypertensive (⩾160/95 mmHg.) | | Treated hypertensive (on medication) | |
|---|---|---|---|---|---|---|---|---|
| **Blood Pressure Category HALS2 (1991/2)** | | | | | | | | |
| | Males | Females | Males | Females | Males | Females | Males | Females |
| Normotensive (⩽140/90 mmHg.) | +4.4 | +5.8 | +2.1 | +0.8 | +2.7 | +1.0 | −1.1 | +1.0 |
| Borderline (141/91 to 159/94 mmHg.) | +3.3 | +5.7 | +2.9 | +0.1 | +1.1 | +0.1 | +1.2 | +1.3 |
| Untreated hypertensive (⩾160/95 mmHg.) | +5.5 | +6.7 | +1.0 | −1.2 | +0.9 | −1.2 | − | 12.3 |
| Treated hypertensive (on medication) | +2.8 | +3.7 | −1.6 | +1.6 | +0.1 | +2.3 | +0.5 | +1.3 |
| (Mean changes by HALS1 categories) | (+4.2) | (+5.8) | (+1.4) | (+1.1) | (+1.1) | (+0.6) | (+0.4) | (+0.7) |
| *Base* = *100%* | 1223 | 1654 | 93 | 67 | 33 | 12 | 6 | 8 |
| | 122 | 93 | 60 | 41 | 28 | 28 | 5 | 4 |
| | 40 | 32 | 30 | 23 | 33 | 20 | − | 6 |
| | 42 | 64 | 31 | 49 | 53 | 48 | 93 | 124 |
| | (1427) | (1843) | (214) | (180) | (147) | (108) | (104) | (142) |

**Table 5.6**     **Blood pressure categories in middle aged and elderly respondents: analysed by age at Survey: percentage of age group**

| | Age at survey | | | | | |
|---|---|---|---|---|---|---|
| | 40-59 | 60-79 | 80+ | 40-59 | 60-79 | 80+ |
| **Blood Pressure Category** | | | | | | |
| **HALS1 (1984/5)** | | Males | | | Females | |
| Normotensive (≤140/90 mmHg.) | 69 | 44 | 43 | 77 | 47 | 39 |
| Borderline (141/91 to 159/94 mmHg.) | 14 | 21 | 24 | 9 | 17 | 19 |
| Untreated hypertensive (≥160/95 mmHg.) | 10 | 15 | 11 | 5 | 16 | 15 |
| Treated hypertensive | 6 | 16 | 16 | 7 | 18 | 23 |
| Normotensive but on drugs with anti-hypertensive effects (≤140/90 mmHg.) | 1 | 4 | 6 | 1 | 3 | 5 |
| (Mean age in years) | (49.2) | (67.9) | (82.6) | (48.8) | (67.6) | (83.5) |
| *Base = 100%* | *1068* | *746* | *63* | *1306* | *858* | *109* |
| | | | | | | |
| **HALS2 (1991/2)** | | | | | | |
| Normotensive (≤140/90 mmHg.) | 76 | 46 | 35 | 81 | 46 | 25 |
| Borderline (141/91 to 159/94 mmHg.) | 11 | 16 | 15 | 5 | 15 | 16 |
| Untreated hypertensive (≥160/95 mmHg.) | 5 | 7 | 13 | 3 | 6 | 12 |
| Treated hypertensive | 7 | 25 | 23 | 8 | 28 | 30 |
| Normotensive but on drugs with anti-hypertensive effects (≤140/90 mmHg.) | 2 | 6 | 15 | 3 | 6 | 17 |
| (Mean age in years) | (48.8) | (68.2) | (83.6) | (48.7) | (68.3) | (84.1) |
| *Base = 100%* | *829* | *586* | *83* | *1118* | *630* | *106* |

**Table 5.7** **Hypertensive respondents: proportions of those untreated and treated in HALS1 and HALS2, by age at Survey: percentage of age group**

| | Age at Survey | | | | | |
|---|---|---|---|---|---|---|
| | 30-39 | 40-49 | 50-59 | 60-69 | 70-79 | 80+ |
| Hypertensive category | | | | | | |
| **HALS1 (1984/5)** | | | **Males** | | | |
| Untreated (≥160/95 mmHg.) | 85 | 73 | 56 | 45 | 53 | 41 |
| Treated (on drugs for high BP) | 15 | 27 | 44 | 55 | 47 | 59 |
| *Base = 100%* | *33* | *63* | *110* | *135* | *102* | *17* |
| **HALS2 (1991/2)** | | | | | | |
| Untreated (≥160/95 mmHg.) | (9) | 56 | 36 | 21 | 19 | 11 |
| Treated (on drugs for high BP) | (3) | 44 | 64 | 79 | 81 | 63 |
| *Base = 100%* | *12* | *43* | *56* | *103* | *84* | *30* |
| **HALS1 (1984/5)** | | | **Females** | | | |
| Untreated (≥160/95 mmHg.) | (8) | 42 | 44 | 44 | 49 | 39 |
| Treated (on drugs for high BP) | (6) | 58 | 56 | 56 | 51 | 61 |
| *Base = 100%* | *14* | *48* | *117* | *144* | *142* | *41* |
| **HALS2 (1991/2)** | | | | | | |
| Untreated (≥160/95 mmHg.) | (7) | 29 | 21 | 17 | 18 | 29 |
| Treated (on drugs for high BP) | (3) | 71 | 79 | 83 | 82 | 71 |
| *Base = 100%* | *10* | *38* | *81* | *110* | *100* | *45* |

**Table 5.8**   **Blood pressure levels at measurement in drug treated hypertensive men and women, analysed by age at Survey: percentage of age group**

| | Age at Survey | | | | | |
|---|---|---|---|---|---|---|
| | 40-59 | 60-79 | 80+ | 40-59 | 60-79 | 80+ |
| Blood pressure levels | | | | | | |
| **HALS1 (1984/5)** | | Males | | | Females | |
| Hypertensive by measurement ($\geqslant$160/95 mmHg.) | 24 | 25 | – | 19 | 29 | 36 |
| Borderline by measurement (141/91 to 159/94 mmHg.) | 33 | 34 | (5) | 20 | 29 | 32 |
| Normotensive by measurement ($\leqslant$140/90 mmHg.) | 42 | 41 | (5) | 61 | 42 | 32 |
| *Base = 100%* | *66* | *122* | *10* | *94* | *153* | *25* |
| **HALS2 (1991/2)** | | | | | | |
| Hypertensive by measurement ($\geqslant$160/95 mmHg.) | 14 | 21 | 11 | 12 | 14 | 22 |
| Borderline by measurement (141/91 to 159/94 mmHg.) | 24 | 27 | 26 | 12 | 32 | 31 |
| Normotensive by measurement ($\leqslant$140/90 mmHg.) | 62 | 52 | 63 | 76 | 54 | 47 |
| *Base = 100%* | *55* | *149* | *19* | *91* | *173* | *32* |

**Table 5.9    Percentage of normotensive subjects analysed by Body Mass Index (BMI) category and age group at Survey**

| Body Mass Index category (BMI) | Age at Survey | | | | | |
|---|---|---|---|---|---|---|
| | 40-59 | 60-79 | 80+ | 40-59 | 60-79 | 80+ |
| **HALS1 (1984/5)** | **Males** | | | **Females** | | |
| Acceptable weight | 75 | 46 | 46 | 86 | 53 | 32 |
| Overweight | 66 | 44 | 36 | 76 | 46 | 47 |
| Obese | 51 | 41 | – | 57 | 37 | 29 |
| *Base = 100%* | *447* | *313* | *22* | *582* | *297* | *41* |
| | *465* | *322* | *25* | *432* | *349* | *34* |
| | *108* | *64* | *3* | *248* | *171* | *24* |
| **HALS2 (1991/2)** | | | | | | |
| Acceptable weight | 83 | 53 | 43 | 89 | 60 | 36 |
| Overweight | 74 | 44 | 33 | 84 | 40 | 10 |
| Obese | 60 | 30 | – | 62 | 33 | 28 |
| *Base = 100%* | *304* | *219* | *35* | *441* | *212* | *39* |
| | *390* | *278* | *33* | *418* | *236* | *39* |
| | *111* | *64* | *6* | *242* | *163* | *18* |

**Table 5.10  Blood pressure categories analysed by socio-economic group (manual and non-manual) and by age at Survey: percentage of age group**

|  | Age at Survey | | | | | | | | | | | |
|---|---|---|---|---|---|---|---|---|---|---|---|---|
|  | 40-59 | 60-79 | 80+ | 40-59 | 60-79 | 80+ | 40-59 | 60-79 | 80+ | 40-59 | 60-79 | 80+ |
| **Blood pressure category** | **Males** | | | | | | **Females** | | | | | |
| **HALS1 (1984/5)** | **Non-manual** | | | **Manual** | | | **Non-manual** | | | **Manual** | | |
| Normotensive (≤140/90 mmHg.) | 70 | 50 | (8) | 68 | 41 | 51 | 79 | 49 | 47 | 76 | 45 | 33 |
| Borderline (141/91 to 159/94 mmHg.) | 13 | 19 | (5) | 14 | 22 | 24 | 8 | 18 | 16 | 10 | 16 | 21 |
| Untreated hypertensive (≥160/95 mmHg.) | 10 | 12 | (5) | 10 | 18 | 14 | 5 | 15 | 13 | 6 | 16 | 16 |
| Treated hypertensive | 7 | 17 | (5) | 7 | 16 | 14 | 7 | 16 | 13 | 8 | 20 | 27 |
| Normotensive but on drugs with anti-hypertensive effects (≤140/90 mmHg.) | 2 | 3 | (2) | 1 | 4 | 5 | 1 | 2 | 11 | 1 | 3 | 2 |
| *Base = 100%* | *460* | *279* | *25* | *607* | *465* | *37* | *629* | *341* | *38* | *665* | *502* | *67* |
| **HALS2 (1991/2)** | | | | | | | | | | | | |
| Normotensive (≤140/90 mmHg.) | 76 | 53 | 29 | 75 | 41 | 40 | 83 | 49 | 28 | 80 | 43 | 24 |
| Borderline (141/91 to 159/94 mmHg.) | 12 | 14 | 9 | 10 | 18 | 19 | 4 | 12 | 25 | 6 | 7 | 10 |
| Untreated hypertensive (≥160/95 mmHg.) | 6 | 6 | 9 | 4 | 7 | 17 | 3 | 8 | 6 | 2 | 4 | 16 |
| Treated hypertensive | 5 | 22 | 34 | 8 | 28 | 13 | 7 | 25 | 25 | 8 | 30 | 34 |
| Normotensive but on drugs with anti-hypertensive effects (≤140/90 mmHg.) | (2) | 5 | 20 | 3 | 7 | 11 | 3 | 6 | 17 | 3 | 6 | 16 |
| *Base = 100%* | *417* | *238* | *35* | *411* | *346* | *47* | *571* | *280* | *36* | *537* | *344* | *68* |

**Table 5.11**    **Blood pressure categories analysed by north/south region of residence and by age at Survey: percentage of age group**

| | Age at Survey | | | | | | | | | | | |
|---|---|---|---|---|---|---|---|---|---|---|---|---|
| | 40-59 | 60-79 | 80+ | 40-59 | 60-79 | 80+ | 40-59 | 60-79 | 80+ | 40-59 | 60-79 | 80+ |
| Blood pressure category | | | | | | | | | | | | |
| | **Males** | | | | | | **Females** | | | | | |
| **HALS1 (1984/5)** | **North** | | | **South** | | | **North** | | | **South** | | |
| Normotensive (≤140/90 mmHg.) | 67 | 39 | 38 | 71 | 48 | 47 | 76 | 46 | 37 | 79 | 48 | 40 |
| Borderline (141/91 to 159/94 mmHg.) | 15 | 20 | 21 | 13 | 21 | 27 | 8 | 17 | 21 | 9 | 17 | 18 |
| Untreated hypertensive (≥160/95 mmHg.) | 12 | 19 | 10 | 8 | 12 | 12 | 6 | 16 | 14 | 5 | 15 | 16 |
| Treated hypertensive | 6 | 17 | 24 | 7 | 16 | 9 | 9 | 16 | 27 | 6 | 19 | 19 |
| Normotensive but on drugs with anti-hypertensive effects (≤140/90 mmHg.) | 1 | 4 | 7 | 2 | 3 | 6 | 1 | 4 | 2 | 1 | 1 | 7 |
| *Base = 100%* | *540* | *345* | *29* | *528* | *401* | *34* | *706* | *450* | *52* | *600* | *408* | *57* |
| **HALS2 (1991/2)** | | | | | | | | | | | | |
| Normotensive (≤140/90 mmHg.) | 75 | 38 | 25 | 77 | 52 | 41 | 78 | 41 | 24 | 85 | 51 | 26 |
| Borderline (141/91 to 159/94 mmHg.) | 11 | 19 | 31 | 11 | 14 | 4 | 6 | 17 | 15 | 4 | 13 | 18 |
| Untreated hypertensive (≥160/95 mmHg.) | 6 | 8 | 9 | 5 | 5 | 16 | 3 | 5 | 9 | 2 | 7 | 16 |
| Treated hypertensive | 7 | 27 | 19 | 5 | 25 | 26 | 10 | 30 | 31 | 6 | 25 | 29 |
| Normotensive but on drugs with anti-hypertensive effects (≤140/90 mmHg.) | 2 | 9 | 16 | 2 | 4 | 14 | 3 | 7 | 22 | 3 | 5 | 12 |
| *Base = 100%* | *436* | *259* | *32* | *393* | *327* | *51* | *582* | *341* | *55* | *536* | *289* | *51* |

**Table 5.12**    **Mean pulse rate in relation to body size and smoking habits in HALS2 (1991/2) (excluding those on medication for cardiac problems or hypertension)**

| | Males | | | | Females | | | |
|---|---|---|---|---|---|---|---|---|
| | Acceptable weight | Over- weight | Obese | All | Acceptable weight | Over- weight | Obese | All |
| | Mean pulse rate with standard error of the mean (S.E.M.) | | | | | | | |
| Non-smoker | 65.0 ±0.7 | 66.2 ±0.7 | 71.3 ±1.4 | 66.3 ±0.5 | 68.7 ±0.4 | 69.7 ±0.5 | 70.8 ±0.7 | 69.6 ±0.3 |
| Ex-smoker | 65.7 ±0.6 | 66.6 ±0.6 | 68.9 ±1.1 | 66.6 ±0.4 | 68.4 ±0.6 | 69.2 ±0.6 | 70.2 ±0.8 | 69.1 ±0.4 |
| Regular smoker | 70.3 ±0.7 | 70.5 ±0.7 | 74.6 ±1.5 | 70.8 ±0.5 | 73.1 ±0.6 | 73.5 ±0.7 | 73.7 ±0.9 | 73.4 ±0.4 |
| All | 67.2 ±0.4 | 67.6 ±0.4 | 71.1 ±0.8 | 67.9 ±0.3 | 69.9 ±0.3 | 70.6 ±0.3 | 71.3 ±0.5 | 70.5 ±0.2 |
| Base | 246 | 233 | 64 | 543 | 455 | 384 | 263 | 1102 |
| | 263 | 363 | 104 | 730 | 247 | 256 | 152 | 655 |
| | 301 | 254 | 62 | 617 | 283 | 231 | 117 | 631 |
| | 810 | 850 | 230 | 1890 | 985 | 871 | 532 | 2388 |

**Table 5.13a  Respiratory function: seven year changes in mean forced expiratory volume in one second (FEV1) (± Standard error of the mean (S.E.M.), and mean percentage of predicted values of FEV1 for age and percentage of each group reported to be on broncho-dilators or anti-asthmatic medication**

Males

Columns are defined by cohort, with each cohort's age at HALS1 (top header row) and at HALS2 (bottom header row). The "HALS2 sub-sample" rows show the same individuals measured at HALS1 (under the HALS1-age reading) and at HALS2 (under the HALS2-age reading).

| | | | | | | | | | |
|---|---|---|---|---|---|---|---|---|---|
| **HALS1 age** | 18-24 | 25-31 | 32-38 | 39-45 | 46-52 | 53-59 | 60-66 | 67-73 | >73 |
| **HALS2 age** | 25-31 | 32-38 | 39-45 | 46-52 | 53-59 | 60-66 | 67-73 | 74-80 | >80 |
| **FEV1 mean in litres** | | | | | | | | | |
| HALS1 sample | 3.95 ±0.03 | 3.87 ±0.04 | 3.68 ±0.04 | 3.37 ±0.04 | 3.05 ±0.04 | 2.68 ±0.04 | 2.42 ±0.04 | 2.04 ±0.05 | 1.66 ±0.04 |
| HALS2 sub-sample (HALS1-age reading) | 3.98 ±0.04 | 3.86 ±0.05 | 3.63 ±0.04 | 3.33 ±0.05 | 3.07 ±0.05 | 2.76 ±0.05 | 2.44 ±0.05 | 2.23 ±0.06 | 1.82 ±0.07 |
| HALS2 sub-sample (HALS2-age reading) | 3.88 ±0.05 | 3.69 ±0.05 | 3.41 ±0.05 | 3.17 ±0.04 | 2.84 ±0.05 | 2.49 ±0.05 | 2.24 ±0.05 | 1.99 ±0.06 | 1.62 ±0.07 |
| **Mean % of predicted FEV1** | | | | | | | | | |
| HALS1 sample | 97.4 ±0.7 | 97.8 ±0.8 | 96.9 ±0.7 | 93.4 ±1.0 | 89.9 ±1.1 | 87.2 ±1.3 | 86.6 ±1.3 | 83.7 ±1.9 | 83.2 ±2.2 |
| HALS2 sub-sample (HALS1-age reading) | 97.9 ±0.9 | 95.9 ±1.1 | 92.9 ±1.1 | 90.6 ±1.4 | 89.9 ±1.6 | 89.1 ±1.9 | 90.3 ±2.7 | 90.9 ±3.8 | 92.9 ±4.5 |
| HALS2 sub-sample (HALS2-age reading) | 97.8 ±1.2 | 94.5 ±0.9 | 93.9 ±1.0 | 90.1 ±1.4 | 86.8 ±1.6 | 89.8 ±2.5 | 90.9 ±2.7 | 92.9 ±3.8 | 98.6 ±4.5 |
| **% on broncho-dilators etc.** | | | | | | | | | |
| HALS1 sample | 2.7 | 2.8 | 0.9 | 1.4 | 3.8 | 3.8 | 4.2 | 6.1 | 9.6 |
| HALS2 sub-sample (HALS1-age reading) | 2.7 | 2.7 | 1.3 | 1.6 | 3.6 | 2.3 | 4.6 | 3.6 | 10.8 |
| HALS2 sub-sample (HALS2-age reading) | 5.8 | 2.2 | 2.6 | 2.0 | 4.0 | 10.0 | 10.3 | 7.1 | 10.8 |
| **Base = 100%** | | | | | | | | | |
| HALS1 | 398 | 360 | 454 | 362 | 311 | 315 | 308 | 228 | 197 |
| HALS2 | 226 | 186 | 310 | 254 | 224 | 220 | 195 | 112 | 65 |

**Table 5.13b  Respiratory function: seven year changes in mean forced expiratory volume in one second (FEV1) (± Standard error of the mean (S.E.M.), and mean percentage of predicted values of FEV1 for age and percentage of each group reported to be on broncho-dilators or anti-asthmatic medication**

| | Females | | | | | | | | |
|---|---|---|---|---|---|---|---|---|---|
| **HALS1 age** | 18-24 | 25-31 | 32-38 | 39-45 | 46-52 | 53-59 | 60-66 | 67-73 | >73 |
| **HALS2 age** | 25-31 | 32-38 | 39-45 | 46-52 | 53-59 | 60-66 | 67-73 | 74-80 | >80 |
| **FEV1 mean in litres** | | | | | | | | | |
| HALS1 sample | 2.87 ±0.03 | 2.80 ±0.02 | 2.70 ±0.02 | 2.54 ±0.02 | 2.30 ±0.02 | 1.99 ±0.03 | 1.75 ±0.02 | 1.50 ±0.03 | 1.27 ±0.03 |
| HALS2 sub-sample | 2.87 ±0.04 | 2.85 ±0.03 | 2.79 ±0.03 | 2.72 ±0.03 | 2.55 ±0.02 | 2.39 ±0.03 | 2.31 ±0.03 | 2.10 ±0.03 | 2.00 ±0.03 |
| | 1.85 ±0.03 | 1.80 ±0.03 | 1.58 ±0.04 | 1.59 ±0.04 | 1.42 ±0.04 | 1.33 ±0.05 | 1.17 ±0.05 | | |
| **Mean % of predicted FEV1** | | | | | | | | | |
| HALS1 sample | 97.4 ±0.8 | 96.3 ±0.7 | 96.3 ±0.6 | 95.9 ±0.8 | 94.8 ±0.9 | 91.0 ±1.2 | 90.5 ±1.2 | 89.4 ±1.8 | 91.4 ±1.9 |
| HALS2 sub-sample | 97.2 ±1.1 | 97.6 ±1.0 | 96.3 ±0.9 | 97.2 ±0.8 | 96.2 ±0.7 | 97.6 ±1.0 | 97.0 ±1.0 | 95.0 ±1.2 | 95.0 ±1.3 |
| | 91.7 ±1.5 | 94.2 ±1.4 | 93.5 ±1.5 | 92.6 ±2.3 | 94.5 ±2.3 | 94.5 ±3.4 | 96.7 ±3.6 | 96.3 | 95.7 |
| **% on broncho-dilators etc.** | | | | | | | | | |
| HALS1 sample | 3.1 | 1.7 | 1.3 | 1.3 | 2.1 | 1.5 | 2.1 | 1.9 | 4.2 | 2.1 |
| HALS2 sub-sample | 3.9 | 5.4 | 1.0 | 1.3 | 1.3 | 3.6 | 1.8 | 2.7 | 2.1 | 4.0 | 2.9 | 7.7 | 1.3 | 7.1 | 2.7 | 5.4 | 3.6 | 4.8 |
| **Base = 100%** | | | | | | | | | |
| HALS1 | 415 | 484 | 623 | 466 | 410 | 333 | 365 | 237 | 241 |
| HALS2 | 204 | 204 | 305 | 305 | 446 | 446 | 329 | 329 | 284 | 284 | 209 | 209 | 226 | 226 | 112 | 112 | 83 | 83 |

**Table 5.14  Respiratory function categories by age at HALS1 and HALS2: percentages of age category with proportion of each category reported to be on broncho-dilators or anti-asthmatic medication as percentages in brackets**

| | Males | | | | | |
|---|---|---|---|---|---|---|
| **HALS**<br>**Age** | **1**<br>18-38 | **2**<br>(25-45) | **1**<br>39-59 | **2**<br>(46-66) | **1**<br>60+ | **2**<br>(67+) |
| Respiratory function category | | | | | | |
| Excellent (above predicted value) | 46 (1%) | 42 (2%) | 37 (0) | 37 (0) | 39 (1%) | 42 (3%) |
| Good (within 2 SD of predicted value) | 50 (3%) | 53 (5%) | 51 (2%) | 49 (3%) | 40 (5%) | 36 (5%) |
| Fair to poor (up to 4 SD below predicted value) | 4 (4%) | 4 (6%) | 9 (6%) | 12 (21%) | 18 (13%) | 17 (21%) |
| * Very poor (over 4 SD below predicted value) | (1) | (2) | 3 (28%) | 3 (44%) | 3 (18%) | 5 (61%) |
| *Base = 100%* | *722* | *722* | *698* | *698* | *372* | *372* |

| | Females | | | | | |
|---|---|---|---|---|---|---|
| Excellent (above predicted value) | 46 (φ) | 46 (1%) | 46 (1%) | 45 (1%) | 44 (1%) | 44 (2%) |
| Good (within 2 SD of predicted value) | 49 (3%) | 49 (4%) | 44 (2%) | 45 (4%) | 40 (2%) | 39 (5%) |
| Fair to poor (up to 4 SD below predicted value) | 5 (9%) | 5 (22%) | 8 (7%) | 8 (20%) | 14 (5%) | 13 (16%) |
| * Very poor (over 4 SD below predicted value) | (2) | – | 2 (13%) | 2 (18%) | 3 (9%) | 3 (36%) |
| *Base = 100%* | *955* | *955* | *822* | *822* | *421* | *421* |

* Includes those unable to perform measurement due to severe chronic respiratory problems
φ = less than 1%

**Table 5.15** **Respiratory function by smoking categories at Survey: mean percentage of predicted values of forced expiratory volume in one second (FEV1) (± Standard error of the mean (S.E.M.)) (Includes only respondents measured in both Surveys but excludes those on broncho-dilators or anti-asthmatic medication)**

| | Males | | Females | | All | |
|---|---|---|---|---|---|---|
| | HALS1 | HALS2 | HALS1 | HALS2 | HALS1 | HALS2 |
| Age | 25-75 | (32-82) | 25-75 | (32-82) | 25-75 | (32-82) |
| Non-smoker | 98.4 | 97.9 | 98.8 | 99.8 | 98.7 | 99.2 |
| | ±0.96 | ±0.96 | ±0.62 | ±0.65 | ±0.52 | ±0.54 |
| Ex-smoker | 95.2 | 95.7 | 98.4 | 98.7 | 96.8 | 97.1 |
| | ±0.93 | ±0.84 | ±0.91 | ±0.76 | ±0.65 | ±0.57 |
| Light regular smoker (1-15/day) | 91.8 | 90.3 | 94.7 | 93.4 | 93.3 | 91.9 |
| | ±1.14 | ±1.22 | ±1.02 | ±1.11 | ±0.76 | ±0.83 |
| Heavy regular smoker (16+/day) | 88.8 | 88.4 | 88.4 | 85.4 | 88.6 | 87.0 |
| | ±1.08 | ±1.11 | ±1.07 | ±1.28 | ±0.76 | ±0.85 |
| All * | 94.2 | 94.2 | 96.7 | 96.9 | 95.6 | 95.7 |
| | ±0.50 | ±0.51 | ±0.43 | ±0.43 | ±0.32 | ±0.33 |
| *Base* | *344* | *352* | *817* | *789* | *1161* | *1141* |
| | *416* | *571* | *410* | *515* | *826* | *1086* |
| | *275* | *247* | *295* | *269* | *570* | *516* |
| | *262* | *213* | *230* | *203* | *492* | *416* |
| | *\* 1391* | *1391* | *1792* | *1792* | *3183* | *3183* |

* Includes occasional smokers (small group: 24 in HALS2)

**Table 5.16** Changes in respiratory function for males and females together in relation to changes in smoking behaviour from HALS1 to HALS2: Mean percentage of predicted values of forced expiratory volume in one second (FEV1) (± Standard error of the mean (S.E.M.)) and mean percentage change (includes only respondents aged 25-75 at HALS1 measured in both Surveys but excludes those on broncho-dilators or anti-asthmatic medication)

| HALS1 smoking category | HALS1* group mean | HALS1 subgroup mean | Mean change | HALS2 subgroup mean | HALS2 smoking category |
|---|---|---|---|---|---|
| Non-smoker | 98.7 ±0.5 | 98.7 | +0.7 ±0.5 | 99.4 | Non-smoker |
| Ex-smoker | 96.8 ±0.7 | 97.0 | +1.2 ±0.5 | 98.2 | Ex-smoker |
| Light regular (1-15/day) | 93.3 ±0.8 | 94.9 | +0.5 ±1.1 | 95.4 | Ex-smoker |
| | | 92.4 | 0.0 ±0.8 | 92.4 | Light regular |
| | | 94.0 | − 3.9 ±1.4 | 90.1 | Heavy regular |
| Heavy regular (16 + /day) | 88.6 ±0.8 | 84.1 | +1.9 ±1.6 | 86.0 | Ex-smoker |
| | | 90.8 | − 1.9 ±1.3 | 88.9 | Light regular |
| | | 88.8 | − 3.2 ±0.6 | 85.6 | Heavy regular |
| Base | 1161 | 1108 | | 1108 | |
| | 826 | 771 | | 771 | |
| | 570 | 140 | | 140 | |
| | | 342 | | 342 | |
| | | 81 | | 81 | |
| | 492 | 67 | | 67 | |
| | | 107 | | 107 | |
| | | 318 | | 318 | |

* Includes all respondents of that original HALS1 smoking category measured in HALS2

**Table 5.17** **Respiratory function categories analysed both by socio-economic group (non-manual (NM), manual (M)) and by smoking category in those respondents whose smoking habits have not changed from HALS1 to HALS2 in two age groups (men and women combined)**

### Age HALS1 18-38 (HALS2 25-45)

| Respiratory function category | Non-smokers | | | | Ex-smokers | | | | Light regular | | | | Heavy regular | | | |
|---|---|---|---|---|---|---|---|---|---|---|---|---|---|---|---|---|
| | NM | | M | | NM | | M | | NM | | M | | NM | | M | |
| HALS | 1 | 2 | 1 | 2 | 1 | 2 | 1 | 2 | 1 | 2 | 1 | 2 | 1 | 2 | 1 | 2 |
| Excellent (above predicted value) | 53 | 52 | 50 | 53 | 54 | 53 | 53 | 52 | 44 | 45 | 41 | 36 | 25 | 27 | 26 | 18 |
| Good (within 2 SD of predicted value) | 43 | 44 | 46 | 43 | 44 | 45 | 43 | 47 | 51 | 51 | 54 | 55 | 73 | 71 | 69 | 69 |
| Fair to very poor (more than 2 SD below predicted value) | 4 | 4 | 4 | 4 | 3 | 2 | 3 | 2 | 5 | 4 | 5 | 9 | 2 | 2 | 5 | 13 |
| *Base = 100%* | *348* | | *335* | | *115* | | *118* | | *78* | | *112* | | *60* | | *104* | |

### Age HALS1 39-59 (HALS2 46-66)

| Respiratory function category | Non-smokers | | | | Ex-smokers | | | | Light regular | | | | Heavy regular | | | |
|---|---|---|---|---|---|---|---|---|---|---|---|---|---|---|---|---|
| | NM | | M | | NM | | M | | NM | | M | | NM | | M | |
| HALS | 1 | 2 | 1 | 2 | 1 | 2 | 1 | 2 | 1 | 2 | 1 | 2 | 1 | 2 | 1 | 2 |
| Excellent (above predicted value) | 51 | 58 | 46 | 44 | 58 | 58 | 39 | 42 | 51 | 36 | 30 | 34 | 24 | 16 | 25 | 13 |
| Good (within 2 SD of predicted value) | 45 | 38 | 42 | 42 | 37 | 37 | 51 | 49 | 36 | 53 | 57 | 50 | 57 | 59 | 57 | 64 |
| Fair to very poor (more than 2 SD below predicted value) | 4 | 4 | 11 | 13 | 5 | 5 | 10 | 9 | 14 | 12 | 13 | 16 | 19 | 25 | 18 | 23 |
| *Base = 100%* | *285* | | *205* | | *180* | | *193* | | *59* | | *93* | | *63* | | *111* | |

# CHANGES IN BODY MEASUREMENTS | 6

**Brian D Cox**

In recent years the two principal studies on body sizes of British adults have been those of Knight (1984) and Cox et al. (1987). Many small scale studies had been undertaken in various parts of the country, but these were the first nationally based ones. Knight (1984) studied the distribution of several body measurements, including height and weight, in adults aged 16 to 64 years. The HALS study (Cox et al. 1987) included individuals aged 18 years and over, with no upper age limit. The second HALS study in 1991/2 (HALS2) which re-measured 4480 of the original respondents who were measured in HALS1 has given an opportunity to assess the changes that have taken place in body size over the seven-year period since HALS1.

## Method

Respondents were weighed on portable electronic scales, and an estimate of the weight of clothing worn was made to allow for a subsequent correction for nude weight. Weight was taken in stockinged feet with jacket or coat removed. Heights were measured without shoes using a stadiometer reading to 1mm. Girth was measured using a tape placed midway between the top of the hip bone and the lowest rib. The measurement at the hips was made at the widest part of the pelvis. The weights, girths and hip measurements of pregnant women were not recorded.

## Heights, weights and body mass index (BMI)

Table 6.1a and 6.1b show the mean values obtained for height, weight, and body mass index. The heights and weights were used to calculate an index of adiposity, as weight unrelated to height, has obvious limitations as a measure. In this survey the body mass index was employed, since it is the most commonly used measure of adiposity. For estimating the body mass index (BMI) (which is also known as Quetelet's index (1869)), the formula: weight (in kilograms) divided by height (in metres) squared ($W/H^2$) is used.

The data are presented as means of the whole HALS1 measured population and the means of the HALS2 sample (which is a sub-sample of the HALS1 population) at both sampling times. The presentation in these tables of the mean values of both the whole HALS1 population and those of the group who were seen exactly seven years later at HALS2 as well as at HALS1, enables an assessment to be made of how representative of the whole HALS1 sample is the HALS2 sub-set. The use of seven-year age bands also enables a comparison to be made of the HALS2 1991/2 results with the values obtained for the next older age group at HALS1.

In both men and women aged under 21 at HALS1 there has been a small increase in mean height in the seven years to HALS2 and this is reflected in the small increase in mean height in the first seven-year age band (Tables 6.1a and 6.1b). As in the study by Knight (1984) the mean height values by decade for the HALS1 population showed a decrease with age. In HALS1 it was suggested that the apparent decline in mean height with age could be caused by a combination of two factors, the thinning of the intervertebral discs and a cohort effect, since in past years relatively poor nutrition may have resulted in many individuals not achieving their genetic potential for height (Cox et al.1987: Rona 1981). This indeed appears to be the case. From age 32-38 for men and age 39-45 for women, a small decrease in height over the seven years between HALS1 and HALS2 was observed in each age group. The cumulative decreases were 3.1 cm and 4.6 cm for men and women respectively, supporting the hypothesis that thinning of the intervertebral discs has occurred. On the other hand the decrease in height after seven years that was seen at HALS2 was in many cases less than would be expected from the values obtained for the HALS1 sample at the same age, strongly supporting the cohort effect hypothesis. The difference between the mean height values at HALS1 for men respondents aged between 25 and 80 was 7.0 cm. The cumulative seven-year changes for men respondents seen at HALS2 amounts to only 3.1 cm. For women between 25 and 80 the difference between the mean height values at HALS1 are 6.3 cm and the cumulative seven-year change is 4.6 cm.

In HALS1 it was found that mean weight increased in both sexes with each age group until the 60s and thereafter declined. This pattern is repeated in HALS2 but in both men and women the seven-year changes in weight are greater than would be expected. Thus, overall, the population has increased in weight and this is also reflected in the mean BMI figures.

## Girth, hip and girth/hip ratio

The changes in girth, hip and girth/ratio are demonstrated in Tables 6.2a and 6.2b. Reflecting the changes in the weight measurements, the increases in girth and hip over the seven-year period are greater than would have been anticipated. Girth/ hip ratio, an index which has been shown to be related to cardio-vascular risk factors (Larsson et al. 1984), in that an increase in this ratio reflects an increased deposition of adipose tissue centrally, has increased very much in line with what would have been expected from the HALS1 values. In HALS1 the hip measurements were only made on the final two-thirds of the population and so full comparative data

are not available. However, the results do tend to show that, although overall body size has increased, the relative distribution of adipose tissue has not changed very much. As shown in HALS1 the maximum mean BMI values occurred in those aged 50-59 in both sexes (Tables 6.1a and 6.1b), and thereafter declined, whereas the girth/hip ratio continued to increase (Tables 6.2a and 6.2b), indicating a redistribution of body tissue in later life.

## Body mass index categories

Using the BMI values obtained, respondents were divided into four categories: underweight, acceptable or normal weight, overweight and obese. There are two main sets of criteria which categorise adiposity by BMI values. One devised in 1979 by the Fogarty Conference in the USA (Bray, 1979) was also later adopted by the Royal College of Physicians (1983). However, the OPCS study (Knight, 1984) used different criteria in categorising females. For the HALS surveys the recommendations of the Royal College of Physicians and the Fogarty conference in the USA have been used.

|   | | *Males* | *Females* |
|---|---|---|---|
| 1 | Underweight | $\leqslant 20.0$ | $\leqslant 18.6$ |
| 2 | Acceptable/Normal | $20.1 - 25.0$ | $18.7 - 23.8$ |
| 3 | Overweight | $25.1 - 29.9$ | $23.9 - 28.5$ |
| 4 | Obese | $\geqslant 30.0$ | $\geqslant 28.6$ |

In Table 6.3 is shown the percentage of men and women in these BMI categories by seven-year age bands at HALS1 and HALS2. The percentage of both men and women in the 'acceptable' weight category has declined from HALS1 to HALS2 in all but the older age groups. At the same time there has been a dramatic increase in the proportion classified as 'obese' in both sexes, especially in the younger and middle-aged groups where over 25% of the women over the age of 50 fall into this classification at HALS2. Another observation is that there is a marked decrease in the number of people who are underweight in the younger age groups but a rise in the older men and women. Being underweight in the middle-aged or older age groups is predictive of mortality (Chapter 3).

The movement between BMI categories from HALS1 to HALS2 in three age groups is shown in Table 6.4, where it can be seen that in the younger

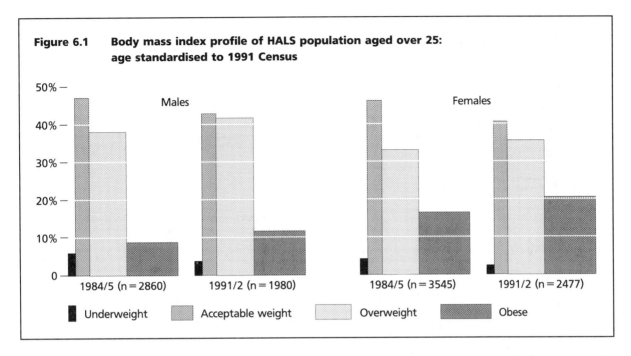

**Figure 6.1    Body mass index profile of HALS population aged over 25: age standardised to 1991 Census**

age groups (aged 18-38 and 39-59 at HALS1) there is considerable movement from the acceptable weight to the overweight category, and a similar move from being overweight to being obese.

In the older age group (aged 60 and over at HALS1) the trends for these categories are tending to reverse and more of the obese are losing weight and moving into the 'overweight' category.

The body mass index profiles of the HALS1 and HALS2 population aged over 25 at both surveys, age standardised to the 1991 Census, are shown in Figure 6.1. These profiles indicate that the British population is becoming increasingly overweight. For men aged 25 or over at HALS1 47% were overweight or obese, for men aged 25 or over at HALS2 the comparative figure is 53%. For women the figures are 50% and 57% respectively with an increase from 17% to 21% in the obese category.

## Body measurements and socio-economic group

In HALS1 several anthropometric differences were identified between household non-manual and manual socio-economic groups (Cox et al. 1987). There were differences between non-manual and manual mean height such that in men in non-manual groups the mean height was greater (1.3 cm in those aged 18-29 and 3.5 cm in those aged 40-49). Men in

non-manual occupations were heavier, but this is a reflection of their greater height since the mean BMI was approximately the same as in the manual group. Amongst women the mean weight of those in manual social classes was generally greater than in the non-manual, although the mean height was less. Mean girth in both socio-economic groups of men was similar but the women of all ages in the manual groups had a greater mean girth than those in the non-manual social classes. A similar pattern was found for hip measurements and the girth/hip ratio. In HALS1 mean values of BMI for men in either non-manual or manual classes varied similarly with age, but at all ages women in manual groups had higher mean BMI values when compared with non-manual.

Table 6.5 demonstrates the mean weight of the respondents at HALS1 with the mean changes in weight that had occurred in the seven years between HALS1 and HALS2. The mean ages of the groups show that there was not a great age disparity between the socio-economic groups. In the men, the mean weight at HALS1 was greater in the non-manual than in the manual groups but the mean changes in weight were similar. Only in the younger age group (aged 18-38 at HALS1) do men in the non-manual groups appear to have put on more weight (5.3 kg as compared to 4.2 kg). The women in the younger age manual groups have a higher mean weight than in the non-manual groups but the

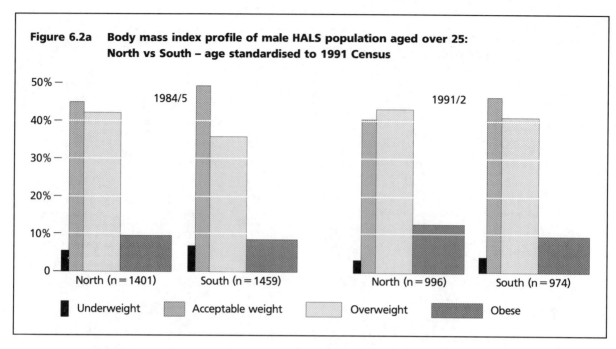

Figure 6.2a    Body mass index profile of male HALS population aged over 25:
North vs South – age standardised to 1991 Census

1984/5      1991/2

North (n = 1401)    South (n = 1459)    North (n = 996)    South (n = 974)

■ Underweight    ▨ Acceptable weight    ▥ Overweight    ▦ Obese

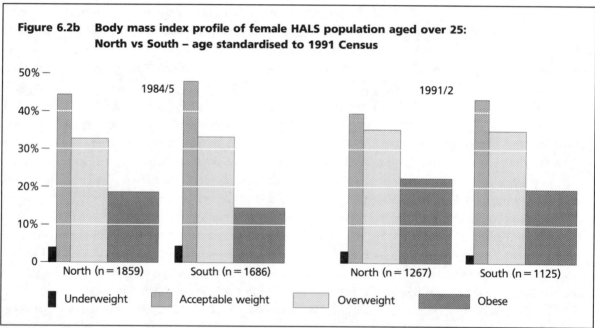

Figure 6.2b    Body mass index profile of female HALS population aged over 25:
North vs South – age standardised to 1991 Census

1984/5      1991/2

North (n = 1859)    South (n = 1686)    North (n = 1267)    South (n = 1125)

■ Underweight    ▨ Acceptable weight    ▥ Overweight    ▦ Obese

changes over seven years are very similar. In both men and women over the age of 60 at HALS1 there has been a mean reduction in weight in the following seven years.

## Body mass index profiles and region of residence

The reduction in the sample size (HALS1 to HALS2) has meant that meaningful simple analysis cannot be carried out by Standard Region as in HALS1, so a dichotomised variable – North/South – has been

used where the Standard regions Scotland, North, North West, Yorks/Humber, Wales and West Midlands are combined as the 'North' and the East Midlands, East Anglia, South West, South East, and Greater London are combined as the 'South'.

The BMI profiles of those aged 25 or over at both Surveys, age standardised to the 1991 Census are demonstrated in Figures 6.2a and 6.2b. At both Surveys the southern men and women have a greater proportion who are of 'acceptable' weight. The northern women have the highest proportion of obese respondents at both Surveys – 19% at HALS1 and 23% at HALS2 – compared to 15% and 20% for the southern women. In HALS1 44% of southern men were overweight or obese compared to 50% for the north. In HALS2 the figures are 50% and 56% respectively.

## BMI category changes by region and by socio-economic groups

Since many of the differences that are seen between the North and South of Britain relate in major part to the disparate distribution of socio-economic groups, it is important to take this factor into consideration when examining differences which occur between northern and southern populations.

The changes in BMI categories that have occurred from HALS1 to HALS2 by North/South division and by non-manual and manual socio-economic groups are shown in Table 6.6, which also demonstrates the higher proportion of men and women in non-manual groups in the south, and men and women in manual groups in the north. The changes are similar in each group but the non-manual groups in both regions and in both sexes are less likely to be overweight or obese than the manual groups. Similarly there is a north/south difference in that all socio-economic and sex groups in the south show less obesity in both Surveys than those in the north. The highest percentage of acceptable weight respondents are found in the non-manual groups in both men and women in the south.

## Weight change and smoking

In HALS1 the regular smokers were found to have a lower BMI than the non-smokers whilst ex-smokers had higher values. This observation was independent of age but was accentuated with increasing age. Between HALS1 and HALS2 changes in smoking behaviour often occurred. The predominant change was for regular smokers to become ex-smokers, although some ex-smokers took up regular smoking again.

The association between smoking habit and change in weight is shown in Table 6.7. In HALS1 the highest mean weight was recorded in the ex-smokers and the lowest in the regular smokers. The mean change in weight from HALS1 to HALS2 was similar in those who remained non-smokers, regular smokers and ex-smokers. However, in those men and women who were regular smokers at HALS1 and who had become ex-smokers by HALS2 there was a great increase in weight especially in those aged 18-38 at HALS1. The mean change in weight for those who did not change smoking behaviour in this age group was 4.9 kg, 3.7 kg, and 4.1 kg for the non-smoking, ex-smoking and regular smoking men respectively. For the women the comparable figures were 4.1 kg, 4.2 kg and 3.8 kg. For those who had changed from regular smoking to become ex-smokers the mean change in weight was 7.4 kg for the men and 8.2 kg for the women. A small number of men and women changed from the ex-smokers category to regular smokers and in these subjects the mean change was 3.0 kg and 3.2 kg in the 18-38 age band but in the 39-59 age band there was a reduction of 0.4 kg and 2.0 kg respectively.

A confirmation of the changes in body size observed in those who had changed smoking habit is seen in Table 6.8 where the mean changes in girth that have occurred from HALS1 to HALS2 are shown. Those who were ex-smokers at HALS1 show the highest values at HALS1 but the largest increases in girth are seen in those respondents who had changed from being regular smokers to ex-smokers.

The time interval since the changes in smoking habits occurred could be from one week to nearly seven years and so it is likely that in those who changed soon after HALS1 the order of magnitude of the mean body size changes will be greater than in those who have changed recently. These changes will be examined in greater detail and with more sophisticated analysis at a later time.

## Summary

Since HALS1 the body dimensions of the HALS respondents have changed considerably, with an increase in weight, girth, hip, and body mass index, particularly in the younger population, which is greater than would be expected from the observed relationship of age to these measures as seen in HALS1. These increases have not been restricted to any one socio-economic group or to the north or south of Great Britain. The implications for the future health of the population of this large increase in the overweight and obese are potentially serious, bearing in mind the association of obesity with arthritic conditions, diabetes and circulatory disorders (Garrow 1981).

Height has decreased with age but not as much as would have been expected from the observed relationship with age seen in HALS1. This adds weight to the argument that there is a strong cohort effect in the height/age relationship.

Changes in smoking behaviour have been shown to be associated with major changes in body size. The cessation of regular smoking has been shown in Chapter 5 to be associated with a decrease in resting pulse rate below the non-smoking values; this probably reflects a lowering of basal metabolic rate, which would make an increase in weight likely if there were no change in dietary intake.

**References**

Bray, G.A. (1979), (ed), 'Obesity in America', Proceedings of the 2nd Fogarty International Centre Conference on Obesity, No. 79, US DHEW, Washington USA.

Cox, B.D. et al. (1987), 'The Health and Lifestyle Survey, Preliminary report of a nationwide survey of the physical and mental health, attitudes and lifestyle of a random sample of 9,003 British adults', Health Promotion Research Trust, London.

Garrow, J.S. (1981), 'Treat Obesity Seriously,' Churchill Livingston, London.

Knight, I. (1984), 'The Heights and Weights of Adults in Great Britain', OPCS, HMSO, London.

Larsson, B. et al. (1984), 'Abdominal adipose tissue distribution, obesity and risk of cardiovascular disease and death: 13 year follow-up of participants in the study of men born in 1913', British Medical Journal, 288, 1401-1404.

Quetelet, L.A.J. (1869), 'Physique Sociale', C. Muquardt, Brussels, 2, 92.

Royal College of Physicians, (1983), 'Obesity report', Journal of the Royal College of Physicians, London, 17, 5-65.

Rona, R. (1981), 'Genetic and Environmental Factors in the Control of Growth in Childhood', British Medical Bulletin, 37, 265-272.

**Table 6.1a    Changes in height, weight and body mass index (BMI) by age in males. HALS1 full sample in comparison to HALS2 sub-sample in 1984/5 and 1991/2 (Mean and standard error of the mean (S.E.M.))**

| | | | | | Age | | | | |
|---|---|---|---|---|---|---|---|---|---|
| **HALS1** | 18-24 | 25-31 | 32-38 | 39-45 | 46-52 | 53-59 | 60-66 | 67-73 | >73 |
| **HALS2** | 25-31 | 32-38 | 39-45 | 46-52 | 53-59 | 60-66 | 67-73 | 74-80 | >80 |
| **Height mean (cm)** | | | | | | | | | |
| HALS1 sample | 175.8 | 175.3 | 175.2 | 174.3 | 174.1 | 172.2 | 171.5 | 169.6 | 168.0 |
| S.E.M. | ±0.3 | ±0.3 | ±0.3 | ±0.3 | ±0.4 | ±0.4 | ±0.4 | ±0.4 | ±0.5 |
| HALS2 sub-sample | 176.0 | 175.4 | 175.0 | 174.9 | 174.5 | 172.6 | 171.7 | 170.7 | 168.3 |
| S.E.M. | ±0.4 | ±0.5 | ±0.4 | ±0.4 | ±0.4 | ±0.4 | ±0.4 | ±0.6 | ±0.8 |
| **Weight mean (kg.)** | | | | | | | | | |
| HALS1 sample | 70.3 | 73.9 | 76.4 | 76.5 | 78.5 | 76.7 | 75.0 | 72.7 | 69.5 |
| S.E.M. | ±0.5 | ±0.6 | ±0.5 | ±0.6 | ±0.7 | ±0.7 | ±0.6 | ±0.7 | ±0.9 |
| HALS2 sub-sample | 75.6 | 79.2 | 80.0 | 79.1 | 80.8 | 78.0 | 75.5 | 74.0 | 67.4 |
| S.E.M. | ±0.8 | ±0.9 | ±0.7 | ±0.8 | ±0.8 | ±0.8 | ±0.7 | ±1.0 | ±1.5 |
| **Body Mass Index** | | | | | | | | | |
| HALS1 sample | 22.7 | 24.0 | 24.9 | 25.2 | 25.9 | 25.8 | 25.5 | 25.2 | 24.5 |
| S.E.M. | ±0.2 | ±0.2 | ±0.2 | ±0.2 | ±0.2 | ±0.2 | ±0.2 | ±0.2 | ±0.3 |
| HALS2 sub-sample | 24.3 | 25.7 | 26.1 | 26.6 | 26.2 | 25.7 | 25.8 | 25.4 | 23.9 |
| S.E.M. | ±0.2 | ±0.3 | ±0.2 | ±0.3 | ±0.3 | ±0.2 | ±0.2 | ±0.3 | ±0.4 |
| *Base* | *442* | *413* | *512* | *412* | *357* | *356* | *339* | *258* | *213* |
| | *240* | *203* | *341* | *280* | *242* | *248* | *220* | *125* | *71* |

**Table 6.1b    Changes in height, weight and body mass index (BMI) by age in females. HALS1 full sample in comparison to HALS2 sub-sample in 1984/5 and 1991/2 (Mean and standard error of the mean (S.E.M.))**

| | 18-24 | 25-31 | 32-38 | 39-45 | 46-52 | 53-59 | 60-66 | 67-73 | >73 |
|---|---|---|---|---|---|---|---|---|---|
| HALS1 | | 25-31 | 32-38 | 39-45 | 46-52 | 53-59 | 60-66 | 67-73 | 74-80 | >80 |
| HALS2 (age) | 25-31 | 32-38 | 39-45 | 46-52 | 53-59 | 60-66 | 67-73 | 74-80 | >80 |
| **Height mean (cm)** | | | | | | | | | |
| HALS1 sample | 162.1 | 161.7 | 161.9 | 161.9 | 160.9 | 159.9 | 158.9 | 157.0 | 155.5 |
| S.E.M. | ±0.3 | ±0.3 | ±0.3 | ±0.3 | ±0.3 | ±0.3 | ±0.3 | ±0.4 | ±0.4 |
| HALS2 sub-sample | 162.2 / 162.3 | 161.8 / 161.6 | 162.0 / 162.3 | 162.1 / 161.2 | 160.6 / 160.0 | 159.3 / 158.9 | 157.5 / 157.1 | 155.6 / 155.5 | 153.0 |
| S.E.M. | ±0.4 / ±0.4 | ±0.5 / ±0.3 | ±0.4 / ±0.4 | ±0.3 / ±0.4 | ±0.3 / ±0.4 | ±0.4 / ±0.3 | ±0.4 / ±0.6 | ±0.4 / ±0.8 | ±0.7 |
| **Weight mean (kg.)** | | | | | | | | | |
| HALS1 sample | 59.4 | 60.4 | 62.3 | 63.5 | 65.6 | 65.5 | 64.1 | 62.2 | 60.9 |
| S.E.M. | ±0.5 | ±0.5 | ±0.4 | ±0.5 | ±0.6 | ±0.6 | ±0.6 | ±0.7 | ±0.7 |
| HALS2 sub-sample | 59.3 / 64.5 | 60.7 / 62.0 | 66.4 / 63.5 | 67.5 / 65.8 | 66.8 / 65.5 | 64.0 / 64.0 | 63.2 / 62.1 | 61.0 / 58.4 | |
| S.E.M. | ±0.6 / ±0.8 | ±0.5 / ±0.6 | ±0.6 / ±0.7 | ±0.6 / ±0.7 | ±0.8 / ±0.8 | ±0.8 / ±0.7 | ±0.9 / ±0.9 | ±0.8 / ±1.2 | |
| **Body Mass Index** | | | | | | | | | |
| HALS1 sample | 22.6 | 23.1 | 23.7 | 24.2 | 25.4 | 25.6 | 25.4 | 25.2 | 25.2 |
| S.E.M | ±0.2 | ±0.2 | ±0.2 | ±0.2 | ±0.2 | ±0.2 | ±0.2 | ±0.3 | ±0.3 |
| HALS2 sub-sample | 22.6 / 24.5 | 23.2 / 23.6 | 24.8 / 24.2 | 25.3 / 25.7 | 25.3 / 26.4 | 25.7 / 26.2 | 25.4 / 25.8 | 25.4 / 25.4 | 24.4 |
| S.E.M. | ±0.2 / ±0.3 | ±0.2 / ±0.2 | ±0.3 / ±0.2 | ±0.2 / ±0.3 | ±0.2 / ±0.2 | ±0.2 / ±0.3 | ±0.3 / ±0.3 | ±0.4 / ±0.3 | ±0.5 |
| *Base* | 446 | 522 | 668 | 530 | 469 | 388 | 418 | 279 | 271 |
| | 201 / 201 | 304 / 304 | 473 / 473 | 372 / 372 | 323 / 323 | 243 / 243 | 250 / 250 | 135 / 135 | 92 / 92 |

**Table 6.2a**  Changes in girth, hips and girth/hip ratio by age in males. HALS1 full sample in comparison to HALS2 sub-sample in 1984/5 and 1991/2 (Mean and standard error of the mean (S.E.M.)) Only 2 waves of sample had hip measurement in 1984/5 so the base numbers for the HALS1 sample are less for hips and girth/hip ratio

In the table below each column is a cohort followed longitudinally. The **HALS1** row gives the age band in 1984/5; the **HALS2** row gives the age band of the same cohort in 1991/2.

| Age | | | | | | | | | | |
|---|---|---|---|---|---|---|---|---|---|
| **HALS1** | 18-24 | 25-31 | 32-38 | 39-45 | 46-52 | 53-59 | 60-66 | 67-73 | >73 |
| **HALS2** | 25-31 | 32-38 | 39-45 | 46-52 | 53-59 | 60-66 | 67-73 | 74-80 | >80 |

**Girth mean (cm)**

| | 18-24/25-31 | 25-31/32-38 | 32-38/39-45 | 39-45/46-52 | 46-52/53-59 | 53-59/60-66 | 60-66/67-73 | 67-73/74-80 | >73/>80 |
|---|---|---|---|---|---|---|---|---|---|
| HALS1 sample | 81.5 | 85.3 | 88.3 | 89.6 | 92.4 | 93.3 | 93.3 | 94.5 | 94.2 |
| S.E.M. | ±0.4 | ±0.5 | ±0.4 | ±0.5 | ±0.5 | ±0.6 | ±0.5 | ±0.6 | ±0.8 |
| HALS2 sub-sample (1984/5) | 80.8 | 85.9 | 88.3 | 89.6 | 92.5 | 93.3 | 93.6 | 95.8 | 93.8 |
| S.E.M. | ±0.5 | ±0.6 | ±0.5 | ±0.6 | ±0.6 | ±0.7 | ±0.7 | ±0.8 | ±1.3 |
| HALS2 sub-sample (1991/2) | 86.9 | 91.4 | 93.0 | 93.6 | 97.2 | 97.2 | 96.6 | 96.7 | 96.6 |
| S.E.M. | ±0.6 | ±0.7 | ±0.5 | ±0.6 | ±0.7 | ±0.8 | ±0.7 | ±0.9 | ±1.4 |
| *Base* HALS1 | *440* | *410* | *507* | *410* | *356* | *355* | *339* | *258* | *211* |
| *Base* HALS2 | *241* | *205* | *341* | *281* | *244* | *251* | *222* | *126* | *70* |

**Hips mean (cm)**

| | 18-24/25-31 | 25-31/32-38 | 32-38/39-45 | 39-45/46-52 | 46-52/53-59 | 53-59/60-66 | 60-66/67-73 | 67-73/74-80 | >73/>80 |
|---|---|---|---|---|---|---|---|---|---|
| HALS1 sample | 93.6 | 96.3 | 97.5 | 98.7 | 100.5 | 101.8 | 101.2 | 101.9 | 103.7 |
| S.E.M. | ±0.5 | ±0.5 | ±0.4 | ±0.5 | ±0.5 | ±0.5 | ±0.5 | ±0.7 | ±0.8 |
| HALS2 sub-sample (1984/5) | 92.9 | 97.2 | 97.8 | 98.9 | 100.9 | 102.0 | 101.3 | 102.9 | 105.1 |
| S.E.M. | ±0.5 | ±0.6 | ±0.5 | ±0.5 | ±0.6 | ±0.6 | ±0.6 | ±0.9 | ±1.3 |
| HALS2 sub-sample (1991/2) | 98.8 | 101.7 | 101.8 | 102.1 | 103.8 | 103.7 | 103.4 | 104.3 | 103.1 |
| S.E.M. | ±0.8 | ±0.5 | ±0.6 | ±0.4 | ±0.5 | ±0.6 | ±0.5 | ±0.8 | ±1.2 |

**Girth/Hip ratio**

| | 18-24/25-31 | 25-31/32-38 | 32-38/39-45 | 39-45/46-52 | 46-52/53-59 | 53-59/60-66 | 60-66/67-73 | 67-73/74-80 | >73/>80 |
|---|---|---|---|---|---|---|---|---|---|
| HALS1 sample | 87.1 | 88.5 | 90.3 | 91.2 | 91.8 | 92.3 | 92.2 | 92.6 | 93.2 |
| S.E.M. | ±0.3 | ±0.3 | ±0.3 | ±0.3 | ±0.4 | ±0.4 | ±0.4 | ±0.4 | ±0.5 |
| HALS2 sub-sample (1984/5) | 86.7 | 88.7 | 90.3 | 91.4 | 92.0 | 92.0 | 92.4 | 92.8 | 93.0 |
| S.E.M. | ±0.4 | ±0.4 | ±0.3 | ±0.4 | ±0.4 | ±0.4 | ±0.4 | ±0.5 | ±0.9 |
| HALS2 sub-sample (1991/2) | 87.9 | 89.9 | 91.2 | 91.6 | 93.5 | 93.2 | 93.3 | 92.6 | 92.7 |
| S.E.M. | ±0.4 | ±0.4 | ±0.3 | ±0.4 | ±0.4 | ±0.4 | ±0.4 | ±0.5 | ±0.7 |
| *Base* HALS1 | *247* | *254* | *312* | *257* | *217* | *224* | *220* | *156* | *134* |
| *Base* HALS2 | *152* | *135* | *221* | *188* | *165* | *160* | *151* | *89* | *47* |

**Table 6.2b**  Changes in girth, hips and girth/hip ratio by age in women. HALS1 full sample in comparison to HALS2 sub-sample in 1984/5 and 1991/2 (Mean and standard error of the mean (S.E.M.)) Only 2 waves of sample had hip measurement in 1984/5 so the base numbers for the HALS1 sample are less for hips and girth/hip ratio

| | | | | | Age | | | | | |
|---|---|---|---|---|---|---|---|---|---|---|
| **HALS1** | 18-24 | 25-31 | 32-38 | 39-45 | 46-52 | 53-59 | 60-66 | 67-73 | >73 | |
| **HALS2** | | 25-31 | 32-38 | 39-45 | 46-52 | 53-59 | 60-66 | 67-73 | 74-80 | >80 |
| **Girth mean (cm)** | | | | | | | | | | |
| HALS1 sample | 71.5 | 74.1 | 74.4 | 76.1 | 78.9 | 80.9 | 82.2 | 82.9 | 85.4 | |
| S.E.M. | ±0.5 | ±0.5 | ±0.4 | ±0.5 | ±0.5 | ±0.6 | ±0.6 | ±0.7 | ±0.7 | |
| HALS2 sub-sample (1984/5) | 71.4 | 74.7 | 74.0 | 75.9 | 79.1 | 80.6 | 81.3 | 82.4 | 84.6 | |
| S.E.M. | ±0.6 | ±0.6 | ±0.4 | ±0.5 | ±0.6 | ±0.7 | ±0.7 | ±0.9 | ±0.9 | |
| HALS2 sub-sample (1991/2) | | 77.3 | 78.4 | 79.7 | 80.7 | 83.7 | 84.2 | 84.5 | 84.7 | 87.9 |
| S.E.M. | | ±0.7 | ±0.6 | ±0.5 | ±0.6 | ±0.7 | ±0.7 | ±0.9 | ±0.9 | ±1.2 |
| Base HALS1 | 458 | 533 | 665 | 530 | 468 | 386 | 419 | 278 | 270 | |
| Base HALS2 | 231 | 339 | 488 | 483 | 394 | 325 | 273 | 256 | 146 | 95 |
| **Hips mean (cm)** | | | | | | | | | | |
| HALS1 sample | 91.7 | 92.5 | 93.8 | 96.6 | 98.4 | 100.1 | 100.1 | 99.6 | 100.9 | |
| S.E.M. | ±0.6 | ±0.5 | ±0.4 | ±0.6 | ±0.6 | ±0.6 | ±0.6 | ±0.8 | ±0.8 | |
| HALS2 sub-sample (1984/5) | 91.6 | 92.9 | 93.4 | 96.5 | 98.8 | 99.9 | 99.6 | 98.9 | 100.2 | |
| S.E.M. | ±0.8 | ±0.6 | ±0.5 | ±0.6 | ±0.7 | ±0.7 | ±0.7 | ±0.9 | ±0.8 | |
| HALS2 sub-sample (1991/2) | | 99.2 | 100.0 | 101.1 | 102.5 | 104.1 | 103.7 | 103.1 | 102.1 | 102.5 |
| S.E.M. | | ±0.7 | ±0.6 | ±0.7 | ±0.7 | ±0.8 | ±0.8 | ±0.9 | ±1.1 | ±1.1 |
| Base HALS1 | 261 | 343 | 459 | 332 | 312 | 244 | 284 | 172 | 171 | |
| Base HALS2 | 136 | 220 | 227 | 335 | 350 | 258 | 373 | 246 | 256 | 138 |
| **Girth/Hip ratio** | | | | | | | | | | |
| HALS1 sample | 78.2 | 78.6 | 78.3 | 78.3 | 78.3 | 80.7 | 82.0 | 82.7 | 84.5 | |
| S.E.M. | ±0.4 | ±0.3 | ±0.3 | ±0.3 | ±0.3 | ±0.4 | ±0.4 | ±0.4 | ±0.4 | |
| HALS2 sub-sample (1984/5) | 78.2 | 79.0 | 78.4 | 78.7 | 79.3 | 80.3 | 81.3 | 82.2 | 84.8 | |
| S.E.M. | ±0.4 | ±0.3 | ±0.3 | ±0.4 | ±0.4 | ±0.4 | ±0.4 | ±0.5 | ±0.5 | |
| HALS2 sub-sample (1991/2) | | 77.8 | 78.3 | 78.2 | 79.3 | 80.2 | 81.2 | 81.9 | 82.9 | 85.8 |
| S.E.M. | | ±0.4 | ±0.4 | ±0.3 | ±0.4 | ±0.4 | ±0.4 | ±0.5 | ±0.9 | ±0.8 |
| Base HALS1 | 261 | 343 | 459 | 332 | 312 | 244 | 284 | 172 | 171 | |
| Base HALS2 | 136 | 220 | 227 | 335 | 350 | 258 | 373 | 246 | 256 | 72 | 70 |

**Table 6.3    Changes in body mass index categories by age: HALS1 to HALS2: percentage of age group**

| HALS1 age (HALS2 age) | 18-24 (25-31) | | 25-31 (32-38) | | 32-38 (39-45) | | 39-45 (46-52) | | 46-52 (53-59) | | 53-59 (60-66) | | 60-66 (67-73) | | 67-73 (74-80) | | >73 (>80) | |
|---|---|---|---|---|---|---|---|---|---|---|---|---|---|---|---|---|---|---|
| HALS | 1 | 2 | 1 | 2 | 1 | 2 | 1 | 2 | 1 | 2 | 1 | 2 | 1 | 2 | 1 | 2 | 1 | 2 |
| **Body mass index category** | | | | | | | | | | | | | | | | | | |
| *Males* | | | | | | | | | | | | | | | | | | |
| Underweight | 20 | 6 | 7 | 1 | 6 | 2 | 4 | 3 | 3 | 4 | 5 | 5 | 2 | 2 | – | 3 | 6 | 14 |
| Acceptable weight | 67 | 58 | 61 | 47 | 54 | 42 | 50 | 38 | 38 | 34 | 40 | 35 | 37 | 38 | 47 | 51 | 42 | 45 |
| Overweight | 11 | 29 | 25 | 39 | 33 | 43 | 41 | 48 | 47 | 46 | 42 | 47 | 52 | 53 | 45 | 38 | 45 | 38 |
| Obese | 2 | 8 | 7 | 12 | 8 | 13 | 5 | 12 | 12 | 17 | 12 | 13 | 9 | 8 | 8 | 8 | 7 | 3 |
| *Base = 100%* | 240 | | 203 | | 341 | | 280 | | 242 | | 248 | | 220 | | 125 | | 71 | |
| *Females* | | | | | | | | | | | | | | | | | | |
| Underweight | 8 | 3 | 4 | 3 | 4 | 1 | 4 | 1 | 5 | 2 | 1 | 3 | 3 | 3 | 2 | 4 | 2 | 7 |
| Acceptable weight | 66 | 50 | 60 | 48 | 58 | 45 | 52 | 41 | 41 | 32 | 36 | 34 | 33 | 34 | 36 | 39 | 30 | 41 |
| Overweight | 21 | 32 | 26 | 30 | 28 | 36 | 31 | 37 | 34 | 38 | 40 | 37 | 42 | 38 | 41 | 32 | 45 | 38 |
| Obese | 6 | 15 | 10 | 18 | 9 | 18 | 13 | 21 | 20 | 28 | 23 | 26 | 22 | 26 | 22 | 25 | 23 | 14 |
| *Base = 100%* | 201 | | 304 | | 473 | | 372 | | 323 | | 243 | | 250 | | 135 | | 91 | |

**Table 6.4** **Change in BMI categories HALS1 to HALS2 as percentage of HALS1 BMI categories:**
**Analysed by sex and three age groups**

| | HALS1 (1984/5) categories and age at HALS1 | | | | | | | | | | | |
| --- | --- | --- | --- | --- | --- | --- | --- | --- | --- | --- | --- | --- |
| | 18-38 | | | | 39-59 | | | | 60 + | | | |
| | Under weight | Accept-able weight | Over-weight | Obese | Under weight | Accept-able weight | Over-weight | Obese | Under weight | Accept-able weight | Over-weight | Obese |
| **HALS2 (1991/2) categories** | | | | | | | | **Males** | | | | |
| Underweight | 22 | 1 | 0 | 0 | 65 | 3 | 0 | 0 | (5) | 7 | (1) | 0 |
| Acceptable weight | 77 | 66 | 4 | 0 | 35 | 69 | 10 | 0 | (3) | 78 | 21 | (1) |
| Overweight | (1) | 32 | 77 | (2) | 0 | 27 | 77 | 23 | 0 | 15 | 75 | 34 |
| Obese | 0 | 1 | 20 | 96 | 0 | 2 | 13 | 77 | 0 | 0 | 3 | 63 |
| *Base = 100%* | *82* | *465* | *189* | *47* | *31* | *332* | *333* | *74* | *8* | *170* | *203* | *35* |
| | | | | | | | | **Females** | | | | |
| Underweight | 29 | 1 | 0 | 0 | 36 | 1 | 0 | 0 | (7) | 6 | (1) | 0 |
| Acceptable weight | 69 | 68 | 11 | 0 | 58 | 67 | 12 | 0 | (5) | 75 | 23 | 4 |
| Overweight | (1) | 28 | 58 | 11 | (2) | 30 | 64 | 12 | 0 | 17 | 62 | 21 |
| Obese | 0 | 3 | 31 | 89 | 0 | 1 | 24 | 88 | 0 | 1 | 15 | 76 |
| *Base = 100%* | *49* | *591* | *256* | *82* | *33* | *415* | *321* | *169* | *12* | *158* | *200* | *106* |

**Table 6.5**      **Mean changes in weight from HALS1 to HALS2 by non-manual/manual socio-economic group. Mean weight in kilograms (kg) at HALS1 with mean change in kg ± Standard Error of the Mean (S.E.M.)**

| | HALS1 Age group | | | | | |
| | 18-38 | 39-59 | 60+ | 18-38 | 39-59 | 60+ |
| | | Males | | | Females | |
|---|---|---|---|---|---|---|
| **Non-manual HALS1** | | | | | | |
| Weight | 75.2 | 77.7 | 75.5 | 60.3 | 63.8 | 63.1 |
| Change | +5.3 | +1.9 | −1.1 | +4.6 | +2.8 | −1.0 |
| S.E.M. | ±0.3 | ±0.3 | ±0.4 | ±0.3 | ±0.3 | ±0.4 |
| **Manual HALS1** | | | | | | |
| Weight | 73.0 | 76.9 | 74.0 | 61.7 | 65.8 | 63.1 |
| Change | +4.2 | +2.1 | −0.8 | +4.4 | +2.9 | −0.3 |
| S.E.M. | ±0.3 | ±0.3 | ±0.4 | ±0.3 | ±0.3 | ±0.3 |
| Mean age | 30.3 | 48.3 | 67.4 | 30.4 | 47.9 | 66.9 |
| | 28.2 | 49.1 | 67.2 | 29.8 | 48.1 | 67.8 |
| Base | 343 | 355 | 171 | 442 | 466 | 203 |
| | 430 | 414 | 243 | 525 | 463 | 271 |

**Table 6.6**      **Change in BMI categories HALS1 to HALS2 by North/South regions and non-manual and manual socio-economic groups for respondents under 60 years at HALS1**

| | Males | | | | | | | | Females | | | | | | | |
| | Non-manual | | | | Manual | | | | Non-manual | | | | Manual | | | |
| | North | | South | | North | | South | | North | | South | | North | | South | |
| HALS | 1 | 2 | 1 | 2 | 1 | 2 | 1 | 2 | 1 | 2 | 1 | 2 | 1 | 2 | 1 | 2 |
|---|---|---|---|---|---|---|---|---|---|---|---|---|---|---|---|---|
| Underweight | 4 | 2 | 8 | 3 | 7 | 3 | 8 | 4 | 4 | 2 | 5 | 2 | 4 | 2 | 3 | 2 |
| Acceptable weight | 50 | 38 | 53 | 45 | 49 | 40 | 52 | 44 | 57 | 44 | 59 | 48 | 43 | 35 | 52 | 41 |
| Overweight | 38 | 46 | 34 | 44 | 35 | 43 | 30 | 38 | 28 | 35 | 27 | 34 | 34 | 36 | 33 | 35 |
| Obese | 8 | 13 | 5 | 8 | 9 | 14 | 10 | 14 | 11 | 18 | 10 | 16 | 19 | 27 | 12 | 22 |
| Base = 100% | 333 | | 383 | | 504 | | 362 | | 431 | | 495 | | 596 | | 417 | |

**Table 6.7**   **Mean changes in weight from HALS1 to HALS2 analysed by smoking habits and age and sex. Mean weight in kilograms (kg) at HALS1 with mean change in kg ± Standard Error of the Mean (S.E.M.)**

| Smoking categories | HALS1 Age group | | | | | |
|---|---|---|---|---|---|---|
| | 18-38 | 39-59 | 60+ | 18-38 | 39-59 | 60+ |
| | | Men | | | Women | |
| **HALS1 – HALS2** | | | | | | |
| **Non-smoking – Non-smoking** | | | | | | |
| HALS1 weight | 73.6 | 76.1 | 76.7 | 61.2 | 65.3 | 64.4 |
| Change | +4.9 | +1.3 | +0.0 | +4.6 | +3.1 | –1.2 |
| S.E.M. | ±0.3 | ±0.4 | ±0.6 | ±0.3 | ±0.3 | ±0.3 |
| **Ex-smoking – Ex-smoking** | | | | | | |
| HALS1 weight | 77.3 | 80.0 | 75.5 | 63.8 | 65.5 | 64.1 |
| Change | +3.7 | +1.6 | –1.5 | +4.2 | +2.8 | –0.6 |
| S.E.M. | ±0.7 | ±0.4 | ±0.4 | ±0.5 | ±0.5 | ±0.6 |
| **Regular – Regular** | | | | | | |
| HALS1 weight | 71.9 | 76.2 | 71.1 | 59.4 | 63.7 | 58.8 |
| Change | +4.1 | +1.6 | –1.7 | +3.8 | +2.1 | –0.8 |
| S.E.M. | ±0.3 | ±0.4 | ±0.6 | ±0.4 | ±0.4 | ±0.6 |
| **Ex-smoking – Regular** | | | | | | |
| HALS1 weight | 78.4 | 79.6 | 77.4 | 61.1 | 67.7 | 56.9 |
| Change | +3.0 | –0.4 | –4.6 | +3.2 | –2.0 | –3.6 |
| S.E.M. | ±1.0 | – | – | ±1.9 | ±1.5 | – |
| **Regular – Ex-smoking** | | | | | | |
| HALS1 weight | 72.4 | 75.0 | 75.4 | 62.1 | 62.2 | 57.0 |
| Change | +7.4 | +5.7 | +1.1 | +8.2 | +5.9 | +6.6 |
| S.E.M. | ±1.0 | ±0.7 | ±1.1 | ±1.1 | ±0.8 | ±1.8 |
| *Base* | *305* | *160* | *64* | *429* | *410* | *241* |
| | *99* | *229* | *180* | *138* | *186* | *121* |
| | *248* | *235* | *99* | *284* | *229* | *65* |
| | *15* | *8* | *2* | *19* | *13* | *3* |
| | *40* | *83* | *39* | *46* | *56* | *23* |

**Table 6.8**     **Mean changes in girth from HALS1 to HALS2 by smoking habits and by age and sex: mean girth in centimetres (cm) at HALS1 with mean change in cm ± Standard Error of the Mean (S.E.M.)**

| | HALS1 Age group | | | | | |
| | 18-38 | 39-59 | 60+ | 18-38 | 39-59 | 60+ |
| Smoking categories | | Males | | | Females | |
| **HALS1 – HALS2** **Non-smoking – Non-smoking** | | | | | | |
| HALS1 girth | 84.8 | 89.7 | 94.9 | 72.8 | 78.1 | 82.9 |
| Change | +6.0 | +3.8 | +2.7 | +5.4 | +4.8 | +2.9 |
| S.E.M. | ±0.4 | ±0.5 | ±0.7 | ±0.4 | ±0.4 | ±0.5 |
| **Ex-smoking – Ex-smoking** | | | | | | |
| HALS1 girth | 88.3 | 93.3 | 95.3 | 75.4 | 78.2 | 81.8 |
| Change | +4.6 | +4.5 | +1.3 | +4.5 | +3.7 | +3.2 |
| S.E.M. | ±0.7 | ±0.6 | ±0.5 | ±0.6 | ±0.5 | ±0.8 |
| **Regular – Regular** | | | | | | |
| HALS1 girth | 84.4 | 91.1 | 92.0 | 72.4 | 77.7 | 79.0 |
| Change | +5.2 | +3.9 | +1.4 | +5.4 | +4.9 | +3.6 |
| S.E.M. | ±0.4 | ±0.5 | ±0.8 | ±0.5 | ±0.5 | ±1.0 |
| **Ex-smoking – Regular** | | | | | | |
| HALS1 girth | 87.7 | 93.2 | 94.2 | 75.9 | 80.1 | 83.7 |
| Change | +4.2 | +2.9 | –1.0 | +1.4 | +3.3 | –5.0 |
| S.E.M. | ±1.2 | – | – | ±1.8 | ±2.2 | – |
| **Regular – Ex-smoking** | | | | | | |
| HALS1 girth | 84.5 | 90.9 | 96.4 | 73.2 | 75.2 | 76.3 |
| Change | +7.8 | +7.9 | +3.9 | +10.3 | +8.1 | +11.7 |
| S.E.M. | ±1.0 | ±0.8 | ±0.9 | ±1.2 | ±1.1 | ±2.0 |
| *Base* | *302* | *159* | *64* | *428* | *408* | *239* |
| | *99* | *227* | *179* | *138* | *183* | *120* |
| | *247* | *233* | *98* | *277* | *228* | *64* |
| | *15* | *8* | *2* | *22* | *13* | *3* |
| | *38* | *83* | *40* | *45* | *56* | *23* |

# PRESCRIBED MEDICATIONS | 7

## Brian D Cox

Information concerning medicines on prescription was obtained by the interviewers, who asked in both HALS1 and HALS2 the same question, 'At the moment do you have anything on prescription?' There were no supplementary questions in the questionnaire about what the prescribed medication was, or for what it had been prescribed. However the respondents who took part in the measurement section of the Survey were also asked by the visiting nurse whether they were presently taking any prescribed medications including, in the case of women of appropriate age, hormone replacement therapy (HRT). Questions were asked as to which drugs were being taken, and for what purpose did the respondents think they had been prescribed.

These questions, in both parts of the Surveys, enabled some assessment of the proportion of respondents who were on prescribed medication at the time of interview and measurement to be made, together with some idea of the various drugs concerned and the medical condition or conditions for which they were being taken.

Table 7.1 shows the percentage taking prescribed medications in both HALS1 and HALS2. The data are presented as percentages of the whole HALS1 measured population and the HALS2 sample (which is a sub-sample of the HALS1 population) at both sampling times. The presentation in these tables of the percentage mean values for both the whole HALS1 population and those for the group who were also seen exactly seven years later at HALS2, enables an assessment to be made of how representative of the whole HALS1 sample is the HALS2 sub-set. The use of seven year age bands also enables a comparison to be made of the HALS2 1991/2 results with the values obtained for those who were the same age at HALS1. For prescribed medications the HALS2 sub-sample at HALS1 can be seen to be representative of the whole HALS1 sample in the younger age bands. In both men and women the percentage of the HALS2 sub-sample at HALS1 on prescribed medications starts to diverge from the whole HALS1 population in those aged 53-59 at HALS1. From that age band onwards a greater proportion of those respondents not seen at HALS2 were on medication at HALS1, reflecting the probability that there are amongst them a higher proportion with severe diseases or conditions many of whom will have died in the succeeding seven year interval.

The percentage on prescribed medications rises with age in HALS1 and in HALS2, but it is also noticeable that for men in all but the youngest age group, and women in all age groups, at HALS2 there is a higher percentage of respondents on prescribed medications than would be expected for the seven year interval between the Surveys. These differences become most marked in the men aged over 60 and the women aged over 46 at HALS2.

Since in some instances patients are advised to take, or are prescribed by their GP, tonics or vitamin supplements, a question about taking tonics or vitamin supplements was asked in the question-naire, and the responses to this question are shown in Table 7.2. These supplements may be self-prescribed for health promoting reasons or be suggested by the GP, but it is not possible to decide between these alternatives from the question. In HALS1 the percentage of women taking these supplements did not increase with increasing age, although in the men there was a slight increase in the older groups. However women under the age of 67 at HALS1 were much more likely to have been taking the supplements than men. At HALS2 there has been a considerable increase across all age bands and within both sexes, amounting to an overall increase of 53% in the men and 56% in the women.

Many medications are prescribed for a limited period to treat a short-term condition or problem, especially in the young. In the older population, with the development of chronic conditions continuous or long-term medication is necessary in many instances. Table 7.3 shows the proportions by HALS1 age group of those respondents who were being treated with prescribed medications at the times of both Surveys. The table gives the proportions who were on medication at one Survey only or not on any medications at either time, in the whole population and non-manual and manual socio-economic groups. With increasing age the proportion who were on medication in both Surveys increases, the highest proportion being amongst the elderly manual women. The group with the highest proportion not on medication at either Survey was the young non-manual men.

A similar format is used to display the distribution of prescribed medications at both Surveys by North/South region of residence (Table 7.4). In this instance the northern women show the highest percentage on medication at both Surveys but the northern men overall have the highest proportion free of medication at both Surveys.

As the percentage of respondents on prescribed medication rises with increasing age, some of the changes that have occurred can only be examined by comparing proportions on prescribed medications in populations of the same age at Survey. This is demonstrated in Table 7.5 for all respondents, by non-manual and manual socio-economic divisions and by north and south region of residence. The increases in the proportions of respondents at HALS2 on prescribed medications in the same age bands are seen in all socio-economic and regional groups.

## Specific medications

The nurse asked each respondent the reason any medication was being taken. It was evident that in some cases, especially in the elderly, the respondents themselves were unclear why they were taking the medication, and gave completely inappropriate answers in relation to the nature of the drug as identified by the nurse. Furthermore, many generic therapeutic agents have an application for more than one medical condition, so that identifying the reason for the prescription without more extensive probing was impossible in the time available for the interview. In order to overcome these problems to some extent the drugs are reported under headings which relate either to their mode of action or to the physiological system on which they more commonly act.

More elaborate and detailed recording of the medications was made in HALS2 than in HALS1, so the results presented here relate specifically to HALS2 (1991/2). Table 7.6 gives the percentage distribution by age and sex of the principal drug types being taken by the respondents at HALS2.

For respiratory problems there is a high proportion in the youngest age band – 25-29 years – who were being treated with broncho-dilators and anti-asthmatic preparations, reflecting the great increase of asthma in the young as reported in Chapter 4. There is also a high proportion in the over 60s who are being treated with these medications: this reflects the increasing frequency of chronic bronchitis in the elderly (Chapter 4).

Drugs acting on the cardiovascular system are reported in several ways, since many types of drugs have specific effects on the heart, whilst others are not so selective and have in addition an effect on the circulatory system. Firstly in Table 7.6 are reported the percentages of the respondents taking all drugs which have anti-hypertensive effects. The prescription of these compounds increases with age so that, in the over 60s more than 30% of the measured population at HALS2 were being treated with drugs with anti-hypertensive effects.

Diuretics, which have an effect on the fluid balance within the body, are used for the treatment of hypertension and also to remove fluid which accumulates in the case of cardiac insufficiency, a complication of congestive cardiac failure. These drugs are also prescribed with increasing frequency with advancing age. ß-blockers, which are used alone or in combination with other drugs, in a single medication for the treatment of hypertension, angina, cardiac arrhythmias, and other unrelated conditions such as migraine, were more likely to be used by women than by men. Calcium ion (Ca++) antagonists which are also often given for the treatment of angina, cardiac arrhythmias and hypertension were more likely to be prescribed for men except in the over-80s. There were no consistent sex differences in the prescribing pattern for angiotensin converting enzyme (ACE) inhibitors. These are relatively new drugs developed for the treatment of hypertension and cardiac conditions, and have fewer of the side effects associated with some of the other compounds used to treat hypertension. Cardio-selective drugs such as digoxin (developed from Digitalis, the foxglove) have a specific effect on controlling the rhythm of the heart and were much more likely to be prescribed for men than women except in the over-80s.

Aspirin was used principally as an analgesic and an anti-inflammatory drug for many years for the treatment of conditions such as arthritis. Its use as a prescribed medication in these roles has almost disappeared nowadays with the development of new analgesics and non-steroidal anti-inflammatory medications (NSAIDs). Aspirin has acquired a major new role in the prevention of circulatory problems because of its effect in reducing the 'stickiness' of blood platelets and helping prevent the formation of blood clots. Its prescription to subjects in the HALS Survey is associated with reporting circulatory or cardiac problems by the respondents. In those respondents under the age of 80, twice as many men as women have been prescribed aspirin.

Many drugs affecting the central nervous system can be prescribed for a variety of conditions. A mild tranquilliser may be prescribed at night to aid sleep or for day-time use for an anxiety state. All drugs which have a psychotrophic effect are reported two ways in Table 7.6, both combined and separated into those which have primarily an anti-depressant or tranquilliser effect and those which are used mainly to assist sleep – the hypnotics. Women are more likely be treated with psychotrophic drugs than men and there is a steady increase in treatment with age. The sleep-

assisting drugs are only prescribed to any extent in the over-60-year-old measured population at HALS2 and there is no consistent male/female pattern of prescription.

The other prescribed medications which were being taken to any significant extent by the population measured at HALS2 are grouped under the heading 'Miscellaneous'. The anti-inflammatory agents include steroids as well as the non-steroidal medications (NSAIDs). The non-steroidal drugs are the principal anti-inflammatory agents on prescription and steroids are no longer prescribed as frequently as in HALS1 for inflammatory conditions, such as rheumatoid arthritis: this is reflected in the low prescription rate for these substances. (An estimate of the proportion of respondents on anti-inflammatory steroids can be made by subtracting the percentage for NSAIDs from the percentage on any anti-inflammatory drug.) Surprisingly there does not seem to be a preponderance of women taking anti-inflammatory drugs, which might be expected since rheumatoid arthritis is much more common in women than in men. There has been an increase in the percentage of younger men reporting 'painful joints' at HALS2 (Chapter 4). However there is a steady increase with age in the percentage taking these types of medication in both sexes.

Analgesics show a similar pattern of prescription to that for the anti-inflammatory drugs shown in Table 7.6b: there is no obvious male/female trend and there is an increase in prescription with age.

A higher proportion of women than of men in the younger age groups were taking antibiotics at the time of Survey.

Prescribed gastric preparations – antacids etc. – do not reflect the true usage of these substances, which are bought over the counter by many individuals without prescription. Nevertheless they are more frequently taken by the older respondents, as are anti-ulcer drugs, which a few of the respondents reported that they were taking because of the side effects of large doses of NSAIDs.

There is a definite preponderance of women being treated with thyroid preparations (2.5% overall), whereas very few men were receiving these medications (0.6% overall),

Usage of oral hypoglycaemic agents (blood-sugar-lowering anti-diabetic drugs), increases with age and reflects the increasing prevalence of Type 2 diabetes with age. Diabetics in the younger age groups are likely to suffer from Type 1 diabetes, for which insulin replacement therapy is the only treatment. In the older age groups Type 2 diabetes becomes more common and oral medication is often effective in controlling blood-sugar levels.

Hormone replacement therapy (HRT) for women during the menopause is becoming much more common and this is reflected in the finding that over 15% of the women aged 50-59 were receiving this treatment. Except as replacement therapy following hysterectomy in younger women this treatment was not mentioned by female respondents in the HALS1 Survey (1984/5).

## Socio-economic patterns of prescription

Since there appear to be socio-economic differences in patterns of health (Chapter 4), the prescription patterns for major drug groups by non-manual and manual groups are presented in Table 7.7. In all groups except the 70-84 year-old men there is a higher percentage of respondents in the manual groups of both sexes who are taking drugs with cardiovascular effects. This is also the case when only those drugs with anti-hypertensive effects are examined. There is no discernible trend with respect to broncho-dilators or anti-asthmatic preparations. However, in men of all ages, the non-manual groups are more likely to be on psychotrophic drugs, but there is no consistent pattern for the women. Except in the oldest men (aged 70-84), manual groups of both sexes are more likely to be taking prescribed analgesics or anti-inflammatory medications and this is especially evident in the women.

## Smoking and prescribed medications

Smoking has many deleterious effects on health, so that smoking often results in the early development of health problems which for the non-smoking population occur at a later stage in life. The relationship of smoking to prescribed medications is examined in Table 7.8. Many smokers give up the habit because of the development of health problems (see Chapter 12), and this is reflected in the finding

that in the male ex-smokers the percentage taking medications for cardio-vascular problems is at most ages greater than that of the non-smokers or the regular smokers. In women, where heart disease constitutes less of a problem at present and the levels of smoking are lower, the percentage on these medications is not as high in the regular smokers or the ex-smokers as in the non-smokers. When drugs with anti-hypertensive effects alone are examined the proportion of ex-smoking men found to be taking these preparations is also higher than in the other groups.

Drugs for respiratory problems are taken more frequently by ex-smoking men and by regular smokers of both sexes than by non-smokers except in the youngest age group (aged 25-39).

Except in the youngest men and women (aged 25-39) a higher percentage of smokers of both sexes are taking psychotrophic drugs, and this rate is more than double that of non-smokers in the 70-84 age group.

An unexpected finding is that in most age groups and both sexes the smokers and ex-smokers are more likely to be taking analgesics. In the men aged 55-69 and the women aged 40-54 the regular smokers are twice as likely as the non-smokers to be taking these medications.

## Number of medications

The range of individual medications taken by the sample measured at HALS2 is too great to be listed here. The number of prescribed medications taken by any one individual ranged from 1 to 8. The frequency of numbers of medications by age group and sex is shown in Table 7.9. In the youngest age group (aged 25-39) 25% of the men and 22% of the women on prescribed medications were taking more than one drug and this had risen to 33% for both sexes in the 40-54 age group, and to 56% and 50% for men and women respectively in those aged 55-69. In the group aged 70 and over 40% of the men and 33% of the women on medication were taking 3 drugs or more on prescription.

# Summary

In the seven years between HALS1 (1984/5) and HALS2 (1991/2) there has been a considerable increase in the proportion of respondents being treated with prescribed medications. These increases are not restricted to any one age/sex group, socio-economic group or regional division. The more detailed recording of specific types of drug at HALS2 has enabled the pattern of drug prescribing in terms of age, sex, social group and smoking behaviour to be revealed in the sample measured. A higher proportion of the manual than non-manual socio-economic groups were being treated with analgesics and anti-inflammatory drugs, and drugs affecting the cardiovascular system, and in the older respondents, smokers, and to a certain extent ex-smokers, were more likely to be being treated with anti-depressants, tranquillisers and analgesics.

It may well be that the increase in prescribed medications reflects the current trend of monitoring the middle-aged and elderly population by GP practices in 'well person' clinics, so that asymptomatic conditions such as hypertension which would previously have gone undiagnosed are now being actively treated with prescribed medications.

**Table 7.1**  **Percentage taking prescribed medications (excluding oral contraceptives) analysed by age in HALS1 full sample, and HALS2 sub-sample at HALS1 and HALS2: Percentage of age group**

| Age at HALS1 | 18-24 | | 25-31 | | 32-38 | | 39-45 | | 46-52 | | 53-59 | | 60-66 | | 67-73 | | >73 | | All | |
| --- | --- | --- | --- | --- | --- | --- | --- | --- | --- | --- | --- | --- | --- | --- | --- | --- | --- | --- | --- | --- |
| Age at HALS2 | | 25-31 | | 32-38 | | 39-45 | | 46-52 | | 53-59 | | 60-66 | | 67-73 | | 74-80 | | >80 | | |
| **Males** | | | | | | | | | | | | | | | | | | | | |
| HALS1 sample | 17 | | 17 | | 17 | | 20 | | 25 | | 42 | | 45 | | 62 | | 57 | | 30 | |
| HALS2 sub-sample | 17 | 19 | 18 | 21 | 17 | 22 | 20 | 27 | 27 | 44 | 39 | 55 | 41 | 70 | 57 | 77 | 47 | 68 | 28 | 39 |
| *Base = 100%* | *534* | | *489* | | *573* | | *474* | | *419* | | *417* | | *412* | | *314* | | *273* | | *3905* | |
| | *299* | *299* | *241* | *241* | *383* | *383* | *324* | *324* | *280* | *280* | *278* | *278* | *259* | *259* | *148* | *148* | *88* | *88* | *2300* | *2300* |
| **Females** | | | | | | | | | | | | | | | | | | | | |
| HALS1 sample | 21 | | 26 | | 24 | | 32 | | 38 | | 47 | | 53 | | 64 | | 64 | | 38 | |
| HALS2 sub-sample | 21 | 23 | 28 | 27 | 24 | 35 | 31 | 49 | 39 | 57 | 45 | 67 | 52 | 69 | 59 | 79 | 61 | 81 | 36 | 49 |
| *Base = 100%* | *626* | | *672* | | *766* | | *618* | | *576* | | *486* | | *553* | | *391* | | *410* | | *5098* | |
| | *311* | *311* | *394* | *394* | *545* | *545* | *432* | *432* | *391* | *391* | *315* | *315* | *327* | *327* | *191* | *191* | *146* | *146* | *3052* | *3052* |

**Table 7.2**  **Percentage taking tonics or vitamins analysed by age in HALS1 full sample, and HALS2 sub-sample at HALS1 and HALS2: Percentage of age group**

| Age at HALS1 | 18-24 | | 25-31 | | 32-38 | | 39-45 | | 46-52 | | 53-59 | | 60-66 | | 67-73 | | >73 | | All | |
| --- | --- | --- | --- | --- | --- | --- | --- | --- | --- | --- | --- | --- | --- | --- | --- | --- | --- | --- | --- | --- |
| Age at HALS2 | | 25-31 | | 32-38 | | 39-45 | | 46-52 | | 53-59 | | 60-66 | | 67-73 | | 74-80 | | >80 | | |
| **Males** | | | | | | | | | | | | | | | | | | | | |
| HALS1 sample | 10 | | 11 | | 11 | | 12 | | 11 | | 14 | | 13 | | 17 | | 19 | | 13 | |
| HALS2 sub-sample | 10 | 15 | 11 | 15 | 11 | 15 | 12 | 20 | 12 | 25 | 11 | 20 | 12 | 24 | 16 | 23 | 20 | 18 | 12 | 19 |
| *Base = 100%* | *534* | | *489* | | *573* | | *474* | | *419* | | *417* | | *412* | | *314* | | *273* | | *3905* | |
| | *299* | *299* | *241* | *241* | *383* | *383* | *324* | *324* | *280* | *280* | *278* | *278* | *259* | *259* | *148* | *148* | *88* | *88* | *2300* | *2300* |
| **Females** | | | | | | | | | | | | | | | | | | | | |
| HALS1 sample | 20 | | 21 | | 22 | | 20 | | 21 | | 21 | | 18 | | 16 | | 23 | | 20 | |
| HALS2 sub-sample | 19 | 23 | 20 | 24 | 22 | 31 | 18 | 41 | 21 | 35 | 24 | 32 | 18 | 38 | 15 | 36 | 18 | 16 | 20 | 32 |
| *Base = 100%* | *626* | | *672* | | *766* | | *618* | | *576* | | *486* | | *553* | | *391* | | *410* | | *5098* | |
| | *311* | *311* | *394* | *394* | *545* | *545* | *432* | *432* | *391* | *391* | *315* | *315* | *327* | *327* | *191* | *191* | *146* | *146* | *3052* | *3052* |

**Table 7.3**     **Respondents on prescribed medications at Survey (excluding oral contraceptives), analysed by age and socio-economic group: Percentage of each group**

| Age HALS1 (Age HALS2) | 18-38 (25-45) | 39-59 (46-66) | 60+ (67+) | 18-38 (25-45) | 39-59 (46-66) | 60+ (67+) | 18-38 (25-45) | 39-59 (46-66) | 60+ (67+) |
|---|---|---|---|---|---|---|---|---|---|
| | **All males** | | | **Non-manual males** | | | **Manual males** | | |
| On medication HALS1 & HALS2 | 8 | 20 | 42 | 7 | 18 | 44 | 9 | 21 | 41 |
| Medication HALS2 not HALS1 | 13 | 22 | 29 | 13 | 18 | 27 | 13 | 25 | 31 |
| Medication HALS1 not HALS2 | 9 | 9 | 4 | 10 | 11 | 5 | 9 | 6 | 4 |
| Not on medication HALS1 or 2 | 70 | 50 | 24 | 71 | 53 | 24 | 69 | 48 | 24 |
| *Base = 100%* | *920* | *882* | *495* | *393* | *405* | *196* | *513* | *476* | *296* |

| | **All females** | | | **Non-manual females** | | | **Manual females** | | |
|---|---|---|---|---|---|---|---|---|---|
| On medication HALS1 & HALS2 | 12 | 28 | 48 | 11 | 24 | 43 | 13 | 33 | 51 |
| Medication HALS2 not HALS1 | 17 | 29 | 27 | 18 | 31 | 29 | 16 | 26 | 25 |
| Medication HALS1 not HALS2 | 13 | 9 | 8 | 14 | 9 | 8 | 12 | 9 | 8 |
| Not on medication HALS1 or 2 | 58 | 34 | 18 | 57 | 36 | 20 | 59 | 32 | 16 |
| *Base = 100%* | *1250* | *1138* | *659* | *577* | *558* | *274* | *657* | *567* | *376* |

**Table 7.4**     **Respondents on prescribed medications at Survey (excluding oral contaceptives), analysed by age and north/south region of residence: Percentage of each group**

| Age HALS1 (Age HALS2) | North 18-38 (25-45) | 39-59 (46-66) | 60+ (67+) | South 18-38 (25-45) | 39-59 (46-66) | 60+ (67+) | North 18-38 (25-45) | 39-59 (46-66) | 60+ (67+) | South 18-38 (25-45) | 39-59 (46-66) | 60+ (67+) |
|---|---|---|---|---|---|---|---|---|---|---|---|---|
| | **Males** | | | | | | **Females** | | | | | |
| On medication HALS1 & HALS2 | 7 | 21 | 47 | 9 | 19 | 39 | 13 | 32 | 53 | 12 | 23 | 42 |
| Medication HALS2 not HALS1 | 13 | 25 | 23 | 12 | 19 | 34 | 17 | 27 | 23 | 18 | 31 | 30 |
| Medication HALS1 not HALS2 | 7 | 6 | 5 | 13 | 12 | 4 | 10 | 9 | 7 | 16 | 10 | 9 |
| Not on medication HALS1 or 2 | 73 | 49 | 26 | 66 | 51 | 23 | 61 | 33 | 16 | 55 | 36 | 19 |
| *Base = 100%* | *515* | *439* | *215* | *405* | *443* | *280* | *670* | *626* | *353* | *580* | *512* | *306* |

**Table 7.5** **Respondents on prescribed medications analysed by age at Survey (excluding oral contraceptives), and by socio-economic group and region of residence: Percentage of each group on prescribed medications**

| | Males | | | | | | | | Females | | | | | | | |
|---|---|---|---|---|---|---|---|---|---|---|---|---|---|---|---|---|
| Age at Survey | 25-39 | | 40-54 | | 55-69 | | 70-84 | | 25-39 | | 40-54 | | 55-69 | | 70-84 | |
| Survey | 1 | 2 | 1 | 2 | 1 | 2 | 1 | 2 | 1 | 2 | 1 | 2 | 1 | 2 | 1 | 2 |
| All respondents | 17 | 20 | 23 | 26 | 48 | 54 | 58 | 73 | 25 | 26 | 37 | 44 | 53 | 62 | 64 | 77 |
| **Socio-economic group** | | | | | | | | | | | | | | | | |
| Non-manual | 16 | 20 | 24 | 23 | 45 | 49 | 61 | 75 | 24 | 25 | 32 | 45 | 49 | 58 | 60 | 74 |
| Manual | 18 | 20 | 23 | 30 | 49 | 58 | 56 | 72 | 26 | 26 | 41 | 44 | 56 | 65 | 66 | 80 |
| **Region** | | | | | | | | | | | | | | | | |
| North | 14 | 18 | 22 | 29 | 52 | 57 | 63 | 71 | 24 | 25 | 39 | 45 | 59 | 66 | 70 | 79 |
| South | 20 | 22 | 25 | 23 | 44 | 51 | 55 | 75 | 27 | 27 | 34 | 43 | 46 | 57 | 57 | 76 |
| *Base = 100%* | 1134 | 583 | 929 | 733 | 853 | 608 | 441 | 350 | 1525 | 775 | 1248 | 1013 | 1083 | 746 | 573 | 459 |
| | 522 | 218 | 418 | 370 | 322 | 262 | 156 | 135 | 726 | 337 | 609 | 498 | 437 | 365 | 205 | 193 |
| | 592 | 351 | 510 | 363 | 527 | 344 | 284 | 214 | 771 | 426 | 625 | 505 | 629 | 373 | 353 | 260 |
| | 561 | 332 | 490 | 384 | 399 | 297 | 207 | 144 | 787 | 432 | 674 | 535 | 591 | 402 | 299 | 252 |
| | 573 | 251 | 439 | 349 | 454 | 311 | 234 | 206 | 738 | 343 | 574 | 478 | 492 | 344 | 274 | 207 |

**Table 7.6a    Prescribed medications reported by measured sample at HALS2 analysed by age: Percentage of each group**

| Drug type | | 25-29 | 30-39 | 40-49 | 50-59 | 60-69 | 70-79 | 80-99 | ALL |
|---|---|---|---|---|---|---|---|---|---|
| | | | | | Age at HALS2 | | | | |
| **Respiratory system** | | | | | | | | | |
| Broncho-dilators and | Males | 5.8 | 2.9 | 1.7 | 3.6 | 8.8 | 10.7 | 9.4 | 5.3 |
| anti-asthmatic medications | Females | 6.2 | 1.7 | 2.8 | 3.3 | 7.0 | 5.4 | 4.7 | 3.9 |
| **Cardiovascular system** | | | | | | | | | |
| Drugs with anti-hypertensive effects | Males | (1) | 1.0 | 4.0 | 13.4 | 26.6 | 37.8 | 36.5 | 14.4 |
| (all types combined) | Females | 0.0 | 1.5 | 6.5 | 17.5 | 30.4 | 38.1 | 47.7 | 15.9 |
| Diuretics | Males | (1) | 0.0 | 1.3 | 4.7 | 11.6 | 22.3 | 27.1 | 7.1 |
| (hypertension and fluid balance) | Females | 0.0 | 1.0 | 3.6 | 9.8 | 17.6 | 23.5 | 37.4 | 9.6 |
| ß-Blockers | Males | 0.0 | (1) | 2.8 | 7.2 | 11.1 | 10.3 | 5.9 | 5.5 |
| (hypertension and angina) | Females | 0.0 | 1.0 | 3.3 | 8.1 | 12.7 | 15.4 | 10.3 | 6.5 |
| Ca++ antagonists | Males | (1) | (1) | (3) | 5.8 | 7.9 | 12.2 | 5.9 | 4.4 |
| (hypertension, angina and arrhythmia) | Females | 0.0 | 0.0 | (4) | 3.1 | 6.5 | 6.9 | 9.3 | 2.9 |
| ACE inhibitors | Males | 0.0 | (1) | 1.1 | 1.7 | 2.8 | 3.4 | 4.7 | 1.7 |
| (hypertension and cardiac conditions) | Females | 0.0 | 0.0 | 1.0 | 1.5 | 3.0 | 3.5 | (1) | 1.4 |
| Cardio-selective drugs | Males | 0.0 | (1) | 1.1 | 3.6 | 11.0 | 12.4 | 11.8 | 4.9 |
| (digoxin & glyceryl tri-nitrate) | Females | 0.0 | 0.0 | 1.2 | 2.9 | 5.4 | 7.3 | 20.6 | 3.3 |
| Anti-platelet aspirin | Males | 0.0 | 0.0 | 1.1 | 2.8 | 8.2 | 10.3 | 7.1 | 3.7 |
| | Females | 0.0 | 0.0 | (2) | 1.0 | 2.2 | 5.0 | 8.4 | 1.4 |
| *Base = 100%* | *Males* | *171* | *308* | *470* | *359* | *353* | *233* | *85* | *1979* |
| | *Females* | *161* | *469* | *642* | *481* | *369* | *260* | *107* | *2489* |

**Table 7.6b    Prescribed medications reported by measured sample at HALS2 analysed by age: Percentage of each group**

| Drug type | | 25-29 | 30-39 | 40-49 | 50-59 | 60-69 | 70-79 | 80-99 | ALL |
|---|---|---|---|---|---|---|---|---|---|
| | | | | | Age at HALS2 | | | | |
| **Central nervous system** | | | | | | | | | |
| All psychotrophic drugs | Males | (2) | 2.9 | 2.1 | 4.2 | 4.3 | 6.9 | 10.6 | 3.8 |
| | Females | (2) | 5.3 | 3.1 | 6.0 | 9.5 | 7.7 | 14.0 | 5.9 |
| Tranquilisers and anti-depressants | Males | 0.0 | 2.0 | 2.1 | 3.9 | 3.7 | 6.0 | 7.1 | 3.2 |
| | Females | (2) | 3.6 | 2.7 | 5.4 | 8.4 | 7.7 | 13.1 | 5.1 |
| Hypnotics (Nitrazepam, Mogadon, etc.) | Males | 0.0 | 0.0 | 0.0 | (1) | 1.1 | 3.0 | 4.7 | 0.8 |
| | Females | 0.0 | 0.0 | (4) | 1.2 | 2.4 | 1.9 | 9.3 | 1.4 |
| **Miscellaneous** | | | | | | | | | |
| Anti-inflammatory agents (all) | Males | 0.0 | 1.9 | 3.8 | 4.7 | 8.2 | 13.7 | 10.6 | 5.6 |
| | Females | 0.0 | 1.7 | 2.8 | 6.7 | 10.6 | 10.4 | 14.0 | 5.6 |
| Non-steroidal anti-inflammatory agents (NSAIDs) | Males | 0.0 | 1.6 | 3.2 | 4.5 | 7.9 | 8.6 | 8.2 | 4.6 |
| | Females | 0.0 | 1.7 | 2.8 | 5.2 | 8.9 | 8.1 | 11.2 | 4.7 |
| Analgesics | Males | (1) | 1.3 | 1.5 | 4.7 | 3.7 | 6.0 | 11.8 | 3.3 |
| | Females | (2) | 1.7 | 1.7 | 4.6 | 7.3 | 9.2 | 11.2 | 4.3 |
| Antibiotics | Males | (2) | 1.0 | (3) | 1.7 | (1) | 1.3 | 2.4 | 1.0 |
| | Females | 3.7 | 1.5 | 1.0 | 1.7 | 1.6 | 1.9 | 0.0 | 1.5 |
| Gastric preparations (antacids etc.) | Males | 0.0 | (1) | (2) | 2.0 | 2.0 | 2.6 | 10.6 | 1.6 |
| | Females | 0.0 | (4) | 1.7 | 1.0 | 3.8 | 6.2 | 8.4 | 2.4 |
| Anti-ulcer | Males | 0.0 | (1) | (3) | 2.5 | 4.5 | 3.9 | 3.5 | 2.1 |
| | Females | 0.0 | (2) | (4) | 2.1 | 4.1 | 3.8 | 8.4 | 2.1 |
| Thyroid preparations (Thyroxine etc.) | Males | 0.0 | (1) | 0.0 | (2) | 1.1 | 1.3 | 1.2 | 0.6 |
| | Females | 0.0 | 1.7 | 1.3 | 3.1 | 4.9 | 3.8 | 3.7 | 2.5 |
| Insulin (diabetes) | Males | 2.3 | 0.0 | (3) | 1.4 | (3) | (2) | 0.0 | 0.9 |
| | Females | (1) | (1) | (4) | (4) | (1) | (1) | 0.0 | 0.4 |
| Oral hypoglycaemic agents (diabetes) | Males | 0.0 | 0.0 | (2) | 1.1 | 3.4 | 5.2 | 5.9 | 1.8 |
| | Females | 0.0 | 0.0 | (1) | (4) | (4) | 1.9 | 3.7 | 0.7 |
| Hormone replacement therapy (HRT) | Females | 0.0 | (3) | 7.2 | 15.4 | 2.7 | 0.0 | 0.0 | – |
| *Base = 100%* | Males | 171 | 308 | 470 | 359 | 353 | 233 | 85 | 1979 |
| | Females | 161 | 469 | 642 | 481 | 369 | 260 | 107 | 2489 |

**Table 7.7** **Respondents on prescribed medications analysed by type of medication and socio-economic group: Percentage of each group on particular medication type**

| Age at Survey | | Males | | | | Females | | | |
|---|---|---|---|---|---|---|---|---|---|
| Drug type | Socio-economic group | 25-39 | 40-54 | 55-69 | 70-84 | 25-39 | 40-54 | 55-69 | 70-84 |
| Cardiovascular agents (cardiac, anti- | non-manual | (1) | 6.0 | 24.3 | 45.2 | (1) | 8.2 | 26.4 | 40.4 |
| hypertensive & circulatory medications) | manual | 1.1 | 9.8 | 33.4 | 41.6 | 1.9 | 11.5 | 30.2 | 51.9 |
| Drugs with anti-hypertensive | non-manual | (1) | 3.9 | 19.5 | 38.1 | (1) | 7.5 | 23.7 | 37.0 |
| effects | manual | 1.1 | 6.7 | 27.0 | 36.8 | 1.7 | 10.0 | 28.2 | 43.3 |
| Broncho-dilators and anti- | non-manual | 4.4 | 1.8 | 5.7 | 11.1 | 3.1 | 3.4 | 4.7 | 4.6 |
| asthmatic preparations | manual | 3.9 | 1.9 | 8.9 | 10.0 | 2.8 | 2.7 | 6.0 | 5.7 |
| Psychotrophic drugs (anti- | non-manual | 1.6 | 3.0 | 3.9 | 7.1 | 3.1 | 2.1 | 6.0 | 8.6 |
| depressants, tranquilisers, etc.) | manual | 1.1 | 2.5 | 3.3 | 5.8 | 3.0 | 4.1 | 9.3 | 9.5 |
| Analgesics (pain killers) and | non-manual | 1.6 | 6.0 | 9.1 | 18.3 | 1.9 | 4.1 | 10.7 | 13.9 |
| anti-inflammatory drugs | manual | 2.1 | 7.0 | 10.9 | 17.4 | 3.3 | 7.0 | 17.6 | 23.3 |
| *Base = 100%* | | *184* | *333* | *230* | *126* | *259* | *438* | *299* | *151* |
| | | *283* | *315* | *302* | *190* | *362* | *442* | *301* | *210* |

**Table 7.8** **Respondents on prescribed medications analysed by type of medication and smoking behaviour at HALS2: Percentage of each group on particular medication type**

| Age at Survey | | Males | | | | Females | | | |
|---|---|---|---|---|---|---|---|---|---|
| Drug type | Smoking group | 25-39 | 40-54 | 55-69 | 70-84 | 25-39 | 40-54 | 55-69 | 70-84 |
| Cardiovascular agents | Non-smokers | (1) | 5.3 | 26.2 | 38.0 | 1.4 | 11.8 | 31.1 | 49.2 |
| (cardiac,anti-hypertensive & | Ex-smokers | 2.6 | 11.2 | 29.4 | 45.3 | (1) | 9.0 | 30.1 | 50.0 |
| circulatory medications) | Regular smokers | (1) | 6.9 | 31.3 | 40.5 | 1.4 | 8.5 | 22.4 | 31.8 |
| Drugs with anti-hypertensive | Non-smokers | (1) | 4.2 | 22.3 | 32.0 | 1.4 | 11.1 | 28.1 | 41.7 |
| effects | Ex-smokers | 2.6 | 7.6 | 24.8 | 39.6 | 0.0 | 7.9 | 28.4 | 42.5 |
| | Regular smokers | (1) | 3.9 | 22.9 | 35.1 | 1.4 | 7.0 | 20.4 | 31.8 |
| Broncho-dilators and anti- | Non-smokers | 3.7 | 0.0 | 3.9 | 6.0 | 3.6 | 2.6 | 3.7 | 4.0 |
| asthmatic preparations | Ex-smokers | 10.3 | 3.2 | 7.6 | 12.0 | 3.1 | 3.3 | 5.1 | 5.0 |
| | Regular smokers | 1.1 | 2.1 | 9.6 | 9.5 | 1.4 | 3.9 | 7.9 | 9.0 |
| Psychotrophic drugs (anti- | Non-smokers | 1.8 | 1.1 | 2.9 | 4.0 | 4.3 | 3.2 | 4.8 | 6.5 |
| depressants, tranquilisers, etc.) | Ex-smokers | 0.0 | 2.7 | 3.4 | 5.6 | 3.1 | 1.7 | 8.5 | 10.8 |
| | Regular smokers | 1.1 | 4.3 | 4.2 | 8.1 | 1.4 | 4.3 | 11.8 | 15.9 |
| Analgesics | Non-smokers | (1) | 1.1 | 1.9 | 6.0 | 1.8 | 1.6 | 6.7 | 7.0 |
| | Ex-smokers | 1.3 | 2.7 | 4.2 | 8.9 | 0.0 | 1.7 | 4.5 | 13.3 |
| | Regular smokers | 1.7 | 3.0 | 5.4 | 5.4 | 2.4 | 4.3 | 8.6 | 13.6 |
| *Base = 100%* | | *218* | *189* | *103* | *50* | *281* | *380* | *270* | *199* |
| | | *78* | *223* | *262* | *192* | *129* | *242* | *176* | *120* |
| | | *177* | *315* | *166* | *74* | *212* | *258* | *152* | *44* |

**Table 7.9      Number of prescribed medications taken by respondents at HALS2: Percentage of each age group**

| Age at Survey | Males | | | | Females | | | |
|---|---|---|---|---|---|---|---|---|
| | 25-39 | 40-54 | 55-69 | 70-84 | 25-39 | 40-54 | 55-69 | 70-84 |
| **Number of medications** | | | | | | | | |
| Nil | 86.4 | 78.7 | 50.7 | 31.3 | 74.8 | 64.0 | 42.1 | 30.5 |
| 1 | 10.9 | 14.2 | 21.5 | 27.7 | 19.7 | 23.6 | 29.1 | 25.6 |
| 2 | 1.7 | 4.0 | 13.5 | 14.8 | 4.1 | 7.4 | 14.5 | 20.7 |
| 3 | (2) | 1.7 | 6.2 | 10.7 | 1.0 | 2.1 | 6.8 | 13.1 |
| 4 | (1) | (3) | 4.1 | 8.8 | (2) | 1.8 | 3.8 | 6.5 |
| 5 | (1) | (5) | 3.2 | 3.5 | (1) | (5) | 2.0 | 1.9 |
| 6 | (1) | (1) | (2) | 2.5 | 0.0 | (2) | 1.3 | (3) |
| 7 | 0.0 | 0.0 | (2) | (3) | 0.0 | (2) | (2) | (2) |
| 8 | 0.0 | 0.0 | 0.0 | 0.0 | 0.0 | 0.0 | 0.0 | (1) |
| *Base = 100%* | *479* | *648* | *534* | *318* | *630* | *887* | *605* | *367* |

# PSYCHOLOGICAL

# HEALTH

# LONGITUDINAL CHANGES IN MENTAL STATE AND PERSONALITY MEASURES | 8

### Felicia A Huppert and Joyce E Whittington

It has become generally accepted that there is an important relationship between physical health and mental health and personality. Illness can affect an individual's mood and behaviour, and in addition there is some evidence that certain personality traits or behaviour patterns are predictors of specific forms of disease. An example is the claim that Type A behaviour, which is characterised by extreme competitiveness, ambition and time urgency, is associated with increased likelihood of coronary heart disease (CHD) (Jenkins et al. 1974; Haynes et al. 1978, 1980).

There is evidence too, that mental state and personality may be related to prognosis. Anxiety and depression have been implicated as specific predictors of an unfavourable outcome in certain forms of cancer (Lancet, 1979) or following cardiac surgery (Kimball, 1969). This accords with the popular view that physical illness or disability can be overcome more effectively by patients who are in the right 'frame of mind'.

There are many ways in which personality and health may interact. Personality variables may predispose people to certain forms of lifestyle or certain types of disease; conversely, circumstances, lifestyle or poor health may influence personality.

Mental health is usually conceptualised in terms of an individual's current state, and it is acknowledged that this state can be influenced by environmental factors (e.g. housing conditions), work and social relationships, as well as physical health and lifestyle (e.g. alcohol consumption, participation in leisure activities). In contrast to mental state, personality is regarded as an enduring trait of an individual, which is stable over time and consistent across situations. From this perspective, longitudinal changes in personality should not occur. However, there are two principal reasons why it is worth looking at personality variables in a longitudinal study. First, personality has come to be reified in terms of what personality tests measure, and an individual's measurement may change over time even if the underlying personality trait does not. Second, the assumption that there exist enduring traits which do not change over time or across situations, may be wrong. For example, individuals who are shy or reserved in some social contexts, or at some period in their life, may be confident and outgoing in other contexts or at other times. Observations of this type clearly raise questions about the extent to which a person's behaviours are determined by intrinsic traits or personality type and the extent to which they represent adaptive responses to different situations.

## Psychological measures

Three measures of personality and a measure of mental health were selected for the Surveys. The mental health measure was the number of psychiatric symptoms reported using the General Health Questionnaire (GHQ) of Goldberg (1972), in the 30-item version. The GHQ is concerned with a person's current mental state. The 30 questions deal with psychiatric symptoms which have been present over the past few weeks. Symptoms include depression, anxiety, sleep disturbance, social functioning and general life satisfaction. The GHQ has been used extensively in Britain and elsewhere, both in community and patient samples. It has been shown to be a useful screen for possible psychiatric illness (Tarnopolsky et al. 1979) and it is also used as a descriptive measure of psychiatric symptoms (e.g. Huppert and Weinstein Garcia, 1991).

Anxiety as a personality trait was measured using the neuroticism scale of the Eysenck Personality Inventory (EPI), which has been widely used in this country (Eysenck and Eysenck, 1964). In broad terms, the neuroticism scale is intended to measure a person's emotionality, on a scale of stability to instability. The resulting score is assumed to reflect an underlying personality trait which is largely independent of the person's current mood state. However, as with all such instruments, scores are affected to some degree by the presence of clinically significant depression and anxiety (Kerr et al. 1970) and cautious interpretation of the findings is required. The EPI also provides a measure of extraversion, i.e., the extent to which a person is sociable, outgoing and impulsive. Extraversion has been associated with health-related behaviour, e.g. smoking (Smith, 1970) and is likely to play a major role in social integration, which is in turn related to morbidity and mortality (House et al. 1988).

We also measured the Type A behaviour pattern using a scale based on that used in the Framingham Heart Study (Haynes et al. 1978). Type A behaviour is the term used to describe people who are ambitious, competitive, pressed for time, etc (see Appendix A). Several studies, chiefly in the United States, have reported a relationship between this type of behaviour and heart disease (Jenkins et al. 1974; Haynes et al. 1978, 1980). Women and men with high Type A scores are more likely to have or to develop CHD than those with lower scores. Although these findings have excited great interest, some doubts have arisen about the generality of the relationship between CHD and Type A behaviour. Among middle-aged males, the effect is seen only in white-collar workers (Haynes et al. 1980). It is not evident among retired people (Haynes et al. 1978, 1980), and its applicability to a young sample is not known. Further doubts have been raised in a report about British civil servants. The study showed that Type A behaviour was more prevalent in the higher grades of the civil service, while coronary heart

disease was more prevalent in the lower grades (Marmot et al. 1983). Although the present Survey does not include objective data about heart disease, it provides the opportunity to describe the distribution and correlates of Type A behaviour in a representative sample of the British adult population, and the way in which it changes over time.

The measures to be described were all obtained by self-report. At the conclusion of the nurse's visit (see Chapter 1), the questionnaires were left behind to be completed and mailed back in a prepaid envelope. The response rate was quite high – 81.5% of the respondents who had returned the self-report questionnaire at HALS1 and were given a similar questionnaire by a nurse at HALS2, returned them. The age and sex distribution of this sub-sample was almost identical to that of the HALS1 sample who returned the questionnaire. However, comparing the HALS1 distribution with the population distribution at the 1981 census, it appears that men aged 18-24 and women aged 75+ were slightly under-represented in our sample.

## Psychiatric symptoms – the GHQ-30

The General Health Questionnaire (Goldberg, 1972) was scored in the usual dichotomous way (see Appendix A), such that for each question the symptom was rated as either present or absent, to produce a maximum score of 30.

In accordance with previous reports, Table 8.1 shows a large sex difference, women having higher scores than men at both HALS1 and HALS2. The mean values in Table 8.1 are similar to those reported by Goldberg (1972) and reviewed by Goldberg and Williams (1988). The work of Jenkins (1985) suggests that the large difference in psychiatric symptoms between women and men is unlikely to reflect fundamental constitutional differences between the sexes. The differences are more likely to be related to different socialisation patterns and the different tendencies of men and women to express emotional difficulties (Brisco, 1982).

Validation studies of the GHQ have suggested that a cutoff between scores of 4 and 5 is a useful first-stage screen for possible cases of psychiatric disorder (Tarnopolsky et al. 1979). When this value is applied to the Survey data, the proportion of respondents who could be considered possible cases of minor

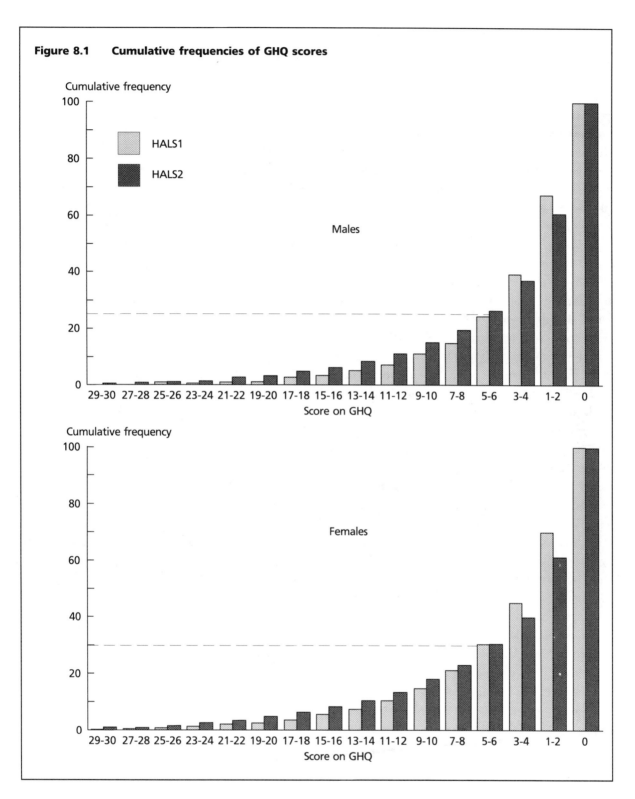

**Figure 8.1    Cumulative frequencies of GHQ scores**

psychiatric illness is very high, an average of 25% for men and 30% for women (Table 8.1). This is certainly an overestimate of the true prevalence of psychiatric disorder. It highlights the problem that a threshold value which has been validated in a general practice setting may not be appropriate for a community Survey (Tarnopolsky et al. 1979). Figure 8.1 shows the cumulative frequency of GHQ scores in the sample which was followed up. From this figure, it is possible to examine the effect of different cut-points on the estimated population prevalence of minor psychiatric disorder.

There does not appear to be a consistent relationship between age and GHQ measures at HALS1 or HALS2 (Table 8.1), nor a consistent, age-related change in scores. While the mean number of psychiatric symptoms increased slightly for both men and women, men also show an average 2% increase in the percentage above threshold, while for women the average figure does not change. However, there are significant increases in GHQ scores in the older sub-groups (mean difference greater than two standard errors of the difference). Among men aged 65-74, the increase is presumably related to a large increase in illness symptoms (see Chapter 4) which are strongly related to mental health (Table 8.3), a detailed discussion of which is presented below. A similar effect among men aged 75+ does not reach statistical significance because of the relatively small number remaining in the sample. The largest increase in psychiatric symptoms is seen among women aged 75+ at HALS1, where the mean score is almost doubled, and 37% are above threshold. This effect results from a combination of factors, including the high rate of illness (Table 8.4), and from widowhood (Table 8.6). Although most of the mean difference scores are within two standard errors of the group mean difference, there are some patterns of change which are worthy of comment. Among the men, the only group which shows a decrease in psychiatric symptoms at HALS2, is men aged 25-34 at HALS1, and this effect is borne out by the large drop in the percentage above threshold in this group. The most likely explanation for this improvement in mental health is that a large number of this group were married between HALS1 and HALS2, and marriage generally appears to be good for mental health (see Table 8.6 and detailed discussion below). A similar explanation may apply to the decreased GHQ scores among women aged 18-24 at HALS1, since women tend to marry at a younger age than men. A moderate improvement in GHQ scores is also seen among women aged 45-64 at HALS1, the explanation for which is likely to be complex. The 35-44 age band, which had consistently low GHQ scores at HALS1 for both men and women, do not retain their good mental health over the seven-year period to HALS2.

A very interesting pattern emerges when we examine the relationship of socio-economic group to GHQ scores (Table 8.2). Although there is no simple association with socio-economic group, young men aged 18-39 in the highest socio-economic group (professional/employers/managers) have the highest GHQ scores, while men aged 65+ in the semi-skilled/unskilled manual group, have the lowest. In contrast, women aged 65+ in the unskilled manual category, have by far the higher GHQ scores: even the mean GHQ is well above the 5+ cutpoint, and 48% of this group can be regarded as possible cases of psychiatric disorder at HALS2. The healthiest group of women (i.e. with the lowest GHQ scores) are those aged 65+ in the highest socio-economic group. Further exploration is required to understand why being in a higher socio-economic group is favourable for mental health in women but unfavourable for men, while being in a low socio-economic group is advantageous for mental health in men but disadvantageous for women.

Although there is a large cross-sectional association between socio-economic group and GHQ measures, socio-economic group does not seem to be related to change in GHQ scores. The only large changes which can be seen in Table 8.2 are for elderly men and women in the 'other non-manual' category, who show a substantial increase in psychiatric symptoms. However, the numbers in these groups are quite low. The only consistent decrease is seen in the percentage of young and middle-aged women in both manual groups, who exceed the GHQ threshold.

## Physical illness and psychiatric symptoms

As part of the HALS1 and HALS2 interviews, subjects rated the presence or absence of physical illness symptoms (e.g. back pain, trouble with eyes, breathlessness), presented as a checklist. On the basis of the total number of symptoms endorsed, subjects were divided into illness categories: low (0-1 symptoms), medium (2-3), and high (4+). Although it cannot be assumed that a large number of symptoms is necessarily more of a problem than one or two severe or frequent symptoms, this measure has proved to be quite informative (e.g. Blaxter, 1990).

As a measure of change in illness symptoms, we categorised individuals according to whether they had moved into a higher illness category ('more illness'), a lower illness category ('less illness') or remained in the same category ('no change'). Table 8.3 presents the percentage of subjects obtaining scores above the standard GHQ threshold, by change in illness symptoms. In the 'no change' groups, the well-known relationship between physical illness and psychiatric symptoms is clearly reproduced. For most age groups and both sexes, the percentage above threshold increases as the number of physical illness symptoms increases. Of those in the high illness category at both HALS1 and HALS2, approximately half are above the GHQ threshold. The association between illness symptoms and GHQ scores differs across age groups. The relationship between low or medium numbers of symptoms and GHQ is considerably greater among young and middle-aged groups than among the elderly. This probably reflects social expectations; illness symptoms are more common among older people, and consequently the association between low or medium numbers of symptoms and mood or mental health is less strong in this group.

In accordance with predictions, subjects who report more illness and are in a higher illness category at HALS2 compared with HALS1 show an increase in the percentage scoring above threshold. Subjects who are in a lower illness category at HALS2 compared with HALS1 show a reduction in the percentage scoring above threshold, in the young and middle-aged groups. However, among older adults, a reduction in illness symptoms is not associated with improved mental health as measured by the GHQ. This may reflect the greater severity or frequency of illness symptoms among older adults.

A different measure of physical illness and its relationship to the GHQ is presented in Table 8.4. This measure is based on the presence or absence of any chronic condition or long-standing illness at HALS1 or HALS2. It can be seen that the absence of long-standing illness at both Surveys is associated with a low percentage of above-threshold scores, and the presence of long-standing illness at both Surveys is associated with a high percentage of above-threshold scores. As predicted, individuals who developed a chronic condition between the Surveys show an increase in the percentage above threshold (except for females, aged 18-39). In accordance with

predictions, young people who recovered from long-standing illness show a decrease in the percentage above threshold but, perhaps surprisingly, middle-aged and older adults do not show this effect. The explanation may reside in the increase in symptoms of physical illness and their effect on GHQ scores in this age group. It is worth commenting on the fact that most groups who had a long-standing illness at both HALS1 and HALS2 show a reduction in the percentage scoring above threshold. This may reflect a decreasing severity of the condition, or perhaps more likely, adaptation to the condition.

Further inspection of Table 8.4 suggests that findings may be influenced by reporting bias. At HALS1, one might expect to find similar percentages above GHQ threshold for the two groups in whom a long-standing illness was absent, and likewise for the two groups in whom a long-standing illness was present. However, the absent-absent group scores considerably lower at HALS1 than the absent-present group for all ages and both sexes. Similarly, the present-present group scores considerably higher at HALS1 then the present-absent group, for all ages and both sexes. Thus, a high prevalence of psychiatric symptoms at HALS2 appears to be more strongly related to the prevalence of psychiatric symptoms at HALS1 then to the presence or absence of long-standing illness.

## Social factors and mental health

The relationship between mental health, as measured by the GHQ, and a number of social factors which may contribute to impaired mental health, is described in Table 8.5 to Table 8.7. First, the effects of employment status in young and middle-aged men is examined, since there has been much concern recently about the effects of unemployment, and its deleterious consequences on mental health. It can be seen in Table 8.5 that men who were employed at both HALS1 and HALS2 have a relatively low percentage of scores above the GHQ threshold. Although the HALS2 sample was large, the number of men whose employment status changed between the Surveys, or who were unemployed at both Surveys, was too small to allow firm conclusions to be drawn about the effects of unemployment.

Table 8.5 also presents data on the effect of retirement on men aged 40-64 at HALS1. Among those who retired between the Surveys, there is only a small increase in the percentage above GHQ threshold. A large increase is seen among those who remained retired. This group comprises men who retired early (under 64 years at HALS1), and the result may reflect increasing dissatisfaction with, or social changes resulting from, being retired (e.g. reduced income), or it may be the consequence of factors which are causally related to early retirement (e.g. health conditions).

The relationship between GHQ and marital status is described in Table 8.6. For young men and women, being married is associated with the best mental health at HALS1 and HALS2, and becoming married is associated with an improvement in mental health. Marriage is also good for middle-aged and older adults, but staying single is a little better for both men and women. Becoming widowed is associated with a massive rise in the percentage over threshold in both men and women. In contrast, becoming divorced has adverse effects on men, but produces no change or a small improvement in women's mental health. Not surprisingly, individuals who divorced between the Surveys had higher GHQ levels at HALS1 than did other groups. This is probably due to psychological symptoms related to a high level of marital friction prior to the divorce.

The mental health problems of older adults are of growing concern in developed countries like Britain where the proportion of elderly people in the population is growing rapidly. Elderly people living alone generally have a higher prevalence of physical and mental ill-health than elderly people living with their spouse or other adults (e.g. Taylor and Ford, 1983). This was confirmed in the analysis of HALS1 data (Huppert et al. 1987) where men and women aged 65 + who lived alone had the highest rates of GHQ scores exceeding the threshold (40% for men; 38% for women). Table 8.7 presents GHQ data by change in household type, for the sub-sample of those aged 65 + at HALS1, who participated in HALS2. It can be seen that elderly men who live alone at both Surveys have poorer mental health than those living with their spouse or other adults. The most dramatic change for both men and women is seen in those who begin to live alone between the Surveys, where there is a twofold increase in the percentage exceeding the GHQ threshold. This is undoubtedly related to the fact that the majority are living alone because they have become widowed (see Table 8.6).

## Neuroticism

The neuroticism scale of the Eysenck Personality Inventory (EPI) is designed to measure emotional stability. Low scores indicate stability, high scores indicate instability (being 'neurotic'). Neuroticism is regarded as a personality trait, i.e. the habitual way in which an individual responds to situations. Although trait theory has had a profound effect in shaping current views of behaviour, it is an empirical question whether behaviours such as emotional stability are enduring or not. Following up the HALS1 sample provides an opportunity to test the theory.

Over the seven-year period between HALS1 and HALS2, neuroticism scores show no overall change for men, and a small but significant overall decrease for women (Table 8.8). The striking exception among women is the group aged 75 and over, whose neuroticism scores increase. A similar increase is seen among elderly men, but the increases in the oldest group of men and women fail to reach statistical significance because of the small number of respondents who completed both Surveys. These findings lend limited support to the notion that neuroticism is an enduring trait.

Central to the study of personality, is the concept of individual differences and of differences between certain groups of individuals. Table 8.8 shows both sex and age differences in neuroticism scores. Women obtain consistently higher scores than men, the average being 8.0 for men and 10.5 for women. For both sexes, the youngest group has the highest score and the oldest group the lowest score, suggesting that emotional stability tends to increase across the lifespan.

Cross-sectional analysis of the full HALS1 data (Huppert et al. 1987) showed a clear relationship between neuroticism score and socio-economic group. The highest scores, indicating least emotional stability, were obtained by those in semi-skilled or unskilled manual groups, and the lowest scores, indicating high emotional stability, were obtained by the professional/managerial group. The same relationship prevails for women at HALS2 but a different pattern is seen for men (Table 8.9). The highest overall level of emotional stability for men is in the other non-manual group, and the most emotionally stable group is the semi-skilled/unskilled manual group aged 65 + at HALS1. There appears therefore to have been selective attrition of men with high neuroticism scores, who were predominantly in the manual and 'other non-manual' categories.

It is instructive to compare scores on the hypothesised trait of emotional instability (high neuroticism scores) with scores on the current state of emotional instability, as measured by high scores on the GHQ. First, these two measures are highly correlated, both at HALS1 and HALS2 (0.49 and 0.52 respectively). This association is also seen in Figure 8.2 which presents neuroticism scores at HALS1 and HALS2 against change in GHQ scores. Among individuals whose GHQ category remained constant, those who scored below the GHQ threshold (less than 5) showed low neuroticism scores at both Surveys, while those who scored above the GHQ threshold had high neuroticism scores at both Surveys. This association could be taken to mean that neuroticism exerts an influence on mental state or that the GHQ measures trait emotionality. However, the data in Figure 8.2 demonstrate that the reverse may be true. Among individuals whose GHQ category changed between the Surveys, those who moved from the low to the high GHQ category showed a corresponding increase in their neuroticism scores; those who moved from the high to the low GHQ category showed a corresponding decrease in their neuroticism score. This trend can be seen in all age groups and both sexes.

It must, therefore, be concluded that present mental state exerts an influence on how individuals respond on the neuroticism scale of the EPI. If neuroticism or emotional stability is defined in terms of what the neuroticism scale measures, then neuroticism is not an enduring trait. On the other hand, the neuroticism scale may be an imperfect measure of a genuine trait which underlies human emotional behaviour. Then the most we can conclude is that performance on this imperfect measure is affected by present emotional state, and that the scores obtained should be interpreted with great caution.

## Extraversion

The extraversion scale of the EPI is designed to measure the extent to which a person is sociable, outgoing and impulsive (Eysenck and Eysenck, 1964). Extraversion is regarded as a personality trait which is orthogonal to (or independent of) the trait of neuroticism. As a personality trait, extraversion should be an enduring characteristic of an individual and scores on the extraversion scale should be stable over time. However the data in Table 8.10 clearly show that extraversion scores are not stable over a seven-year period. Scores decrease significantly for men and women overall, and a decrease is seen in every age group. This evidence of longitudinal change is consistent with the cross-sectional data, which show that extraversion scores are highest among young people and are progressively lower in older age groups.

It appears from these data that across the lifespan, and as individuals age, they are less likely to do things regarded as evidence of extraversion (e.g. 'let yourself go and enjoy yourself a lot at a lively party', 'do almost anything for a dare'). Thus it may be concluded, as it was for neuroticism, that extraversion, as measured by the EPI, is not a stable personality trait. Extraversion appears to be even less stable than neuroticism over the seven-year period of our study.

There do not appear to be sex differences in extraversion scores (Table 8.10), but there is an association with socio-economic group (Table 8.11). Manual groups have higher scores than non-manual groups at both HALS1 and HALS2.

## Type A Behaviour

The Surveys employed 9 of the 10 items of the Type A Behaviour Pattern scale used in the Framingham Heart Study (Haynes et al. 1978). The omitted item covered the same information as one of the other items, but was more difficult for respondents to interpret. Table 8.12 presents the mean scores (multiplied by 100) by age and sex. Men have higher scores than women, and younger people have higher scores than older people at both Surveys. There is a small but significant tendency for Type A scores to decrease over the seven-year period. The only reversal of this trend is among men and women aged 18-24 at HALS1, who show an increase in Type

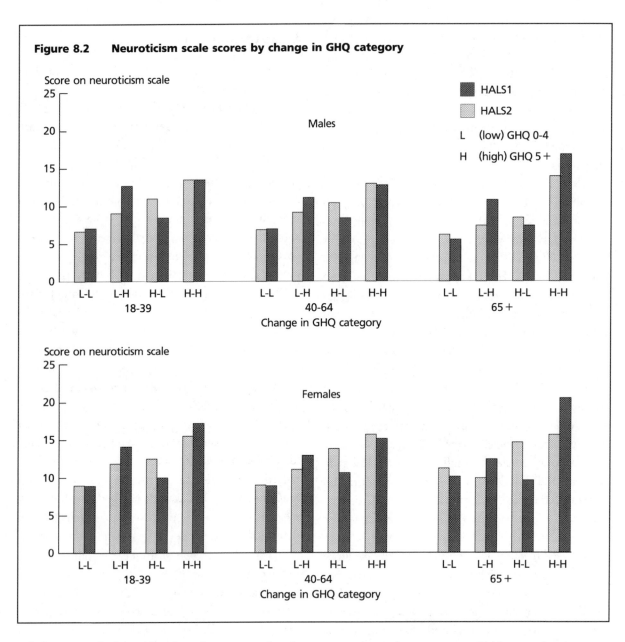

**Figure 8.2    Neuroticism scale scores by change in GHQ category**

A behaviour, which could perhaps be associated with establishing a career. The longitudinal changes, together with the age-related cross-sectional differences in Type A behaviour, show that this behaviour is at least in part under the influence of environmental factors, and is not simply intrinsic to the individual.

To the extent that Type A attributes such as ambition, competitiveness and time-pressure, are career-related, an association with education and socio-economic group might be expected. This is confirmed in Table 8.13 and Table 8.14. In general. Type A scores increase in both men and women with increasing level of education. The one exception is young men with either no qualification or a work-related qualification, whose scores are as high as the most educated young group. Table 8.14 shows a very strong effect of socio-economic group among men, with professional/employers/managers having the highest scores in every age level, and scores decreasing steadily across categories. It is interesting that the relationship between Type A behaviour and occupation is still evident in the oldest group even though they were aged 72 and over at HALS2 and therefore the majority would have retired long since. However, women do not show a parallel effect in relation to socio-economic group, a categorisation which is based on the occupation of the head of the household (assumed to be the man, if present). For women in all age-bands, the highest Type A scores are found in the 'other non-manual' category.

# Summary

It is generally accepted that there are relationships between physical health, mental health and personality factors. Physical and mental health are hypothesised to influence each other, while personality, a collection of enduring traits, may influence physical and mental health but, at least over the short-term, should not be changed by them. Mental health, usually conceptualised in terms of an individual's current state, is also hypothesised to be influenced by environmental factors, such as work and social relationships. Some of these claims were investigated using data from the HALS1 and HALS2 Surveys.

Mental health, or current mental state, was measured by the General Health Questionnaire (GHQ). Distribution of scores on the GHQ is very skewed, and an alternative measure is obtained by considering scores above and below a threshold value. A cut-off between scores of 4 and 5 is often used as an indicator of mild psychiatric disorder. In the HALS2 Survey, this cut-off resulted in over 30% of women and 25% of men being classified as possible 'cases'.

There was a strong relationship between physical and mental health. The number of physical illness symptoms was directly related to the percentage of GHQ scores over the threshold, for all ages and both sexes. Where there was a marked change in illness symptoms between the Surveys, GHQ scores rose and fell with illness symptoms. Similar relationships were found when physical illness was assessed by presence or absence of a long-standing health condition. One notable exception was that, for respondents who reported a long-standing condition at both Surveys, the percentage over the GHQ threshold fell, rather than remaining stable. This may reflect habituation to, or improvement in, the condition over the intervening years.

In agreement with other studies, women had higher GHQ scores than men, at both Surveys. Mean scores at HALS2 were higher for the oldest age groups of both sexes, and this was conjectured to be due in large part to illness and widowhood. However, there was a drop in scores for men aged 25-34 and women aged 18-25 at HALS1. Changes in GHQ were associated with changes in marital status; namely, a fall in GHQ followed a change from single to married (young groups) and a rise in GHQ followed a change from married to widowed (older groups). This latter was also reflected in the finding that, in the over 65s, a change to living alone (usually as a result of widowhood) was associated with a rise in GHQ. Associations with employment status were investigated for men aged under 65 at HALS1, but numbers changing status were disappointingly small and the hypothesised relationship could not be confirmed.

Of the personality variables (neuroticism, extraversion, Type A behaviour), only neuroticism was found to be associated with mental health. Neuroticism and GHQ correlated 0.49 and 0.52 at HALS1 and HALS2 respectively. Also, changes in GHQ between the Surveys were mirrored by changes in neuroticism scores.

For all three personality measures, individual scores were found to have changed a great deal between the Surveys, casting doubt on the stability of hypothesised traits. (On extraversion, 12% changed scores by five or more, out of 24, and 20% changed similarly on neuroticism.) The decline in extraversion scores with increasing age was conjectured to reflect, in part, the increasing inapplicability to older people of items on the scale. The data for Type A behaviour suggest that it may be related to work situation, rather than being a characteristic of an individual. It was found that men had higher scores than women at both Surveys, that scores declined with age, and that scores were strongly related to socio-economic group and less strongly to education.

### References

Blaxter, M. (1990), Health and Lifestyles, London, Tavistock/Routledge.

Brisco, M. (1982), Sex differences in psychological well-being, Pyschological Medicine, Monograph Supplement 7.

Goldberg, D.P. (1972), The detection of psychiatric illness by questionnaire, London: Oxford University Press.

Goldberg, D.P. and Williams, P. (1988), A user's guide to the general health questionnaire, Windsor: NFER-Nelson.

Eysenck, H.J. and Eysenck, B.G. (1964), Manual of the Eysenck Personality Inventory, London: Hodder and Stoughton.

Haynes, S.G., Feinleib, M., Levine, S., Scotch N. and Kannel, W.B. (1978), The Relationship of psychosocial factors to coronary heart disease in the Framingham study, II: Prevalence of Coronary Heart Disease, American Journal of Epidemiology, 107, 384-402.

Haynes, S.G., Feinleib, M. and Kannel, W.B. (1980), The relationship of psychosocial factors to coronary heart disease in the Framingham study, III: Eight-year incidence of coronary heart disease, American Journal of Epidemiology, 111, 37-57.

House, J.S., Landis, K.R. and Umberson, D. (1988), Social relationships and health science, 241, 540-545.

Huppert, F.A., Roth, M. and Gore, M. (1987), 'Psychological Factors' In: Cox, B.D. et al. The Health and Lifestyle Survey: Preliminary Report of a Nationwide Survey of the Physical and Mental Health, Attitudes and Lifestyle of a Random Sample of 9003 British Adults, London, Health Promotion Research Trust.

Huppert F.A. and Weinstein Garcia, A. (1991), Qualitative differences in psychiatric symptoms between high risk groups assessed on a screening test (GHQ-30), Soc Psychiatry Psychiatr Epidemiol, 26, 252-258.

Jenkins, C.D., Rosenman, R.H. and Zyzanski S.J. (1974), Prediction of clinical coronary heart disease by a test of the coronary-prone behaviour pattern, New England Journal of Medicine 290, 1271-1275.

Jenkins, R. (1985), Sex differences in minor psychiatric morbidity, Psychological Medicine, Monograph Supplement 7.

Kerr, T.A., Schapira, K., Rother, M. and Garside, R.F. (1970), The relationship between the Maudsley Personality Inventory and the course of affective disorders, Brit. J. Psychiat. 116, 11-19.

Kimball, C.P. (1969), Psychological responses to the experience of open-heart surgery, Am. J. Psychiatry, 126, 348-349.

Lancet, (1979), Mind and cancer, 1, 706.

Marmot, M.G. (1983), Stress, social and cultural variations in heart disease, J. Psychosomatic Res., 27, 377-384.

Smith, G.K., (1970), Personality and smoking: A review of the empirical literature, In: Hunt, W.A. (Ed.) Learning Mechanisms in Smoking, Chicago, pp. 42-61.

Tarnopolsky, A. et al. (1979), Validity and use of a screening questionnaire (GHQ) in the community, British J. of Psychiatry, 125, 508-515.

Taylor, R.C. and Ford, E.G. (1983), The elderly at risk: A critical examination of commonly identified risk groups, Journal of the Royal College of Practitioners, 33, 699-705.

**Table 8.1    Scores on 30-item General Health Questionnaire by age and sex**

| | Males | | | Females | | | Base numbers | |
|---|---|---|---|---|---|---|---|---|
| | HALS1 | HALS2 | Difference (±SEM) | HALS1 | HALS2 | Difference (±SEM) | Males | Females |
| **Age at HALS1** | | | **Mean GHQ Score (Max 30)** | | | | | |
| **18-24** | 3.2 | 4.1 | +0.9 (±0.5) | 4.3 | 4.1 | −0.2 (±0.5) | 173 | 163 |
| **25-34** | 3.3 | 3.2 | −0.1 (±0.3) | 4.2 | 4.4 | +0.2 (±0.3) | 237 | 433 |
| **35-44** | 3.1 | 3.7 | +0.6 (±0.3) | 3.5 | 4.1 | +0.6 (±0.3) | 338 | 519 |
| **45-54** | 3.3 | 3.9 | +0.6 (±0.4) | 4.3 | 4.0 | −0.3 (±0.3) | 284 | 361 |
| **55-64** | 3.3 | 3.3 | 0 (±0.3) | 3.9 | 3.6 | −0.3 (±0.3) | 307 | 328 |
| **65-74** | 2.6 | 3.5 | +0.9 (±0.3) | 4.0 | 4.4 | +0.4 (±0.4) | 165 | 183 |
| **75+** | 2.9 | 3.6 | +0.7 (±0.7) | 3.4 | 6.4 | +3.0 (±0.8) | 40 | 46 |
| **All ages** | 3.2 | 3.6 | +0.4 (±0.2) | 3.9 | 4.2 | +0.3 (±0.2) | 1544 | 2033 |
| | | | **Percentage scoring 5+** | | | | | |
| **18-24** | 27 | 31 | +4 | 37 | 30 | −7 | 173 | 163 |
| **25-34** | 27 | 21 | −6 | 33 | 32 | −1 | 237 | 433 |
| **35-44** | 21 | 26 | +5 | 27 | 29 | +2 | 338 | 519 |
| **45-54** | 27 | 30 | +3 | 33 | 30 | −3 | 284 | 361 |
| **55-64** | 24 | 25 | +1 | 29 | 27 | −2 | 307 | 328 |
| **65-74** | 19 | 22 | +3 | 27 | 34 | +7 | 165 | 183 |
| **75+** | 25 | 30 | +5 | 24 | 37 | +13 | 40 | 46 |
| **All ages** | 24 | 26 | +2 | 30 | 30 | 0 | 1544 | 2033 |

**Table 8.2a    Mean scores on the General Health Questionnaire by socio-economic group (males)**

| | Household socio-economic group at HALS1 | | | | | | | | | | | | Base numbers | | | |
| | Professional/employers/managers | | | Other non-manual | | | Skilled manual/own account trades | | | Semi-skilled and unskilled manual | | | | | | |
| Age at HALS1 | HALS1 | HALS2 | Difference (±SEM) | HALS1 | HALS2 | Difference (±SEM) | HALS1 | HALS2 | Difference (±SEM) | HALS1 | HALS2 | Difference (±SEM) | Prof | Other n-m | Skilled | Semi |
|---|---|---|---|---|---|---|---|---|---|---|---|---|---|---|---|---|
| **Mean GHQ Score** | | | | | | | | | | | | | | | | |
| 18-39 | 4.1 | 4.3 | +0.2 (±0.5) | 2.7 | 3.2 | +0.5 (±0.5) | 2.9 | 3.2 | +0.3 (±0.3) | 3.6 | 3.4 | −0.2 (±0.6) | 128 | 130 | 220 | 102 |
| 40-64 | 3.3 | 3.4 | +0.1 (±0.4) | 3.3 | 3.9 | +0.6 (±0.5) | 3.3 | 3.9 | +0.6 (±0.4) | 3.1 | 3.8 | +0.7 (±0.4) | 208 | 133 | 258 | 141 |
| 65+ | 2.5 | 3.5 | +1.0 (±0.7) | 2.6 | 4.9 | +2.3 (±0.8) | 3.1 | 3.7 | +0.6 (±0.5) | 1.9 | 2.3 | +0.4 (±0.6) | 51 | 31 | 80 | 42 |
| All Ages | 3.5 | 3.7 | +0.2 (±0.3) | 3.0 | 3.7 | +0.7 (±0.3) | 3.1 | 3.6 | +0.5 (±0.3) | 3.1 | 3.4 | +0.3 (±0.3) | 387 | 294 | 558 | 285 |
| **Percentage scoring 5+** | | | | | | | | | | | | | | | | |
| 18-39 | 33 | 33 | 0 | 20 | 27 | +7 | 21 | 21 | 0 | 30 | 26 | −4 | | | | |
| 40-64 | 24 | 23 | −1 | 27 | 28 | +1 | 24 | 30 | +6 | 23 | 28 | +5 | | | | |
| 65+ | 20 | 26 | +6 | 23 | 32 | +9 | 24 | 23 | −1 | 12 | 14 | +2 | | | | |
| All Ages | 26 | 27 | +1 | 23 | 28 | +5 | 23 | 25 | +2 | 24 | 25 | +1 | | | | |

**Table 8.2b   Mean scores on the General Health Questionnaire by socio-economic group (females)**

| | Household socio-economic group at HALS1 | | | | | | | | | | | | Base numbers | | | |
| | Professional/employers/managers | | | Other non-manual | | | Skilled manual/own account trades | | | Semi-skilled and unskilled manual | | | | | | |
| | HALS1 | HALS2 | Difference (±SEM) | HALS1 | HALS2 | Difference (±SEM) | HALS1 | HALS2 | Difference (±SEM) | HALS1 | HALS2 | Difference (±SEM) | | | | |
|---|---|---|---|---|---|---|---|---|---|---|---|---|---|---|---|---|
| **Mean GHQ Score** | | | | | | | | | | | | | | | | |
| **Age at HALS1** | | | | | | | | | | | | | | | | |
| 18-39 | 3.3 | 4.0 | +0.7 (±0.5) | 4.2 | 4.0 | -0.2 (±0.4) | 3.8 | 4.1 | +0.3 (±0.4) | 4.9 | 5.2 | +0.3 (±0.5) | 182 | 231 | 295 | 173 |
| 40-64 | 3.3 | 3.6 | +0.3 (±0.3) | 3.5 | 3.8 | +0.3 (±0.5) | 4.2 | 4.0 | -0.2 (±0.3) | 4.3 | 3.7 | -0.6 (±0.5) | 279 | 176 | 291 | 159 |
| 65+ | 3.1 | 3.4 | +0.3 (±0.7) | 3.0 | 4.9 | +1.9 (±1.0) | 3.7 | 4.3 | +0.6 (±0.7) | 5.4 | 6.8 | +1.4 (±0.8) | 61 | 36 | 71 | 59 |
| All Ages | 3.3 | 3.7 | +0.4 (±0.3) | 3.8 | 4.0 | +0.2 (±0.4) | 4.0 | 4.1 | +0.1 (±0.3) | 4.7 | 4.9 | +0.2 (±0.4) | 522 | 443 | 657 | 391 |
| **Percentage scoring 5+** | | | | | | | | | | | | | | | | |
| 18-39 | 26 | 28 | +2 | 32 | 32 | 0 | 32 | 28 | -4 | 39 | 38 | -1 | 182 | 231 | 295 | 173 |
| 40-64 | 24 | 28 | +4 | 28 | 31 | +3 | 33 | 30 | -3 | 33 | 27 | -6 | 279 | 176 | 291 | 159 |
| 65+ | 18 | 31 | +13 | 22 | 33 | +11 | 25 | 28 | +3 | 41 | 48 | +7 | 61 | 36 | 71 | 59 |
| All Ages | 24 | 28 | +4 | 30 | 32 | +2 | 32 | 29 | -3 | 37 | 35 | -2 | 522 | 443 | 657 | 391 |

**Table 8.3**    **Relationship between mental health and physical illness. Percentage scoring 5+ on the GHQ by changes in physical illness symptoms**

| | | Age at HALS1 | | | | | | | | | Base numbers | | |
| | | 18-39 | | | 40-64 | | | 65+ | | | | | |
| | | HALS1 | HALS2 | Diff. | HALS1 | HALS2 | Diff. | HALS1 | HALS2 | Diff. | | | |
| **Change in illness category** | | | | | **Males** | | | | | | | | |
| More illness | | 24 | 30 | +6 | 27 | 34 | +7 | 29 | 29 | 0 | 161 | 209 | 52 |
| Less illness | | 26 | 23 | −3 | 19 | 18 | −1 | 24 | 27 | +3 | 153 | 161 | 55 |
| No change: low | | 21 | 19 | −2 | 16 | 16 | 0 | 4 | 8 | +4 | 177 | 199 | 48 |
| medium | | 32 | 26 | −6 | 33 | 30 | −3 | 4 | 4 | 0 | 80 | 103 | 26 |
| high | | 42 | 58 | +16 | 43 | 54 | +11 | 42 | 54 | +12 | 26 | 70 | 24 |
| | | | | | **Females** | | | | | | | | |
| More illness | | 31 | 36 | +5 | 29 | 32 | +3 | 22 | 35 | +13 | 233 | 236 | 72 |
| Less illness | | 33 | 27 | −6 | 33 | 26 | −7 | 28 | 38 | +10 | 248 | 209 | 29 |
| No change: low | | 21 | 22 | +1 | 10 | 13 | +3 | 9 | 3 | −6 | 197 | 163 | 32 |
| medium | | 37 | 29 | −8 | 24 | 26 | +2 | 22 | 32 | +10 | 143 | 142 | 40 |
| high | | 52 | 54 | +2 | 50 | 46 | −4 | 45 | 51 | +6 | 71 | 162 | 55 |

**Table 8.4**    **Percentage scoring 5+ on the General Health Questionnaire in relation to chronic conditions or long-standing illness**

| | | Age at HALS1 | | | | | | | | | Base numbers | | |
| | | 18-39 | | | 40-64 | | | 65+ | | | | | |
| | | HALS1 | HALS2 | Diff. | HALS1 | HALS2 | Diff. | HALS1 | HALS2 | Diff. | | | |
| **Long-standing illness state** | | | | | | | | | | | | | |
| HALS1 | HALS2 | | | | **Males** | | | | | | | | |
| Absent | Absent | 21 | 24 | +3 | 18 | 19 | +1 | 12 | 13 | +1 | 393 | 330 | 77 |
| Absent | Present | 26 | 31 | +5 | 27 | 34 | +7 | 18 | 33 | +15 | 78 | 131 | 33 |
| Present | Absent | 29 | 18 | −11 | 19 | 23 | +4 | 14 | 28 | +14 | 51 | 79 | 29 |
| Present | Present | 43 | 32 | −11 | 35 | 38 | +3 | 33 | 30 | −3 | 75 | 202 | 66 |
| | | | | | **Females** | | | | | | | | |
| Absent | Absent | 29 | 29 | 0 | 23 | 22 | −1 | 21 | 32 | +11 | 631 | 468 | 75 |
| Absent | Present | 41 | 33 | −8 | 36 | 41 | +5 | 31 | 46 | +15 | 93 | 153 | 54 |
| Present | Absent | 37 | 24 | −13 | 29 | 28 | −1 | 17 | 24 | +7 | 68 | 86 | 29 |
| Present | Present | 41 | 45 | +4 | 40 | 37 | −3 | 33 | 31 | −2 | 100 | 205 | 70 |

**Table 8.5**    **Percentage scoring 5+ on the General Health Questionnaire by employment status for males**

| | | 18-39 | | | 40-64 | | | Base numbers | |
|---|---|---|---|---|---|---|---|---|---|
| | | HALS1 | HALS2 | Difference | HALS1 | HALS2 | Difference | | |
| **Employment Status** | | | | | | | | | |
| **HALS2** | **HALS1** | | | | | | | | |
| Employed | Employed | 23 | 23 | 0 | 20 | 21 | +1 | *492* | *381* |
| Employed | Unemployed | 35 | 35 | 0 | (47) | (58) | (+11) * | *20* | *19* |
| Unemployed | Employed | 36 | 33 | −3 | (47) | (20) | (−27) | *36* | *15* |
| Employed | Retired | − | − | − | 21 | 23 | +2 | − | *159* |
| Retired | Retired | − | − | − | 18 | 25 | +7 | − | *61* |

*Age at HALS1*

* Percentages are in brackets where base numbers are below 20. Numbers in other categories were too small for inclusion.

**Table 8.6**    **Relationship between mental health and marital status. Percentage scoring 5+ on the GHQ by changes in marital status**

| | | 18-39 | | | 40-64 | | | 65+ | | | Base numbers | | |
|---|---|---|---|---|---|---|---|---|---|---|---|---|---|
| | | HALS1 | HALS2 | Diff. | HALS1 | HALS2 | Diff. | HALS1 | HALS2 | Diff. | | | |
| **Marital Status** | | | | | **Males** | | | | | | | | |
| **HALS2** | **HALS1** | | | | | | | | | | | | |
| Single | Single | 26 | 31 | +5 | 23 | 21 | −2 | (0) | (25) | (+25) * | *108* | *43* | *8* |
| Married | Married | 21 | 22 | +1 | 24 | 26 | +2 | 22 | 21 | −1 | *333* | *619* | *134* |
| W | W | − | − | − | (46) | (46) | (0) | 25 | 21 | −4 | − | *13* | *28* |
| S/W/D | Married | 31 | 23 | −8 | − | − | − | − | − | − | *93* | − | − |
| M/D | Widowed | − | − | − | 26 | 56 | +30 | 17 | 37 | +20 | − | *27* | *30* |
| M/S | Divorced | 39 | 46 | +7 | (25) | (42) | (+17) | − | − | − | *41* | *12* | − |
| | | | | | **Females** | | | | | | | | |
| Single | Single | 42 | 40 | −2 | 24 | 30 | +6 | (12) | (23) | (+11) | *84* | *37* | *17* |
| Married | Married | 29 | 28 | −1 | 29 | 28 | −1 | 27 | 33 | +6 | *602* | *668* | *84* |
| W | W | − | − | − | 29 | 20 | −9 | 32 | 33 | +1 | − | *66* | *84* |
| S/W/D | Married | 34 | 30 | −4 | (45) | (18) | (−27) | − | − | − | *96* | *11* | − |
| M/D | Widowed | − | − | − | 25 | 37 | +12 | 19 | 40 | +21 | − | *65* | *37* |
| M/S | Divorced | 45 | 40 | −5 | (37) | (37) | (0) | − | − | − | *65* | *19* | − |

*Age at HALS1*

S = Single  M = Married  D = Divorced  W = Widowed

* Percentages are in brackets where base numbers are below 20. Numbers in other categories were too small for inclusion.

**Table 8.7**  **Percentage scoring 5+ on the GHQ by changes in household type for those aged 65+ at HALS1**

| | | Males | | | Females | | | Base numbers | |
|---|---|---|---|---|---|---|---|---|---|
| | | HALS1 | HALS2 | Difference | HALS1 | HALS2 | Difference | Males | Females |
| **Household Type** | | | | | | | | | |
| **HALS1** | **HALS2** | | | | | | | | |
| Lives alone | Lives alone | 26 | 26 | 0 | 27 | 29 | +2 | 23 | 84 |
| Not alone | Not alone | 20 | 19 | −1 | 26 | 33 | +7 | 139 | 99 |
| Not alone | Lives alone | 12 | 25 | +13 | 0 | 33 | +33 | 32 | 38 |

Numbers in other categories were too small for inclusion.

**Table 8.8**  **Mean scores on the neuroticism scale of the Eysenck Personality Inventory by age and sex**

| | Males | | | Females | | | Base numbers | |
|---|---|---|---|---|---|---|---|---|
| | HALS1 | HALS2 | Difference (±SEM) | HALS1 | HALS2 | Difference (±SEM) | Males | Females |
| **Age at HALS1** | | | | | | | | |
| **18-24** | 8.6 | 8.6 | 0 (±0.3) | 11.3 | 11.1 | −0.2 (±0.4) | 173 | 163 |
| **25-34** | 8.4 | 8.3 | −0.1 (±0.2) | 10.7 | 10.5 | −0.2 (±0.2) | 239 | 429 |
| **35-44** | 8.0 | 8.1 | +0.1 (±0.2) | 10.6 | 10.1 | −0.5 (±0.2) | 341 | 516 |
| **45-54** | 7.9 | 7.9 | 0 (±0.2) | 10.7 | 10.3 | −0.4 (±0.2) | 282 | 360 |
| **55-64** | 8.2 | 8.1 | −0.1 (±0.2) | 10.6 | 10.2 | −0.4 (±0.2) | 308 | 325 |
| **65-74** | 7.2 | 7.3 | +0.1 (±0.3) | 10.1 | 10.1 | 0 (±0.2) | 167 | 177 |
| **75+** | 6.0 | 6.6 | +0.6 (±0.4) | 8.0 | 8.6 | +0.6 (±0.5) | 41 | 45 |
| **All ages** | 8.0 | 8.0 | 0 (±0.1) | 10.6 | 10.3 | −0.3 (±0.1) | 1551 | 2015 |

**Table 8.9 Mean scores on the neuroticism scale of the Eysenck Personality Inventory by socio-economic group**

| Age at HALS1 | Professional/employers/managers | | | Other non-manual | | | Skilled manual/own account trades | | | Semi-skilled and unskilled manual | | | Base numbers | | | |
|---|---|---|---|---|---|---|---|---|---|---|---|---|---|---|---|---|
| | HALS1 | HALS2 | Difference (±SEM) | HALS1 | HALS2 | Difference (±SEM) | HALS1 | HALS2 | Difference (±SEM) | HALS1 | HALS2 | Difference (±SEM) | | | | |
| **Males** | | | | | | | | | | | | | | | | |
| 18-39 | 8.8 | 9.0 | +0.2 (±0.3) | 8.0 | 7.6 | −0.4 (±0.4) | 8.0 | 8.2 | +0.2 (±0.3) | 8.7 | 8.5 | −0.2 (±0.4) | 130 | 132 | 222 | 103 |
| 40-64 | 7.9 | 7.5 | −0.4 (±0.3) | 7.6 | 7.6 | 0 (±0.3) | 8.4 | 8.5 | +0.1 (±0.2) | 8.4 | 8.3 | −0.1 (±0.3) | 207 | 133 | 258 | 140 |
| 65+ | 7.5 | 7.3 | −0.2 (±0.4) | 7.0 | 7.7 | +0.7 (±0.7) | 7.3 | 7.4 | +0.1 (±0.4) | 6.0 | 6.0 | 0 (±0.6) | 52 | 31 | 82 | 42 |
| All Ages | 8.1 | 8.0 | −0.1 (±0.2) | 7.7 | 7.6 | −0.1 (±0.2) | 8.1 | 8.2 | +0.1 (±0.2) | 8.1 | 8.0 | −0.1 (±0.2) | 389 | 296 | 562 | 285 |
| **Females** | | | | | | | | | | | | | | | | |
| 18-39 | 10.3 | 9.9 | −0.4 (±0.3) | 10.5 | 10.0 | −0.5 (±0.3) | 10.8 | 10.4 | −0.4 (±0.3) | 12.0 | 12.1 | +0.1 (±0.4) | 181 | 227 | 293 | 172 |
| 40-64 | 9.9 | 9.5 | −0.4 (±0.2) | 10.6 | 10.6 | 0 (±0.3) | 10.6 | 10.3 | −0.3 (±0.2) | 11.3 | 10.9 | −0.4 (±0.3) | 279 | 174 | 289 | 159 |
| 65+ | 8.6 | 8.6 | 0 (±0.4) | 10.7 | 10.4 | −0.3 (±0.4) | 9.7 | 10.0 | +0.3 (±0.4) | 10.2 | 10.5 | +0.3 (±0.4) | 61 | 33 | 69 | 57 |
| All Ages | 9.9 | 9.5 | −0.4 (±0.2) | 10.6 | 10.3 | −0.3 (±0.2) | 10.6 | 10.3 | −0.3 (±0.2) | 11.4 | 11.4 | 0 (±0.2) | 521 | 434 | 651 | 388 |

**Table 8.10**    **Mean scores on the extraversion scale of the Eysenck Personality Inventory by age and sex**

| | Males | | | Females | | | Base numbers | |
|---|---|---|---|---|---|---|---|---|
| | HALS1 | HALS2 | Difference (±SEM) | HALS1 | HALS2 | Difference (±SEM) | Males | Females |
| **Age at HALS1** | | | | | | | | |
| **18-24** | 14.5 | 13.7 | − 0.8 (±0.3) | 13.6 | 13.3 | − 0.3 (±0.3) | 174 | 160 |
| **25-34** | 12.4 | 11.7 | − 0.7 (±0.2) | 12.2 | 12.0 | − 0.2 (±0.2) | 239 | 423 |
| **35-44** | 11.8 | 11.3 | − 0.5 (±0.2) | 11.1 | 10.7 | − 0.4 (±0.1) | 338 | 515 |
| **45-54** | 10.6 | 10.5 | − 0.1 (±0.2) | 10.5 | 10.4 | − 0.1 (±0.2) | 284 | 359 |
| **55-64** | 10.6 | 10.6 | 0 (±0.2) | 10.1 | 9.9 | − 0.2 (±0.2) | 302 | 321 |
| **65-74** | 10.0 | 9.4 | − 0.6 (±0.2) | 10.1 | 9.9 | − 0.2 (±0.2) | 168 | 180 |
| **75+** | 9.5 | 9.4 | − 0.1 (±0.4) | 9.3 | 8.7 | − 0.6 (±0.4) | 40 | 44 |
| **All ages** | 11.5 | 11.1 | − 0.4 (±0.1) | 11.1 | 10.9 | − 0.2 (±0.1) | 1545 | 2002 |

**Table 8.11  Mean scores on the extraversion scale of the Eysenck Personality Inventory by socio-economic group**

| | Household socio-economic group at HALS1 | | | | | | | | | | | | Base numbers | | | |
| | Professional/employers/managers | | | Other non-manual | | | Skilled manual/own account trades | | | Semi-skilled and unskilled manual | | | | | | |
| Age at HALS1 | HALS1 | HALS2 | Difference (±SEM) | HALS1 | HALS2 | Difference (±SEM) | HALS1 | HALS2 | Difference (±SEM) | HALS1 | HALS2 | Difference (±SEM) | | | | |
|---|---|---|---|---|---|---|---|---|---|---|---|---|---|---|---|---|
| **Males** | | | | | | | | | | | | | | | | |
| 18-39 | 11.8 | 11.2 | -0.6 (±0.3) | 12.7 | 11.8 | -0.9 (±0.3) | 13.1 | 12.7 | -0.4 (±0.2) | 13.8 | 13.0 | -0.8 (±0.3) | 129 | 131 | 223 | 103 |
| 40-64 | 10.7 | 10.4 | -0.3 (±0.2) | 10.0 | 9.5 | -0.5 (±0.2) | 11.3 | 11.2 | -0.1 (±0.2) | 10.9 | 11.2 | +0.3 (±0.3) | 206 | 131 | 258 | 137 |
| 65+ | 8.8 | 8.7 | -0.1 (±0.4) | 9.5 | 8.4 | -1.1 (±0.6) | 10.5 | 9.7 | -0.8 (±0.3) | 10.4 | 10.7 | +0.3 (±0.4) | 52 | 31 | 81 | 43 |
| All Ages | 10.8 | 10.4 | -0.4 (±0.2) | 11.2 | 10.4 | -0.8 (±0.2) | 11.9 | 11.6 | -0.3 (±0.1) | 11.9 | 11.8 | -0.1 (±0.2) | 387 | 293 | 562 | 283 |
| **Females** | | | | | | | | | | | | | | | | |
| 18-39 | 11.5 | 10.7 | -0.8 (±0.3) | 12.1 | 11.4 | -0.7 (±0.2) | 12.0 | 12.1 | +0.1 (±0.2) | 12.4 | 12.4 | 0 (±0.2) | 180 | 224 | 292 | 166 |
| 40-64 | 10.1 | 9.9 | -0.2 (±0.2) | 10.2 | 9.9 | -0.3 (±0.2) | 10.8 | 10.7 | -0.1 (±0.2) | 11.3 | 11.0 | -0.3 (±0.2) | 277 | 174 | 288 | 158 |
| 65+ | 10.2 | 9.2 | -1.0 (±0.4) | 9.3 | 9.6 | +0.3 (±0.5) | 10.2 | 10.1 | -0.1 (±0.4) | 9.7 | 9.4 | -0.3 (±0.4) | 61 | 34 | 70 | 57 |
| All Ages | 10.6 | 10.1 | -0.5 (±0.1) | 11.1 | 10.7 | -0.4 (±0.2) | 11.3 | 11.3 | 0 (±0.1) | 11.6 | 11.4 | -0.2 (±0.1) | 518 | 432 | 650 | 381 |

**Table 8.12    Mean scores on Type A behaviour scale (x 100) by age and sex**

| | Males | | | Females | | | Base numbers | |
|---|---|---|---|---|---|---|---|---|
| | HALS1 | HALS2 | Difference (±SEM) | HALS1 | HALS2 | Difference (±SEM) | Males | Females |
| **Age at HALS1** | | | | | | | | |
| **18-24** | 52 | 56 | +4 (±2) | 50 | 52 | +2 (±2) | 174 | 162 |
| **25-34** | 55 | 53 | −2 (±1) | 51 | 51 | 0 (±1) | 238 | 435 |
| **35-44** | 55 | 53 | −2 (±1) | 50 | 49 | −1 (±1) | 339 | 520 |
| **45-54** | 51 | 49 | −2 (±1) | 50 | 47 | −3 (±1) | 283 | 361 |
| **55-64** | 49 | 46 | −3 (±1) | 45 | 41 | −4 (±1) | 307 | 319 |
| **65-74** | 48 | 43 | −5 (±1) | 43 | 39 | −4 (±2) | 163 | 180 |
| **75+** | 38 | 34 | −4 (±2) | 38 | 33 | −5 (±2) | 40 | 42 |
| **All ages** | 51 | 50 | −1 (±0) | 48 | 47 | −1 (±0) | 1544 | 2019 |

**Table 8.13     Mean scores on Type A behaviour scale (x 100) by education**

| | Highest educational qualification at HALS 1 | | | | | | | | | | | |
|---|---|---|---|---|---|---|---|---|---|---|---|---|
| | None/work related | | | GCSE/O-level | | | A-level/professional/degree | | | Base numbers | | |
| | HALS1 | HALS2 | Differ. (±SEM) | HALS1 | HALS2 | Differ. (±SEM) | HALS1 | HALS2 | Differ. (±SEM) | | | |
| **Age at HALS1** | | | | | **Males** | | | | | | | |
| **18-39** | 56 | 53 | − 3 (±1) | 52 | 54 | + 2 (±1) | 56 | 56 | 0 (±1) | 172 | 177 | 252 |
| **40-64** | 47 | 46 | − 1 (±1) | 55 | 51 | − 4 (±2) | 55 | 53 | − 2 (±1) | 444 | 77 | 218 |
| **65 +** | 44 | 40 | − 4 (±1) | (46) | (41) * | − 5 (±3) | 50 | 45 | − 5 (±2) | 146 | 12 | 48 |
| **All ages** | 48 | 46 | − 2 (±1) | 53 | 53 | 0 (±1) | 55 | 54 | − 1 (±1) | 762 | 266 | 515 |
| | | | | | **Females** | | | | | | | |
| **18-39** | 47 | 47 | 0 (±1) | 49 | 51 | + 2 (±1) | 54 | 54 | 0 (±1) | 323 | 273 | 296 |
| **40-64** | 45 | 42 | − 3 (±1) | 51 | 49 | − 2 (±1) | 53 | 51 | − 2 (±1) | 515 | 112 | 277 |
| **65 +** | 40 | 36 | − 4 (±1) | (44) | (38) | − 6 (±5) | 50 | 45 | − 5 (±3) | 167 | 13 | 42 |
| **All ages** | 45 | 43 | − 2 (±1) | 50 | 50 | 0 (±1) | 54 | 52 | − 2 (±1) | 1005 | 398 | 615 |

* Percentages are in brackets when base numbers are below 20.

**Table 8.14 Mean scores on Type A behaviour scale (x 100) by socio-economic group**

| | Household socio-economic group at HALS 1 | | | | | | | | | | | | Base numbers | | | |
| | Professional/employers/managers | | | Other non-manual | | | Skilled manual/own account trades | | | Semi-skilled and unskilled manual | | | | | | |
| Age at HALS1 | HALS1 | HALS2 | Difference (±SEM) | HALS1 | HALS2 | Difference (±SEM) | HALS1 | HALS2 | Difference (±SEM) | HALS1 | HALS2 | Difference (±SEM) | | | | |
|---|---|---|---|---|---|---|---|---|---|---|---|---|---|---|---|---|
| **Males** | | | | | | | | | | | | | | | | |
| 18-39 | 63 | 63 | 0 (±1) | 53 | 56 | +3 (±1) | 54 | 52 | −2 (±1) | (48) | (49)* | +1 (±2) | 129 | 133 | 221 | 12 |
| 40-64 | 60 | 56 | −4 (±1) | 50 | 49 | −1 (±1) | 47 | 45 | −2 (±1) | 43 | 43 | 0 (±1) | 204 | 134 | 258 | 141 |
| 65+ | 50 | 48 | −2 (±2) | 48 | 44 | −4 (±2) | 46 | 40 | −6 (±2) | 38 | 34 | −4 (±3) | 51 | 31 | 78 | 42 |
| All Ages | 60 | 57 | −3 (±1) | 51 | 52 | +1 (±1) | 50 | 47 | −3 (±1) | 44 | 44 | 0 (±1) | 384 | 298 | 557 | 285 |
| **Females** | | | | | | | | | | | | | | | | |
| 18-39 | 51 | 52 | +1 (±1) | 52 | 53 | +1 (±1) | 49 | 49 | 0 (±1) | 50 | 49 | −1 (±1) | 181 | 231 | 298 | 173 |
| 40-64 | 49 | 48 | −1 (±1) | 51 | 49 | −2 (±1) | 46 | 43 | −3 (±1) | 46 | 42 | −4 (±1) | 278 | 174 | 286 | 158 |
| 65+ | 43 | 38 | −5 (±2) | 46 | 41 | −5 (±3) | 42 | 35 | −7 (±2) | 39 | 39 | 0 (±2) | 61 | 36 | 66 | 57 |
| All Ages | 49 | 48 | −1 (±1) | 51 | 50 | −1 (±1) | 47 | 45 | −2 (±1) | 47 | 45 | −2 (±1) | 520 | 441 | 650 | 388 |

* Percentages are in brackets when base numbers are below 20.

# CHANGES IN COGNITIVE FUNCTION IN A POPULATION SAMPLE | 9

Felicia A Huppert and Joyce E Whittington

Surveys of health and lifestyle in the general adult population rarely include measures of cognitive function, yet cognitive function is an important part of an individual's ability to respond effectively to both internal and external factors. Cognitive processes include the ability to pay attention, to learn and remember, to draw inferences, make decisions and react appropriately. Although individuals may not be equally endowed with respect to their cognitive abilities, there are undoubtedly variations between individuals and within individuals which are primarily environmental in character. Physical illness and depressed mood impair cognitive functioning (Schaie, 1983; Holland and Rabbitt, 1990; Weingartner et al. 1981), as do lack of sleep (Webb, 1985) and other health-related behaviours. Many commonly used forms of medication have adverse effects on cognition. These include sleeping pills (hypnotics) and the minor tranquillizers (e.g. Librium, Valium) which are taken by a high percentage of adults (Brosen et al. 1986).

In addition to the influence which health, behaviour and circumstances can exert on cognitive functioning, cognitive functioning may itself exert an influence on health. A high level of functioning may be associated with the avoidance of accidents, with health-seeking behaviour, and with the ability to benefit from health education. Conversely, impaired cognitive function may be associated with increased risks to health and a reduced ability to benefit from advice about health practices.

In view of the integral role played by cognitive functioning in relation to health, tests of cognitive function were included in the Health and Lifestyle Surveys (HALS1 in 1984/5 and HALS2 in 1991/2). These yield, for the first time, information about cognitive change on a representative national sample which can be related to the wealth of other measures available on the same subjects.

The tests of cognitive function were administered by a nurse in the respondent's home, at the conclusion of the physiological measurements (see Chapter 1). Because of the limited time available, the tests were confined to simple measures of mental speed, memory and reasoning. Two measures of mental speed were employed. Speed of response (psychomotor speed) was assessed by measuring reaction time to the appearance of a visual stimulus. Decision speed was assessed by a measure of choice reaction time i.e. the time taken to choose the correct response when several choices are available. The choice reaction time task also provides a measure of response accuracy.

Memory was selected for investigation because it plays a central part in all aspects of our daily lives. The particular type of memory examined in the Survey is the ability to recall recently acquired information. In clinics and psychological laboratories, this is conventionally tested by having subjects recall lists of random words. For the Survey, it was thought preferable to use a test which more closely resembles real-life memory performance. Accordingly, a brief memory test using material which was health-related was designed for the Survey.

Like memory, the ability to reason or solve simple problems is utilized in many areas of daily life. Many standard tests of reasoning can be readily recognised as intelligence tests and it was felt that respondents would be unwilling to participate in such a test. A reasoning test of a different kind, requiring subjects to make inferences about the number of blocks depicted in drawings of block piles was chosen (see below).

Most of the data reported below are for the sub-sample of individuals who were successfully tested at both HALS1 and HALS2. At the end of the chapter detailed comparisons of this sub-sample and the original HALS1 population are presented, both to examine selective attrition and to compare age effects with cohort effects.

## Reaction time

Reaction time was measured by using a small battery-operated machine which was designed for the survey (see Appendix B). Simple reaction time (psychomotor speed) was the time taken for the subject to press a key as quickly as possible after a particular digit appeared on a screen. Choice reaction time (decision speed) was the time taken to press one of four keys corresponding to one of four digits that could appear on the screen. For both simple and choice reaction time, the mean time and the standard deviation were recorded for each individual in milliseconds (msec). In the case of choice reaction time, the number of errors was also recorded. The reaction time values given in the following tables are for correct responses only.

The well-known finding that older subjects respond more slowly than younger subjects (Birren et al. 1980) is confirmed both in HALS1 and HALS2 (Table 9.1, Table 9.3 and Table 9.14). For simple reaction time, the response slowing is minimal until age 45-54. Thereafter, responses become progressively slower with a marked deterioration at age 75 +.

Table 9.1 shows an impressive consistency in mean reaction time (RT) over a seven-year period. The difference within an age group is usually within two standard errors of the difference, indicating that the differences are not significant, except for males aged 65-74. However there is an interesting pattern of differences across age. The mean RT of the younger groups is slightly faster (negative sign) at HALS2 compared with HALS1, while the mean RT of the older groups is slightly slower (positive sign) at HALS2 compared with HALS1. Information about change is presented in a different way in Table 9.2, which shows the percentage of individuals who have changed by more than their standard deviation at

HALS1. Overall, approximately 30% of subjects change by more than their standard deviation; the majority of these become slower, particularly in the two older age groups.

Similar effects are observed in relation to choice reaction time (Table 9.3). There are large age differences at both HALS1 and HALS2 and the slowing is a continuous rising function of age. There is reasonable consistency in choice reaction time means over the seven-year interval for all age groups up to age 55; the mean differences are within two standard errors of the difference except in females aged 18-34 who respond significantly faster at HALS2 than at HALS1. From age 55, however, the differences in the means at HALS1 and HALS2 are very large, and increase markedly with advancing age. As with simple reaction time, the direction of difference scores changes with age. The youngest groups show a tendency to respond faster in HALS2 than in HALS1 (negative sign) while older groups respond more slowly in HALS2 compared with HALS1. The percentage of individuals who changed by more than their standard deviation at HALS1 was very low (11%), so Table 9.4 presents the percentage changing by more than half their standard deviation at HALS1. The percentage changing by this amount increases with age, the majority of the older groups becoming slower.

In the choice reaction time test it was possible to make errors by pressing the wrong response key. There was very little variation in the mean number of errors made. The range was 0.97 to 1.90 in different age bands at HALS1, and 0.98 to 2.85 at HALS2. Accordingly, error data are reported in terms of the percentage of each group who made no errors.

The error data in Table 9.3 show that, overall, the youngest group is the most likely to make errors. This is an example of the trade-off between speed and accuracy. Young subjects respond rapidly, at the cost of being inaccurate, whereas middle-aged and older subjects tend to respond more accurately at the cost of being slower. This trade-off does not, however, account for all the data. Among males, those aged 75 + are the most likely to make errors and also have the slowest reaction times. Among females, those aged 25-34 and those aged 65-74 are least likely to make errors, but differ markedly in their reaction time.

While all studies of reaction time find an age-related decline in performance, sex differences are not usually reported. Table 9.1 and Table 9.3 show consistent but very small sex differences in reaction time means. Combining HALS1 and HALS2 data, women are on average 12 msec slower on simple reaction time (motor speed) but only 3 msec slower on choice reaction time (decision speed). On the other hand, there is a substantial sex difference in accuracy, with a higher percentage of women than men making no errors on the choice reaction time task (42% vs 36% on average). This may indicate a difference in response strategy, with males tending to maximise speed and females tending to maximise accuracy. There do not appear to be sex differences in relation to change in reaction time over seven years, but there is a sex difference in changes in accuracy, at least in the older age groups. Men aged 65-74 show a marked decrease in accuracy (40% to 28% with error-free performance), while women in this age group show an increase in accuracy (42% to 51% error-free performance).

It has been claimed that mental speed is closely related to intelligence (Jensen, 1982), although this suggestion has aroused some opposition (Mackintosh, 1981). If the claim is correct, a strong association between reaction time and educational qualifications would be expected. An association is indeed found (Table 9.5 and Table 9.6) in both HALS1 and HALS2. Individuals with no educational qualification or a work-related qualification have much slower mean reaction times than the remaining groups. The direction of causality is of course unclear. If mental speed is an intrinsic part of intellectual capacity, individuals with slow mental speed may have difficulty at school and obtain no educational qualifications. On the other hand, it is possible that the mental challenge of occupations which follow the attainment of educational qualifications may produce or maintain fast mental speed. If this is the case, then mental speed could be modified by appropriate training.

There is little evidence from our data that changes in reaction time are associated with educational attainment. The data, therefore, do not support the hypothesis that cognitive decline is slower in better educated or more intellectually able individuals (Christensen and Henderson, 1991).

## Memory

A list of 10 common foods was read out to the respondent, who was asked to say which of the foods contained dietary fibre. A few minutes later, without prior warning, the subject was asked to recall the words. This differs from most conventional memory tests where subjects are instructed to remember the information. Our measure of 'incidental' memory was chosen to reflect the fact that usually when we remember something, it is not information which we deliberately set out to learn; it is information we acquired incidentally in the course of our normal lives by seeing it, hearing it, etc.

The mean number of foods correctly recalled out of 10, by the whole sample, was 6.7 and 6.8 at HALS1 and HALS2 respectively, with a median of 7 on both occasions. Figure 9.1 shows that the data are normally distributed, avoiding both ceiling and floor effects.

Table 9.7 and Table 9.8 show the expected strong relationship between age and memory (Huppert, 1991) in both HALS1 and HALS2. There is an impressive degree of consistency in the mean number of items recalled at HALS1 and HALS2. The difference within an age group is within two standard errors of the group mean. However the pattern of the difference scores across age resembles that seen in the reaction time measures; for young groups HALS2 performance is slightly better than HALS1, while for older groups HALS2 performance is slightly worse than HALS1.

The age effect is highlighted by examining the percentage obtaining high scores (8-10 correct out of 10) on the memory test (Table 9.8). The percentage drops dramatically with advancing age in both HALS1 and HALS2, particularly among the males. The effect is even more striking if the percentage obtaining high scores in both Surveys is compared. Twenty per cent of the youngest group of males attain this criterion, compared with 0% of the oldest group, and a similar trend is seen for females.

Table 9.9 presents the percentage of individuals whose performance changes by more than one item recalled. The scores of 39% of males and 26% of females change by more than this amount and, overall, the percentage whose scores decline is equal

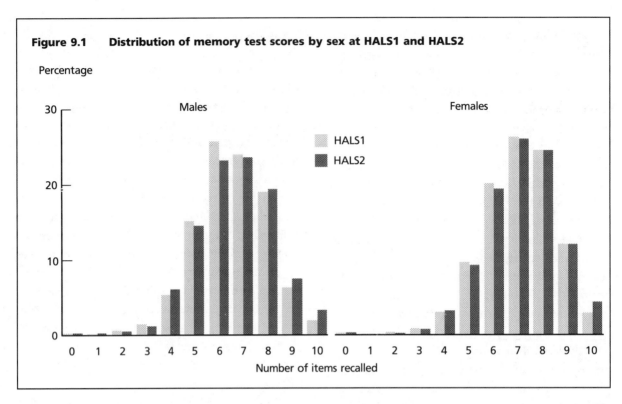

**Figure 9.1    Distribution of memory test scores by sex at HALS1 and HALS2**

to the percentage whose scores improve. However, the pattern differs across age. The percentage showing decline increases steadily with age, while the percentage showing improvement tends to decrease with age.

The data also reveal a small but consistent sex difference; women recall more items at every age than men do. A sex difference has rarely been reported on memory tests. This could be because small numbers of subjects are normally tested, even in such famous studies as the normalisation sample of the Wechsler Memory Scale – Revised (Wechsler, 1987), where the number in each 10-year age band was 50-55. The possibility should also be considered that some particular feature of our test, or the test material itself, might be responsible for this difference. The foods in the original list were all very common, so it is unlikely that there would be a sex bias in familiarity. Another possibility is that women are more interested than men in food, and this is reflected in their incidental memory. However, there are now a few reports of a female superiority in memory tests where the items were neutral words which were unlikely to be of more interest to one sex (Delis et al. 1987).

Performance in memory tests is known to be related to level of education. The expected association between memory and education can be

seen in Table 9.10, particularly if one compares the group with no qualifications or work-related qualifications with the other two groups. This table also provides information about whether sex and age differences are present in groups with comparable educational qualifications. The educational groupings in this table are relatively crude. The various changes in the education system which have taken place this century make impossible a valid comparison of older and younger people. Nevertheless, it can be seen that there are sizeable age and sex differences within each educational category. As was the case with reaction time, education does not appear to be related to the degree of change in memory over the seven-year interval.

## Reasoning

A measure of visuospatial reasoning was obtained using the block counting test (see Appendix A). Respondents were shown drawings representing three-dimensional piles of blocks, and were instructed to record the number of blocks contained in each pile. The correct answers could only be calculated by making inferences about the three-dimensional structure of the piles and counting the blocks which were hidden from view as well as those which were visible. This widely used test is sometimes regarded as a measure of spatial visualisation but correct responses do not require the ability to visualise.

The score was the total number of correct answers. Almost half the sample (47%) made no errors and a further 28% made only one error, those figures being virtually identical for HALS1 and HALS2. A very small percentage of subjects made no correct response (2.3% at HALS1, 3.3% at HALS2). The overall mean was 4.97 and the median 5.

The range of possible scores on the block-counting test is very small (0-6), and although mean values are presented the percentage making 5 or 6 correct responses is a more sensitive measure of performance. Table 9.11 shows a very small age effect on mean values, a substantial difference appearing only in the oldest age group (75 + at HALS1). The pattern of change in the difference scores mimics that seen for reaction time and memory; younger subjects tend to perform better at HALS2 than at HALS1, while older subjects perform more poorly at HALS2 than at HALS1.

Table 9.12 shows that the percentage scoring 5 or 6 correct (out of 6) decreases with age, and the effect is particularly marked among women. It is interesting that, on this test, peak performance at HALS1 was found, not in the youngest age group, but in those aged 25-44, in both sexes. It was originally hypothesised (Huppert, 1987) that this might indicate the operation of a cohort effect (see below), with this group differing from the others in education or experience, in ways which affect their performance on this task. However, the large improvement seen in the performance of the youngest group over the seven-year period suggests that the effect is an age effect or an effect of variables associated with the ageing process. From age 55, it can be seen that the proportion of subjects obtaining high scores at HALS2 drops markedly compared to HALS1. This is confirmed in Table 9.13, which presents the percentage of individuals whose score changes by more than 1 point, between HALS1 and HALS2. A ceiling effect makes it difficult to compare the percentage whose score improves, but a dramatic effect of age can be seen on the percentage whose score declines.

These are startling results, since one might have expected a reasoning test of this type to measure 'crystallized intelligence' i.e. an intellectual ability which is likely to be retained over time. Not only do 15% of men and 26% of women change their scores by more than 1 point, but older adults show very marked impairment over a seven-year period on this relatively simple test of reasoning.

In psychological tests of spatial ability, males tend to perform better than females (e.g. Maccoby and Jacklin, 1978). The measure of reasoning used in the survey has a large spatial component (making inferences about 3-dimensional space). The expected sex difference can be clearly seen in Table 9.11 and Table 9.12. It is also known that performance on tests of visuospatial domain processing tends to decline with age (Flicker et al. 1988), and it may be the fact that the reasoning task was in the visuospatial, rather than the verbal domain, which accounts for the age-related decline we observe.

## Age versus cohort effects

In addition to considering the many variables which may influence an individual's cognitive functioning, there may also be variables which influence the functioning of whole cohorts of individuals. Generational changes in education, smoking habits, nutrition and exposure to different diseases may result in cohort differences in cognitive functioning. The possibility of cohort difference must be considered when interpreting cross-sectional results of the kind reported here.

Table 9.14 to Table 9.16 present data on the cognitive tests by seven-year cohorts. This allows us to compare cognitive performance both across age groups (cross-sectional comparison) and within age cohorts as the individuals grow older (longitudinal comparison). In these tables, we also present the scores of the parent population sample (HALS1) as well as the sub-sample who were tested at both HALS1 and HALS2.

On all cognitive measures, the selected sub-sample tended to perform better than the population sample. However, within age and sex groups there were exceptions to this overall picture for all but the blocks test measures. The overall tendency for the retested group to out-perform the original cross-sectional sample is consistent with evidence from other studies showing that initial cognitive performance is lower among those who die prior to testing or refuse to be retested (e.g. Riegel and Riegel, 1972).

Improvements within cohorts are matched by improvements between cohorts for the younger groups. But whereas there are decrements in performance within cohorts from middle age for all measures, the improvement between cohorts is evident on all measures; at each chronological age, later-born cohorts generally perform better than earlier-born cohorts. The greater improvement of the younger subjects results in the highest performance at HALS2 by the same age groups that achieved the highest performance at HALS1. This implies that the highest achievement is age-related and not a cohort effect.

The finding that younger groups improved on all measures over the seven-year period is unexpected. It is not feasible that a practice effect would be evident over a seven-year interval, although it is possible that some respondents remembered that an unexpected memory test previously followed the questions about fibre in food, so the memory test was not unexpected in HALS2 (i.e. learning was intentional rather than incidental). However, no similar explanation can be given for the improvement in reaction time or blocks test performance.

## Summary

Cognitive functioning is related to health in two major ways. First, cognitive functioning may be impaired by illness or by adverse lifestyle or circumstances, and conversely, cognitive functioning may be improved or at least maintained in later life by good health or by favourable lifestyle or circumstances. Second, the level of cognitive functioning may influence health; people who are functioning well may be less likely to have accidents or enter stressful situations and may be more likely to understand health promotion messages and engage in health protective behaviour.

Simple measures of cognitive function were administered as part of the Survey. They included tests of reaction time, memory and reasoning. Little is known about the demographic characteristics of cognitive functions. Information about how performance is distributed throughout the population is a prerequisite for examining relationships between cognitive variables and health and lifestyle variables. This chapter presents the basic demographic findings on which subsequent analysis of these relationships can be based.

On most measures, the effects of age and education are very marked. In general, older groups perform more poorly than younger groups. The largest educational differences are seen when comparing groups with no educational qualification and groups with some qualification. At all ages, those with no educational qualifications tend to perform poorly on the cognitive measures. Neither education nor sex are predictors of subsequent decline, although age is a strong predictor. Younger groups show little change, or even an improvement on the cognitive tests over a seven-year interval, while older groups show a consistent decline which increases with advancing age. The data also show evidence of cohort effects. Among middle-aged and older adults, later-born cohorts tend to perform better than earlier-born cohorts, although in the youngest groups, age effects predominate over cohort effects.

### References

Birren, J.E., Woods, A.M. and Williams, M.V. (1980), Behavioural slowing with age; causes, organisation and consequences, In L.W. Poon (Ed.) Ageing in the 1980s. Washington D.C: American Psychological Association.

Brosen, L., Broadbent, D., Nutt, D. and Broadbent, M. (1986), Performance effects of diazepam during and after prolonged administration, Psychological Medicine 16, 561-571.

Christensen, H. and Henderson, A.S. (1991), Is age kinder to the initially more able? A study of eminent scientists and academics, Psychological Medicine, 21, 935-946.

Delis, D.C., Kramer, J.H., Kaplan, E., Obler, B.A. (1987), Manual of the California Verbal Learning Test, (Research Edition), Adult Version, San Antonio: Psychological Corporation.

Flicker, C., Ferris, S.H., Crook, T., Reisberg, B. and Bartus, R.T. (1988), Equivalent spatial-rotation deficits in normal aging and Alzheimer's Disease, Journal of Clinical and Experimental Neuropsychology, 10, 4, 387-399.

Holland, C.A. and Rabbitt, P.M.A. (1990), The course and causes of cognitive change with advancing age, Reviews in Clinical Gerontology, 1, 81-96.

Huppert, F.A. (1987), 'Cognitive Function' in: Cox, B.D. et al. The Health and Lifestyle Survey: Preliminary Report of a Nationwide Survey of the Physical and Mental Health, Attitudes and Lifestyle of a Random Sample of 9003 British Adults, London: Health Promotion Research Trust.

Huppert, F.A. (1991), Age-related changes in memory: Learning and remembering new information, In: F. Boller and J. Grafman (Eds.) Handbook of Neuropsychology. Elsevier Science Publishers. Amsterdam: 5, 7, 123-147.

Jensen, A.R. (1982), Reaction time and psychometric g, In: H.J. Eysenck (Ed.) A Model for Intelligence, Berlin: Springer-Verlag.

Maccoby, E.E. and Jacklin, C.N. (1978), The Psychology of Sex Differences, London: Oxford University Press.

Mackintosh, N.J. (1981), A new measure of intelligence? Nature, 289, 529-530.

Riegel, K.F., and Riegel, R.M. (1972), Development, drop and death, Development Psycology, 6, 2, 306-319.

Schaie, K.W. (1983), The Seattle Longitudinal Study: A twenty-one year exploration of psychometric intelligence in adulthood. In K.W. Schaie (Ed.), New York: Guilford, Longitudinal Studies of Adult Psychological Development.

Webb, W.B. (1985), A further analysis of age and sleep deprivation effect, Psychophysiology, 22, 156-161.

Wechsler, D.A. (1987), Wechsler Memory Scale – Revised (WMS-R), Harcourt Brace Jovanovich: The Psychological Corporation.

Weingartner, H., Cohen, R.M., Murphy, D.L., Martello, J. and Gerdt, C. (1981), Cognitive processes in depression, Archives of General Psychiatry, 38, 42-47.

**Table 9.1**    **Simple reaction time changes by age and sex. Mean (±SEM) in milliseconds**

| | Males | | | Females | | | Base numbers | |
|---|---|---|---|---|---|---|---|---|
| | HALS1 | HALS2 | Difference | HALS1 | HALS2 | Difference | Males | Females |
| **Age at HALS1** | | | | | | | | |
| **18-24** | 297 | 293 | − 4 (±5) | 318 | 309 | − 9 (±7) | 235 | 216 |
| **25-34** | 300 | 290 | − 10 (±4) | 314 | 309 | − 5 (±4) | 324 | 511 |
| **35-44** | 297 | 301 | + 4 (±4) | 311 | 310 | − 1 (±5) | 446 | 613 |
| **45-54** | 320 | 320 | 0 (±6) | 332 | 328 | − 4 (±5) | 339 | 430 |
| **55-64** | 343 | 339 | − 4 (±8) | 347 | 359 | + 12 (±8) | 344 | 353 |
| **65-74** | 377 | 405 | + 28 (±12) | 408 | 432 | + 24 (±14) | 189 | 200 |
| **75+** | 475 | 498 | + 23 (±36) | 482 | 535 | + 53 (±40) | 48 | 60 |
| **All ages** | 322 | 323 | + 1 (±3) | 333 | 336 | + 3 (±3) | 1925 | 2383 |

**Table 9.2**    **Changes in simple reaction time by age and sex. Percentage changing by more than their own standard deviation at (s.d.) HALS1**

| | Males | | | Females | | | Base numbers | |
|---|---|---|---|---|---|---|---|---|
| | Faster | Within 1 s.d. | Slower | Faster | Within 1 s.d. | Slower | Males | Females |
| **Age at HALS1** | | | | | | | | |
| **18-24** | 9 | 76 | 15 | 11 | 71 | 18 | 235 | 216 |
| **25-34** | 11 | 73 | 16 | 12 | 73 | 15 | 324 | 511 |
| **35-44** | 7 | 75 | 18 | 11 | 74 | 15 | 446 | 613 |
| **45-54** | 9 | 72 | 19 | 12 | 72 | 16 | 339 | 430 |
| **55-64** | 16 | 64 | 20 | 13 | 63 | 24 | 344 | 353 |
| **65-74** | 12 | 59 | 29 | 13 | 62 | 25 | 189 | 200 |
| **75+** | 6 | 65 | 29 | 10 | 55 | 35 | 48 | 60 |
| **All ages** | 10 | 71 | 19 | 12 | 70 | 18 | 1925 | 2383 |

**Table 9.3    Choice reaction time changes by age and sex**

| | Males | | | Females | | | Base numbers | |
|---|---|---|---|---|---|---|---|---|
| | HALS1 | HALS2 | Difference | HALS1 | HALS2 | Difference | Males | Females |
| **Age at HALS1** | | | Mean (±SEM) in milliseconds | | | | | |
| **18-24** | 567 | 560 | − 7 (±4) | 594 | 581 | − 13 (±4) | *231* | *215* |
| **25-34** | 593 | 588 | − 5 (±5) | 605 | 593 | − 12 (±3) | *318* | *508* |
| **35-44** | 616 | 617 | + 1 (±4) | 618 | 616 | − 2 (±3) | *444* | *608* |
| **45-54** | 657 | 664 | + 7 (±4) | 664 | 667 | + 3 (±4) | *334* | *428* |
| **55-64** | 691 | 717 | + 26 (±5) | 698 | 725 | + 27 (±6) | *343* | *351* |
| **65-74** | 748 | 802 | + 54 (±10) | 773 | 827 | + 54 (±9) | *184* | *196* |
| **75+** | 836 | 910 | + 74 (±24) | 829 | 931 | + 102 (±23) | *47* | *57* |
| **All ages** | 645 | 656 | + 11 (±2) | 651 | 658 | + 7 (±2) | *1901* | *2363* |
| | | | Percentage making no errors | | | | | |
| **18-24** | 28 | 35 | + 7 | 36 | 27 | − 9 | *231* | *215* |
| **25-34** | 36 | 46 | + 10 | 46 | 42 | − 4 | *318* | *508* |
| **35-44** | 35 | 39 | + 4 | 43 | 42 | − 1 | *444* | *608* |
| **45-54** | 36 | 37 | + 1 | 40 | 40 | 0 | *334* | *428* |
| **55-64** | 36 | 34 | − 2 | 40 | 36 | − 4 | *343* | *351* |
| **65-74** | 40 | 28 | − 12 | 42 | 51 | + 9 | *184* | *196* |
| **75+** | 25 | 29 | + 4 | 39 | 49 | + 10 | *47* | *57* |
| **All ages** | 35 | 37 | + 2 | 42 | 41 | − 1 | *1901* | *2363* |

**Table 9.4** Changes in choice reaction time by age and sex. Percentage changing by more than 0.5 of their own standard deviation (s.d.) at HALS1

| | Males | | | Females | | | Base numbers | |
|---|---|---|---|---|---|---|---|---|
| | Faster | Within 0.5 s.d. | Slower | Faster | Within 0.5 s.d. | Slower | Males | Females |
| **Age at HALS1** | | | | | | | | |
| **18-24** | 20 | 63 | 17 | 21 | 66 | 13 | 231 | 215 |
| **25-34** | 18 | 68 | 14 | 22 | 65 | 18 | 318 | 507 |
| **35-44** | 17 | 65 | 18 | 17 | 65 | 18 | 443 | 609 |
| **45-54** | 15 | 63 | 22 | 15 | 64 | 21 | 334 | 428 |
| **55-64** | 12 | 59 | 29 | 12 | 62 | 26 | 343 | 351 |
| **65-74** | 10 | 55 | 35 | 11 | 57 | 32 | 184 | 196 |
| **75+** | 17 | 35 | 48 | 9 | 42 | 49 | 46 | 57 |
| **All ages** | 16 | 62 | 22 | 17 | 63 | 20 | 1899 | 2363 |

**Table 9.5** Changes in simple reaction time by education. Mean (±SEM) in milliseconds

| | Highest Educational Qualification | | | | | | | | | | | |
|---|---|---|---|---|---|---|---|---|---|---|---|---|
| | None/work related | | | GCSE/O-level | | | A-level/professional/degree | | | | | |
| Age at HALS1 | HALS1 | HALS2 | Diff. | HALS1 | HALS2 | Diff. | HALS1 | HALS2 | Diff. | Base numbers | | |
| **Males** | | | | | | | | | | | | |
| **18-39** | 319 | 302 | − 17 (±6) | 295 | 294 | − 1 (±5) | 284 | 281 | − 3 (±4) | 240 | 234 | 332 |
| **40-64** | 340 | 340 | 0 (±6) | 311 | 319 | + 8 (±8) | 295 | 298 | + 3 (±7) | 526 | 101 | 254 |
| **65+** | 418 | 441 | + 23 (±15) | 335 | 374 | + 39 (±22) | 332 | 370 | + 38 (±22) | 177 | 13 | 47 |
| **All ages** | 350 | 349 | − (±5) | 301 | 304 | + 3 (±4) | 292 | 295 | + 3 (±4) | 943 | 348 | 633 |
| **Females** | | | | | | | | | | | | |
| **18-39** | 339 | 330 | − 9 (±7) | 305 | 299 | − 6 (±4) | 295 | 296 | + 1 (±4) | 411 | 322 | 343 |
| **40-64** | 349 | 355 | + 6 (±6) | 311 | 308 | − 3 (±6) | 304 | 302 | − 2 (±5) | 609 | 121 | 316 |
| **65+** | 441 | 469 | + 28 (±17) | 468 | 479 | + 11 (±41) | 336 | 392 | + 56 (±31) | 201 | 16 | 43 |
| **All ages** | 361 | 365 | + 4 (±5) | 313 | 308 | − 5 (±4) | 301 | 304 | + 3 (±4) | 1221 | 459 | 702 |

**Table 9.6**     **Changes in choice reaction time by education. Mean (±SEM) in milliseconds**

| | Highest Educational Qualification | | | | | | | | | | | |
| | None/work-related | | | GCSE/O-level | | | A-level/professional/degree | | | Base numbers | | |
| | HALS1 | HALS2 | Diff. | HALS1 | HALS2 | Diff. | HALS1 | HALS2 | Diff. | | | |
| **Age at HALS1** | | | | | Males | | | | | | | |
| **18-39** | 625 | 619 | − 6 (±6) | 576 | 572 | − 4 (±4) | 570 | 565 | − 5 (±4) | 240 | 229 | 326 |
| **40-64** | 688 | 705 | + 17 (±4) | 641 | 660 | + 19 (±8) | 626 | 634 | + 8 (±4) | 521 | 100 | 253 |
| **65+** | 783 | 846 | + 63 (±11) | 725 | 786 | + 61 (±24) | 714 | 777 | + 63 (±23) | 172 | 13 | 46 |
| **All ages** | 689 | 708 | + 19 (±4) | 601 | 606 | + 5 (±4) | 604 | 609 | + 5 (±3) | 933 | 342 | 625 |
| | | | | | Females | | | | | | | |
| **18-39** | 637 | 625 | − 12 (±4) | 586 | 575 | − 11 (±3) | 587 | 581 | − 6 (±4) | 408 | 317 | 342 |
| **40-64** | 689 | 702 | + 13 (±4) | 638 | 641 | + 3 (±7) | 629 | 637 | + 8 (±4) | 605 | 121 | 316 |
| **65+** | 806 | 869 | + 63 (±10) | 795 | 850 | + 55 (±24) | 685 | 774 | + 89 (±25) | 195 | 16 | 42 |
| **All ages** | 690 | 703 | + 13 (±3) | 607 | 602 | − 5 (±3) | 612 | 618 | + 6 (±3) | 1208 | 454 | 700 |

**Table 9.7**    **Changes in memory test scores by age and sex. Mean number correct out of 10**

| | Males | | | Females | | | Base numbers | |
|---|---|---|---|---|---|---|---|---|
| | HALS1 | HALS2 | Difference (±SEM) | HALS1 | HALS2 | Difference (±SEM) | Males | Females |
| **Age at HALS1** | | | | | | | | |
| **18-24** | 6.9 | 7.1 | +0.2 (±0.1) | 7.0 | 7.4 | +0.4 (±0.1) | 235 | 217 |
| **25-34** | 6.8 | 7.0 | +0.2 (±0.1) | 7.2 | 7.4 | +0.3 (±0.1) | 326 | 513 |
| **35-44** | 6.7 | 7.0 | +0.2 (±0.1) | 7.2 | 7.3 | +0.1 (±0.1) | 452 | 621 |
| **45-54** | 6.6 | 6.5 | −0.3 (±0.1) | 7.1 | 7.0 | −0.1 (±0.1) | 336 | 438 |
| **55-64** | 6.2 | 6.3 | +0.1 (±0.1) | 6.8 | 6.9 | +0.1 (±0.1) | 353 | 362 |
| **65-74** | 6.0 | 5.7 | −0.3 (±0.1) | 6.4 | 6.2 | −0.2 (±0.1) | 188 | 210 |
| **75+** | 5.4 | 5.2 | −0.2 (±0.3) | 6.1 | 5.5 | −0.6 (±0.2) | 49 | 69 |
| **All ages** | 6.5 | 6.6 | +0.1 (±0.0) | 7.0 | 7.1 | +0.1 (±0.0) | 1939 | 2430 |

**Table 9.8**    **Changes in memory test scores by age and sex. Percentage scoring 8-10 correct out of 10 at HALS1, HALS2 and at both Surveys**

| | Males | | | | Females | | | | Base numbers | |
|---|---|---|---|---|---|---|---|---|---|---|
| | HALS1 | HALS2 | Difference | HALS1 and HALS2 | HALS1 | HALS2 | Difference | HALS1 and HALS2 | Males | Females |
| **Age at HALS1** | | | | | | | | | | |
| **18-24** | 38 | 42 | +4 | 20 | 35 | 47 | +12 | 21 | 235 | 217 |
| **25-34** | 33 | 38 | +5 | 18 | 45 | 48 | +3 | 27 | 326 | 513 |
| **35-44** | 30 | 37 | +7 | 16 | 45 | 47 | +2 | 28 | 452 | 621 |
| **45-54** | 27 | 29 | +2 | 13 | 44 | 40 | −4 | 23 | 336 | 438 |
| **55-64** | 20 | 22 | +2 | 6 | 32 | 34 | +2 | 15 | 353 | 362 |
| **65-74** | 16 | 11 | −5 | 2 | 28 | 21 | −7 | 10 | 188 | 210 |
| **75+** | 4 | 6 | +2 | 0 | 14 | 9 | −5 | 1 | 49 | 69 |
| **All ages** | 27 | 30 | +3 | 13 | 40 | 41 | +1 | 22 | 1939 | 2430 |

**Table 9.9** **Changes in memory test scores by age and sex. Percentage changing by more than one item correct**

| | Males | | | Females | | | Base numbers | |
|---|---|---|---|---|---|---|---|---|
| | Better | Little change | Worse | Better | Little change | Worse | Males | Females |
| **Age at HALS1** | | | | | | | | |
| **18-24** | 20 | 65 | 15 | 14 | 80 | 6 | *235* | *217* |
| **25-34** | 21 | 66 | 13 | 12 | 79 | 9 | *326* | *513* |
| **35-44** | 24 | 61 | 15 | 14 | 74 | 12 | *452* | *621* |
| **45-54** | 18 | 61 | 21 | 12 | 77 | 11 | *336* | *438* |
| **55-64** | 21 | 60 | 19 | 10 | 78 | 12 | *353* | *362* |
| **65-74** | 17 | 56 | 27 | 13 | 57 | 30 | *188* | *210* |
| **75+** | 16 | 57 | 27 | 12 | 52 | 36 | *49* | *69* |
| **All ages** | 21 | 61 | 18 | 13 | 74 | 13 | *1939* | *2430* |

**Table 9.10** **Changes in memory test scores by education. Mean number correct out of 10**

| | Highest Educational Qualification | | | | | | | | | | | |
|---|---|---|---|---|---|---|---|---|---|---|---|---|
| | None/work related | | | GCSE/O-level | | | A-level/professional/degree | | | Base numbers | | |
| | HALS1 | HALS2 | Diff. (±SEM) | HALS1 | HALS2 | Diff. (±SEM) | HALS1 | HALS2 | Diff. (±SEM) | | | |
| **Age at HALS1** | | | | **Males** | | | | | | | | |
| **18-39** | 6.5 | 6.8 | +0.3 (±0.1) | 6.9 | 7.1 | +0.2 (±0.1) | 7.1 | 7.2 | +0.1 (±0.1) | *247* | *231* | *333* |
| **40-64** | 6.2 | 6.4 | +0.2 (±0.1) | 6.2 | 6.7 | +0.5 (±0.2) | 6.9 | 6.8 | −0.1 (±0.1) | *528* | *101* | *261* |
| **65+** | 5.8 | 5.5 | −0.3 (±0.1) | 6.1 | 5.4 | −0.7 (±0.4) | 6.0 | 5.6 | −0.4 (±0.3) | *174* | *13* | *50* |
| **All ages** | 6.2 | 6.3 | +0.1 (±0.1) | 6.6 | 6.9 | +0.3 (±0.1) | 6.9 | 6.9 | 0.0 (±0.1) | *949* | *345* | *644* |
| | | | | **Females** | | | | | | | | |
| **18-39** | 6.9 | 7.1 | +0.2 (±0.1) | 7.2 | 7.6 | +0.4 (±0.1) | 7.5 | 7.5 | 0.0 (±0.1) | *415* | *324* | *347* |
| **40-64** | 6.8 | 6.8 | 0.0 (±0.1) | 7.4 | 7.1 | −0.3 (±0.1) | 7.4 | 7.4 | 0.0 (±0.1) | *624* | *121* | *319* |
| **65+** | 6.3 | 6.0 | −0.3 (±0.1) | 6.3 | 6.4 | +0.1 (±0.5) | 6.8 | 6.4 | −0.4 (±0.2) | *217* | *17* | *45* |
| **All ages** | 6.7 | 6.8 | +0.1 (±0.1) | 7.3 | 7.4 | +0.1 (±0.1) | 7.4 | 7.4 | 0.0 (±0.1) | *1256* | *462* | *711* |

**Table 9.11**  **Changes in block counting test scores by age and sex. Mean number correct out of 6**

| | Males | | | Females | | | Base numbers | |
|---|---|---|---|---|---|---|---|---|
| | HALS1 | HALS2 | Difference (±SEM) | HALS1 | HALS2 | Difference (±SEM) | Males | Females |
| **Age at HALS1** | | | | | | | | |
| **18-24** | 5.1 | 5.3 | +0.2 (±0.1) | 4.7 | 5.0 | +0.3 (±0.1) | 241 | 222 |
| **25-34** | 5.4 | 5.4 | 0.0 (±0.1) | 4.8 | 4.9 | +0.1 (±0.1) | 329 | 517 |
| **35-44** | 5.4 | 5.5 | +0.1 (±0.1) | 4.8 | 4.9 | +0.1 (±0.1) | 457 | 628 |
| **45-54** | 5.1 | 5.2 | +0.1 (±0.1) | 4.8 | 4.8 | 0.0 (±0.1) | 344 | 444 |
| **55-64** | 5.1 | 5.0 | −0.1 (±0.1) | 4.5 | 4.5 | 0.0 (±0.1) | 356 | 366 |
| **65-74** | 5.0 | 4.7 | −0.3 (±0.1) | 4.5 | 3.9 | −0.6 (±0.1) | 192 | 210 |
| **75+** | 4.7 | 3.9 | −0.8 (±0.2) | 3.8 | 2.8 | −1.0 (±0.3) | 53 | 74 |
| **All ages** | 5.2 | 5.2 | 0.0 (±0.0) | 4.7 | 4.7 | 0.0 (±0.0) | 1972 | 2461 |

**Table 9.12**  **Changes in block counting test scores by age and sex. Percentage scoring 5 or 6 correct out of 6 at HALS1, HALS2 and both Surveys**

| | Males | | | | Females | | | | Base numbers | |
|---|---|---|---|---|---|---|---|---|---|---|
| | HALS1 | HALS2 | Difference | HALS1 and HALS2 | HALS1 | HALS2 | Difference | HALS1 and HALS2 | Males | Females |
| **Age at HALS1** | | | | | | | | | | |
| **18-24** | 83 | 88 | +5 | 77 | 68 | 77 | +9 | 60 | 241 | 222 |
| **25-34** | 90 | 90 | 0 | 84 | 72 | 75 | +3 | 61 | 329 | 517 |
| **35-44** | 89 | 90 | +1 | 83 | 74 | 76 | +2 | 61 | 457 | 628 |
| **45-54** | 83 | 84 | +1 | 75 | 71 | 75 | +4 | 59 | 344 | 444 |
| **55-64** | 82 | 81 | −1 | 70 | 67 | 64 | −3 | 52 | 356 | 366 |
| **65-74** | 77 | 69 | −8 | 57 | 62 | 50 | −12 | 37 | 192 | 210 |
| **75+** | 68 | 43 | −25 | 38 | 45 | 27 | −18 | 19 | 53 | 74 |
| **All ages** | 84 | 84 | 0 | 75 | 69 | 70 | +1 | 56 | 1972 | 2461 |

**Table 9.13** **Changes in block counting test scores by age and sex. Percentage changing by more than one item**

| | Males | | | Females | | | Base numbers | |
|---|---|---|---|---|---|---|---|---|
| | Better | Little change | Worse | Better | Little change | Worse | Males | Females |
| **Age at HALS1** | | | | | | | | |
| **18-24** | 8 | 88 | 4 | 26 | 62 | 12 | *241* | *222* |
| **25-34** | 5 | 91 | 4 | 19 | 66 | 15 | *329* | *517* |
| **35-44** | 6 | 91 | 3 | 18 | 67 | 15 | *457* | *628* |
| **45-54** | 9 | 85 | 6 | 16 | 67 | 17 | *344* | *444* |
| **55-64** | 9 | 80 | 11 | 19 | 63 | 18 | *356* | *366* |
| **65-74** | 9 | 72 | 19 | 18 | 60 | 22 | *192* | *210* |
| **75+** | 6 | 68 | 26 | 10 | 58 | 32 | *53* | *74* |
| **All ages** | 7 | 85 | 7 | 18 | 65 | 17 | *1972* | *2461* |

**Table 9.14** **Simple reaction time and choice reaction time measures by age and sex: 7-year cohorts at HALS1 and HALS2 (sub-sample) and population sample at HALS1**

| | HALS1 age 18-24 | | 25-31 | | 32-38 | | 39-45 | | 46-52 | | 53-59 | | 60-66 | | 67-73 | | 74+ | | All ages | |
| --- | --- | --- | --- | --- | --- | --- | --- | --- | --- | --- | --- | --- | --- | --- | --- | --- | --- | --- | --- | --- |
| | HALS2 age | | 25-31 | | 32-38 | | 39-45 | | 46-52 | | 53-59 | | 60-66 | | 67-73 | | 74-80 | | 81+ | | All ages |

**Mean simple reaction time in milliseconds**

**Males**

| | | | | | | | | | | | | | | | | | | | | |
| --- | --- | --- | --- | --- | --- | --- | --- | --- | --- | --- | --- | --- | --- | --- | --- | --- | --- | --- | --- | --- |
| HALS1 | 291 | | 308 | | 298 | | 302 | | 320 | | 347 | | 345 | | 376 | | 476 | | 329 | |
| HALS2 | 297 | 293 | 308 | 294 | 293 | 290 | 297 | 297 | 317 | 319 | 349 | 340 | 339 | 340 | 358 | 412 | 490 | 496 | 322 | 323 |

**Females**

| | | | | | | | | | | | | | | | | | | | | |
| --- | --- | --- | --- | --- | --- | --- | --- | --- | --- | --- | --- | --- | --- | --- | --- | --- | --- | --- | --- | --- |
| HALS1 | 315 | | 321 | | 312 | | 319 | | 335 | | 347 | | 366 | | 431 | | 560 | | 350 | |
| HALS2 | 318 | 309 | 319 | 314 | 310 | 307 | 310 | 310 | 331 | 328 | 339 | 332 | 365 | 385 | 402 | 442 | 480 | 524 | 334 | 336 |

| | | | | | | | | | | | | | | | | | | | | |
| --- | --- | --- | --- | --- | --- | --- | --- | --- | --- | --- | --- | --- | --- | --- | --- | --- | --- | --- | --- | --- |
| Base nos | 440 | | 412 | | 503 | | 406 | | 352 | | 355 | | 337 | | 253 | | 208 | | 3266 | |
| | 235 | 235 | 200 | 200 | 334 | 334 | 271 | 271 | 237 | 237 | 245 | 245 | 213 | 213 | 123 | 123 | 67 | 67 | 1925 | 1925 |
| | 469 | | 562 | | 672 | | 526 | | 461 | | 382 | | 408 | | 269 | | 256 | | 4005 | |
| | 216 | 216 | 332 | 332 | 473 | 473 | 367 | 367 | 311 | 311 | 235 | 235 | 243 | 243 | 129 | 129 | 77 | 77 | 2383 | 2383 |

**Choice reaction time. Mean time in milliseconds**

**Males**

| | | | | | | | | | | | | | | | | | | | | |
| --- | --- | --- | --- | --- | --- | --- | --- | --- | --- | --- | --- | --- | --- | --- | --- | --- | --- | --- | --- | --- |
| HALS1 | 573 | | 589 | | 603 | | 629 | | 672 | | 688 | | 698 | | 775 | | 875 | | 657 | |
| HALS2 | 567 | 560 | 592 | 589 | 600 | 595 | 628 | 632 | 655 | 662 | 690 | 703 | 691 | 729 | 753 | 807 | 836 | 915 | 645 | 657 |

**Females**

| | | | | | | | | | | | | | | | | | | | | |
| --- | --- | --- | --- | --- | --- | --- | --- | --- | --- | --- | --- | --- | --- | --- | --- | --- | --- | --- | --- | --- |
| HALS1 | 591 | | 605 | | 611 | | 633 | | 638 | | 691 | | 741 | | 805 | | 926 | | 671 | |
| HALS2 | 594 | 580 | 605 | 590 | 611 | 604 | 624 | 625 | 661 | 665 | 682 | 698 | 726 | 755 | 768 | 839 | 822 | 920 | 651 | 658 |

| | | | | | | | | | | | | | | | | | | | | |
| --- | --- | --- | --- | --- | --- | --- | --- | --- | --- | --- | --- | --- | --- | --- | --- | --- | --- | --- | --- | --- |
| Base nos | 438 | | 409 | | 501 | | 406 | | 352 | | 350 | | 334 | | 250 | | 202 | | 3242 | |
| | 231 | 231 | 196 | 196 | 333 | 333 | 269 | 269 | 235 | 235 | 241 | 241 | 213 | 213 | 119 | 119 | 65 | 65 | 1902 | 1902 |
| | 469 | | 557 | | 667 | | 523 | | 460 | | 377 | | 407 | | 265 | | 249 | | 3974 | |
| | 215 | 215 | 330 | 330 | 470 | 470 | 365 | 365 | 310 | 310 | 233 | 233 | 242 | 242 | 126 | 126 | 73 | 73 | 2364 | 2364 |

**Percentage making no errors**

**Males**

| | | | | | | | | | | | | | | | | | | | | |
| --- | --- | --- | --- | --- | --- | --- | --- | --- | --- | --- | --- | --- | --- | --- | --- | --- | --- | --- | --- | --- |
| HALS1 | 25 | | 33 | | 38 | | 37 | | 38 | | 38 | | 39 | | 31 | | 35 | | 35 | |
| HALS2 | 28 | 36 | 31 | 46 | 37 | 41 | 37 | 40 | 35 | 34 | 37 | 36 | 38 | 35 | 34 | 24 | 33 | 36 | 35 | 37 |

**Females**

| | | | | | | | | | | | | | | | | | | | | |
| --- | --- | --- | --- | --- | --- | --- | --- | --- | --- | --- | --- | --- | --- | --- | --- | --- | --- | --- | --- | --- |
| HALS1 | 35 | | 47 | | 46 | | 42 | | 39 | | 40 | | 45 | | 41 | | 42 | | 42 | |
| HALS2 | 36 | 36 | 48 | 40 | 47 | 44 | 39 | 39 | 40 | 39 | 36 | 41 | 44 | 38 | 40 | 51 | 37 | 51 | 42 | 41 |

| | | | | | | | | | | | | | | | | | | | | |
| --- | --- | --- | --- | --- | --- | --- | --- | --- | --- | --- | --- | --- | --- | --- | --- | --- | --- | --- | --- | --- |
| Base nos | 436 | | 409 | | 496 | | 404 | | 350 | | 349 | | 333 | | 247 | | 201 | | 3225 | |
| | 230 | 230 | 197 | 197 | 330 | 330 | 269 | 269 | 234 | 234 | 240 | 240 | 212 | 212 | 118 | 118 | 66 | 66 | 1896 | 1896 |
| | 468 | | 557 | | 660 | | 522 | | 459 | | 374 | | 407 | | 264 | | 249 | | 3957 | |
| | 215 | 215 | 330 | 330 | 465 | 465 | 363 | 363 | 310 | 310 | 230 | 230 | 241 | 241 | 125 | 125 | 73 | 73 | 2352 | 2352 |

**Table 9.15    Memory test score by age and sex: 7-year cohorts at HALS1 (sample) and HALS2 (sub-sample) and population sample at HALS1**

| HALS1 age | 18-24 | | 25-31 | | 32-38 | | 39-45 | | 46-52 | | 53-59 | | 60-66 | | 67-73 | | 74+ | | All ages | |
|---|---|---|---|---|---|---|---|---|---|---|---|---|---|---|---|---|---|---|---|---|
| HALS2 age | | 25-31 | | 32-38 | | 39-45 | | 46-52 | | 53-59 | | 60-66 | | 67-73 | | 74-80 | | 81+ | | All ages |

**Mean number correct**

**Males**

| | 18-24 | 25-31 | 25-31 | 32-38 | 32-38 | 39-45 | 39-45 | 46-52 | 46-52 | 53-59 | 53-59 | 60-66 | 60-66 | 67-73 | 67-73 | 74-80 | 74+ | 81+ | All | All |
|---|---|---|---|---|---|---|---|---|---|---|---|---|---|---|---|---|---|---|---|---|
| HALS1 | 6.8 | | 6.8 | | 6.7 | | 6.7 | | 6.4 | | 6.2 | | 6.2 | | 5.7 | | 5.2 | | 6.4 | |
| HALS2 | 6.9 | 7.1 | 6.8 | 7.1 | 6.7 | 7.0 | 6.8 | 6.9 | 6.6 | 6.6 | 6.2 | 6.4 | 6.3 | 6.2 | 5.8 | 5.6 | 5.6 | 5.3 | 6.5 | 6.6 |

**Females**

| | | | | | | | | | | | | | | | | | | | | |
|---|---|---|---|---|---|---|---|---|---|---|---|---|---|---|---|---|---|---|---|---|
| HALS1 | 7.2 | | 7.2 | | 7.3 | | 7.1 | | 7.0 | | 7.0 | | 6.5 | | 6.2 | | 5.7 | | 6.9 | |
| HALS2 | 7.0 | 7.4 | 7.2 | 7.4 | 7.2 | 7.3 | 7.2 | 7.2 | 7.1 | 7.0 | 6.9 | 6.9 | 6.6 | 6.7 | 6.5 | 6.3 | 6.1 | 5.5 | 7.0 | 7.1 |

| Base nos | | | | | | | | | | | | | | | | | | | | |
|---|---|---|---|---|---|---|---|---|---|---|---|---|---|---|---|---|---|---|---|---|
| | 435 | | 408 | | 506 | | 406 | | 351 | | 354 | | 337 | | 252 | | 210 | | 3259 | |
| | 235 | 235 | 200 | 200 | 339 | 339 | 275 | 275 | 234 | 234 | 248 | 248 | 218 | 218 | 124 | 124 | 66 | 66 | 1939 | 1939 |
| | 474 | | 556 | | 682 | | 527 | | 465 | | 380 | | 413 | | 278 | | 265 | | 4040 | |
| | 217 | 217 | 332 | 332 | 480 | 480 | 370 | 370 | 320 | 320 | 239 | 239 | 249 | 249 | 136 | 136 | 87 | 87 | 2430 | 2430 |

**Percentage scoring 8-10 correct**

**Males**

| | | | | | | | | | | | | | | | | | | | | |
|---|---|---|---|---|---|---|---|---|---|---|---|---|---|---|---|---|---|---|---|---|
| HALS1 | 37 | | 35 | | 31 | | 32 | | 28 | | 19 | | 20 | | 11 | | 7 | | 27 | |
| HALS2 | 38 | 42 | 32 | 40 | 30 | 37 | 33 | 36 | 28 | 30 | 18 | 25 | 23 | 17 | 13 | 9 | 9 | 9 | 27 | 30 |

**Females**

| | | | | | | | | | | | | | | | | | | | | |
|---|---|---|---|---|---|---|---|---|---|---|---|---|---|---|---|---|---|---|---|---|
| HALS1 | 42 | | 43 | | 46 | | 41 | | 44 | | 39 | | 25 | | 25 | | 14 | | 38 | |
| HALS2 | 35 | 47 | 45 | 49 | 45 | 48 | 44 | 45 | 46 | 41 | 38 | 34 | 27 | 33 | 32 | 24 | 14 | 8 | 40 | 41 |

| Base nos | | | | | | | | | | | | | | | | | | | | |
|---|---|---|---|---|---|---|---|---|---|---|---|---|---|---|---|---|---|---|---|---|
| | 435 | | 408 | | 506 | | 406 | | 351 | | 354 | | 337 | | 252 | | 210 | | 3259 | |
| | 235 | 235 | 200 | 200 | 339 | 339 | 275 | 275 | 234 | 234 | 248 | 248 | 218 | 218 | 124 | 124 | 66 | 66 | 1939 | 1939 |
| | 474 | | 556 | | 682 | | 527 | | 465 | | 380 | | 413 | | 278 | | 265 | | 4040 | |
| | 217 | 217 | 332 | 332 | 480 | 480 | 370 | 370 | 320 | 320 | 239 | 239 | 249 | 249 | 136 | 136 | 87 | 87 | 2430 | 2430 |

**Table 9.16** **Block counting test score by age and sex: 7-year cohorts at HALS1 (sample) and HALS2 (subsample) and population sample at HALS1**

| | 18-24 | | 25-31 | | 32-38 | | 39-45 | | 46-52 | | 53-59 | | 60-66 | | 67-73 | | 74+ | | All ages | |
|---|---|---|---|---|---|---|---|---|---|---|---|---|---|---|---|---|---|---|---|---|
| **HALS1 age** | 18-24 | | 25-31 | | 32-38 | | 39-45 | | 46-52 | | 53-59 | | 60-66 | | 67-73 | | 74+ | | All ages | |
| **HALS2 age** | | 25-31 | | 32-38 | | 39-45 | | 46-52 | | 53-59 | | 60-66 | | 67-73 | | 74-80 | | 81+ | | All ages |
| **Mean number correct** | | | | | | | | | | | | | | | | | | | | |
| **Males** | | | | | | | | | | | | | | | | | | | | |
| HALS1 | 5.1 | | 5.2 | | 5.3 | | 5.4 | | 5.0 | | 5.1 | | 5.1 | | 4.8 | | 4.4 | | 5.1 | |
| HALS2 | 5.1 | 5.3 | 5.3 | 5.4 | 5.4 | 5.5 | 5.5 | 5.5 | 5.1 | 5.2 | 5.1 | 5.0 | 5.2 | 5.0 | 5.0 | 4.7 | 4.6 | 4.0 | 5.2 | 5.2 |
| **Females** | | | | | | | | | | | | | | | | | | | | |
| HALS1 | 4.6 | | 4.7 | | 4.8 | | 4.7 | | 4.6 | | 4.5 | | 4.4 | | 4.2 | | 3.5 | | 4.5 | |
| HALS2 | 4.6 | 5.0 | 4.7 | 4.9 | 4.8 | 5.0 | 4.9 | 4.9 | 4.8 | 4.8 | 4.7 | 4.8 | 4.5 | 4.4 | 4.5 | 3.8 | 4.0 | 2.9 | 4.7 | 4.7 |
| *Base nos* | 443 | | 414 | | 511 | | 410 | | 353 | | 359 | | 336 | | 257 | | 212 | | 3295 | |
| | 241 | 241 | 203 | 203 | 341 | 341 | 279 | 279 | 240 | 240 | 251 | 251 | 219 | 219 | 126 | 126 | 72 | 72 | 1972 | 1972 |
| | 479 | | 563 | | 685 | | 532 | | 469 | | 388 | | 418 | | 272 | | 260 | | 4066 | |
| | 222 | 222 | 334 | 334 | 484 | 484 | 375 | 375 | 323 | 323 | 243 | 243 | 252 | 252 | 135 | 135 | 93 | 93 | 2461 | 2461 |
| **Percentage scoring 5-6 correct** | | | | | | | | | | | | | | | | | | | | |
| **Males** | | | | | | | | | | | | | | | | | | | | |
| HALS1 | 83 | | 85 | | 88 | | 89 | | 79 | | 81 | | 82 | | 71 | | 60 | | 82 | |
| HALS2 | 83 | 88 | 88 | 89 | 89 | 90 | 92 | 90 | 81 | 84 | 80 | 80 | 84 | 81 | 77 | 70 | 65 | 49 | 84 | 84 |
| **Females** | | | | | | | | | | | | | | | | | | | | |
| HALS1 | 67 | | 68 | | 74 | | 71 | | 67 | | 65 | | 63 | | 54 | | 40 | | 66 | |
| HALS2 | 68 | 77 | 69 | 74 | 74 | 77 | 74 | 74 | 71 | 75 | 69 | 70 | 65 | 60 | 62 | 50 | 48 | 28 | 69 | 70 |
| *Base nos* | 443 | | 414 | | 511 | | 410 | | 353 | | 359 | | 336 | | 257 | | 212 | | 3295 | |
| | 241 | 241 | 203 | 203 | 341 | 341 | 279 | 279 | 240 | 240 | 251 | 251 | 219 | 219 | 126 | 126 | 72 | 72 | 1972 | 1972 |
| | 479 | | 563 | | 685 | | 532 | | 469 | | 388 | | 418 | | 272 | | 260 | | 4066 | |
| | 222 | 222 | 334 | 334 | 484 | 484 | 375 | 375 | 323 | 323 | 243 | 243 | 252 | 252 | 135 | 135 | 93 | 93 | 2461 | 2461 |

# THE IMPACT OF LIFE EVENTS ON WELL BEING

**10**

### Joyce E Whittington and Felicia A Huppert

There is a large and growing volume of literature linking stressful life events to deterioration in physical health (e.g. Harris, 1989) and mental health (e.g. Cohen, 1988; Thoits, 1983; Paykel, 1974). Originating from different traditions in the 1930s, when Hans Selye suggested stress as a factor in physical illness and Franz Alexander suggested personality-related reactions as a factor in mental illness, there is now emerging a common aetiological model. The model suggests that the onset of illness is associated with a number of factors, including the presence of stressful environmental conditions, perception by the individual that such conditions are stressful, the relative ability to cope with or adapt to these conditions, genetic predisposition to a disease, and the presence of a disease agent.

It is therefore appropriate in any study of health to try to measure the experience of adverse life events and the amount of stress thereby caused to individuals. Accordingly, a measure of life events was added to the measures used in HALS2.

The instrument used in HALS2 was developed by Huppert and colleagues for the Healthy Ageing Study funded by the Economic and Social Research Council. It was based on the scales used in the West of Scotland Twenty-07 Study of Health in the Community, and The National Survey of Health and Development (see Appendix A). The life events instrument comprises 25 adverse events covering six salient areas of everyday experience: health, death, work, housing, relationships, social problems, and also an open-ended question about 'other serious upsets'. For each event experienced, respondents are asked to rate the degree to which the event disrupted or changed their life and the amount of worry or stress they felt, each on a three-point scale: none, some, a great deal. The list was presented as part of the interview stage of HALS2.

Although the form of the instrument was dictated in part by practical considerations (it had to be short and simple enough to be completed in about ten minutes), theoretical considerations were most important in its construction. First, it concentrates on the occurrence of 'adverse' events (i.e. events usually rated 'adverse' by a majority of people), since there is evidence that positive events may not add to stress and may in fact help to alleviate it (Reich and Zautra, 1988). However, the HALS2 instrument does conclude with an open-ended question about the occurrence of positive events.

Second, respondents are asked to rate the change and stress caused by each event they have experienced, i.e. a subjective measure is used. It thus combines a traditional checklist approach (Holmes and Rahe, 1967; Paykel et al. 1971) with a subjective component, the importance of which has been demonstrated by Brown and Harris (1989). This is both in the spirit of the aetiological model (in which the subjective experience of stress is a contributory factor) and in the spirit of HALS (in which self-ratings, e.g. of health, are regarded as important variables). This leaves open the options for scoring – a simple additive measure of the number of events, a weighted measure using standard, independently-derived weights for a given event, or a measure based on the respondent's own subjective ratings.

Third, the period covered is the twelve months prior to the interview. Although some researchers consider that event reporting is unreliable over periods of more than six months, there is evidence that when information is collected in an interview, rather than a self-completion checklist, reporting is adequate over a longer period (Funch and Marshall, 1984; Paykel, 1983). In order to cover the period from HALS1, the occurrence of some events is also ascertained over the intervening seven years, but only if no such event is reported in the last twelve months. However, the seven-year data are bound to be less reliable than the twelve-month data.

Reliability and validity data are not available for the present instrument. However, data for similar interview measures suggest that both will be higher than for the most widely-used self-completion checklists, the Schedule of Recent Experience (SRE) and the Social Readjustment Rating Scale (SRRS), which have test-retest correlations varying from 0.26 to 0.90 (Rahe, 1974). The frequency distribution of remembered events over time shows a fall-off of 5% per month for self-completion questionnaires (such as the SRE and SRRS), but only 2% per month for interview methods (Funch and Marshall, 1984; Paykel, 1983). Validity can be checked for some events, from data collected in other parts of the HALS study. In general, agreements between self-reporting of events and reporting by a 'significant other' have been found to be quite high (Paykel, 1983; Yager et al. 1981).

Most studies of life events and their effect on health have been conducted on selected, usually relatively small groups, typically comparing patient and control groups. Little is known about the frequency and impact of life events in a general population sample, or about the variables which mediate their impact. The introduction of a life events instrument into the HALS2 interview provided the opportunity both to obtain data on a large population sample and to examine the associates and precursors of the impact of life events.

## Occurrence and impact of adverse life events

Table 10.1 shows the frequencies with which each of the 25 adverse events was experienced in the last year, and the proportions of such events which respondents said had caused 'a great deal' of disruption or change and the proportion which had caused 'a great deal' of worry or stress.

The most frequently reported event was 'serious problem with health of family member or close friend', which was twice as frequent as the next most frequently reported events, 'death of close family member' and 'death of close friend'. The only other frequencies of occurrence which were above 10% in the population were: 'serious difficulty with children', 'serious illness/handicap developed', 'major financial problems' 'house occupants changed' and 'family member left home or new person moved in'. Among working men and women there was also a greater than 10% incidence of job change and job loss (or impending loss), and for women with working partners, a high incidence of job crisis for their partner. The lowest frequency was 'divorced/ separated' which occurred in 2% of the sample in the previous 12 months.

The most disruptive events, i.e. those rated as causing 'a great deal' of disruption or change to their life by those who experienced them, were 'divorced/ separated', 'retirement', 'serious illness/handicap developed' and 'serious financial problems'.

The most stressful events, i.e. those rated as causing 'a great deal' of worry or stress by those reporting the event, were 'divorced/separated', 'major financial problems' and 'serious difficulty with children'. Ranked not far behind these, were 'problems with officials/the law' and 'serious disagreements with partner/feeling betrayed or disappointed by partner'. All these events were rated as considerably more stressful by women than by men.

There is some confounding in the literature of the amount of life change caused by an event and the amount of stress experienced. Table 10.1 shows that, while respondents rated divorce/separation as both the most disruptive and the most stressful, they rated retirement, job change, and their own health conditions as causing large changes but not so much stress. In contrast, difficulties with children was a cause of great stress but not so much change.

Sex differences were very small in relation to the occurrence of adverse life events, with the exception of 'serious difficulty with children' which was reported by 15% of fathers and 21% of mothers. Although a higher percentage of women than men reported moving to a new area, the total number who moved house in the last year is too small to make this difference reliable.

However, there are large sex differences in the ratings of the degree of disruption and stress caused by life events. In general, a higher proportion of women than men report a great deal of disruption to their life, and a great deal of worry or stress. The differences are particularly marked for moving house, disagreements with partner, and major financial problems. In addition, 'divorced/separated' and 'serious difficulty with children' are rated as equally disruptive by men and women, but cause much more worry and stress for women than for men.

The types of events included in the life events list suggest that there will be age differences in the frequencies with which events are reported. Questions relating to work are largely inapplicable to the oldest age group, but even where questions can apply to all ages, some differences may be expected. For example, there are likely to be more health problems and more deaths among friends and family for the older groups. Predictions about age differences in the percentage reporting great change and great stress are less easy to make.

As expected, events relating to one's own health were more frequent in the older groups, although the middle-aged and oldest groups differed very little from one another. Death of a friend was also higher in the older groups, while the frequency of death of a close family member showed little association with age. All other events had a higher frequency in the younger groups than in the oldest group. The youngest group had the highest frequency of problems with relationships, housing and finances, while the middle-aged group had the higher frequency of a change in the occupants of their house.

The data are summarised in Figure 10.1 and Table 10.2. Figure 10.1 presents the frequency distribution of the number of life events reported in the past 12 months. Values ranged from 0-14, with one event being the most common response, and women reporting more events than men. Table 10.2 presents the mean number of life events and their impact, by age and sex. It can be seen that the number of adverse life events reported in the last year decreases with age, but for those individuals who have experienced the events, the degree of disruption and stress is

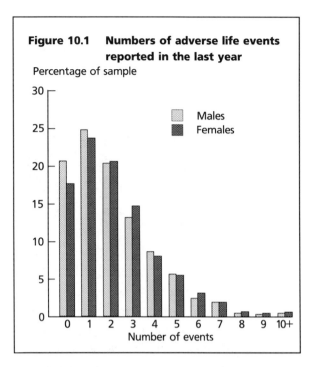

**Figure 10.1    Numbers of adverse life events reported in the last year**

roughly comparable across age groups. Although the low number of life events reported by those aged 65 and over may, in part, reflect the poorer memory of this group (see Chapter 9), there is a negligible correlation between the number of events reported and scores on the memory test. The difference probably results mainly from the relative absence of work-related events in this group, along with the interesting finding that the oldest group reports very few problems with relationships.

A summary of the data on stressful life events is presented in Figure 10.2. A higher percentage of men than women report either no events or events which caused no stress. For women, the most frequent response in the two younger age groups was that they had experienced at least one event in the past year which caused great stress. For both men and women, the percentage reporting stressful events decreased with age.

For selected events (15 out of 25), subjects who had not experienced the event in the past 12 months were asked if it had happened in the past 7 years, and if it still caused disruption or stress. Table 10.3 compares the frequencies with which each of the events (excluding 'other upsets') was reported for the previous year, and the previous seven years (when no such event had occurred in the previous year).

Comparison of event frequencies shows that most

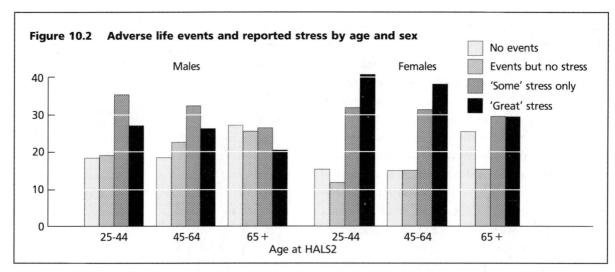

**Figure 10.2   Adverse life events and reported stress by age and sex**

events are under-reported over the seven-year period. For example, unemployment and economic difficulties would need to be growing out of control to account for the reporting of fewer job losses and financial difficulties over a six-year period compared with the last year. In general, it can be seen that no event frequency for the seven-year period begins to approach the increase over the one-year frequencies which would be expected if reporting was reliable. Comparison of change and stress ratings suggests that the events which take longest for recovery are not necessarily those which initially caused most change and stress. For example, the rating of 'great change' caused by recent divorce/separation, compared with that for divorce/separation occurring more than a year ago, shows a large fall over time, whereas the 'great change' caused by the development or worsening of a health condition falls very much less over time. Clearly, some events, though catastrophic at the time, are in many cases without long-term consequences (e.g. operations such as appendectomy), whereas others may lead to chronic conditions which last for years (e.g. physical handicap, financial difficulties such as bankruptcy). For all events, the proportion of individuals rating events in the more remote period as continuing to cause great disruption or great stress is much smaller than for more recent events. This could be regarded as the 'time as healer' effect.

## Positive events

Table 10.4 shows the percentage of respondents who reported a 'nice' event in the past year, or in the past seven years (if none was recorded in the past year).

'Nice' events reported by respondents covered a wide range of areas of experiences, the most common being the birth of children or grandchildren, holidays and special occasions such as golden wedding anniversaries. It is quite surprising that fewer than half the respondents reported such an event in the past year, and altogether, fewer than three-quarters of all respondents reported a nice event in the past seven years.

Women tended to report more nice events than men, and the younger groups reported more than the oldest group, where only 35% of males and 44% of females reported a nice event in the past year.

Table 10.5 shows a relationship between socio-economic groups (manual/non-manual categories) and the reporting of 'nice' events in the last year. For all age groups and both sexes, the non-manual group reports a higher frequency of 'nice' events.

## Adverse life events, social class and residential neighbourhood

In contrast to the clear relationship between socio-economic group and reporting of positive events (Table 10.5), it is less easy to discern an association with the reporting of adverse life events and their impact (Table 10.6). An exception is the social problems category where the impact is greater in the manual group for women in the two older age-bands, even though the frequency of occurrence in the 65 + age group is considerably higher in the non-manual category.

The possibility that life events may be more frequent or more disturbing among respondents living in poor housing conditions is addressed in

Table 10.7. It is clear that most large differences between groups are between those living in high-rise developments and all other neighbourhood categories. Five of the seven categories of events show such differences. Of these, death events and social problems are more frequent for those living in high-rise developments in both socio-economic groups. But for two other event categories (health and housing), there are interactions with socio-economic group. Thus, health events and housing events are increased in the manual group but decreased in the non-manual group for high-rise residents, compared to other residential categories.

There is also a sizeable difference in the frequencies of reporting social problems between the socio-economic groups residing in country districts (12% manual, 21% non-manual). Further analysis showed that two events, 'assault/robbery' and 'financial problems', were responsible for this difference.

## Life events and physical illness

The relationship between the number of life events experienced and subsequent illness is examined in Table 10.8 and Table 10.9. Table 10.8 shows that, for all age groups and both sexes, the percentage reporting four or more illness symptoms 'in the past month' at HALS2 rises with the number of adverse life events (excluding 'own health' events) reported 'in the past year'. This gives support to the aetiological model in which adverse life events are hypothesised as being a precipitating factor in the onset of illness. The strength of the relationship in Table 10.8 is an important result, because it has been established in a general population sample. Many previous studies, mainly in the USA, have found a similar relationship, but their samples tend to have been restricted to particular sections of the population (e.g. naval recruits, post-retirement age groups).

Table 10.9 utilises the seven-year life event data in conjunction with the one-year data to examine the relationship between the development of specific health conditions since HALS1 and the number of life events experienced (excluding 'own health' events) in the intervening seven years. Only respondents who did not have any of these health conditions at HALS1 were included. This selection resulted in very small numbers in the oldest group, which has therefore

been omitted from the table. Although the numbers developing the health conditions are small, even in the younger groups, there is a tendency for the onset of depression and migraine to increase with increasing number of life events experienced. For females only, there is also a tendency for bronchitis/other chest conditions and rheumatism/arthritis to increase with increasing number of life events, and for males in the middle-aged group there is a similar tendency for the incidence of heart trouble to increase with increasing number of life events.

## Life events and psychiatric symptoms

Most researchers in the field of life events endorse the view that particular forms of psychiatric illness (e.g. depression) are often triggered by one or more stressful life events. However, there is a difference of opinion about the number and nature of events necessary before such a trigger is activated. The relationship between life events in the past year and current psychiatric symptoms is explored in Table 10.10 to Table 10.13. Table 10.10 shows a strong relationship between the number of life events reported in the previous year and the number of psychiatric symptoms, expressed as the percentage of each group exceeding the standard threshold (5 or more symptoms) for possible psychiatric disorder on the General Health Questionnaire of Goldberg (1972). On average, it can be seen that the percentage of respondents who exceed the GHQ threshold is two to three times higher in those reporting four or more life events compared with those reporting 0 or 1 life events. The association between the number of life events and GHQ scores is particularly strong in the middle-aged group. Again, the finding of such a relationship between life events and psychiatric symptoms is important because of the representativeness of the population sample.

Some idea of the relative importance of the total number of events experienced, compared with the stress produced by the events, can be gleaned from Table 10.11. The first two columns compare events with little or no associated stress (no events vs one or more events), while columns three to five compare the effects of different numbers of stressful events (events that caused 'a great deal' of worry or stress). Some caution is needed in the interpretation of this association, since number of stressful events is confounded with total number of events (correlation 0.68). However, taken in conjunction with Table 10.10, the data in Table 10.11 suggest that both the total number of events experienced, whether or not they are felt to be stressful, and the number of events felt to cause great stress are related to the presence of psychiatric symptoms, as measured by the GHQ. There is support in Table 10.11 for the argument advanced by Brown and Harris (1986), that one stressful event may be enough to produce psychiatric symptoms. The doubling of percentages over the GHQ threshold between no stressful events and one stressful event strongly supports this position.

However, an interpretative problem remains which is shared by much life event research, concerning the direction of causality of the observed associations. Life events, and particularly stressful life events, may play a role in the development of psychiatric symptoms, but the presence of psychiatric disorder or symptoms may result in certain life events, namely those over which the individual can exert some control. These could include problems with work, housing, relationships, or finance. In the HALS investigation, information about the sequence in which symptoms appeared and events occurred is insufficient to tease apart the causal relationship.

While there is a strong association between the events and psychiatric symptoms, it is clear that some people experience many events, even many stressful events, without any evidence of psychiatric symptoms. This has led to the development of hypotheses about factors which may protect against or modify the psychological effect of adverse life events. A number of possible modifiers have been proposed, including locus of control, coping strategies and personality variables. The experience of positive events and a high level of social support, have also been proposed as possible modifiers of the impact of negative events (Reich and Zautra; 1988, Brown and Harris, 1989). These claims are examined in Table 10.12 and Table 10.13. Table 10.12 shows that for individuals reporting 4 or more adverse life events, the percentage above the GHQ threshold is lower for those who also report a positive event in the past year, compared with those who report no positive event. This trend is less obvious among respondents who report 0-3 adverse life events. Interpretation of this result is not straightforward. It

could be taken at face value, as evidence that the occurrence of a positive event alleviates the deleterious effects of adverse events. However, there is also evidence that people who are depressed fail to recall positive events (e.g., Lloyd and Lishman, 1975; Teasdale and Fogarty, 1979), and so would report no nice event; or that they experience the same 'nice events' as people who are not depressed, but fail to see them as nice events.

Table 10.13 examines the relationship between perceived social support at HALS2 and percentage over the GHQ threshold at HALS2. Perceived social support at HALS2 is taken as a proxy for social support over the last year, when the events were experienced. The table shows the predicted trend, with the percentage of people over the GHQ threshold falling with increasing degrees of perceived social support, both for few and for many experienced life events in the past year. It is interesting that in all groups the majority of respondents report a high level of perceived social support, even when they have experienced many adverse events.

Again, interpretation is not straightforward. It would be necessary to show that subjective assessment of social support does not differ between the two GHQ categories in order to conclude with confidence that social support does ameliorate the effects of adverse events. It could be that the same friendly overtures are seen as 'help and support' by respondents with low GHQ scores (few or no psychiatric symptoms) and as 'interference' by respondents with high GHQ scores.

## Summary

Frequencies of the occurrence and subjectively rated impact of 25 adverse life events over the previous year were calculated for the HALS2 population. Information about 15 of these over the previous seven years was also obtained, as well as information about the occurrence of positive events over the previous year and previous seven years. Population frequencies for the various events in the past year ranged from 37% (serious problem with health of family member or close friend) to 2% (divorce/ separation). The percentage of individuals who said a given event had caused 'a great deal' of disruption or change ranged from 73% (divorce/separation) to 10%

(death of a close friend) and similar ratings for 'a great deal' of stress ranged from 57% (divorce/separation) to 10% (partner's retirement). The data suggest that people can and do draw a distinction between the amount of change or disruption caused by an event and the amount of worry or stress caused by that event. Not surprisingly, however, events that cause change or disruption usually also cause stress; the correlation between the numbers of great change and great stress ratings was 0.82.

The total number of adverse life events reported in the previous year ranged from none (19% of the HALS2 population) to 14 events (one person). In general, the number of events reported declined with age, as did change and stress ratings. Overall, women reported more events and gave higher change and stress ratings than did men.

There was gross under-reporting of events over the seven-year interval between the surveys, compared to the reporting of events for the previous year. The only event which reached anything near the frequency expected over seven years was retirement. Major financial problems and serious problems with officials/the law were actually less frequently reported for the seven-year period. Positive ('nice') events were reported by a surprisingly low percentage of respondents: fewer than 50% reported a positive event in the previous year, and fewer than 50% of the remainder reported one in the previous seven years.

The relationship between life events and illness was explored, and a positive relationship was found between the number of adverse life events in the previous year and illness symptoms in the previous month. Development of specific health conditions in the seven years between HALS1 and HALS2 was related to adverse life events in the same period, particularly for depression and migraine. There was also a positive relationship with chest conditions and rheumatic conditions in women and with heart troubles in men aged 40 and over.

The number of life events experienced was positively associated with the number of psychiatric symptoms endorsed on the General Health Questionnaire. The number of very stressful events was even more strongly related to GHQ score, and even one very stressful event was enough to show an increase in the percentage with high GHQ scores.

Both the occurrence of a positive event and a high degree of social support were associated with low GHQ scores, even in groups reporting a high number of adverse life events. While this is consistent with the hypothesis that such variables may exert a modifying effect on mental health, other explanations were also considered.

### References

Brown, G.W. and Harris, T.O. (1989) Life Events and Illness, London: Unwin Hyman Limited.

Cohen, L.H. (1988) Life Events and Psychological Functioning, London: Sage.

Funch, D. and Marshall, J. (1984) Measuring life stress. Journal of Health and Social Behaviour, 25, 453-464.

Goldberg, D.P. (1972). The detection of psychiatric illness by questionnaire. London: Oxford University Press

Harris, T.O. (1989) Physical Illness; An Introduction. In Brown, G.W. and Harris, T.O. (Eds) Life Events and Illness, London: Unwin Hyman.

Holmes, T.H. and Rahe, R.H. (1967) The Social Readjustment Rating Scale. Journal of Psychosomatic Research, 11, 213-218.

Lloyd, G.G and Lishman, W.A. (1975) Effect of Depression on the speed of recall of pleasant and unpleasant experiences. Psychological Medicine, 5, 173-180.

Paykel, E.S., Prussof, B.A. and Uhlenhuth, E.H. (1971) Scaling of Life Events. Archives of General Psychiatry, 25, 340-347.

Paykel, E.S. (1974) Life stress and psychiatric disorder. In Dohrenwend, B.S. and Dohrenwend, B.P. (Eds) Stressful life events: their nature and effects, New York, John Wiley.

Paykel, E.S. (1983) Methodological aspects of life events research. Journal of Psychosomatic Research, 29, 341-352.

Rahe, R. (1974) In Dohrenwend, B.S. and Dohrenwend, B.P. (Eds) Stressful life events: their nature and effects, New York: Wiley

Reich, J.W. and Zautra, A.J. (1988) Direct and Stress-moderating effects of positive life experiences. In Cohen, L.H. (Ed) Life Events and Psychological Functioning, London: Sage.

Teasdale, J.D. and Fogarty, S.J. (1979) Differential Effects of induced mood on retrieval of pleasant and unpleasant events from episodic memory. Journal of Abnormal Psychology, 88, 248-252.

Thoits, P. (1983) Dimensions of life events that influence psychological distress: an evaluation and synthesis of the Literature. Psychological Stress: Trends and Research, New York: Academic Press.

Yager, J., Grant, I., Sweetwood, H. and Gerst, M. (1981) Life event reports by psychiatric patients, non-patients, and their partners. Archives of General Psychiatry, 38, 343-347.

**Table 10.1** **Individual life events presented by age and sex. Percentage reporting that the event occurred in last 12 months, and percentage rating the event as causing a great deal of change and/or a great deal of stress.**

| Age at HALS2 | | 25-44 | 45-64 | 65+ | All ages | Base numbers | | | |
|---|---|---|---|---|---|---|---|---|---|
| | | | | **Health events** | | | | | |

**Severe illness/handicap developed or got worse**

| | | | | | | | | | |
|---|---|---|---|---|---|---|---|---|---|
| Males: | Occurrence | 6 | 15 | 17 | 12 | 846 | 863 | 577 | 2286 |
| | Great change | 31 | 34 | 44 | 37 | 52 | 125 | 98 | 275 |
| | Great stress | 17 | 24 | 27 | 24 | 52 | 124 | 98 | 274 |
| Females: | Occurrence | 8 | 14 | 20 | 13 | 1163 | 1137 | 738 | 3038 |
| | Great change | 34 | 32 | 46 | 38 | 88 | 160 | 149 | 397 |
| | Great stress | 40 | 37 | 34 | 36 | 87 | 159 | 148 | 394 |

**Serious accident/injury/operation/hospitalization**

| | | | | | | | | | |
|---|---|---|---|---|---|---|---|---|---|
| Males: | Occurrence | 9 | 8 | 11 | 9 | 846 | 860 | 577 | 2283 |
| | Great change | 24 | 31 | 15 | 24 | 79 | 68 | 61 | 208 |
| | Great stress | 18 | 27 | 17 | 21 | 77 | 68 | 59 | 204 |
| Females: | Occurrence | 12 | 10 | 11 | 11 | 1163 | 1136 | 739 | 3038 |
| | Great change | 19 | 26 | 29 | 24 | 138 | 112 | 79 | 329 |
| | Great stress | 21 | 27 | 31 | 26 | 136 | 112 | 77 | 325 |

**Painful or upsetting treatment of condition**

| | | | | | | | | | |
|---|---|---|---|---|---|---|---|---|---|
| Males: | Occurrence | 8 | 11 | 10 | 10 | 844 | 861 | 575 | 2280 |
| | Great change | 25 | 20 | 19 | 21 | 63 | 91 | 57 | 211 |
| | Great stress | 23 | 22 | 16 | 21 | 65 | 90 | 57 | 212 |
| Females: | Occurrence | 9 | 9 | 9 | 9 | 1160 | 1136 | 737 | 3033 |
| | Great change | 20 | 29 | 40 | 28 | 101 | 96 | 63 | 260 |
| | Great stress | 30 | 35 | 38 | 34 | 100 | 96 | 61 | 257 |

**Health problem of family/close friend**

| | | | | | | | | | |
|---|---|---|---|---|---|---|---|---|---|
| Males: | Occurrence | 37 | 37 | 29 | 35 | 845 | 863 | 573 | 2281 |
| | Great change | 18 | 17 | 25 | 19 | 308 | 318 | 166 | 792 |
| | Great stress | 24 | 26 | 27 | 25 | 307 | 317 | 166 | 790 |
| Females: | Occurrence | 40 | 39 | 33 | 38 | 1161 | 1136 | 736 | 3033 |
| | Great change | 20 | 30 | 22 | 24 | 462 | 433 | 236 | 1131 |
| | Great stress | 36 | 42 | 38 | 39 | 455 | 432 | 235 | 1122 |

| Age at HALS2 | | 25-44 | 45-64 | 65+ | All ages | | Base numbers | | | *Table 10.1 continued...* |
|---|---|---|---|---|---|---|---|---|---|---|
| | | | | **Death events** | | | | | | |
| **Death of close family member** | | | | | | | | | | |
| Males: | Occurrence | 15 | 18 | 18 | 17 | 846 | 863 | 576 | 2285 | |
| | Great change | 18 | 22 | 15 | 19 | 128 | 151 | 102 | 381 | |
| | Great stress | 20 | 21 | 18 | 20 | 126 | 151 | 101 | 378 | |
| Females: | Occurrence | 19 | 21 | 19 | 20 | 1162 | 1135 | 738 | 3035 | |
| | Great change | 29 | 28 | 29 | 29 | 222 | 235 | 136 | 593 | |
| | Great stress | 33 | 31 | 33 | 32 | 221 | 231 | 134 | 586 | |
| **Death of close friend** | | | | | | | | | | |
| Males: | Occurrence | 11 | 20 | 23 | 18 | 838 | 855 | 572 | 2265 | |
| | Great change | 10 | 8 | 7 | 8 | 95 | 172 | 128 | 395 | |
| | Great stress | 5 | 9 | 9 | 8 | 94 | 168 | 128 | 390 | |
| Females: | Occurrence | 12 | 19 | 23 | 17 | 1159 | 1131 | 733 | 3023 | |
| | Great change | 16 | 11 | 11 | 12 | 137 | 211 | 170 | 518 | |
| | Great stress | 18 | 16 | 12 | 15 | 134 | 210 | 165 | 509 | |
| | | | | **Work events** | | | | | | |
| **Job change** | | | | | | | | | | |
| Males: | Occurrence | 15 | 8 | 8 | 12 | 800 | 698 | 66 | 1564 | |
| | Great change | 41 | 41 | (40)* | 41 | 120 | 54 | 5 | 179 | |
| | Great stress | 13 | 13 | (20) | 14 | 120 | 53 | 5 | 178 | |
| Females: | Occurrence | 16 | 10 | 5 | 13 | 07 | 721 | 37 | 1448 | |
| | Great change | 28 | 33 | (0) | 29 | 145 | 69 | 2 | 216 | |
| | Great stress | 10 | 15 | (0) | 11 | 145 | 69 | 2 | 216 | |
| **Job loss (actual or pending)** | | | | | | | | | | |
| Males: | Occurrence | 19 | 16 | 10 | 18 | 800 | 698 | 69 | 1567 | |
| | Great change | 28 | 32 | (40) | 29 | 153 | 114 | 5 | 272 | |
| | Great stress | 28 | 24 | (20) | 26 | 153 | 113 | 5 | 271 | |
| Females: | Occurrence | 12 | 13 | 13 | 12 | 908 | 723 | 38 | 1669 | |
| | Great change | 21 | 27 | (0) | 23 | 106 | 94 | 5 | 205 | |
| | Great stress | 18 | 20 | (0) | 19 | 105 | 93 | 5 | 203 | |
| **Job crisis/serious disappointment** | | | | | | | | | | |
| Males: | Occurrence | 11 | 11 | 4 | 11 | 802 | 699 | 67 | 1568 | |
| | Great change | 25 | 23 | (33) | 25 | 87 | 77 | 3 | 167 | |
| | Great stress | 28 | 40 | (67) | 34 | 87 | 75 | 3 | 165 | |
| Females: | Occurrence | 8 | 6 | 10 | 7 | 911 | 722 | 39 | 1672 | |
| | Great change | 28 | 29 | (50) | 29 | 69 | 45 | 4 | 118 | |
| | Great stress | 40 | 42 | (75) | 42 | 68 | 45 | 4 | 117 | |

* Percentages are given in brackets where base numbers are below 20.

*Table 10.1 continued...*

| Age at HALS2 | | 25-44 | 45-64 | 65+ | All ages | Base numbers | | | |
|---|---|---|---|---|---|---|---|---|---|

**Work events cont.**

**Retired**

| | | 25-44 | 45-64 | 65+ | All ages | | | | |
|---|---|---|---|---|---|---|---|---|---|
| Males: | Occurrence | 0 | 5 | 29 | 4 | 800 | 703 | 68 | 1571 |
| | Great change | – | 66 | (53)* | 61 | 0 | 35 | 19 | 54 |
| | Great stress | – | 17 | (5) | 13 | 0 | 36 | 19 | 55 |
| Females: | Occurrence | 1 | 5 | 30 | 3 | 909 | 726 | 43 | 1678 |
| | Great change | (50) | 59 | (46) | 55 | 6 | 39 | 13 | 58 |
| | Great stress | (17) | 16 | (15) | 16 | 6 | 38 | 13 | 57 |

**Partner job crisis/serious disappointment**

| | | | | | | | | | |
|---|---|---|---|---|---|---|---|---|---|
| Males: | Occurrence | 9 | 9 | 2 | 9 | 502 | 510 | 58 | 1070 |
| | Great change | 28 | 25 | (0) | 26 | 46 | 44 | 1 | 91 |
| | Great stress | 24 | 16 | (0) | 20 | 46 | 44 | 1 | 91 |
| Females: | Occurrence | 19 | 15 | 11 | 17 | 887 | 706 | 53 | 1646 |
| | Great change | 42 | 43 | (17) | 42 | 166 | 106 | 6 | 278 |
| | Great stress | 48 | 43 | (17) | 46 | 164 | 106 | 6 | 276 |

**Partner retired**

| | | | | | | | | | |
|---|---|---|---|---|---|---|---|---|---|
| Males: | Occurrence | < 1 | 3 | 4 | 2 | 641 | 723 | 243 | 1607 |
| | Great change | (0) | 17 | (11) | 15 | 1 | 23 | 9 | 33 |
| | Great stress | (100) | 13 | (0) | 12 | 1 | 23 | 9 | 33 |
| Females: | Occurrence | < 1 | 7 | 12 | 4 | 932 | 792 | 82 | 1806 |
| | Great change | (50) | 26 | (9) | 24 | 2 | 53 | 11 | 66 |
| | Great stress | (50) | 13 | (0) | 12 | 2 | 53 | 10 | 65 |

**Housing events**

**Moved house**

| | | | | | | | | | |
|---|---|---|---|---|---|---|---|---|---|
| Males: | Occurrence | 10 | 2 | 3 | 5 | 845 | 863 | 577 | 2285 |
| | Great change | 26 | 30 | (29) | 27 | 77 | 20 | 14 | 111 |
| | Great stress | 12 | 5 | (15) | 11 | 77 | 20 | 13 | 110 |
| Females: | Occurrence | 9 | 3 | 4 | 6 | 1163 | 1137 | 739 | 3039 |
| | Great change | 37 | 48 | 41 | 40 | 102 | 31 | 27 | 160 |
| | Great stress | 21 | 23 | 15 | 21 | 103 | 31 | 26 | 160 |

**Moved to new area**

| | | | | | | | | | |
|---|---|---|---|---|---|---|---|---|---|
| Males: | Occurrence | 17 | 33 | (25) | 21 | 81 | 21 | 16 | 118 |
| | Great change | (9) | (33) | (0) | 15 | 11 | 6 | 3 | 20 |
| | Great stress | (10) | (17) | (0) | 11 | 10 | 6 | 3 | 19 |
| Females: | Occurrence | 34 | 36 | 30 | 33 | 107 | 31 | 30 | 168 |
| | Great change | 25 | (54) | (33) | 32 | 36 | 11 | 9 | 56 |
| | Great stress | 14 | (46) | (22) | 22 | 35 | 11 | 9 | 55 |

* Percentages are given in brackets where base numbers are below 20.

*Table 10.1 continued...*

| Age at HALS2 | | 25-44 | 45-64 | 65+ | All ages | Base numbers | | | |
|---|---|---|---|---|---|---|---|---|---|
| | | | | Housing events cont. | | | | | |

**Worry about housing**

| | | | | | | | | | |
|---|---|---|---|---|---|---|---|---|---|
| Males: | Occurrence | 11 | 7 | 7 | 8 | 841 | 863 | 575 | 2279 |
| | Great change | 30 | 34 | 24 | 30 | 89 | 62 | 37 | 188 |
| | Great stress | 34 | 40 | 38 | 37 | 89 | 62 | 37 | 188 |
| Females: | Occurrence | 12 | 9 | 9 | 10 | 1157 | 1134 | 736 | 3027 |
| | Great change | 31 | 31 | 29 | 31 | 142 | 98 | 68 | 308 |
| | Great stress | 45 | 47 | 40 | 45 | 141 | 98 | 68 | 307 |

**Family member left home/new person moved in**

| | | | | | | | | | |
|---|---|---|---|---|---|---|---|---|---|
| Males: | Occurrence | 10 | 17 | 4 | 11 | 840 | 858 | 577 | 2275 |
| | Great change | 40 | 17 | 29 | 26 | 80 | 140 | 21 | 241 |
| | Great stress | 17 | 7 | 14 | 11 | 78 | 139 | 21 | 238 |
| Females: | Occurrence | 12 | 16 | 1 | 11 | 1160 | 1136 | 738 | 3034 |
| | Great change | 25 | 23 | (33)* | 24 | 143 | 180 | 9 | 332 |
| | Great stress | 16 | 16 | (11) | 16 | 142 | 178 | 9 | 329 |

**Relationships**

**Divorced/separated**

| | | | | | | | | | |
|---|---|---|---|---|---|---|---|---|---|
| Males: | Occurrence | 4 | 1 | <1 | 2 | 704 | 820 | 551 | 2075 |
| | Great change | 80 | (50) | (100) | 74 | 25 | 8 | 1 | 34 |
| | Great stress | 44 | (38) | (100) | 44 | 25 | 8 | 1 | 34 |
| Females: | Occurrence | 4 | 1 | 0 | 2 | 164 | 1099 | 683 | 2846 |
| | Great change | 81 | (46) | – | 73 | 42 | 13 | 0 | 55 |
| | Great stress | 64 | (69) | – | 66 | 42 | 13 | 0 | 55 |

**Serious disagreements with partner/felt betrayed or disappointed by partner**

| | | | | | | | | | |
|---|---|---|---|---|---|---|---|---|---|
| Males: | Occurrence | 10 | 4 | 1 | 5 | 702 | 818 | 548 | 2068 |
| | Great change | 34 | 23 | (0) | 29 | 67 | 35 | 4 | 106 |
| | Great stress | 37 | 26 | (25) | 33 | 67 | 35 | 4 | 106 |
| Females: | Occurrence | 12 | 6 | 2 | 7 | 1063 | 1098 | 683 | 2844 |
| | Great change | 39 | 37 | (15) | 37 | 129 | 65 | 13 | 207 |
| | Great stress | 47 | 54 | (23) | 48 | 126 | 65 | 13 | 204 |

**Serious difficulty with children**

| | | | | | | | | | |
|---|---|---|---|---|---|---|---|---|---|
| Males: | Occurrence | 17 | 16 | 9 | 15 | 575 | 754 | 465 | 1794 |
| | Great change | 30 | 20 | 29 | 25 | 99 | 121 | 42 | 262 |
| | Great stress | 35 | 35 | 48 | 37 | 99 | 120 | 42 | 261 |
| Females: | Occurrence | 26 | 23 | 10 | 21 | 926 | 1031 | 595 | 2552 |
| | Great change | 33 | 27 | 21 | 29 | 231 | 233 | 58 | 522 |
| | Great stress | 51 | 54 | 48 | 52 | 231 | 233 | 59 | 523 |

* Percentages are given in brackets where base numbers are below 20.

| Age at HALS2 | | 25-44 | 45-64 | 65+ | All ages | Base numbers | | | |
|---|---|---|---|---|---|---|---|---|---|
| | | | | **Relationships (cont.)** | | | | | |

**Serious difficulty with friend or relative/felt betrayed**

| | | 25-44 | 45-64 | 65+ | All ages | | | | |
|---|---|---|---|---|---|---|---|---|---|
| Males: | Occurrence | 11 | 7 | 3 | 8 | 844 | 862 | 576 | 2282 |
| | Great change | 22 | 21 | (29)* | 22 | 94 | 63 | 14 | 171 |
| | Great stress | 27 | 22 | (23) | 25 | 90 | 64 | 13 | 167 |
| Females: | Occurrence | 15 | 9 | 3 | 10 | 1159 | 1134 | 738 | 3031 |
| | Great change | 23 | 28 | 18 | 24 | 171 | 95 | 22 | 288 |
| | Great stress | 31 | 38 | 36 | 34 | 169 | 95 | 22 | 286 |

**Lost contact with close family/friend**

| | | 25-44 | 45-64 | 65+ | All ages | | | | |
|---|---|---|---|---|---|---|---|---|---|
| Males: | Occurrence | 12 | 7 | 5 | 8 | 845 | 861 | 576 | 2282 |
| | Great change | 7 | 7 | 18 | 9 | 102 | 58 | 28 | 188 |
| | Great stress | 5 | 9 | 21 | 9 | 99 | 58 | 28 | 185 |
| Females: | Occurrence | 11 | 7 | 4 | 8 | 1159 | 1133 | 736 | 3028 |
| | Great change | 11 | 16 | 19 | 14 | 126 | 73 | 32 | 231 |
| | Great stress | 11 | 25 | 25 | 18 | 125 | 72 | 32 | 229 |

**Social problems**

**Assault/robbery**

| | | 25-44 | 45-64 | 65+ | All ages | | | | |
|---|---|---|---|---|---|---|---|---|---|
| Males: | Occurrence | 9 | 6 | 2 | 6 | 846 | 863 | 577 | 2286 |
| | Great change | 12 | 17 | (17) | 14 | 74 | 54 | 12 | 140 |
| | Great stress | 16 | 17 | (25) | 17 | 74 | 54 | 12 | 140 |
| Females: | Occurrence | 7 | 6 | 4 | 6 | 1163 | 1137 | 738 | 3038 |
| | Great change | 30 | 22 | 10 | 24 | 78 | 63 | 29 | 170 |
| | Great stress | 36 | 27 | 28 | 31 | 78 | 62 | 29 | 169 |

**Major financial problems**

| | | 25-44 | 45-64 | 65+ | All ages | | | | |
|---|---|---|---|---|---|---|---|---|---|
| Males: | Occurrence | 14 | 10 | 2 | 9 | 846 | 863 | 577 | 2286 |
| | Great change | 33 | 33 | (29) | 32 | 119 | 83 | 14 | 216 |
| | Great stress | 36 | 42 | (50) | 39 | 118 | 83 | 14 | 215 |
| Females: | Occurrence | 16 | 10 | 4 | 11 | 1161 | 1136 | 736 | 3033 |
| | Great change | 43 | 41 | 14 | 40 | 180 | 116 | 28 | 324 |
| | Great stress | 54 | 50 | 29 | 50 | 179 | 115 | 28 | 322 |

**Serious problems with officials/the law**

| | | 25-44 | 45-64 | 65+ | All ages | | | | |
|---|---|---|---|---|---|---|---|---|---|
| Males: | Occurrence | 6 | 3 | 2 | 4 | 846 | 863 | 577 | 2286 |
| | Great change | 23 | 21 | (15) | 22 | 47 | 28 | 13 | 88 |
| | Great stress | 35 | 38 | (15) | 33 | 46 | 29 | 13 | 88 |
| Females: | Occurrence | 5 | 3 | 1 | 3 | 1163 | 1137 | 736 | 3036 |
| | Great change | 26 | 31 | (22) | 27 | 54 | 32 | 9 | 95 |
| | Great stress | 48 | 52 | (44) | 49 | 54 | 31 | 9 | 94 |

* Percentages are given in brackets when base numbers are below 20

**Table 10.2    Mean number of adverse life events in the last year and ratings of change and stress presented by age and sex**

| | Mean numbers of events (±SEM) | Percentage causing some change | Percentage causing great change | Percentage causing some stress | Percentage causing great stress | Base numbers |
|---|---|---|---|---|---|---|
| | | | **Males** | | | |
| **Age at HALS2** | | | | | | |
| **25-44** | 2.4 (±0.1) | 33 | 25 | 41 | 23 | 849 |
| **45-64** | 2.3 (±0.1) | 34 | 23 | 40 | 22 | 867 |
| **65+** | 1.5 (±0.1) | 31 | 22 | 34 | 22 | 584 |
| **All ages** | 2.2 (< ±0.1) | 33 | 23 | 39 | 22 | 2300 |
| | | | **Females** | | | |
| **25-44** | 2.7 (±0.1) | 37 | 28 | 41 | 33 | 1167 |
| **45-64** | 2.4 (±0.1) | 36 | 29 | 38 | 34 | 1137 |
| **65+** | 1.6 (±0.1) | 31 | 26 | 40 | 30 | 748 |
| **All ages** | 2.3 (< ±0.1) | 35 | 28 | 39 | 33 | 3052 |

**Table 10.3**   Comparison of one-year and seven-year life event frequencies and subjective ratings. Percentage reporting that event occurred in the last year or in the last 7 years (when no event in last year). Percentage reporting that event (i) caused great change/still affects their life a great deal; (ii) caused/still causes a great deal of stress.

| | Occurrence | | Change | | Stress | | Base numbers | | | |
|---|---|---|---|---|---|---|---|---|---|---|
| | Last year | Last 7 years (not in last year) | Great change (1 year) | Still affects life (7 years) | Great stress (1 year) | Still causes stress (7 years) | Occurrence | | change/stress | |

**Health events**

**Severe illness/handicap developed or got worse**

| | | | | | | | | | | |
|---|---|---|---|---|---|---|---|---|---|---|
| Males: | 12 | 15 | 37 | 26 | 24 | 9 | 2286 | 2006 | 274 | 300 |
| Females: | 13 | 16 | 38 | 23 | 36 | 10 | 3038 | 2634 | 394 | 420 |

**Serious accident/injury/operation/hospitalization**

| | | | | | | | | | | |
|---|---|---|---|---|---|---|---|---|---|---|
| Males: | 9 | 21 | 24 | 10 | 21 | 4 | 2283 | 2071 | 204 | 434 |
| Females: | 11 | 27 | 24 | 9 | 26 | 5 | 3038 | 2695 | 325 | 721 |

**Death events**

**Death of close family member**

| | | | | | | | | | | |
|---|---|---|---|---|---|---|---|---|---|---|
| Males: | 17 | 47 | 19 | 6 | 20 | 4 | 2285 | 1898 | 378 | 878 |
| Females: | 20 | 50 | 29 | 10 | 32 | 7 | 3035 | 2428 | 586 | 1194 |

**Death of close friend**

| | | | | | | | | | | |
|---|---|---|---|---|---|---|---|---|---|---|
| Males: | 18 | 27 | 8 | 2 | 8 | 1 | 2265 | 1848 | 390 | 489 |
| Females: | 17 | 26 | 12 | 4 | 15 | 3 | 3023 | 2485 | 509 | 639 |

**Work events**

**Job change**

| | | | | | | | | | | |
|---|---|---|---|---|---|---|---|---|---|---|
| Male: | 12 | 34 | 41 | 23 | 14 | 6 | 1564 | 1629 | 178 | 549 |
| Female: | 13 | 41 | 29 | 12 | 11 | 2 | 1448 | 1798 | 216 | 721 |

**Job loss (actual or pending)**

| | | | | | | | | | | |
|---|---|---|---|---|---|---|---|---|---|---|
| Male: | 18 | 17 | 29 | 17 | 26 | 8 | 1567 | 1532 | 271 | 251 |
| Female: | 12 | 9 | 23 | 5 | 19 | 5 | 1669 | 1796 | 203 | 166 |

**Job crisis/serious disappointment**

| | | | | | | | | | | |
|---|---|---|---|---|---|---|---|---|---|---|
| Male: | 11 | 10 | 25 | 13 | 34 | 7 | 1568 | 1636 | 165 | 169 |
| Female: | 7 | 7 | 29 | 8 | 42 | 5 | 1672 | 1881 | 117 | 127 |

**Retired**

| | | | | | | | | | | |
|---|---|---|---|---|---|---|---|---|---|---|
| Male: | 4 | 12 | 61 | 28 | 13 | 3 | 1571 | 1773 | 54 | 201 |
| Female: | 3 | 11 | 55 | 24 | 16 | 2 | 1678 | 1981 | 57 | 203 |

| | Occurrence | | Change | | Stress | | Base numbers | | | |
|---|---|---|---|---|---|---|---|---|---|---|
| | Last year | Last 7 years (not in last year) | Great change (1 year) | Still affects life (7 years) | Great stress (1 year) | Still causes strees (7 years) | Occurence | | change/stress | |

### Work events cont.

**Partner job crisis/serious disappointment**

| | | | | | | | | | | |
|---|---|---|---|---|---|---|---|---|---|---|
| Male: | 9 | 8 | 26 | 7 | 20 | 6 | 1070 | 1187 | 91 | 94 |
| Female: | 17 | 19 | 42 | 14 | 46 | 11 | 1646 | 1592 | 276 | 297 |

**Partner retired**

| | | | | | | | | | | |
|---|---|---|---|---|---|---|---|---|---|---|
| Male: | 2 | 6 | 15 | 10 | 12 | 2 | 1607 | 1633 | 33 | 101 |
| Female: | 4 | 11 | 24 | 24 | 12 | 4 | 1806 | 1891 | 65 | 205 |

### Relationships

**Divorced/separated**

| | | | | | | | | | | |
|---|---|---|---|---|---|---|---|---|---|---|
| Male: | 2 | 5 | 74 | 15 | 44 | 12 | 2075 | 2041 | 34 | 96 |
| Female: | 2 | 6 | 73 | 10 | 66 | 9 | 2846 | 2789 | 55 | 156 |

### Social problems

**Assault/robbery**

| | | | | | | | | | | |
|---|---|---|---|---|---|---|---|---|---|---|
| Male: | 6 | 10 | 14 | 2 | 17 | 2 | 2286 | 2135 | 140 | 210 |
| Female: | 6 | 10 | 24 | 6 | 31 | 7 | 3038 | 2842 | 169 | 292 |

**Major financial problems**

| | | | | | | | | | | |
|---|---|---|---|---|---|---|---|---|---|---|
| Male: | 9 | 5 | 32 | 9 | 39 | 5 | 2286 | 2060 | 215 | 101 |
| Female: | 11 | 5 | 40 | 7 | 50 | 8 | 3033 | 2694 | 322 | 132 |

**Serious problems with officials/the law**

| | | | | | | | | | | |
|---|---|---|---|---|---|---|---|---|---|---|
| Male: | 4 | 3 | 22 | 7 | 33 | 7 | 2286 | 2187 | 88 | 71 |
| Female: | 3 | 2 | 27 | 7 | 49 | 11 | 3036 | 2915 | 94 | 46 |

**Table 10.4    Positive life events by age and sex. Percentage reporting a nice event in the last year or in the last seven years**

| | Time of event | | | | Base numbers | | | |
|---|---|---|---|---|---|---|---|---|
| | Last year | Last 7 years (not in last year) | Last year | Last 7 years (not in last year) | Males | | Females | |
| | Males | | Females | | | | | |

**Age at HALS2**

| | | | | | | | | |
|---|---|---|---|---|---|---|---|---|
| **25-44** | 48 | 55 | 46 | 52 | 849 | 444 | 1166 | 632 |
| **45-64** | 46 | 43 | 52 | 49 | 865 | 464 | 1137 | 549 |
| **65+** | 35 | 32 | 44 | 41 | 579 | 373 | 742 | 418 |
| **All ages** | 44 | 44 | 47 | 48 | 2293 | 1281 | 3045 | 1599 |

**Table 10.5** Positive life events by socio-economic group at HALS1. Percentage reporting at least one nice event in the last year

| | Manual | Non-manual | Manual | Non-manual | Base numbers | | | |
|---|---|---|---|---|---|---|---|---|
| | Males | | Females | | Males | | Females | |
| **Age at HALS2** | | | | | | | | |
| **25-44** | 44 | 53 | 42 | 49 | 482 | 339 | 620 | 526 |
| **45-64** | 41 | 52 | 50 | 53 | 460 | 404 | 558 | 566 |
| **65+** | 32 | 39 | 40 | 48 | 340 | 236 | 421 | 311 |
| **All ages** | 40 | 49 | 45 | 50 | 1282 | 979 | 1599 | 1403 |

**Table 10.6** Category of life events by socio-economic group (manual, non-manual) at HALS1. Percentage reporting that at least one adverse event occurred in the category in the last year, and percentage of events reported as causing great changes and/or great stress.

| Age at HALS1 | | 25-44 | | 45-64 | | 65+ | | All ages | | Base numbers | | | | | |
|---|---|---|---|---|---|---|---|---|---|---|---|---|---|---|---|
| | | M | NM | M | NM | M | NM | M | NM | (omitting those for all ages) | | | | | |
| **Health** | | | | | | | | | | | | | | | |
| Males: | Occurrence | 47 | 45 | 55 | 47 | 50 | 49 | 51 | 47 | 480 | 339 | 458 | 404 | 337 | 237 |
| | Great change | 23 | 17 | 28 | 20 | 34 | 28 | 28 | 21 | 224 | 150 | 249 | 190 | 166 | 115 |
| | Great stress | 25 | 22 | 28 | 26 | 31 | 23 | 28 | 24 | 223 | 150 | 248 | 190 | 165 | 115 |
| Females: | Occurrence | 50 | 53 | 54 | 51 | 53 | 50 | 52 | 52 | 618 | 525 | 558 | 566 | 418 | 311 |
| | Great change | 26 | 21 | 36 | 30 | 36 | 34 | 32 | 27 | 312 | 281 | 299 | 284 | 217 | 156 |
| | Great stress | 38 | 36 | 42 | 41 | 43 | 33 | 41 | 37 | 310 | 273 | 299 | 283 | 215 | 153 |
| **Death** | | | | | | | | | | | | | | | |
| Males: | Occurrence | 25 | 20 | 33 | 33 | 32 | 37 | 30 | 30 | 480 | 339 | 458 | 404 | 337 | 237 |
| | Great change | 13 | 18 | 15 | 13 | 17 | 7 | 15 | 13 | 122 | 68 | 150 | 133 | 108 | 87 |
| | Great stress | 12 | 18 | 17 | 12 | 19 | 7 | 16 | 12 | 120 | 67 | 149 | 130 | 108 | 87 |
| Females: | Occurrence | 30 | 25 | 37 | 33 | 38 | 34 | 34 | 30 | 618 | 525 | 558 | 566 | 418 | 310 |
| | Great change | 25 | 24 | 19 | 24 | 19 | 21 | 21 | 23 | 183 | 131 | 205 | 187 | 159 | 105 |
| | Great stress | 25 | 29 | 25 | 25 | 21 | 23 | 24 | 26 | 181 | 129 | 204 | 185 | 155 | 104 |
| **Work** | | | | | | | | | | | | | | | |
| Males: | Occurrence | 32 | 39 | 28 | 34 | 4 | 8 | 24 | 29 | 481 | 339 | 458 | 404 | 337 | 237 |
| | Great change | 32 | 35 | 34 | 35 | (57)* | (39) | 34 | 35 | 155 | 133 | 129 | 133 | 14 | 18 |
| | Great stress | 26 | 26 | 22 | 26 | (14) | (17) | 24 | 25 | 155 | 133 | 128 | 132 | 14 | 18 |
| Females: | Occurrence | 31 | 33 | 27 | 27 | 4 | 4 | 23 | 24 | 618 | 525 | 558 | 566 | 418 | 311 |
| | Great change | 30 | 38 | 37 | 39 | (26) | (29) | 33 | 38 | 192 | 172 | 150 | 153 | 19 | 17 |
| | Great stress | 28 | 34 | 26 | 31 | (28) | (6) | 27 | 31 | 190 | 171 | 150 | 153 | 18 | 17 |

| Age at HALS1 | | 25-44 | | 45-64 | | 65+ | | All ages | | Base numbers | | | | | |
|---|---|---|---|---|---|---|---|---|---|---|---|---|---|---|---|
| | | M | NM | M | NM | M | NM | M | NM | (omitting those for all ages) | | | | | |
| **Housing** | | | | | | | | | | | | | | | |
| Males: | Occurrence | 24 | 24 | 22 | 26 | 11 | 14 | 20 | 22 | 479 | 339 | 458 | 404 | 337 | 237 |
| | Great change | 34 | 32 | 27 | 18 | 33 | 22 | 31 | 24 | 117 | 77 | 99 | 103 | 36 | 32 |
| | Great stress | 23 | 22 | 18 | 15 | 37 | 19 | 23 | 18 | 115 | 78 | 99 | 102 | 35 | 32 |
| Females: | Occurrence | 27 | 28 | 23 | 25 | 13 | 13 | 22 | 24 | 618 | 525 | 558 | 566 | 418 | 311 |
| | Great change | 30 | 41 | 31 | 25 | 37 | 32 | 31 | 33 | 164 | 145 | 127 | 143 | 54 | 41 |
| | Great stress | 30 | 32 | 30 | 23 | 36 | 32 | 31 | 28 | 162 | 145 | 127 | 141 | 53 | 41 |
| **Relationships** | | | | | | | | | | | | | | | |
| Males: | Occurrence | 32 | 30 | 27 | 23 | 12 | 13 | 25 | 23 | 481 | 339 | 458 | 404 | 337 | 237 |
| | Great change | 31 | 24 | 12 | 27 | 30 | 19 | 24 | 25 | 154 | 100 | 122 | 93 | 43 | 31 |
| | Great stress | 32 | 28 | 25 | 30 | 39 | 33 | 31 | 30 | 153 | 99 | 122 | 92 | 43 | 30 |
| Females: | Occurrence | 43 | 38 | 32 | 30 | 16 | 14 | 32 | 29 | 618 | 525 | 558 | 566 | 418 | 311 |
| | Great change | 34 | 30 | 27 | 26 | 23 | 19 | 30 | 28 | 260 | 197 | 176 | 171 | 66 | 41 |
| | Great stress | 43 | 39 | 48 | 52 | 42 | 38 | 45 | 44 | 259 | 195 | 176 | 170 | 66 | 42 |
| **Social problems** | | | | | | | | | | | | | | | |
| Males: | Occurrence | 25 | 21 | 15 | 18 | 6 | 7 | 16 | 16 | 480 | 339 | 458 | 404 | 337 | 237 |
| | Great change | 26 | 24 | 28 | 29 | (16) | (23) | 26 | 26 | 118 | 72 | 68 | 70 | 19 | 17 |
| | Great stress | 29 | 28 | 32 | 37 | (21) | (41) | 30 | 33 | 116 | 72 | 68 | 71 | 19 | 17 |
| Females: | Occurrence | 24 | 21 | 16 | 16 | 7 | 12 | 17 | 17 | 618 | 525 | 558 | 566 | 417 | 311 |
| | Great change | 38 | 37 | 32 | 30 | 21 | 8 | 34 | 30 | 148 | 113 | 91 | 91 | 29 | 36 |
| | Great stress | 49 | 50 | 46 | 36 | 41 | 19 | 47 | 40 | 148 | 112 | 90 | 89 | 29 | 36 |

* Percentages are given in brackets when base numbers are less than 20

M = Manual, NM = Non-manual

**Table 10.7**    **Categories of life events presented by socio-economic group and residential neighbourhood. Percentages reporting at least one event in given event category**

| | Type of neighbourhood | | | | |
| | High-rise development | Built-up area No open space | Built-up area with open space | Country district | All types |
|---|---|---|---|---|---|
| **Category of event** | | | | | |
| **Health:** | | | | | |
| Manual | 60 | 50 | 53 | 50 | 52 |
| Non-manual | 44 | 51 | 50 | 47 | 50 |
| **Death:** | | | | | |
| Manual | 41 | 34 | 31 | 30 | 32 |
| Non-manual | 48 | 29 | 31 | 29 | 30 |
| **Work:** | | | | | |
| Manual | 24 | 22 | 25 | 19 | 23 |
| Non-manual | 20 | 27 | 27 | 26 | 27 |
| **House:** | | | | | |
| Manual | 33 | 22 | 21 | 17 | 21 |
| Non-manual | 8 | 26 | 22 | 23 | 23 |
| **Relationships:** | | | | | |
| Manual | 23 | 30 | 31 | 23 | 29 |
| Non-manual | 32 | 28 | 27 | 25 | 27 |
| **Social problems:** | | | | | |
| Manual | 26 | 20 | 16 | 12 | 17 |
| Non-manual | 28 | 18 | 14 | 21 | 17 |
| *Base numbers* | | | | | |
| *Manual* | *70* | *805* | *1495* | *451* | *2825* |
| *Non-manual* | *25* | *500* | *1294* | *523* | *2354* |

**Table 10.8**     **Relationship between life events and illness symptoms at HALS2. Percentages reporting 4+ illness symptoms**

|  | Number of life events in the last year | | | | Base Numbers | | | |
|---|---|---|---|---|---|---|---|---|
|  | None | One | Two or Three | Four or More |  | | | |
| **Age at HALS2** |  |  | Males | | | | | |
| **25-44** | 8 | 9 | 15 | 28 | 174 | 204 | 280 | 191 |
| **45-64** | 12 | 21 | 24 | 33 | 197 | 226 | 291 | 153 |
| **65+** | 23 | 28 | 31 | 37 | 215 | 200 | 134 | 35 |
| **All ages** | 15 | 19 | 22 | 31 | 586 | 630 | 705 | 379 |
|  |  | | Females | | | | | |
| **25-44** | 15 | 21 | 22 | 36 | 206 | 257 | 404 | 300 |
| **45-64** | 29 | 28 | 34 | 49 | 216 | 286 | 434 | 201 |
| **65+** | 30 | 45 | 52 | 42 | 250 | 240 | 225 | 33 |
| **All ages** | 23 | 30 | 30 | 37 | 667 | 783 | 1063 | 534 |

**Table 10.9** **Development of health condition since HALS1 presented by total number of adverse events experienced between the Surveys. Percentage of respondents free of these conditions at HALS1 who developed the condition by HALS2 (multiple conditions allowed)**

| Age at HALS1 | 18-39 | | | 40-64 | | | 18-39 | 40-64 |
|---|---|---|---|---|---|---|---|---|
| | Number of events | | | | | | | |
| | Up to one | Two or three | Four or more | Up to one | Two or three | Four or more | Numbers developing the condition | |
| **Health condition** | | | | **Males** | | | | |
| Asthma | 1 | 1 | 3 | – | 2 | 5 | 9 | 10 |
| Bronchitis and other chest | 10 | 7 | 11 | 11 | 13 | 11 | 49 | 44 |
| Rheumatism and arthritis | 11 | 10 | 7 | 19 | 15 | 15 | 45 | 61 |
| High blood pressure | 6 | 5 | 7 | 15 | 11 | 12 | 31 | 47 |
| Heart Trouble | 2 | 2 | 2 | 2 | 7 | 11 | 10 | 27 |
| Depression | – | 3 | 5 | 4 | 3 | 10 | 19 | 21 |
| Migraine | 5 | 7 | 7 | 8 | 6 | 10 | 35 | 30 |
| | | | | **Females** | | | | |
| Asthma | – | 3 | 5 | 4 | 4 | 2 | 19 | 10 |
| Bronchitis and other chest | 7 | 11 | 13 | 7 | 11 | 15 | 64 | 39 |
| Rheumatism and arthritis | 5 | 9 | 9 | 17 | 27 | 31 | 46 | 89 |
| High blood pressure | 6 | 9 | 9 | 13 | 15 | 10 | 46 | 42 |
| Heart Trouble | – | 2 | 1 | 7 | 6 | 6 | 7 | 20 |
| Depression | 6 | 10 | 16 | 11 | 12 | 9 | 67 | 35 |
| Migraine | 7 | 15 | 20 | 7 | 9 | 14 | 90 | 36 |
| *Base numbers* | | | | | | | | |
| *Males* | *95* | *183* | *246* | *94* | *157* | *131* | | |
| *Females* | *83* | *211* | *261* | *75* | *138* | *126* | | |

**Table 10.10**  Relationship between adverse life events in the last year and psychiatric symptoms at HALS2. Percentage scoring 5+ on the General Health Questionnaire (GHQ)

| Age at HALS2 | Number of life events | | | | Base numbers | | | |
|---|---|---|---|---|---|---|---|---|
| | 0 events | 1 event | 2-3 events | 4+ events | | | | |
| *Males* | | | | | | | | |
| 25-44 | 17 | 16 | 28 | 42 | 97 | 127 | 196 | 144 |
| 45-64 | 9 | 20 | 28 | 50 | 115 | 144 | 229 | 162 |
| 65+ | 14 | 16 | 34 | 33 | 118 | 142 | 140 | 49 |
| All ages | 13 | 17 | 29 | 45 | 330 | 413 | 565 | 355 |
| *Females* | | | | | | | | |
| 25-44 | 24 | 22 | 28 | 43 | 134 | 169 | 288 | 256 |
| 45-64 | 15 | 24 | 29 | 47 | 123 | 194 | 324 | 206 |
| 65+ | 22 | 26 | 36 | 52 | 121 | 136 | 165 | 65 |
| All ages | 21 | 24 | 30 | 46 | 378 | 499 | 777 | 527 |

**Table 10.11**  Relationship between stressful life events and psychiatric symptoms at HALS2. Percentage scoring 5+ on the General Health Questionnaire

| Age at HALS2 | Number of stressful events | | | | | Base numbers | | | | |
|---|---|---|---|---|---|---|---|---|---|---|
| | No events | Event but no great stress | One great stress event | Two great stress events | More than two great stress events | | | | | |
| *Males* | | | | | | | | | | |
| 25-44 | 17 | 22 | 38 | 40 | 60 | 97 | 316 | 66 | 40 | 45 |
| 45-64 | 9 | 22 | 42 | 54 | 74 | 115 | 350 | 100 | 43 | 42 |
| 65+ | 14 | 19 | 44 | 39 | (69)* | 118 | 243 | 52 | 23 | 13 |
| All ages | 13 | 21 | 41 | 45 | 67 | 330 | 909 | 218 | 106 | 100 |
| *Females* | | | | | | | | | | |
| 25-44 | 24 | 19 | 38 | 45 | 58 | 134 | 371 | 157 | 84 | 101 |
| 45-64 | 15 | 21 | 40 | 38 | 64 | 123 | 382 | 163 | 95 | 84 |
| 65+ | 22 | 24 | 38 | 67 | 64 | 121 | 211 | 85 | 45 | 25 |
| All ages | 21 | 21 | 39 | 46 | 61 | 378 | 964 | 405 | 224 | 210 |

* Percentage given in brackets as base number is less than 20

**Table 10.12**   **Relationship between psychiatric symptoms at HALS2 and adverse life events and positive events in the last 12 months. Percentage scoring 5+ on the General Health Questionnaire**

| | | Number of adverse events | | | | Base numbers | | | |
| | | 0-3 events | 4+ events | 0-3 events | 4+ events | Males | | Females | |
| | | Males | | Females | | | | | |
| **Age at HALS2** | | | | | | | | | |
| 25-44 | Positive event | 24 | 40 | 25 | 42 | 187 | 80 | 235 | 151 |
| | No positive event | 20 | 45 | 25 | 45 | 233 | 64 | 355 | 105 |
| 45-64 | Positive event | 21 | 46 | 22 | 42 | 217 | 82 | 339 | 110 |
| | No positive event | 20 | 54 | 27 | 52 | 270 | 80 | 302 | 96 |
| 65+ | Positive event | 26 | 21 | 26 | 48 | 144 | 28 | 186 | 40 |
| | No positive event | 20 | 48 | 30 | 60 | 255 | 21 | 234 | 25 |
| All ages | Positive event | 23 | 40 | 24 | 43 | 548 | 190 | 760 | 301 |
| | No positive event | 20 | 50 | 27 | 50 | 758 | 165 | 891 | 226 |

**Table 10.13**   **Relationship between adverse life events in the last year, psychiatric symptoms and perceived social support (PSS) at HALS2. Percentage scoring 5+ on the General Health Questionnaire**

| | | Number of adverse events | | | | Base Numbers | | | |
| | | 0-3 events | 4+ events | 0-3 events | 4+ events | Males | | Females | |
| | | Males | | Females | | | | | |
| **Age at HALS2** | **PSS** | | | | | | | | |
| 25-44 | Low | 23 | (36)* | 39 | 52 | 22 | 14 | 41 | 33 |
| | Medium | 18 | 48 | 25 | 34 | 124 | 52 | 122 | 68 |
| | High | 23 | 40 | 24 | 45 | 272 | 77 | 425 | 155 |
| 45-64 | Low | 32 | (67) | 48 | 60 | 47 | 15 | 40 | 20 |
| | Medium | 26 | 47 | 24 | 52 | 124 | 47 | 123 | 50 |
| | High | 19 | 49 | 23 | 43 | 313 | 100 | 473 | 134 |
| 65+ | Low | 31 | (50) | 46 | (71) | 42 | 4 | 26 | 7 |
| | Medium | 25 | (36) | 39 | (71) | 100 | 11 | 84 | 14 |
| | High | 19 | 29 | 24 | 41 | 253 | 34 | 303 | 42 |
| All ages | Low | 30 | 52 | 44 | 57 | 111 | 33 | 107 | 60 |
| | Medium | 22 | 46 | 28 | 45 | 348 | 110 | 329 | 132 |
| | High | 20 | 43 | 23 | 44 | 838 | 211 | 1201 | 331 |

* Percentages given in brackets when base numbers are less than 20

# LIFESTYLE

# CHANGES IN DIETARY HABITS

# 11

Margaret J Whichelow

The questions asked of respondents in the HALS2 Survey about their dietary habits were identical to those used in the first Survey, so that direct comparisons of behaviour can be made between the two. A few items, mainly of convenience foods, were added to the list of foods where the frequency of consumption was recorded (See Appendix C, Q.58) but the responses are not reported in this chapter. Respondents were also asked whether they thought they had changed their diet in the previous seven years and, if so, why. The aims of this chapter are, as in the report of the first Survey (Whichelow 1987;), to describe aspects of eating habits where there appeared to be differences between groups of individuals of different ages, sex, social class or regions of residence and, of more importance in this report, the changes that have occurred between the two Surveys. The wealth of information provided by the Survey dictates that much information has had to be omitted from this overview.

In a survey of this nature it was impossible to assess the amount of any particular food eaten by individual respondents, or the nutrient intake of individuals or groups. This could only have been done by weighing the food consumed over a period of days or by detailed dietary diaries and comparing food portions with food models or photographs. However, the results of the questions about frequency of consumption of food items do give an indication of which groups are eating more or less of any item.

The questions which assessed knowledge of the fibre content of the diet were included because of the current advice to the British population to increase dietary fibre intake. This question is to be found in the 'Measurements' section of Appendix C, as it served a second purpose in the Surveys. It was also used for a memory test as part of the cognitive functioning assessment.

In this chapter only the results at HALS1 and HALS2 for the 5352 respondents interviewed in both Surveys are presented, although analyses of the whole 9003 HALS1 sample have also been made. The values for the whole 9003 HALS1 sample for the Tables where 7 age groups are presented are similar to these of the 5352 sub-sample at HALS1, except in some cases for those over 73 years, so that the HALS2 sub-sample can be taken as representative of the whole sample at that age.

## Medical diets

The number of respondents reporting being 'on a diet', the medical reason for this and the types of diet prescribed are set out in Table 11.1. Although as a percentage of the survey population the proportion on prescribed diets was small in both surveys, for some conditions the number of subjects on diets has increased markedly between HALS1 and HALS2. Obesity, diabetes and hypercholesterolaemia in both sexes and hypertension or heart disease in women are all conditions where the numbers in HALS2 are greater. These changes are too large to be explained solely on the basis that the survey population is seven years older than at HALS1. Since 1984/5 there has been an increase in 'well person clinics', and GPs are now encouraged to measure blood pressure and cholesterol levels. Greater awareness of preventative measures may therefore account for these increased numbers on diets. The increased number of anti-diabetic diets reflects the much higher prevalence of diabetes now than in 1984/5 (see Chapter 4). The mean body mass index has been shown to have increased (see Chapter 6), which may have led to more respondents being recommended to control their food intake.

There have also been changes in the types of diet reported. Low fat diets have become more popular, as have high fibre, low sugar and, to a lesser extent, low salt diets: low carbohydrate diets, on the other hand, are not so common. Some of these changes reflect the recommended changes for diabetic diets, away from regulated carbohydrate portions to low fat and low sugar diets, with a more liberal complex carbohydrate intake.

## Breakfast and breakfast cereal

Respondents were asked 'How soon after rising do you first have something to eat?' rather than 'Do you eat breakfast?' to allow for shift workers. Breakfast was then defined as something to eat within two hours of rising. In the report of the first survey it was shown that the proportion of people eating breakfast was about two thirds in the youngest respondents and rose with age. Table 11.2 shows that this trend is confirmed in the HALS2 sub-sample at both Surveys, and for both sexes. The results are shown by seven year age groups: thus the change in individuals over seven years can be seen and comparisons made of similar age groups in the two Surveys, bearing in mind the limitations on the comparability of the whole 9003 HALS1 sample with the 5352 HALS sub-sample. Although the proportion in each age group not eating breakfast has changed very little, that eating a light breakfast has increased considerably in most age groups. This is at the expense of cooked breakfasts — both daily and at weekends. At all ages and in both Surveys men were more likely than women to eat a cooked breakfast.

The change in the frequent (most or every day) consumption of breakfast cereal, which has implications for dietary fibre intake, is shown in Table 11.3. Overall consumption has increased in both sexes, a finding in agreement with that of the National Food Survey Committee (1991). By 1991/2, in those who were over 45 years old at HALS1, 13% more men and 11% more women were eating breakfast cereal

frequently whereas there was only a 3% increase in the younger respondents. Using the socio-economic group at HALS1, the trends in cereal consumption noted in the previous Survey are confirmed here, with approximately twice as many respondents in the professional groups as in the unskilled groups being frequent cereal consumers at HALS1. In almost all groups there has been an increase in the proportion of frequent cereal consumers at HALS2.

## Bread consumption

The variety of types of bread reported at Q51a (Appendix C) were grouped into 'white' and 'wholemeal/brown', the latter including wholemeal, wheatmeal and granary, as there was no way of being certain that respondents could accurately distinguish between wholemeal and other non-white breads. In both men and women, wholemeal/brown bread consumption was more prevalent amongst the non-manual groups, and more prevalent in women than in men (Table 11.4). There has been an increase in the proportion consuming wholemeal/brown bread in HALS2, which is apparent in both sexes and both socio-economic groups. Thus, although the manual respondents are now more likely to eat wholemeal/brown bread than they were seven years ago, the social class differential has been maintained.

The amount of bread consumed per day was calculated by summing the number of slices eaten and 1.5 times the number of rolls. The daily consumption of bread in the two Surveys is shown in Table 11.5, in relation to the type of bread usually eaten. In both Surveys men eating predominantly white bread tended to eat more bread than did those choosing wholemeal/brown bread. This trend was much less apparent amongst the women, where fewer were eating the equivalent of five or more slices per day. There has been a marked drop in the proportion of men eating over five slices a day of white bread, and only a small drop amongst the other groups. The National Food Survey Committee (1991) has shown a steady decrease of 8% between 1984 and 1990 in the amount of bread eaten, but their studies do not discriminate between individual household members. The fall in bread consumption, even of white bread, might be expected to result in a drop in dietary fibre intake, which has indeed been observed by the National Food Survey Committee since 1986.

## Use of spreads on bread

Since the first Survey in 1984/5 campaigns have continued to exhort the British public to reduce fat intake, and to replace saturated by polyunsaturated fat. Much advertising has promoted low fat and polyunsaturated spreads. The effectiveness of this aspect of health promotion is revealed in the results shown in Table 11.6. The use of butter has declined dramatically, particularly in the men and in all but the older women. The choice of ordinary margarine has also declined even more and it is now the least popular of all the spreads. The use of polyunsaturated margarine and low fat spread has increased at all ages. Low fat polyunsaturated spread was not reported at HALS1, but was being consumed by 10% of the men and 11% of the women by HALS2. The proportions of men and women using the various spreads was very similar. The National Food Survey Committee reports a decrease in butter and margarine consumption since 1984, and an increase in that of low fat spreads.

## Frequency of consumption of foods

For many foods, the respondents were asked in both HALS1 and HALS2 how often they ate the foods in question – 'More than once a day', 'daily', 'most days', 'once or twice a week', 'less than once a week', and 'rarely or never'. These were grouped into 'frequently' which was 'most days' or 'more frequently' for some food items, whilst for others 'frequently' was designated as at least 'once or twice a week', depending on the distribution of responses. Figure 11.1 shows the age distributions in both surveys for the 'frequent' consumption of 15 foods. In the high fat foods (fried food, chips, carcass meat, processed meat including sausages, meat pies and burgers, eggs, cheese, puddings and pies and to a lesser extent, cakes) there has been a marked reduction in 'frequent' consumption. The change has occurred across all age groups and in both sexes. Although the reduction in cheese consumption might be explained, at least in part, by recent concern about listeria and that of eggs by the salmonella issue, the reduction of the intake of other foods is more likely to be related to health campaigns. The findings are in line with some of those of the National Food Survey Committee (1991). The trend towards consuming less

fat in HALS2 is emphasised by the increase in the frequent consumption of poultry, pasta (including rice) and light desserts (such as yoghurt and ice cream) in both sexes and across the whole age range. Once again, the findings follow the annual trends shown by the National Food Survey Committee. It is interesting that where there are age trends in consumption, as with, for instance, chips and light desserts, the changes observed between the two Surveys are greater than would have been expected just because each group is seven years older at HALS2.

For some food items no appreciable change was observed, notably fruit consumption in summer or in winter. This finding is in contrast to the findings of the National Food Survey Committee who report an increase in fruit consumption over the period between the two Surveys. There appeared to be a small overall reduction in frequent salad consumption in summer, but a slight increase in winter, in both sexes. Since almost all respondents were interviewed at the same time of year in both Surveys difference in interview times cannot account for these differences in consumption.

It was shown in the first Survey (Whichelow 1987) that for many foods there were socio-economic differences in the rates of frequent consumption. In both HALS1 and HALS2 non-manual respondents were more likely than manual respondents to be frequent consumers of cheese, poultry, puddings and pies, light desserts, pasta, fresh fruit in summer and winter and salads in summer and winter, but less likely to eat fried food, chips, processed meats and cakes (Table 11.7). There are also differences between the sexes, most noticeably that women are less likely to eat fried food, chips, or processed meats but more likely to eat fresh fruit and salad frequently.

These findings are similar to those of observed by Gregory et al. (1990). In all the foods examined, the changes that have taken place have occurred to approximately the same extent in both sexes and socio-economic groups, so that the differentials between the groups have been maintained.

The dietary patterns of smokers and non-smokers have been reported in the first Health and Lifestyle Survey (Whichelow et al. 1991a) and other studies to show considerable differences (Fehily et al. 1984; Hebert and Kabat, 1990), with more non-smokers

**Figure 11.1    'Frequent' consumption of foods in HALS1 and HALS2. Percentage of each age group**

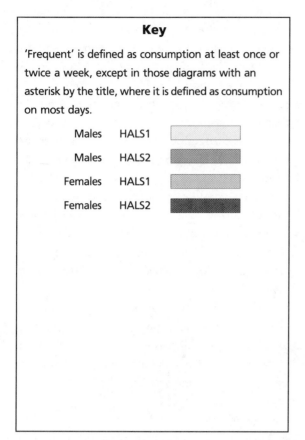

### Key

'Frequent' is defined as consumption at least once or twice a week, except in those diagrams with an asterisk by the title, where it is defined as consumption on most days.

Males     HALS1
Males     HALS2
Females   HALS1
Females   HALS2

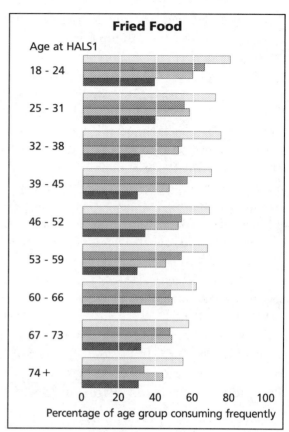

### Fried Food

Age at HALS1

18 - 24
25 - 31
32 - 38
39 - 45
46 - 52
53 - 59
60 - 66
67 - 73
74 +

0    20    40    60    80    100
Percentage of age group consuming frequently

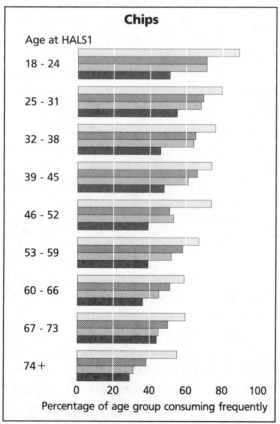

### Chips

Age at HALS1

18 - 24
25 - 31
32 - 38
39 - 45
46 - 52
53 - 59
60 - 66
67 - 73
74 +

0    20    40    60    80    100
Percentage of age group consuming frequently

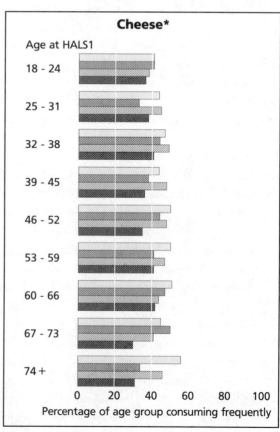

### Cheese*

Age at HALS1

18 - 24
25 - 31
32 - 38
39 - 45
46 - 52
53 - 59
60 - 66
67 - 73
74 +

0    20    40    60    80    100
Percentage of age group consuming frequently

**Figure 11.1   'Frequent' consumption of foods in HALS1 and HALS2. Percentage of each age group**

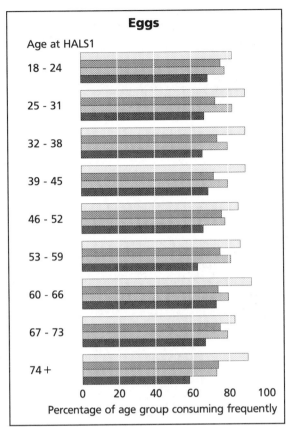

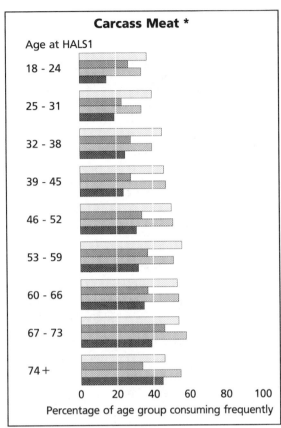

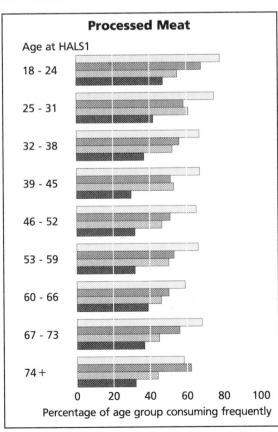

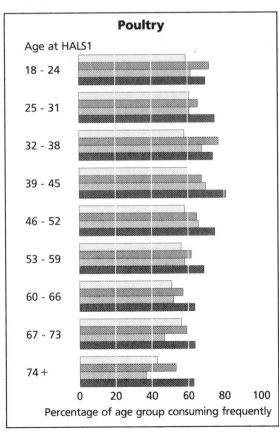

**Figure 11.1 'Frequent' consumption of foods in HALS1 and HALS2. Percentage of each age group**

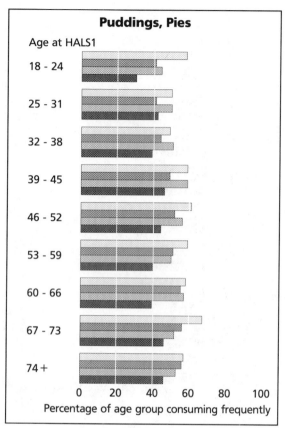

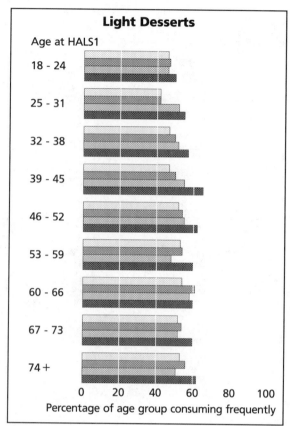

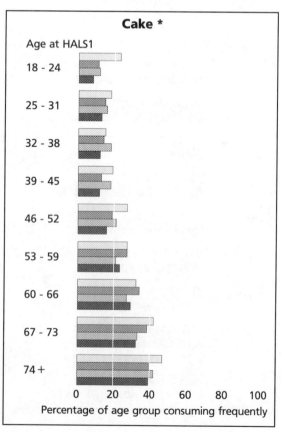

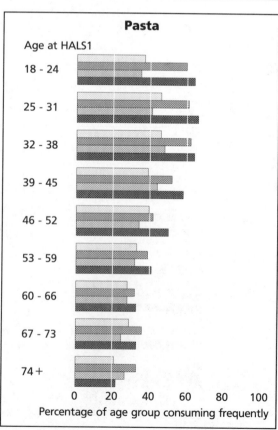

**Figure 11.1    'Frequent' consumption of foods in HALS1 and HALS2. Percentage of each age group**

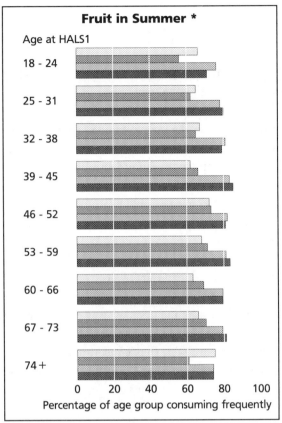

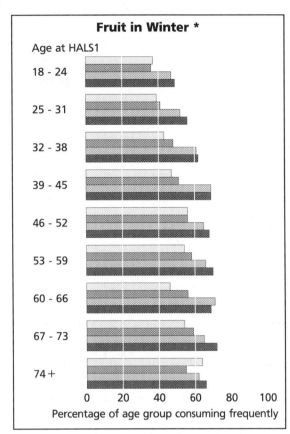

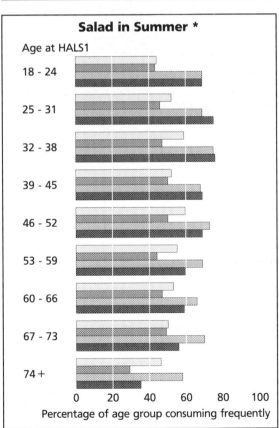

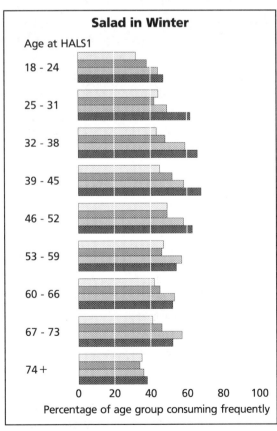

consuming what would be considered a 'healthier' diet in terms of fewer fatty foods and more fruit and salads. The respondents in the two Surveys have been compared by their smoking status at HALS1 and HALS2 in respect of frequent fruit (Table 11.8) and frequent fried food consumption (Table 11.9). The lack of change in frequent fruit consumption, noted in Figure 11.1 and Table 11.7, is also apparent in most of the smoking groups, in the young, middle aged and elderly respondents. The exception is amongst those men and women who have become regular smokers since HALS1 where the proportion eating fruit frequently has dropped by 23% in the men and 10% in the women. At HALS1 the proportions of the 'regular smoker since HALS1' groups eating fruit frequently were very similar to those of the 'always non-smoker' groups, but by HALS2 they were much nearer that of the 'always regular smoker' groups. The proportion of frequent fruit consumers at HALS1 among those who had given up smoking since HALS1 was midway between that of the regular smokers and the non-smokers, and remained essentially unchanged at HALS2. The long-term ex-smokers exhibited values very close to those of the non-smokers. The frequent consumption of fried food is shown in a similar way for the various categories of smokers. Frequent consumption was lower in non-smokers and long-term ex-smokers than in the other groups. The changes between HALS1 and HALS2 are very similar in all categories and at all ages, so that the differentials between the smokers and non-smokers are maintained.

In the report of the first Survey some differences in food consumption between standard regions were shown, and differences in the rates of consumption of many foods were later described, which took account of the sex, age, social class and smoking differences between the regions (Whichelow et al. 1991b). That study revealed particularly large regional variations in the frequent consumption of fried food and salad in winter. The regional changes between HALS1 and HALS2 that have occurred are shown in Table 11.10. There is a tendency in both Surveys for fried food to be consumed less frequently and salads more frequently in the southern part of the country. However, reductions in the frequent consumption of fried food occurred across all regions, with small

increases in salad consumption (except for women in Wales and the North where the increase was larger — over 10%).

As shown in Figure 11.1 the consumption of carcass meat, processed meat and poultry has changed between the two Surveys. Table 11.11 shows the changes in the frequency of eating all meats that have occurred at all levels of consumption for both sexes in the young, middle aged and older respondents. The largest changes are the increased number of people now eating meat 'most days', and the reduced proportion of those eating meat more frequently. The changes are similar in all age groups.

In contrast there have been small changes in vegetable consumption (Table 11.12). With the marked reduction in frequent consumption of chips, and the small reduction in frequent consumption of other forms of potato, the overall consumption of potatoes has been reduced, as was found by the National Food Survey Committee. In both sexes fewer respondents were frequent consumers of pulses at HALS2. These findings add further evidence that dietary fibre intake may have been reduced.

## Sugar in beverages

Although the overall consumption of cups of tea and coffee was only slightly reduced in HALS2 compared to HALS1 there have been changes in the consumption of sugar in these beverages (Table 11.13). More men and women, of all ages, are having tea and coffee without sugar, and there has been a reduction in the proportion taking both 'a lot' and 'some' sugar in these beverages. These findings are once again in accordance with those of the National Food Survey Committee. For both tea and coffee, in all groups, more women than men do not take sugar.

## Attitudes to eating habits

At the end of the section on eating habits in HALS2 the respondents were asked whether or not they had changed their diet in the previous seven years, and the reason for change. As there were no differences in the responses between the men and women, the results from both sexes have been combined. Over half the youngest respondents reported changing their diet, and this proportion decreased with age. The most common reason given by the young was 'health campaigns' and by the middle aged and elderly respondents 'ill health'. 'Change in food preference' and 'to lose weight/improve appearance' featured prominently for the young but not the old, as did 'suiting others in the household' (Table 11.14).

The respondents were also asked how healthy they considered their diet to be. Optimism about the quality of the diet increased markedly with age (Table 11.15). For those over 66 years the majority considered that their diet was 'very healthy'. Only the young admitted having an unhealthy diet. However, opinions about the quality of the diet were not always a reliable reflection of what was eaten. In Table 11.16 the respondents' assessment of their diet is examined in relation to the frequency of consumption of fruit in summer, which could be considered a healthy food, and fried food, which could not. Although a higher proportion of those eating fruit 'frequently' than 'infrequently' reported that their diet was 'very healthy' the differences were not great. Similarly for 'fried food', very few who ate fried food 'frequently' believed their diet to be 'unhealthy'. This is interesting in view of the reduction in the number of people who consume fried food frequently, presumably as a result of health campaigns.

## Knowledge of fibre in foods

In the first survey the questions about whether or not ten foods contained dietary fibre revealed considerable ignorance in the population about the nature of dietary fibre, and a more detailed report on these studies was published later (Whichelow, 1988). The same questions were posed again in HALS2 and the responses in both surveys are shown in Table 11.17. Knowledge about Weetabix (a commercially advertised product) remained high, and for all other fibre containing foods the proportion of respondents giving the correct answer was increased at HALS2, at all ages. For the fibre-free foods, however, there was no change in the pattern of responses. Clearly there is still a great lack of understanding about the nature of dietary fibre, as only just over half the respondents believe that there is no dietary fibre in roast meat or grilled fish. The differences in knowledge about dietary fibre with social class are revealed in the score of correct answers for the fibre-containing and fibre-free foods (Table 11.18). The

proportions of respondents achieving all or nearly all correct responses for both types of food are higher in the non-manual than the manual groups for both sexes. For the fibre-containing foods a higher score of correct answers was achieved for both non-manual and manual groups in HALS2.

## Summary

The major change that has occurred between HALS1 and HALS2 has been a marked reduction in the frequency of consumption of many high-fat foods, by both sexes and non-manual and manual groups and at all ages. Although more respondents correctly identified high-fibre foods as containing dietary fibre, the frequency of consumption of fruit, vegetables and cereal products has not increased.

### References

Fehily, A.M., Phillips, K.M., and Yarnell, J.W.G. (1984), 'Diet, smoking, social class and body mass index in the Caerphilly heart disease study', American Journal of Clinical Nutrition, 40, 827-833.

Gregory, J., Foster, K., Tyler, H., and Wiseman, M. (1990), 'The dietary and nutritional survey of British adults', London: HMSO.

Hebert, J.R., and Kabat, G.C. (1990), 'Differences in dietary intake associated with smoking status'. European Journal of Clinical Nutrition, 44, 185-193.

National Food Survey Committee (1991), 'Household Food Consumption and Expenditure 1990', London: HMSO.

Whichelow, M.J. (1987), 'Dietary Habits', in Cox, B.D. et al., 'The Health and Lifestyle Survey', Preliminary report of a nationwide survey of the physical and mental health, attitudes and lifestyle of a random sample of 9,003 British adults', London: Health Promotion Research Trust.

Whichelow, M.J. (1988), 'Which foods contain dietary fibre?', The beliefs of a random sample of the British population, European Journal of Clinical Nutrition, 42, 945-951.

Whichelow, M.J., Erzinclioglu, S.W. and Cox, B.D. (1991a), 'A comparison of the diets of non-smokers and smokers', British Journal of Addiction, 86, 71-81.

Whichelow, M.J., Erzinclioglu, S.W. and Cox, B.D. (1991b), 'Some regional variations in dietary patterns in a random sample of British adults', European Journal of Clinical Nutrition, 45, 253-262.

**Table 11.1    Numbers of subjects reporting conditions for which a special diet was prescribed and type of diet**

| HALS<br>Medical condition | 1<br>Males | 2 | 1<br>Females | 2 | Type of diet | 1<br>Males | 2 | 1<br>Females | 2 |
|---|---|---|---|---|---|---|---|---|---|
| Obesity | 24 | 34 | 66 | 103 | Low fat | 64 | 111 | 110 | 191 |
| Diabetes | 32 | 61 | 31 | 60 | High fibre | 26 | 41 | 69 | 70 |
| Hypertension/<br>heart disease | 34 | 38 | 37 | 52 | Low sugar | – | 47 | – | 59 |
| High cholesterol | 4 | 24 | 8 | 47 | Low calorie | 21 | 22 | 50 | 51 |
| Ulcers (intestinal) | 16 | 8 | 18 | 21 | No dairy products | 13 | 18 | 23 | 31 |
| Food allergy | 10 | 7 | 20 | 14 | Low carbohydrate | 35 | 11 | 59 | 17 |
| Gall stones | 1 | 5 | 20 | 10 | Low salt | 8 | 12 | 18 | 21 |
| Coeliac disease | 2 | 4 | 12 | 8 | Gluten free | 2 | 4 | 9 | 11 |
| Renal failure | 2 | 5 | 4 | 4 | Low protein | 2 | 1 | 8 | 5 |

**Table 11.2    Change in patterns of breakfast consumption from HALS1 to HALS2. Percentage of age groups and difference (+/−)**

| Age at HALS1 | 18-24 | | 25-31 | | 32-38 | | 39-45 | | 46-52 | | 53-59 | | 60-66 | | 67-73 | | >73 | | Total | |
|---|---|---|---|---|---|---|---|---|---|---|---|---|---|---|---|---|---|---|---|---|
| HALS | 1 | 2 | 1 | 2 | 1 | 2 | 1 | 2 | 1 | 2 | 1 | 2 | 1 | 2 | 1 | 2 | 1 | 2 | 1 | 2 |
| **Males** | | | | | | | | | | | | | | | | | | | | |
| No breakfast | 31 | 34 | 39 | 35 | 34 | 30 | 32 | 30 | 23 | 23 | 23 | 18 | 18 | 10 | 10 | 6 | 5 | 6 | 27 | 24 |
| | (+3) | | (−4) | | (−4) | | (−2) | | (0) | | (−5) | | (−8) | | (−4) | | (+1) | | (−3) | |
| Light breakfast | 39 | 43 | 32 | 48 | 37 | 45 | 35 | 43 | 38 | 50 | 41 | 51 | 46 | 61 | 48 | 64 | 55 | 66 | 39 | 50 |
| | (+4) | | (+16) | | (+8) | | (+8) | | (+12) | | (+10) | | (+15) | | (+16) | | (+11) | | (+11) | |
| Cooked (weekends) | 17 | 15 | 18 | 12 | 18 | 17 | 20 | 19 | 24 | 18 | 22 | 16 | 15 | 14 | 10 | 11 | 13 | 11 | 18 | 16 |
| | (−2) | | (−6) | | (−1) | | (−1) | | (−6) | | (−6) | | (−1) | | (+1) | | (−2) | | (−2) | |
| Cooked (daily) | 13 | 8 | 11 | 5 | 12 | 8 | 13 | 8 | 16 | 10 | 14 | 15 | 21 | 15 | 32 | 19 | 28 | 16 | 16 | 11 |
| | (−5) | | (−6) | | (−4) | | (−5) | | (−6) | | (+1) | | (−6) | | (−13) | | (−12) | | (−5) | |
| *Base = 100%* | *299* | | *241* | | *383* | | *324* | | *280* | | *278* | | *259* | | *148* | | *88* | | *2300* | |
| **Females** | | | | | | | | | | | | | | | | | | | | |
| No breakfast | 36 | 40 | 31 | 33 | 31 | 32 | 24 | 18 | 24 | 20 | 22 | 16 | 13 | 8 | 9 | 6 | 10 | 3 | 24 | 22 |
| | (+4) | | (+2) | | (+1) | | (−6) | | (−4) | | (−6) | | (−5) | | (−3) | | (−7) | | (−2) | |
| Light breakfast | 39 | 45 | 49 | 56 | 47 | 53 | 51 | 65 | 50 | 60 | 49 | 65 | 60 | 69 | 66 | 75 | 66 | 83 | 51 | 61 |
| | (+6) | | (+7) | | (+6) | | (+14) | | (+10) | | (+16) | | (+9) | | (+9) | | (+17) | | (+10) | |
| Cooked (weekends) | 17 | 13 | 16 | 9 | 18 | 13 | 17 | 13 | 16 | 16 | 19 | 9 | 16 | 13 | 11 | 8 | 14 | 4 | 16 | 12 |
| | (−4) | | (−7) | | (−5) | | (−4) | | (0) | | (−10) | | (−3) | | (−3) | | (−10) | | (−4) | |
| Cooked (daily) | 8 | 2 | 5 | 1 | 4 | 2 | 8 | 4 | 9 | 3 | 10 | 10 | 11 | 11 | 14 | 10 | 10 | 9 | 8 | 5 |
| | (−6) | | (−4) | | (−2) | | (−4) | | (−6) | | (0) | | (0) | | (−4) | | (−1) | | (−3) | |
| *Base = 100%* | *311* | | *394* | | *545* | | *432* | | *391* | | *315* | | *327* | | *191* | | *146* | | *3052* | |

**Table 11.3** Frequent (most days or more often) consumption of breakfast cereal in relation to HALS1 socio-economic group and age in HALS1 and HALS2. Percentage of HALS1 age group and difference (+/−)

| | Professional | | Managers | | Other non-manual | | Skilled | | Semi-skilled | | Unskilled | | ALL (includes unclassified etc.) | |
|---|---|---|---|---|---|---|---|---|---|---|---|---|---|---|
| **HALS** | 1 | 2 | 1 | 2 | 1 | 2 | 1 | 2 | 1 | 2 | 1 | 2 | 1 | 2 |
| **HALS1 Age** | | | | | | | **Males** | | | | | | | |
| **18-45** | 55 | 56 | 40 | 43 | 47 | 52 | 36 | 41 | 37 | 32 | 33 | 24 | 40 | 43 |
| | (+1) | | (+3) | | (+5) | | (+5) | | (−5) | | (−9) | | (+3) | |
| **46-99** | 64 | 68 | 49 | 66 | 54 | 60 | 39 | 55 | 46 | 55 | 30 | 54 | 46 | 59 |
| | (+4) | | (+17) | | (+6) | | (+16) | | (+9) | | (+24) | | (+13) | |
| *Base = 100%* | 66 | | 233 | | 239 | | 466 | | 161 | | 54 | | 1247 | |
| | 50 | | 206 | | 187 | | 371 | | 181 | | 54 | | 1053 | |
| | | | | | | | **Females** | | | | | | | |
| **18-45** | 51 | 50 | 45 | 46 | 48 | 52 | 42 | 42 | 31 | 39 | 26 | 41 | 42 | 45 |
| | (−1) | | (+1) | | (+4) | | (0) | | (+8) | | (+15) | | (+3) | |
| **46-99** | 58 | 69 | 48 | 62 | 47 | 61 | 45 | 53 | 53 | 59 | 37 | 47 | 47 | 58 |
| | (+11) | | (+14) | | (+14) | | (+8) | | (+6) | | (+10) | | (+11) | |
| *Base = 100%* | 96 | | 264 | | 427 | | 546 | | 265 | | 58 | | 1682 | |
| | 78 | | 284 | | 256 | | 429 | | 232 | | 73 | | 1370 | |

**Table 11.4** Type of bread usually consumed in 1984/5 compared to that consumed in 1991/2. Percentage of non-manual and manual groups

| | Males | | | | Females | | | |
|---|---|---|---|---|---|---|---|---|
| | Non-manual | | Manual | | Non-manual | | Manual | |
| **HALS** | 1 | 2 | 1 | 2 | 1 | 2 | 1 | 2 |
| Type of bread | | | | | | | | |
| None | 1.1 | 0.1 | 0.5 | 0.2 | 2.1 | 0.4 | 1.5 | 0.6 |
| Wholemeal/brown | 49.2 | 54.7 | 25.8 | 32.6 | 60.5 | 63.8 | 41.0 | 46.2 |
| White | 49.5 | 45.2 | 73.6 | 67.1 | 37.3 | 35.7 | 57.4 | 53.3 |
| *Base = 100%* | 995 | | 1287 | | 1410 | | 1604 | |

**Table 11.5    Daily bread consumption by type of bread usually eaten in HALS1 and HALS2. Percentage of those eating white or wholemeal/brown bread**

| | Males | | | | Females | | | |
| | White | | Wholemeal/brown | | White | | Wholemeal/brown | |
| HALS | 1 | 2 | 1 | 2 | 1 | 2 | 1 | 2 |
| --- | --- | --- | --- | --- | --- | --- | --- | --- |
| Slices bread per day | | | | | | | | |
| <2.5 | 13.2 | 17.9 | 19.2 | 21.6 | 34.0 | 37.9 | 35.3 | 38.3 |
| 3 – 3.5 | 9.6 | 14.3 | 14.1 | 16.1 | 22.8 | 21.2 | 24.9 | 24.8 |
| 4 – 4.5 | 22.8 | 23.0 | 24.7 | 24.7 | 21.8 | 22.5 | 22.5 | 21.6 |
| 5+ | 54.4 | 44.7 | 42.0 | 37.6 | 21.4 | 18.3 | 17.3 | 14.8 |
| Base = 100% | 1451 | 1321 | 829 | 974 | 1465 | 1375 | 1531 | 1654 |

**Table 11.6    Change in type of spread used from HALS1 to HALS2. Percentage of each age group and difference ( +/− )**

| Age at HALS1 | 18-24 | | 25-31 | | 32-38 | | 39-45 | | 46-52 | | 53-59 | | 60-66 | | 67-73 | | >73 | | Total | |
|---|---|---|---|---|---|---|---|---|---|---|---|---|---|---|---|---|---|---|---|---|
| HALS | 1 | 2 | 1 | 2 | 1 | 2 | 1 | 2 | 1 | 2 | 1 | 2 | 1 | 2 | 1 | 2 | 1 | 2 | 1 | 2 |
| **Males** | | | | | | | | | | | | | | | | | | | | |
| Butter | 40 | 23 | 35 | 24 | 34 | 24 | 34 | 24 | 46 | 31 | 44 | 29 | 37 | 29 | 41 | 33 | 53 | 37 | 39 | 27 |
| | (− 17) | | (− 11) | | (− 10) | | (− 10) | | (− 15) | | (− 15) | | (− 8) | | (− 8) | | (− 16) | | (− 12) | |
| Margarine | 39 | 8 | 33 | 15 | 36 | 8 | 35 | 11 | 31 | 10 | 30 | 9 | 32 | 11 | 26 | 14 | 26 | 16 | 33 | 11 |
| | (− 31) | | (− 18) | | (− 28) | | (− 24) | | (− 21) | | (− 21) | | (− 21) | | (− 12) | | (− 10) | | (− 22) | |
| Polyunsatura-ted margarine | 11 | 36 | 15 | 31 | 18 | 31 | 19 | 33 | 15 | 30 | 16 | 26 | 20 | 30 | 21 | 25 | 18 | 26 | 17 | 30 |
| | (+ 25) | | (+ 16) | | (+ 13) | | (+ 14) | | (+ 15) | | (+ 10) | | (+ 10) | | (+ 4) | | (+ 8) | | (+ 13) | |
| Low fat spread | 6 | 19 | 13 | 17 | 8 | 24 | 10 | 16 | 5 | 15 | 8 | 18 | 8 | 17 | 10 | 18 | 1 | 15 | 8 | 18 |
| | (+ 13) | | (+ 4) | | (+ 16) | | (+ 6) | | (+ 10) | | (+ 10) | | (+ 9) | | (+ 8) | | (+ 14) | | (+ 10) | |
| Low fat polyunsaturated spread | 0 | 9 | 0 | 12 | 0 | 8 | 0 | 10 | 0 | 9 | 0 | 15 | 0 | 9 | 0 | 10 | 0 | 2 | 0 | 10 |
| Other/nothing | 3 | 5 | 4 | 2 | 4 | 5 | 3 | 6 | 2 | 6 | 2 | 4 | 3 | 4 | 3 | 2 | 2 | 4 | 3 | 4 |
| *Base = 100%* | 300 | | 241 | | 382 | | 324 | | 279 | | 281 | | 257 | | 147 | | 89 | | 2300 | |
| **Females** | | | | | | | | | | | | | | | | | | | | |
| Butter | 37 | 23 | 36 | 16 | 35 | 17 | 33 | 23 | 44 | 22 | 44 | 26 | 44 | 32 | 45 | 39 | 55 | 53 | 40 | 25 |
| | (− 14) | | (− 20) | | (− 18) | | (− 10) | | (− 22) | | (− 18) | | (− 12) | | (− 6) | | (− 2) | | (− 15) | |
| Margarine | 33 | 10 | 34 | 12 | 30 | 12 | 30 | 6 | 27 | 8 | 18 | 9 | 26 | 7 | 22 | 6 | 24 | 10 | 28 | 9 |
| | (− 23) | | (− 22) | | (− 18) | | (− 24) | | (− 19) | | (− 9) | | (− 19) | | (− 16) | | (− 14) | | (− 19) | |
| Polyunsatura-ted margarine | 10 | 23 | 13 | 30 | 17 | 29 | 19 | 26 | 18 | 30 | 20 | 25 | 14 | 28 | 18 | 29 | 13 | 18 | 16 | 27 |
| | (+ 13) | | (+ 17) | | (+ 12) | | (+ 7) | | (+ 12) | | (+ 5) | | (+ 14) | | (+ 11) | | (+ 5) | | (+ 11) | |
| Low fat spread | 15 | 25 | 11 | 22 | 12 | 22 | 12 | 24 | 6 | 20 | 14 | 21 | 12 | 20 | 11 | 17 | 5 | 10 | 11 | 21 |
| | (+ 10) | | (+ 11) | | (+ 10) | | (+ 12) | | (+ 14) | | (+ 7) | | (+ 8) | | (+ 6) | | (+ 5) | | (+ 10) | |
| Low fat polyunsaturated spread | 0 | 12 | 0 | 11 | 0 | 11 | 0 | 11 | 0 | 12 | 0 | 13 | 0 | 10 | 0 | 6 | 0 | 3 | 0 | 11 |
| Other/nothing | 6 | 8 | 6 | 9 | 6 | 9 | 6 | 9 | 5 | 9 | 5 | 5 | 4 | 4 | 4 | 3 | 3 | 5 | 5 | 7 |
| *Base = 100%* | 310 | | 392 | | 547 | | 435 | | 390 | | 316 | | 324 | | 192 | | 146 | | 3052 | |

**Table 11.7** **Change in 'frequent' consumption of foods in non-manual and manual groups. Percentage of socio-economic group and difference (+/−). 'Frequent' is most days or more often, except for * where 'frequent' is at least once or twice a week**

| HALS | Males | | | | Females | | | |
|---|---|---|---|---|---|---|---|---|
| | Non-manual | | Manual | | Non-manual | | Manual | |
| | 1 | 2 | 1 | 2 | 1 | 2 | 1 | 2 |
| Fried food (excl. chips)* | 63 | 47 | 75 | 60 | 46 | 27 | 56 | 39 |
| | (− 16) | | (− 15) | | (− 19) | | (− 17) | |
| Chips* | 66 | 53 | 78 | 66 | 49 | 32 | 65 | 53 |
| | (− 13) | | (− 12) | | (− 17) | | (− 12) | |
| Cheese | 51 | 43 | 44 | 41 | 51 | 43 | 41 | 33 |
| | (− 8) | | (− 3) | | (− 8) | | (− 8) | |
| Eggs* | 85 | 73 | 89 | 75 | 80 | 67 | 79 | 67 |
| | (− 12) | | (− 14) | | (− 13) | | (− 12) | |
| Carcass meat | 46 | 29 | 48 | 33 | 46 | 26 | 46 | 28 |
| | (− 17) | | (− 15) | | (− 20) | | (− 18) | |
| Processed meat* | 62 | 49 | 72 | 61 | 46 | 31 | 56 | 42 |
| | (− 13) | | (− 11) | | (− 15) | | (− 14) | |
| Poultry* | 60 | 71 | 54 | 62 | 64 | 75 | 58 | 69 |
| | (+ 11) | | (+ 8) | | (+ 11) | | (+ 11) | |
| Puddings, pies* | 59 | 52 | 55 | 46 | 55 | 41 | 51 | 41 |
| | (− 7) | | (− 9) | | (− 14) | | (− 10) | |
| Light desserts* | 52 | 55 | 47 | 49 | 56 | 63 | 49 | 56 |
| | (+ 3) | | (+ 2) | | (+ 7) | | (+ 7) | |
| Cake | 23 | 20 | 26 | 21 | 18 | 18 | 23 | 17 |
| | (− 3) | | (− 5) | | (0) | | (− 6) | |
| Pasta* | 47 | 57 | 30 | 43 | 44 | 60 | 31 | 45 |
| | (+ 10) | | (+ 13) | | (+ 16) | | (+ 14) | |
| Fruit in summer | 74 | 74 | 61 | 60 | 86 | 85 | 75 | 76 |
| | (0) | | (− 1) | | (− 1) | | (+ 1) | |
| Fruit in winter | 53 | 57 | 43 | 45 | 68 | 71 | 56 | 58 |
| | (+ 4) | | (+ 2) | | (+ 3) | | (+ 2) | |
| Salad in summer | 63 | 53 | 46 | 41 | 74 | 72 | 66 | 61 |
| | (− 10) | | (− 5) | | (− 2) | | (− 5) | |
| Salad in winter* | 51 | 54 | 36 | 39 | 61 | 65 | 47 | 53 |
| | (+ 3) | | (+ 3) | | (+ 4) | | (+ 6) | |
| *Base = 100%* | 995 | | 1287 | | 1410 | | 1604 | |

**Table 11.8**    **Frequent fruit consumption (most days or more often) by smoking habit and change in smoking habit. Percentage eating fruit frequently in each age group but numbers (in brackets) where base numbers are <20**

| HALS | Always non-smoker 1 | 2 | Ex-smoker >7 years 1 | 2 | Ex-smoker since HALS1 1 | 2 | Always regular smoker 1 | 2 | Regular smoker since HALS1 1 | 2 |
|---|---|---|---|---|---|---|---|---|---|---|
| **Age at HALS1** | | | | | **Males** | | | | | |
| **18-38** | 69 | 69 | 74 | 71 | 65 | 65 | 56 | 47 | 74 | 48 |
| **39-59** | 79 | 82 | 73 | 78 | 70 | 71 | 49 | 52 | 85 | 70 |
| **60+** | 73 | 85 | 71 | 70 | 65 | 68 | 55 | 55 | (8) | (5) |
| **All** | 73 | 75 | 73 | 74 | 67 | 68 | 53 | 50 | 75 | 52 |
| *Base = 100%* | *358* | | *112* | | *89* | | *289* | | *46* | |
| | *186* | | *259* | | *133* | | *269* | | *20* | |
| | *78* | | *211* | | *72* | | *116* | | *13* | |
| | *622* | | *582* | | *294* | | *674* | | *79* | |
| | | | | | **Females** | | | | | |
| **18-38** | 87 | 85 | 78 | 88 | 76 | 78 | 67 | 61 | 83 | 72 |
| **39-59** | 87 | 89 | 88 | 91 | 77 | 81 | 71 | 68 | (14) | (14) |
| **60+** | 80 | 83 | 80 | 77 | 84 | 86 | 63 | 62 | (10) | (8) |
| **All** | 85 | 86 | 82 | 86 | 77 | 81 | 68 | 64 | 83 | 73 |
| *Base = 100%* | *541* | | *183* | | *91* | | *360* | | *53* | |
| | *475* | | *225* | | *108* | | *293* | | *19* | |
| | *325* | | *167* | | *57* | | *89* | | *10* | |
| | *1341* | | *575* | | *256* | | *742* | | *82* | |

**Table 11.9** Frequent (at least once or twice a week) fried food consumption by smoking habit and change in smoking habit. Percentage eating fried food frequently in each age group and difference (+/−)

| HALS | Always non-smoker | | Ex-smoker >7 years | | Ex-smoker since HALS1 | | Always regular smoker | | Regular smoker since HALS1 | |
|---|---|---|---|---|---|---|---|---|---|---|
| | 1 | 2 | 1 | 2 | 1 | 2 | 1 | 2 | 1 | 2 |
| **Age at HALS1** | | | | | **Males** | | | | | |
| **18-38** | 72 | 51 | 74 | 48 | 78 | 54 | 82 | 71 | 76 | 61 |
| | (− 21) | | (− 26) | | (− 24) | | (− 11) | | (− 15) | |
| **39-59** | 66 | 50 | 65 | 50 | 71 | 58 | 76 | 64 | 55 | 40 |
| | (− 16) | | (− 15) | | (− 13) | | (− 12) | | (− 15) | |
| **60 +** | 55 | 40 | 55 | 41 | 58 | 44 | 71 | 56 | (7) | (7) |
| | (− 15) | | (− 14) | | (− 14) | | (− 15) | | | |
| **All** | 68 | 49 | 63 | 47 | 70 | 53 | 78 | 65 | 67 | 54 |
| | (− 19) | | (− 16) | | (− 17) | | (− 13) | | (− 13) | |
| *Base = 100%* | *358* | | *112* | | *89* | | *289* | | *46* | |
| | *186* | | *259* | | *133* | | *269* | | *20* | |
| | *78* | | *211* | | *72* | | *116* | | *13* | |
| | *622* | | *582* | | *294* | | *674* | | *79* | |
| | | | | | **Females** | | | | | |
| **18-38** | 56 | 29 | 44 | 27 | 59 | 35 | 62 | 50 | 49 | 32 |
| | (− 27) | | (− 14) | | (− 24) | | (− 12) | | (− 17) | |
| **39-59** | 45 | 29 | 42 | 23 | 49 | 31 | 59 | 41 | (9) | (7) |
| | (− 16) | | (− 19) | | (− 18) | | (− 18) | | | |
| **60 +** | 48 | 33 | 46 | 30 | 40 | 35 | 51 | 35 | (5) | (4) |
| | (− 15) | | (− 16) | | (− 5) | | (− 16) | | | |
| **All** | 50 | 30 | 44 | 26 | 51 | 33 | 59 | 45 | 49 | 34 |
| | (− 20) | | (− 18) | | (− 18) | | (− 14) | | (− 15) | |
| *Base = 100%* | *541* | | *183* | | *91* | | *360* | | *53* | |
| | *475* | | *225* | | *108* | | *293* | | *19* | |
| | *325* | | *167* | | *57* | | *89* | | *10* | |
| | *1341* | | *575* | | *256* | | *742* | | *82* | |

**Table 11.10** **Regional variations in the percentage of respondents frequently consuming fried food and salad in winter and difference (+/−) between HALS1 and HALS2**

| HALS | Fried food | | | | Salad in winter | | | | Base = 100% | |
| | Male | | Female | | Male | | Female | | Males | Females |
| | 1 | 2 | 1 | 2 | 1 | 2 | 1 | 2 | | |
|---|---|---|---|---|---|---|---|---|---|---|
| Scotland | 72 | 57 | 55 | 38 | 30 | 32 | 41 | 42 | 249 | 320 |
| | (− 15) | | (− 17) | | (+ 2) | | (+ 1) | | | |
| Wales | 70 | 65 | 56 | 40 | 27 | 32 | 43 | 59 | 136 | 166 |
| | (− 5) | | (− 16) | | (+ 5) | | (+ 16) | | | |
| North | 77 | 57 | 57 | 38 | 33 | 37 | 42 | 53 | 115 | 199 |
| | (− 20) | | (− 190 | | (+ 4) | | (+ 11) | | | |
| North West | 68 | 54 | 48 | 33 | 40 | 48 | 56 | 59 | 250 | 417 |
| | (− 14) | | (− 15) | | (+ 8) | | (+ 3) | | | |
| Yorkshire/Humberside | 76 | 62 | 58 | 44 | 43 | 45 | 52 | 56 | 219 | 274 |
| | (− 16) | | (− 14) | | (+ 2) | | (+ 4) | | | |
| West Midlands | 72 | 53 | 49 | 30 | 40 | 48 | 54 | 63 | 201 | 275 |
| | (− 19) | | (− 19) | | (+ 8) | | (+ 9) | | | |
| East Midlands | 71 | 54 | 56 | 33 | 48 | 55 | 62 | 65 | 193 | 234 |
| | (− 17) | | (− 23) | | (+ 7) | | (+ 3) | | | |
| East Anglia | 71 | 54 | 56 | 32 | 42 | 46 | 68 | 63 | 84 | 131 |
| | (− 17) | | (− 24) | | (+ 4) | | (− 5) | | | |
| South West | 66 | 50 | 47 | 27 | 39 | 42 | 56 | 63 | 187 | 233 |
| | (− 16) | | (− 20) | | (+ 3) | | (+ 7) | | | |
| South East | 65 | 47 | 46 | 25 | 53 | 52 | 58 | 62 | 448 | 539 |
| | (− 18) | | (− 21) | | (− 1) | | (+ 4) | | | |
| Greater London | 68 | 53 | 49 | 35 | 53 | 50 | 58 | 59 | 218 | 264 |
| | (− 15) | | (− 14) | | (− 3) | | (+ 1) | | | |
| All Regions | 70 | 54 | 51 | 33 | 42 | 45 | 54 | 58 | 2300 | 3047 |
| | (− 16) | | (− 18) | | (+ 3) | | (+ 4) | | | |

**Table 11.11** **Frequency of meat (carcass, processed plus poultry) consumption at HALS1 and HALS2. Percentage of each age group eating meat each week and difference (+/–)**

| | Males | | | | | | Females | | | | | |
|---|---|---|---|---|---|---|---|---|---|---|---|---|
| Age at HALS1 | 18-38 | | 39-59 | | 60+ | | 18-38 | | 39-59 | | 60+ | |
| HALS | 1 | 2 | 1 | 2 | 1 | 2 | 1 | 2 | 1 | 2 | 1 | 2 |
| None | 2 | 3 | 1 | 1 | 0 | 1 | 2 | 3 | 1 | 2 | 1 | 1 |
| | (+1) | | (0) | | (+1) | | (+1) | | (+1) | | (0) | |
| 1-3 days | 2 | 6 | 4 | 9 | 4 | 8 | 6 | 9 | 6 | 11 | 7 | 12 |
| | (+4) | | (+5) | | (+4) | | (+3) | | (+5) | | (+5) | |
| Most days | 45 | 56 | 37 | 52 | 41 | 50 | 48 | 59 | 42 | 54 | 38 | 48 |
| | (+11) | | (+15) | | (+9) | | (+11) | | (+12) | | (+10) | |
| Daily | 20 | 13 | 23 | 18 | 27 | 21 | 20 | 15 | 25 | 19 | 29 | 22 |
| | (–7) | | (–5) | | (–6) | | (–5) | | (–6) | | (–7) | |
| > 1/Day | 32 | 22 | 35 | 21 | 28 | 20 | 24 | 13 | 27 | 15 | 26 | 17 |
| | (–10) | | (–14) | | (–8) | | (–11) | | (–12) | | (–9) | |
| *Base = 100%* | 923 | | 882 | | 495 | | 1250 | | 1138 | | 664 | |

**Table 11.12** **Vegetable consumption in 1984/5 and 1991/2. Percentage of males and females eating vegetables on most days or more often**

| | Potatoes (excl. chips) | | Green vegetables | | Pulses | | Root vegetables | | Other vegetables | |
|---|---|---|---|---|---|---|---|---|---|---|
| HALS | 1 | 2 | 1 | 2 | 1 | 2 | 1 | 2 | 1 | 2 |
| Males | 79.8 | 75.7 | 56.8 | 56.9 | 57.1 | 50.5 | 54.0 | 55.0 | 29.2 | 29.7 |
| *Base = 100%* | 2300 | | 2300 | | 2300 | | 2300 | | 2300 | |
| Females | 73.0 | 72.7 | 59.6 | 59.2 | 46.0 | 41.7 | 55.2 | 58.2 | 34.5 | 35.7 |
| *Base = 100%* | 3047 | | 3047 | | 3047 | | 3047 | | 3047 | |

**Table 11.13** **Change in sugar consumption in beverages in those drinking tea or coffee at HALS1 and HALS2. Percentage in each age group and difference (+/−)**

| | Males | | | | | | Females | | | | | |
|---|---|---|---|---|---|---|---|---|---|---|---|---|
| Age at HALS | 18-38 | | 39-59 | | 60+ | | 18-38 | | 39-59 | | 60+ | |
| HALS | 1 | 2 | 1 | 2 | 1 | 2 | 1 | 2 | 1 | 2 | 1 | 2 |
| **Sugar in tea** | | | | | | | | | | | | |
| None | 38 | 50 | 45 | 52 | 41 | 47 | 67 | 72 | 72 | 77 | 68 | 71 |
| | (+12) | | (+7) | | (+6) | | (+5) | | (+5) | | (+3) | |
| Some | 21 | 21 | 19 | 19 | 23 | 24 | 14 | 15 | 13 | 11 | 17 | 16 |
| | (0) | | (0) | | (+1) | | (+1) | | (−2) | | (−1) | |
| A lot | 41 | 29 | 37 | 29 | 36 | 29 | 19 | 14 | 15 | 12 | 15 | 13 |
| | (−12) | | (−8) | | (−7) | | (−5) | | (−3) | | (−2) | |
| Base = 100% | 693 | | 768 | | 466 | | 932 | | 963 | | 630 | |
| **Sugar in coffee** | | | | | | | | | | | | |
| None | 31 | 46 | 40 | 49 | 37 | 41 | 60 | 69 | 66 | 72 | 57 | 60 |
| | (+15) | | (+9) | | (+4) | | (+9) | | (+6) | | (+3) | |
| Some | 41 | 32 | 38 | 36 | 54 | 52 | 26 | 22 | 26 | 23 | 39 | 39 |
| | (−9) | | (−2) | | (−2) | | (−4) | | (−3) | | (0) | |
| A lot | 28 | 21 | 22 | 15 | 10 | 7 | 14 | 9 | 8 | 5 | 4 | 2 |
| | (−7) | | (−7) | | (−3) | | (−5) | | (−3) | | (−2) | |
| Base = 100% | 546 | | 517 | | 252 | | 807 | | 737 | | 368 | |

**Table 11.14**   **Percentages of young, middle aged and elderly respondents (men and women combined) reporting change in diet since 1984-5, and the reasons for change (multiple responses were possible). Percentage of age group**

| Age at HALS2 | 25-45 | 46-66 | 67+ |
|---|---|---|---|
| Change in diet | 59.2 | 48.4 | 37.2 |
| **Reason for change** | | | |
| Health campaigns | 16.9 | 11.5 | 3.9 |
| Illness | 7.1 | 15.0 | 12.0 |
| To lose weight/improve appearance | 10.8 | 8.7 | 3.7 |
| Change in food preference | 8.9 | 6.8 | 4.1 |
| To suit others in household | 11.3 | 5.7 | 3.4 |
| Change in household structure | 7.8 | 4.3 | 6.2 |
| Change in income | 4.2 | 1.7 | 1.1 |
| Convenience | 3.4 | 1.9 | 2.0 |
| Change in working circumstances | 3.0 | 2.5 | 2.3 |
| Change in appetite | 0.6 | 1.8 | 3.0 |
| Food availability | 2.9 | 1.3 | 1.0 |
| *Base = 100%* | *2172* | *2025* | *1150* |

**Table 11.15**   **Male and female respondents' assessment of the quality of their diet. Percentages of age group**

| Age at HALS2 | 25-31 | 32-38 | 39-45 | 46-52 | 53-59 | 60-66 | 67-73 | 74-80 | 80-86 | >86 |
|---|---|---|---|---|---|---|---|---|---|---|
| Diet considered to be: | | | | | | | | | | |
| Very healthy | 10 | 13 | 12 | 22 | 28 | 39 | 51 | 62 | 66 | 78 |
| Quite good | 80 | 77 | 81 | 73 | 69 | 57 | 46 | 36 | 30 | 16 |
| Unhealthy | 10 | 10 | 7 | 5 | 2 | 3 | 1 | 1 | 3 | 0 |
| Don't know | 0 | 0 | 0 | 0 | 0 | 0 | 1 | 1 | 1 | 7 |
| *Base = 100%* | *610* | *633* | *929* | *759* | *669* | *597* | *580* | *338* | *186* | *45* |

**Table 11.16**  **Respondents' assessment of their diet in relation to the frequency of consumption of fruit in summer and of fried food. Percentage in each age group of 'Frequent' and 'Infrequent' consumers, where 'Infrequent' for fruit in summer is never to once or twice a week and for fried food is never to less than once a week. 'Frequent' for fruit in summer is most days or more often and for fried food is once or twice a week or more often**

| Age at HALS2 | Males | | | | | | Females | | | | | |
|---|---|---|---|---|---|---|---|---|---|---|---|---|
| | 25-45 | | 46-66 | | >66 | | 25-45 | | 46-66 | | >66 | |
| | Infr. | Freq. | Infr. | Freq. | Infr. | Freq. | Infr. | Freq. | Infr. | Freq. | Infr. | Freq. |
| **Fruit in Summer** | | | | | | | | | | | | |
| Very healthy | 10 | 12 | 27 | 35 | 56 | 61 | 7 | 13 | 20 | 28 | 48 | 61 |
| Quite good | 74 | 82 | 65 | 62 | 44 | 38 | 74 | 82 | 71 | 71 | 48 | 38 |
| Unhealthy | 15 | 6 | 8 | 3 | 1 | 1 | 19 | 5 | 9 | 1 | 4 | 1 |
| *Base = 100%* | *355* | *567* | *264* | *617* | *154* | *329* | *281* | *967* | *197* | *942* | *133* | *517* |
| **Fried Food** | | | | | | | | | | | | |
| Very healthy | 13 | 11 | 33 | 33 | 60 | 58 | 13 | 10 | 28 | 22 | 61 | 53 |
| Quite good | 80 | 79 | 65 | 61 | 39 | 41 | 82 | 77 | 69 | 75 | 37 | 46 |
| Unhealthy | 8 | 11 | 2 | 6 | 0 | 1 | 6 | 13 | 2 | 4 | 2 | 1 |
| *Base = 100%* | *387* | *534* | *396* | *485* | *262* | *221* | *807* | *441* | *784* | *355* | *436* | *212* |

**Table 11.17** **Percentage of young, middle aged and older respondents giving correct (C), incorrect (I) and Don't Know (DK) answers to whether or not there is fibre in ten foods, in Surveys HALS1 and HALS2**

| | | Males | | | | | | | | | | | Females | | | | | | | | | | | |
|---|---|---|---|---|---|---|---|---|---|---|---|---|---|---|---|---|---|---|---|---|---|---|---|---|
| Age (at HALS1) | | 18-38 | | | 39-59 | | | 60-99 | | | ALL | | | 18-38 | | | 39-59 | | | 60-99 | | | ALL | | |
| Type of Response | | C | I | DK | C | I | DK | C | I | DK | C | I | DK | C | I | DK | C | I | DK | C | I | DK | C | I | DK |
| **Fibre-containing foods** | | | | | | | | | | | | | | | | | | | | | | | | | |
| HALS | | | | | | | | | | | | | | | | | | | | | | | | | |
| Weetabix | 1 | 94 | 3 | 3 | 93 | 4 | 3 | 89 | 5 | 6 | 92 | 4 | 4 | 96 | 2 | 2 | 96 | 2 | 1 | 94 | 2 | 4 | 96 | 2 | 2 |
| | 2 | 98 | 1 | 1 | 97 | 2 | 1 | 91 | 3 | 5 | 96 | 2 | 2 | 99 | 1 | (3) | 98 | 1 | (4) | 92 | 3 | 4 | 97 | 2 | 1 |
| Digestive | 1 | 76 | 16 | 7 | 79 | 14 | 7 | 75 | 17 | 7 | 77 | 16 | 7 | 82 | 13 | 5 | 85 | 11 | 4 | 84 | 10 | 7 | 83 | 11 | 5 |
| biscuits | 2 | 80 | 17 | 4 | 82 | 15 | 3 | 77 | 16 | 7 | 80 | 16 | 4 | 85 | 12 | 3 | 87 | 10 | 4 | 80 | 14 | 6 | 85 | 11 | 4 |
| Potatoes | 1 | 45 | 46 | 8 | 38 | 55 | 7 | 36 | 54 | 9 | 41 | 51 | 8 | 60 | 32 | 8 | 56 | 35 | 9 | 37 | 50 | 13 | 54 | 37 | 9 |
| | 2 | 75 | 20 | 4 | 66 | 29 | 5 | 62 | 30 | 7 | 69 | 26 | 5 | 84 | 14 | 3 | 79 | 17 | 4 | 65 | 26 | 10 | 78 | 17 | 4 |
| White bread | 1 | 45 | 50 | 4 | 44 | 51 | 5 | 46 | 48 | 6 | 45 | 50 | 5 | 40 | 55 | 5 | 37 | 58 | 5 | 34 | 60 | 5 | 38 | 57 | 5 |
| | 2 | 62 | 35 | 3 | 56 | 41 | 3 | 57 | 38 | 5 | 58 | 38 | 3 | 57 | 41 | 2 | 52 | 46 | 2 | 46 | 48 | 6 | 53 | 44 | 3 |
| Apples | 1 | 40 | 48 | 12 | 52 | 39 | 9 | 47 | 43 | 10 | 46 | 43 | 10 | 52 | 38 | 10 | 58 | 35 | 7 | 52 | 39 | 9 | 54 | 37 | 9 |
| | 2 | 56 | 37 | 8 | 65 | 28 | 6 | 61 | 31 | 7 | 60 | 32 | 7 | 64 | 29 | 7 | 68 | 26 | 6 | 64 | 26 | 9 | 66 | 27 | 7 |
| **Fibre-free foods** | | | | | | | | | | | | | | | | | | | | | | | | | |
| Roast meat | 1 | 53 | 32 | 15 | 52 | 34 | 13 | 46 | 36 | 17 | 51 | 34 | 15 | 54 | 30 | 16 | 52 | 32 | 16 | 41 | 39 | 20 | 51 | 32 | 17 |
| | 2 | 56 | 34 | 11 | 50 | 40 | 9 | 41 | 43 | 16 | 50 | 38 | 11 | 58 | 30 | 13 | 50 | 36 | 14 | 38 | 41 | 21 | 51 | 34 | 15 |
| Grilled fish | 1 | 57 | 25 | 19 | 60 | 28 | 12 | 59 | 27 | 13 | 58 | 26 | 15 | 57 | 23 | 20 | 63 | 21 | 16 | 54 | 29 | 16 | 59 | 23 | 17 |
| | 2 | 62 | 26 | 13 | 53 | 34 | 12 | 47 | 41 | 11 | 55 | 32 | 12 | 64 | 22 | 14 | 61 | 27 | 12 | 42 | 41 | 16 | 59 | 28 | 13 |
| Orange juice | 1 | 69 | 19 | 12 | 72 | 19 | 9 | 68 | 20 | 11 | 70 | 19 | 10 | 64 | 23 | 13 | 69 | 22 | 9 | 67 | 22 | 11 | 66 | 22 | 11 |
| | 2 | 69 | 22 | 8 | 70 | 23 | 6 | 65 | 26 | 9 | 69 | 24 | 8 | 62 | 31 | 8 | 66 | 25 | 9 | 58 | 29 | 13 | 63 | 28 | 9 |
| Cheese | 1 | 78 | 10 | 12 | 79 | 12 | 9 | 78 | 15 | 7 | 78 | 12 | 10 | 78 | 10 | 12 | 82 | 9 | 10 | 65 | 23 | 13 | 77 | 12 | 11 |
| | 2 | 85 | 7 | 8 | 82 | 12 | 6 | 63 | 28 | 8 | 79 | 14 | 7 | 86 | 7 | 7 | 85 | 8 | 7 | 60 | 26 | 14 | 80 | 11 | 8 |
| Eggs | 1 | 80 | 12 | 8 | 84 | 8 | 8 | 80 | 11 | 9 | 81 | 10 | 8 | 81 | 9 | 10 | 84 | 6 | 9 | 75 | 12 | 12 | 81 | 9 | 10 |
| | 2 | 84 | 9 | 8 | 85 | 9 | 7 | 73 | 16 | 10 | 82 | 10 | 8 | 85 | 7 | 8 | 85 | 7 | 8 | 69 | 15 | 15 | 82 | 9 | 9 |
| *Base = 100%* | | 784 | | | 773 | | | 420 | | | 1977 | | | 1045 | | | 941 | | | 484 | | | 2470 | | |

**Table 11.18** **Socio-economic variations in number of correct answers to 'Do you think these foods contain dietary fibre?' for 5 fibre-free and 5 fibre-containing foods. Percentage of non-manual and manual group**

| | Males | | | | Females | | | |
| | Non-manual | | Manual | | Non-manual | | Manual | |
| HALS | 1 | 2 | 1 | 2 | 1 | 2 | 1 | 2 |
|---|---|---|---|---|---|---|---|---|
| **Number of correct answers** | | | | Fibre-free foods | | | | |
| 0 | 3 | 2 | 6 | 7 | 3 | 3 | 8 | 7 |
| 1 | 5 | 3 | 12 | 9 | 7 | 4 | 10 | 11 |
| 2 | 9 | 10 | 13 | 14 | 11 | 11 | 14 | 12 |
| 3 | 22 | 25 | 20 | 24 | 21 | 23 | 20 | 22 |
| 4 | 28 | 30 | 26 | 26 | 28 | 31 | 24 | 27 |
| 5 | 34 | 29 | 23 | 19 | 31 | 27 | 24 | 22 |
| **Number of correct answers** | | | | Fibre-containing foods | | | | |
| 0 | 1 | 0 | 3 | 1 | 0 | 0 | 1 | 1 |
| 1 | 5 | 2 | 6 | 3 | 3 | 2 | 5 | 1 |
| 2 | 22 | 10 | 24 | 12 | 16 | 7 | 24 | 12 |
| 3 | 32 | 22 | 39 | 28 | 29 | 20 | 33 | 26 |
| 4 | 28 | 37 | 20 | 36 | 36 | 36 | 29 | 37 |
| 5 | 13 | 29 | 8 | 20 | 16 | 35 | 9 | 23 |
| *Base = 100%* | 869 | | 1085 | | 1139 | | 1294 | |

# ALTERATIONS IN SMOKING PATTERNS | 12

Margaret J Whichelow and Brian D Cox

Tobacco smoking has been identified as being the lifestyle behaviour most implicated in the aetiology of ill-health in Great Britain, with a clearly defined relationship to respiratory and circulatory disease. In the past few years, health professionals have endeavoured to make the population aware of this relationship, and to encourage people to stop smoking. In many places where the habit was previously tolerated, it is now forbidden. The HALS2 survey has given the opportunity to examine in some part the changes that have occurred as a result of these efforts.

In HALS1 the routing of the smoking section of the questionnaire was complex, resulting in interviewers in some cases omitting questions. In order to overcome these difficulties the questions were re-ordered (see Appendix A). In both Surveys the information collected was designed to categorise respondents as life-time non-smokers (those who had never smoked as much as one cigarette a day for six months, or had not regularly smoked pipes or cigars), as ex-smokers (those who did not currently smoke but who used to smoke regularly), occasional smokers (those currently smoking, but fewer than one cigarette per day on average) and current regular smokers (those smoking at least one cigarette, cigar or bowl of pipe tobacco a day). Regular smokers were further divided into light – up to 15 cigarettes per day – and heavy smokers – 16 or more cigarettes per day. Regular pipe or cigar smokers were classified as light smokers, and occasional pipe or cigar smokers as non-smokers. By far the major part of tobacco smoked in this country is in the form of cigarettes. In HALS2 there were no pipe or cigar smokers amongst

the women. The comparatively few men who are, or were, only pipe or cigar smokers are included with the cigarette smokers, as smokers or ex-smokers, for many of the tables. Those analyses where only cigarettes are considered are specified in the table headings. The inclusion of cigar and/or pipe smokers with the cigarette smokers has been done because there is reason to believe that all forms of tobacco are harmful to health (Jarvis and Jackson, 1988).

## Smoking prevalence

Over the past few decades the prevalence of cigarette smoking has been declining steadily in men and somewhat less rapidly in women (Capell, 1978; Smyth and Browne, 1992). A decrease in regular smoking between HALS1 and HALS2 has occurred in both men and women (Table 12.1). The decrease in regular cigarette smoking is apparent at all ages, except for those who were aged 18 to 25 at HALS1. The most striking trend, however, is the decline to almost negligible levels of 1% in both sexes of the occasional smokers, who contribute equally with the regular smokers to the rise in the proportion of ex-smokers by HALS2.

The change in smoking status from HALS1 to HALS2 is shown in Table 12.2. In both sexes and at all ages the few respondents who have taken up smoking since HALS1 have mostly given up again or become light smokers. It was demonstrated previously (Golding, 1987) that the majority of smokers took up the habit in their mid-teens, with very few commencing smoking after age 20, so the small number taking up smoking observed here was to be expected. Overall, 21% of men and 27% of women occasional smokers have become non-smokers – that is, they were occasional smokers who had never regularly smoked. Those occasional smokers who had previously been regular smokers, but who had, by HALS2, stopped altogether have become ex-smokers. Some of the younger men and women have increased their cigarette consumption. A few who were ex-smokers at HALS1 have taken up smoking again, particularly at younger ages, a finding which is not surprising as many smokers give up on numerous occasions and some of those seen in HALS1 had only given up a few days or weeks before interview. Most of the regular smokers at HALS1 had remained as such, but within the regular smoking category more heavy smokers had become light smokers than vice-versa except in the men aged 18-38. The tendency in both men and women has been, with advancing age, to reduce or stop smoking. As might be expected more light than heavy smokers had succeeded in giving up completely.

There is a well-established social class gradient, with the prevalence of smoking much lower in non-manual than manual groups (Golding, 1987; Smyth and Browne, 1992). These trends for both men and women in HALS1 and HALS2 are confirmed in Table 12.3. The decrease in smoking from HALS1 to HALS2, both regular and occasional, has taken place in all socio-economic groups to much the same extent, so that the social class differentials are maintained.

Table 12.4 shows the differences by socio-economic groups in the changes between smoking categories which have occurred between HALS1 and HALS2. More men in non-manual than in manual groups have remained non-smokers, but the difference is not so marked in women. In both sexes more light smokers in the non-manual than the manual groups have given up smoking, as have more women in the non-manual group who were heavy smokers.

Regional variations in socio-economic structure result in the regions in the northern part of the country having a higher proportion of manual workers, but this accounts only in part for the regional variations seen in smoking prevalence (Whichelow et al. 1990). In all regions there has been a drop in smoking prevalence between HALS1

and HALS2, so that the differences between the regions remain (Table 12.5). In most regions the proportion of men who were regular smokers in either Survey exceeds the proportion of women regular smokers, this difference being particularly marked in Wales, East Anglia and the South West. The differences were smaller in London and the South East and non-existent in Scotland and the North.

Table 12.6 separates out cigarette, pipe and cigar smoking for the men only. There was a marked drop in cigar smoking between HALS1 and HALS2 at all ages. There has also been a reduction in pipe smoking, but this was already at a low rate in HALS1. Cigarette smoking has also declined in all but the youngest age group and most noticeably in those aged between 46 and 66 at HALS1 (53 to 73 in HALS2).

There has been little change in the overall consumption of cigarettes by regular smokers between HALS1 and HALS2 (Table 12.7), except amongst the women in non-manual groups, where the proportion of heavy smokers, 16 or more cigarettes per day, has declined. In both non-manual and manual groups there are more men than women who are heavy smokers. Amongst the women, but not the men, the respondents in manual groups are the heavier smokers. There is also a socio-economic group difference in respect of the self-assessed tar level of the cigarettes smoked, with the non-manual women in both Surveys and the non-manual men in HALS1 preferring the lowest tar level brands (Table 12.8). The General Household Survey (Smyth and Browne, 1992) also found that women are more likely than men to choose cigarettes with a low tar content. Since HALS1 there has been a shift, in both sexes, towards low tar cigarettes. This continues a trend in the type of tobacco used that has been evident for some years (Fourth Scarborough Conference on Preventive Medicine, 1985). In HALS1, particularly in the men, smokers in non-manual groups were more likely than those in manual groups to be smoking low/middle or low tar cigarettes, but by HALS2 the difference had been eliminated.

The comparatively large number of respondents who gave up smoking between HALS1 and HALS2 – 524 – enables comparisons to be made of the reasons given by those who gave up more than seven years ago with those who gave up recently (Table 12.9). As might be expected health reasons were frequently cited. In the young 'fear of illness' was more likely to be mentioned especially by young men (42% in HALS1 and 45% in HALS2), whereas in the older groups 'ill health' was predominant (41% and 45% in the men and 35% of the women in both Surveys). In the men the percentage quoting 'social pressure' has doubled and although there has been a smaller increase in women citing this reason it was mentioned more often at both Surveys by those aged over 39 at HALS1. The effects of banning, or limiting, smoking in public places and places of work and the publicity about the hazards of passive smoking have presumably been having some effect. Evidence for this is the fact that in HALS2, but not HALS1, ex-smokers were giving the 'health of others' as a reason for quitting.

In HALS2, those who gave 'ill-health' as a reason for having given up smoking were asked to specify the illness. The results shown in Table 12.10 reveal that lung and chest conditions were the major factor reported, especially amongst the elderly. Heart problems, mostly ischaemic heart disease, as well as transient illnesses such as colds and flu also featured.

## Passive smoking

In recent years the hypothesis that passive smoking may be injurious to health has gained much support (US Surgeon General, 1986), although it is not universally accepted (Lee, 1992). Respondents were asked in HALS1 and HALS2 whether there were smokers other than themselves in the household. The responses in HALS1 were unsatisfactory in many cases, since many respondents clearly misunderstood the question. As the question was posed in another part of the smoking section in HALS2 the responses are more reliable and are presented in Table 12.11. Smokers are more likely to live in a smoking household, particularly if they are in the manual socio-economic groups. Non-smokers in the manual groups are also more likely than those in the non-manual groups to live with smokers. Confirmation of the exposure to passive smoking will be obtained when the cotinine measurements, from saliva collected by the nurse during the physiological measurements session, are available.

## Ill Health and Smoking

Higher levels of malaise and illness symptoms (see Appendix A for definitions) were reported by smokers in HALS1; similarly, in HALS2 a higher proportion of smokers than non-smokers consistently report high levels of malaise and illness symptoms, and these are shown in Table 12.12. There is a tendency for the oldest respondents in most smoking categories to be less likely to report low malaise in HALS2, but otherwise there is little consistent change between the Surveys. The numbers with high levels of illness have risen in the oldest respondents in all smoking groups. In general the proportion of ex-smokers with high and low levels of illness and malaise lie between those of the smokers and the non-smokers.

The levels of respiratory and heart disease reported differ among non-smokers, ex-smokers and regular smokers (Table 12.13). Asthma is more prevalent amongst young ex-smoking men, and, in general, there are fewer asthmatics among the smokers than the non-smokers or ex-smokers. The most notable finding is of an increase in the prevalence of asthma at HALS2 in all ages (see Chapter 4) and in most smoking groups. The proportion suffering from chronic bronchitis, which has changed little between HALS1 and HALS2, is higher amongst the smokers and ex-smokers than among the non-smokers. 'Other' chest conditions are also more common amongst ex-smokers and smokers than among non-smokers. There has been a tendency for an increased proportion of smokers to report that they suffer from 'other' chest conditions, which include emphysema, at HALS2. This is in line with the observation that since HALS1 the lung function of heavy smokers has deteriorated more than would be expected for their age, as reported in Chapter 5. As far as heart disease is concerned, in the oldest men and women (where the disease is more prevalent) the highest proportions are found in the ex-smokers. The most likely explanation for this finding is that those who have heart disease have been encouraged by this experience or by their doctor to stop smoking. The proportion of non-smokers reporting no respiratory problems is consistently higher than the proportion for the smokers and all but the middle aged men who are ex-smokers. At most age groups the smokers are the least likely to be free of respiratory problems. In all groups there is a tendency for the proportion with no respiratory problems to decrease with advancing age.

## Characteristics of those smoking in HALS2

In HALS2 smokers were asked how soon after waking they first smoked. Heavy smokers were, not unexpectedly, more likely than light smokers to have their first smoke immediately on waking (Table 12.14). Very few heavy smokers, particularly women heavy smokers, waited more than an hour before smoking, whereas 53% of the men and 42% of the women who were light smokers did not smoke that early.

A similar difference between light and heavy smokers was found in respect of craving for tobacco (Table 12.15). The significant proportion reporting 'never' experiencing craving includes those, mainly heavy smokers, who said that they were never without tobacco. Those smokers reporting craving 'frequently' or 'always' might be considered to be among the most addicted to smoking, who would find it most difficult to stop.

Nevertheless a high proportion of heavy smokers, of all ages except the elderly men, reported a 'strong' desire to stop. Amongst the men, more light than heavy smokers had no desire to stop (Table 12.16). Although the numbers of pipe and cigar smokers are small, the proportion at all ages who expressed no desire to stop smoking is very high. It may be that pipe and cigar smoking is not perceived being as hazardous to health as cigarette smoking (Jarvis and Jackson, 1988).

Cigarette smokers' opinions at HALS2 as to whether they were smoking more, less or the same amount as at HALS2 were compared with the more objective assessment of change, by comparing the number of cigarettes reportedly smoked at the time of the two Surveys (Table 12.17). For those who reported no change in cigarette consumption only 41%, or less, were actually smoking the same number of cigarettes, whereas those who said they were smoking fewer were more likely to be accurate. Except for the middle-aged women, over two-thirds of those claiming to smoke more had increased their cigarette consumption.

Further evidence of the under-reporting of smoking was revealed when 151 respondents who claimed at HALS2 to be life-time non-smokers were identified from the HALS1 records as having been ex-regular smokers. The characteristics of this group are shown in Table 12.18. In these groups the women out-number the men by 3:1, and they were distributed fairly evenly across the age groups, whereas in the men there was a predominance in the 39-59 year old group. There were no socio-economic group differences.

## Summary

Changes in smoking habits over the seven years between HALS1 and HALS2 have been observed, with an increase in the number of ex-smokers, particularly in those aged between 46 and 66 at HALS1. Although many light, and some heavy smokers have stopped, the more striking finding is that the majority of occasional cigarette smokers and cigar smokers have also given up smoking. There has also been a trend towards low tar cigarettes amongst all groups of smokers. The stigmatisation of smoking seems to be felt as recent ex-smokers are more frequently reporting 'social pressure' and the health of others as reasons for quitting.

### References

Capell, P.J. (1978), 'Trends in cigarette smoking in the UK', Health Trends, 10, 49-54.

Fourth Scarborough Conference on Preventive Medicine (1985) 'Is there a future for lower tar yield cigarettes', Lancet, 2, 1111-1114.

Golding, J.F. (1987), in Cox, B.D. et al. 'The Health and Lifestyle Survey', London, Health Promotion Research Trust.

Jarvis, M. and Jackson, P. (1988), 'Cigar and pipe smoking in Britain: implications for smoking prevalence and cessation', British Journal of Addiction, 83, 323-330.

Lee, P.N. (1992), 'Environmental Tobacco Smoke and Mortality', London, Karger.

Smyth, M. and Browne, F. (1992), 'General Household Survey 1990', London: HMSO.

U.S. Surgeon General (1986), 'The Health Consequences of Involuntary Smoking', Rockville, USA: US Department of Health and Human Services, Public Health Service.

Whichelow, M.J., Erzinclioglu, S.W. and Cox, B.D. (1991), 'Some regional variations in dietary patterns in a random sample of British adults', European Journal of Clinical Nutrition, 45, 253-262.

**Table 12.1** **Smoking habits by age in HALS1 full sample, and HALS2 sub-sample at HALS1 and HALS2. Percentage of age group**

| Age at HALS1 | 18-24 | | 25-31 | | 32-38 | | 39-45 | | 46-52 | | 53-59 | | 60-66 | | 67-73 | | >73 | | All | |
| --- | --- | --- | --- | --- | --- | --- | --- | --- | --- | --- | --- | --- | --- | --- | --- | --- | --- | --- | --- | --- |
| Age at HALS2 | | 25-31 | | 32-38 | | 39-45 | | 46-52 | | 53-59 | | 60-66 | | 67-73 | | 74-80 | | >80 | | |

**Males**

**Never smoked**

| | | | | | | | | | | | | | | | | | | | | | |
| --- | --- | --- | --- | --- | --- | --- | --- | --- | --- | --- | --- | --- | --- | --- | --- | --- | --- | --- | --- | --- | --- |
| HALS1 sample | 49 | | 37 | | 29 | | 19 | | 23 | | 16 | | 13 | | 14 | | 13 | | 25 | |
| HALS2 sub-sample | 55 | 50 | 39 | 39 | 33 | 35 | 22 | 23 | 28 | 28 | 17 | 17 | 18 | 16 | 18 | 17 | 15 | 15 | 29 | 28 |

**Occasional smokers**

| | | | | | | | | | | | | | | | | | | | | | |
| --- | --- | --- | --- | --- | --- | --- | --- | --- | --- | --- | --- | --- | --- | --- | --- | --- | --- | --- | --- | --- | --- |
| HALS1 sample | 7 | | 9 | | 7 | | 8 | | 6 | | 3 | | 4 | | 5 | | 5 | | 6 | |
| HALS2 sub-sample | 5 | 2 | 9 | (1) | 7 | (3) | 8 | (3) | 5 | (1) | 3 | (1) | 5 | (2) | 7 | 0 | 6 | 0 | 6 | 1 |

**Ex-smokers**

| | | | | | | | | | | | | | | | | | | | | | |
| --- | --- | --- | --- | --- | --- | --- | --- | --- | --- | --- | --- | --- | --- | --- | --- | --- | --- | --- | --- | --- | --- |
| HALS1 sample | 6 | | 11 | | 24 | | 25 | | 26 | | 39 | | 42 | | 44 | | 49 | | 27 | |
| HALS2 sub-sample | 6 | 12 | 10 | 20 | 24 | 31 | 28 | 39 | 24 | 41 | 40 | 55 | 41 | 56 | 47 | 60 | 45 | 56 | 27 | 38 |

**Regular smokers**

| | | | | | | | | | | | | | | | | | | | | | |
| --- | --- | --- | --- | --- | --- | --- | --- | --- | --- | --- | --- | --- | --- | --- | --- | --- | --- | --- | --- | --- | --- |
| HALS1 sample | 38 | | 43 | | 41 | | 48 | | 45 | | 42 | | 40 | | 37 | | 33 | | 41 | |
| HALS2 sub-sample | 34 | 36 | 42 | 41 | 36 | 34 | 42 | 38 | 43 | 31 | 40 | 28 | 36 | 27 | 28 | 22 | 34 | 28 | 38 | 33 |

| *Base = 100%* | | | | | | | | | | | | | | | | | | | | | |
| --- | --- | --- | --- | --- | --- | --- | --- | --- | --- | --- | --- | --- | --- | --- | --- | --- | --- | --- | --- | --- | --- |
| *HALS1* | *515* | | *482* | | *549* | | *464* | | *409* | | *408* | | *407* | | *313* | | *270* | | *3817* | |
| *HALS2* | | *299 298* | *241 241* | | *383 383* | | *324 324* | | *280 280* | | *278 278* | | *259 259* | | *148 147* | | *88 87* | | *2300 2297* | |

**Females**

**Never smoked**

| | | | | | | | | | | | | | | | | | | | | | |
| --- | --- | --- | --- | --- | --- | --- | --- | --- | --- | --- | --- | --- | --- | --- | --- | --- | --- | --- | --- | --- | --- |
| HALS1 sample | 53 | | 45 | | 43 | | 42 | | 45 | | 37 | | 42 | | 54 | | 64 | | 46 | |
| HALS2 sub-sample | 51 | 48 | 45 | 42 | 44 | 43 | 44 | 42 | 48 | 47 | 39 | 39 | 45 | 42 | 57 | 54 | 62 | 62 | 47 | 45 |

**Occasional smokers**

| | | | | | | | | | | | | | | | | | | | | | |
| --- | --- | --- | --- | --- | --- | --- | --- | --- | --- | --- | --- | --- | --- | --- | --- | --- | --- | --- | --- | --- | --- |
| HALS1 sample | 4 | | 3 | | 2 | | 3 | | 3 | | 3 | | 2 | | 2 | | 2 | | 3 | |
| HALS2 sub-sample | 4 | 1 | 3 | 2 | 2 | 1 | 3 | (1) | 2 | 1 | 2 | (2) | 2 | (2) | 2 | 2 | 3 | 0 | 3 | 1 |

**Ex-smokers**

| | | | | | | | | | | | | | | | | | | | | | |
| --- | --- | --- | --- | --- | --- | --- | --- | --- | --- | --- | --- | --- | --- | --- | --- | --- | --- | --- | --- | --- | --- |
| HALS1 sample | 8 | | 17 | | 20 | | 22 | | 17 | | 23 | | 25 | | 24 | | 24 | | 20 | |
| HALS2 sub-sample | 10 | 15 | 19 | 24 | 20 | 25 | 24 | 32 | 17 | 24 | 24 | 32 | 28 | 37 | 24 | 30 | 28 | 32 | 21 | 27 |

**Regular smokers**

| | | | | | | | | | | | | | | | | | | | | | |
| --- | --- | --- | --- | --- | --- | --- | --- | --- | --- | --- | --- | --- | --- | --- | --- | --- | --- | --- | --- | --- | --- |
| HALS1 sample | 35 | | 34 | | 35 | | 33 | | 35 | | 38 | | 31 | | 21 | | 10 | | 31 | |
| HALS2 sub-sample | 35 | 36 | 33 | 32 | 33 | 32 | 29 | 26 | 33 | 28 | 35 | 29 | 26 | 20 | 18 | 14 | 5 | 6 | 30 | 27 |

| *Base = 100%* | | | | | | | | | | | | | | | | | | | | | |
| --- | --- | --- | --- | --- | --- | --- | --- | --- | --- | --- | --- | --- | --- | --- | --- | --- | --- | --- | --- | --- | --- |
| *HALS1* | *625* | | *669* | | *759* | | *617* | | *575* | | *484* | | *550* | | *391* | | *405* | | *5073* | |
| *HALS2* | | *311 311* | *394 394* | | *545 545* | | *432 432* | | *391 391* | | *315 315* | | *327 326* | | *191 190* | | *146 143* | | *3052 3047* | |

**Table 12.2** Change in smoking categories from HALS1 to HALS2 in young, middle-aged and elderly respondents. Percentage of HALS1 smoking category

| | HALS1 (1984/5) smoking categories and age at HALS1 | | | | | | | | | | | | | | |
| | 18-38 | | | | | 39-59 | | | | | 60+ | | | | |
| | Non- | Occ. | Ex- | Light | Heavy | Non- | Occ. | Ex- | Light | Heavy | Non- | Occ. | Ex- | Light | Heavy |
| **HALS2 (1991/2) smoking categories** | | | | | | | | Males | | | | | | | |
| Non-smokers | 93 | 31 | – | – | – | 94 | 20 | – | – | – | 90 | 4 | – | – | – |
| Occasional | (3) | (1) | 2 | 1 | 0 | 0 | 2 | (2) | 1 | 0 | 0 | 0 | (1) | 1 | 0 |
| Ex-smokers | 4 | 37 | 84 | 20 | 8 | 5 | 60 | 96 | 32 | 19 | 10 | 64 | 98 | 31 | 22 |
| Light regular | 4 | 23 | 9 | 53 | 23 | (1) | 18 | 3 | 53 | 18 | 0 | 32 | (2) | 64 | 33 |
| Heavy regular | (2) | 8 | 5 | 27 | 68 | (1) | 0 | (1) | 13 | 63 | 0 | 0 | (2) | 4 | 45 |
| *Base = 100%* | *386* | *62* | *133* | *188* | *153* | *197* | *50* | *270* | *182* | *183* | *87* | *28* | *216* | *104* | *58* |
| | | | | | | | | Females | | | | | | | |
| Non-smokers | 94 | 16 | – | – | – | 95 | 36 | – | – | – | 94 | (5) | – | – | – |
| Occasional | (4) | 8 | 3 | 1 | 0 | (2) | 7 | (1) | 2 | 0 | (1) | (1) | 0 | 4 | 0 |
| Ex-smokers | 4 | 35 | 85 | 17 | 9 | 4 | 57 | 93 | 24 | 14 | 6 | (4) | 96 | 29 | 22 |
| Light regular | 1 | 41 | 9 | 61 | 24 | (2) | 0 | 5 | 63 | 23 | 0 | (3) | 4 | 64 | 38 |
| Heavy regular | (3) | 0 | 3 | 22 | 67 | 0 | 0 | 2 | 12 | 64 | 0 | 0 | 0 | 2 | 41 |
| *Base = 100%* | *578* | *37* | *216* | *255* | *164* | *501* | *28* | *243* | *193* | *173* | *345* | *13* | *174* | *90* | *37* |

**Table 12.3** Change in smoking status from HALS1 to HALS2 by HALS1 socio-economic group. Percentage of socio-economic group

| | Males | | | | | | | | Females | | | | | | | |
| | Never smoked | | Occasional smokers | | Ex- smokers | | Regular smokers | | Base = 100% | Never smoked | | Occasional smokers | | Ex- smokers | | Regular smokers | | Base = 100% |
| HALS | 1 | 2 | 1 | 2 | 1 | 2 | 1 | 2 | | 1 | 2 | 1 | 2 | 1 | 2 | 1 | 2 | |
| Professional | 42 | 45 | 10 | 1 | 26 | 33 | 22 | 21 | *116* | 54 | 53 | 3 | 1 | 29 | 33 | 14 | 13 | *174* |
| Empl/managers | 27 | 28 | 8 | 1 | 31 | 42 | 34 | 29 | *439* | 53 | 51 | 2 | 1 | 20 | 26 | 25 | 21 | *548* |
| Other non-manual | 36 | 36 | 7 | 1 | 27 | 38 | 31 | 25 | *426* | 52 | 50 | 4 | 1 | 20 | 27 | 25 | 22 | *683* |
| Skilled manual | 27 | 25 | 5 | 1 | 28 | 39 | 41 | 36 | *837* | 43 | 40 | 2 | 1 | 20 | 27 | 35 | 31 | *975* |
| Semi-skilled | 24 | 20 | 5 | 1 | 24 | 37 | 47 | 42 | *342* | 42 | 39 | 2 | 1 | 22 | 27 | 34 | 33 | *498* |
| Unskilled | 22 | 21 | 7 | 0 | 23 | 35 | 48 | 44 | *108* | 34 | 33 | 3 | 0 | 23 | 28 | 41 | 39 | *131* |

**Table 12.4** **Change in smoking categories from HALS1 to HALS2 in non-manual and manual respondents. Percentage of HALS1 smoking category**

| | HALS1 (1984/5) smoking categories | | | | | | | | | |
|---|---|---|---|---|---|---|---|---|---|---|
| | Non-manual | | | | | Manual | | | | |
| | Non- | Occ. | Ex- | Light | Heavy | Non- | Occ. | Ex- | Light | Heavy |
| **HALS2 (1991/2) smoking categories** | | | | | **Males** | | | | | |
| Non-smokers | 97 | 24 | – | – | – | 89 | 18 | – | – | – |
| Occasional | 0 | 1 | 1 | 2 | 0 | (3) | 2 | (3) | (1) | 0 |
| Ex-smokers | 3 | 53 | 95 | 30 | 13 | 8 | 47 | 93 | 25 | 16 |
| Light regular | (1) | 19 | 3 | 55 | 23 | 2 | 29 | 4 | 56 | 21 |
| Heavy regular | (1) | 3 | (2) | 12 | 64 | (2) | 5 | 2 | 19 | 62 |
| *Base = 100%* | *333* | *75* | *279* | *177* | *130* | *330* | *62* | *338* | *293* | *262* |
| | | | | | **Females** | | | | | |
| Non-smokers | 95 | 21 | – | – | – | 93 | 32 | – | – | – |
| Occasional | (4) | 10 | 1 | 2 | 0 | (3) | 6 | (3) | 2 | 0 |
| Ex-smokers | 3 | 50 | 91 | 26 | 17 | 6 | 32 | 90 | 19 | 10 |
| Light regular | 1 | 19 | 5 | 65 | 24 | (3) | 29 | 7 | 60 | 25 |
| Heavy regular | 0 | 0 | 2 | 7 | 58 | (3) | 0 | 2 | 19 | 65 |
| *Base = 100%* | *740* | *42* | *292* | *208* | *127* | *667* | *34* | *335* | *324* | *240* |

**Table 12.5** Regional variations in changes of smoking habit in those respondents seen in both Surveys. Percentages in each region

| | Scotland | | Wales | | North | | North West | | Yorks./ Humber. | | West Midlands | | East Midlands | | East Anglia | | South West | | South East | | Greater London | |
|---|---|---|---|---|---|---|---|---|---|---|---|---|---|---|---|---|---|---|---|---|---|---|
| HALS | 1 | 2 | 1 | 2 | 1 | 2 | 1 | 2 | 1 | 2 | 1 | 2 | 1 | 2 | 1 | 2 | 1 | 2 | 1 | 2 | 1 | 2 |
| **Males** | | | | | | | | | | | | | | | | | | | | | | |
| Never smoked | 35 | 30 | 29 | 28 | 26 | 28 | 24 | 25 | 28 | 27 | 32 | 33 | 31 | 30 | 25 | 23 | 23 | 23 | 32 | 32 | 28 | 27 |
| Occasional smokers | 4 | 1 | 5 | 0 | 10 | 0 | 5 | 1 | 7 | 0 | 6 | 1 | 5 | 0 | 5 | 0 | 6 | 1 | 8 | 1 | 6 | 3 |
| Ex-smokers | 19 | 33 | 21 | 27 | 25 | 37 | 26 | 36 | 25 | 37 | 25 | 31 | 26 | 37 | 27 | 46 | 32 | 46 | 29 | 44 | 33 | 42 |
| Regular smokers | 42 | 37 | 46 | 45 | 39 | 36 | 45 | 38 | 40 | 36 | 37 | 34 | 38 | 33 | 43 | 30 | 39 | 31 | 28 | 24 | 34 | 29 |
| Base = 100% | 249 | | 136 | | 115 | | 250 | | 219 | | 201 | | 193 | | 84 | | 187 | | 448 | | 218 | |
| **Females** | | | | | | | | | | | | | | | | | | | | | | |
| Never smoked | 48 | 45 | 48 | 46 | 33 | 31 | 44 | 43 | 44 | 42 | 49 | 44 | 50 | 48 | 47 | 44 | 53 | 51 | 51 | 49 | 44 | 43 |
| Occasional smokers | 1 | 1 | 3 | 1 | 1 | 0 | 3 | 1 | 4 | 1 | 2 | (1) | 4 | (1) | 4 | 5 | 2 | 1 | 2 | 1 | 4 | 1 |
| Ex-smokers | 12 | 17 | 15 | 23 | 27 | 32 | 19 | 26 | 23 | 29 | 19 | 28 | 21 | 27 | 25 | 31 | 25 | 29 | 24 | 28 | 20 | 32 |
| Regular smokers | 40 | 38 | 34 | 29 | 40 | 37 | 34 | 31 | 29 | 28 | 31 | 27 | 25 | 25 | 24 | 21 | 19 | 18 | 23 | 21 | 31 | 24 |
| Base = 100% | 320 | | 166 | | 199 | | 417 | | 274 | | 275 | | 234 | | 131 | | 233 | | 539 | | 264 | |

**Table 12.6** Changes in cigarette, cigar and pipe smoking in men from HALS1 to HALS2. (Smoking more than one type of tobacco was possible.) Percentage of age group

| Age at HALS1 | 18-24 | | 25-31 | | 32-38 | | 39-45 | | 46-52 | | 53-59 | | 60-66 | | 67-73 | | >73 | | ALL | |
|---|---|---|---|---|---|---|---|---|---|---|---|---|---|---|---|---|---|---|---|---|
| HALS | 1 | 2 | 1 | 2 | 1 | 2 | 1 | 2 | 1 | 2 | 1 | 2 | 1 | 2 | 1 | 2 | 1 | 2 | 1 | 2 |
| **Smoking type** | | | | | | | | | | | | | | | | | | | | |
| Cigarettes | 33 | 34 | 39 | 36 | 32 | 28 | 35 | 31 | 34 | 25 | 32 | 23 | 27 | 20 | 22 | 17 | 16 | 16 | 32 | 27 |
| | | +1 | | − 3 | | − 4 | | − 4 | | − 9 | | − 9 | | − 7 | | − 5 | | 0 | | − 5 |
| Cigars | 10 | 4 | 15 | 4 | 17 | 5 | 22 | 7 | 18 | 5 | 14 | 4 | 19 | 5 | 15 | 4 | 14 | 3 | 16 | 5 |
| | | − 6 | | − 11 | | − 12 | | − 15 | | − 13 | | − 10 | | − 14 | | − 11 | | − 11 | | − 11 |
| Pipe | 0 | 0 | 2 | (1) | 4 | 3 | 6 | 3 | 10 | 4 | 5 | 3 | 8 | 5 | 5 | 3 | 16 | 11 | 5 | 3 |
| | | | | − 1 | | − 3 | | − 6 | | − 2 | | − 3 | | − 2 | | − 5 | | − 2 | | |
| Base = 100% | 299 | | 241 | | 383 | | 324 | | 280 | | 278 | | 259 | | 148 | | 88 | | 2300 | |

**Table 12.7    Comparison of number of cigarettes smoked by regular smokers in HALS1 and HALS2. Percentage in non-manual and manual groups**

| | Males | | | | Females | | | |
|---|---|---|---|---|---|---|---|---|
| | Non-manual | | Manual | | Non-manual | | Manual | |
| HALS | 1 | 2 | 1 | 2 | 1 | 2 | 1 | 2 |
| **Cigarettes smoked** | | | | | | | | |
| 1-5 per day | 12 | 12 | 8 | 10 | 15 | 19 | 10 | 9 |
| 6-10 per day | 18 | 16 | 19 | 18 | 25 | 22 | 27 | 24 |
| 11-15 per day | 15 | 15 | 19 | 17 | 22 | 26 | 20 | 23 |
| 16-20 per day | 30 | 30 | 37 | 33 | 28 | 25 | 30 | 31 |
| 21-25 per day | 6 | 8 | 6 | 8 | 5 | 2 | 4 | 6 |
| Over 25 per day | 20 | 19 | 11 | 13 | 5 | 6 | 8 | 7 |
| *Base = 100%* | *234* | *190* | *489* | *425* | *338* | *291* | *564* | *520* |

**Table 12.8    Tar level of cigarettes (excluding hand-rolled cigarettes) smoked in HALS1 and HALS2: Percentage of regular smokers**

| | Males | | | | Females | | | |
|---|---|---|---|---|---|---|---|---|
| | Non-manual | | Manual | | Non-manual | | Manual | |
| HALS | 1 | 2 | 1 | 2 | 1 | 2 | 1 | 2 |
| **Tar level** | | | | | | | | |
| High/middle high | 1 | 5 | 2 | 3 | 2 | 2 | 1 | 2 |
| Middle | 46 | 36 | 53 | 35 | 29 | 22 | 39 | 22 |
| Low middle | 42 | 36 | 28 | 35 | 33 | 22 | 38 | 36 |
| Low | 11 | 21 | 13 | 21 | 33 | 51 | 21 | 36 |
| Don't know | 1 | 2 | 3 | 7 | 3 | 2 | 1 | 5 |
| *Base = 100%* | *151* | | *264* | | *256* | | *468* | |

**Table 12.9** **Reasons given for stopping smoking in those who gave up before HALS1 (B = more than 7 years) and those giving up between HALS1 and HALS2 (A = less than 7 years). Percentage of ex-smokers. (Multiple responses were possible.)**

| Age at HALS1 | 18-38 | | 39-59 | | 60 + | | | 18-38 | | 39-59 | | 60 + | |
|---|---|---|---|---|---|---|---|---|---|---|---|---|---|
| Before or after HALS1 | B | A | B | A | B | A | | B | A | B | A | B | A |
| **Reason for stopping** | | | | **Males** | | | | | | | **Females** | | |
| Ill-health | 23 | 24 | 29 | 33 | 41 | 45 | | 15 | 17 | 24 | 33 | 35 | 35 |
| Fear of illness | 42 | 45 | 34 | 33 | 28 | 21 | | 26 | 32 | 29 | 24 | 11 | 19 |
| Expense | 30 | 23 | 33 | 20 | 27 | 21 | | 24 | 17 | 26 | 11 | 33 | 14 |
| Social pressure | 12 | 23 | 5 | 12 | 4 | 8 | | 13 | 18 | 16 | 17 | 10 | 14 |
| Pregnancy | – | – | – | – | – | – | | 22 | 18 | 3 | 5 | 4 | 5 |
| Will power/lost interest | 26 | 18 | 22 | 20 | 15 | 16 | | 26 | 23 | 19 | 28 | 14 | 23 |
| Ill-health of others | 0 | 4 | 0 | 2 | 0 | 0 | | 0 | 2 | 0 | 4 | 0 | 2 |
| *Base = 100%* | *112* | *83* | *259* | *123* | *211* | *62* | | *183* | *91* | *225* | *108* | *167* | *57* |

**Table 12.10** **Health reasons for giving up smoking reported by ex-smokers at HALS2. Percentage of ex-smokers in age group – men and women combined**

| Age at HALS2 | 25-45 | 46-66 | 67 + |
|---|---|---|---|
| **Health reasons** | | | |
| Lung/chest conditions | 8 | 11 | 14 |
| Heart disease | (2) | 4 | 5 |
| Colds/flu | 3 | 4 | 5 |
| Cancer | (1) | (3) | (3) |
| Other – smoking related | 5 | 5 | 5 |
| Other – not smoking related | 2 | 4 | 6 |
| *Base = 100%* | *469* | *715* | *497* |

**Table 12.11    Passive smoking. Percentages of non-smoking and smoking respondents in households with and without other smokers in HALS2**

| | Respondents | | | |
| | Non-manual | | Manual | |
| | Not Current smoker | Current regular smoker | Not Current smoker | Current regular smoker |
|---|---|---|---|---|
| **Males** | | | | |
| Other smokers in household | 15 | 41 | 22 | 46 |
| No smokers in household | 77 | 51 | 68 | 42 |
| Lives alone | 7 | 8 | 10 | 12 |
| *Base = 100%* | *725* | *261* | *789* | *488* |
| **Females** | | | | |
| Other smokers in household | 19 | 42 | 28 | 51 |
| No smokers in household | 66 | 42 | 56 | 37 |
| Lives alone | 15 | 16 | 16 | 13 |
| *Base = 100%* | *1101* | *291* | *1067* | *520* |

**Table 12.12** High and low levels of malaise and illness symptoms at HALS1 and HALS2 in non-smokers, ex-smokers and regular smokers. Percentage in each age/smoking group (medium levels of malaise and illness omitted)

| Age at HALS1 | 18-38 | | 39-59 | | 60+ | | | 18-38 | | 39-59 | | 60+ | |
|---|---|---|---|---|---|---|---|---|---|---|---|---|---|
| HALS | 1 | 2 | 1 | 2 | 1 | 2 | | 1 | 2 | 1 | 2 | 1 | 2 |
| | **Males** | | | | | | | **Females** | | | | | |
| **Low malaise** | | | | | | | | | | | | | |
| Non-smokers | 41 | 42 | 55 | 57 | 62 | 51 | | 37 | 35 | 36 | 37 | 43 | 40 |
| Ex-smokers | 39 | 46 | 49 | 51 | 63 | 58 | | 27 | 35 | 29 | 36 | 38 | 35 |
| Regular smokers | 34 | 37 | 39 | 37 | 51 | 51 | | 20 | 28 | 26 | 27 | 28 | 26 |
| **High malaise** | | | | | | | | | | | | | |
| Non-smokers | 19 | 17 | 16 | 13 | 10 | 14 | | 25 | 26 | 26 | 27 | 25 | 26 |
| Ex-smokers | 20 | 20 | 16 | 20 | 12 | 20 | | 34 | 30 | 35 | 28 | 35 | 36 |
| Regular smokers | 28 | 26 | 27 | 26 | 15 | 18 | | 41 | 40 | 42 | 42 | 39 | 52 |
| **Low illness** | | | | | | | | | | | | | |
| Non-smokers | 58 | 56 | 59 | 53 | 54 | 43 | | 47 | 47 | 41 | 40 | 35 | 30 |
| Ex-smokers | 47 | 49 | 46 | 39 | 40 | 40 | | 36 | 44 | 28 | 33 | 25 | 23 |
| Regular smokers | 54 | 50 | 42 | 42 | 39 | 37 | | 38 | 39 | 30 | 29 | 28 | 20 |
| **High illness** | | | | | | | | | | | | | |
| Non-smokers | 10 | 13 | 10 | 17 | 15 | 25 | | 16 | 18 | 24 | 29 | 30 | 39 |
| Ex-smokers | 13 | 16 | 14 | 24 | 25 | 28 | | 30 | 23 | 33 | 31 | 40 | 46 |
| Regular smokers | 14 | 17 | 21 | 27 | 24 | 29 | | 25 | 24 | 34 | 38 | 34 | 44 |
| *Base = 100%* | | | | | | | | | | | | | |
| Non-smokers | *386* | *377* | *197* | *196* | *87* | *79* | | *578* | *547* | *501* | *485* | *348* | *330* |
| Ex-smokers | *133* | *201* | *270* | *392* | *216* | *283* | | *216* | *274* | *243* | *333* | *176* | *224* |
| Regular smokers | *342* | *335* | *365* | *289* | *164* | *129* | | *419* | *413* | *366* | *312* | *127* | *99* |

**Table 12.13** **Proportion of non-smokers, ex-smokers and regular smokers in HALS1 and HALS2 suffering from chest or heart conditions or with no respiratory problems. Percentage in each age/smoking group**

| Age at HALS1 | 18-38 | | 39-59 | | 60+ | | | 18-38 | | 39-59 | | 60+ | |
|---|---|---|---|---|---|---|---|---|---|---|---|---|---|
| HALS | 1 | 2 | 1 | 2 | 1 | 2 | | 1 | 2 | 1 | 2 | 1 | 2 |
| | | | | Males | | | | | | | Females | | |
| **Asthma** | | | | | | | | | | | | | |
| Non-smokers | 9 | 10 | 9 | 8 | 5 | 10 | | 5 | 9 | 5 | 9 | 6 | 8 |
| Ex-smokers | 14 | 14 | 5 | 8 | 6 | 10 | | 7 | 8 | 7 | 10 | 4 | 8 |
| Regular smokers | 7 | 8 | 4 | 8 | 4 | 6 | | 4 | 9 | 5 | 8 | 3 | 9 |
| **Chronic bronchitis** | | | | | | | | | | | | | |
| Non-smokers | 6 | 7 | 11 | 9 | 13 | 11 | | 5 | 5 | 8 | 10 | 14 | 13 |
| Ex-smokers | 11 | 8 | 10 | 12 | 17 | 20 | | 7 | 9 | 14 | 16 | 19 | 20 |
| Regular smokers | 8 | 8 | 10 | 16 | 18 | 18 | | 6 | 6 | 15 | 19 | 20 | 19 |
| **'Other' chest conditions** | | | | | | | | | | | | | |
| Non-smokers | 11 | 10 | 16 | 18 | 15 | 14 | | 12 | 14 | 15 | 17 | 17 | 18 |
| Ex-smokers | 26 | 20 | 20 | 21 | 22 | 24 | | 13 | 16 | 19 | 19 | 17 | 20 |
| Regular smokers | 17 | 19 | 18 | 26 | 17 | 22 | | 16 | 19 | 22 | 25 | 22 | 27 |
| **No respiratory problems** | | | | | | | | | | | | | |
| Non-smokers | 78 | 79 | 67 | 72 | 78 | 72 | | 82 | 78 | 77 | 71 | 72 | 70 |
| Ex-smokers | 59 | 65 | 69 | 67 | 63 | 59 | | 80 | 73 | 67 | 65 | 69 | 64 |
| Regular smokers | 73 | 70 | 72 | 61 | 67 | 61 | | 76 | 71 | 66 | 62 | 60 | 58 |
| **Heart problems** | | | | | | | | | | | | | |
| Non-smokers | 1 | 0 | 7 | 9 | 16 | 27 | | (5) | (1) | 4 | 5 | 11 | 13 |
| Ex-smokers | 1 | 1 | 6 | 10 | 21 | 24 | | 3 | 2 | 7 | 8 | 13 | 15 |
| Regular smokers | 1 | 2 | 7 | 11 | 9 | 12 | | 2 | 1 | 7 | 7 | 11 | 11 |
| *Base = 100%* | | | | | | | | | | | | | |
| *Non-smokers* | 386 | 377 | 197 | 196 | 87 | 79 | | 578 | 547 | 501 | 485 | 348 | 330 |
| *Ex-smokers* | 133 | 201 | 270 | 392 | 216 | 283 | | 216 | 274 | 243 | 333 | 176 | 224 |
| *Regular smokers* | 342 | 335 | 365 | 289 | 164 | 129 | | 419 | 413 | 366 | 312 | 127 | 99 |

**Table 12.14    Time after waking to first smoke of the day.
Percentage of smoking category at HALS2**

|  | Males | | Females | |
| --- | --- | --- | --- | --- |
| Time until first smoke | Light smokers | Heavy smokers | Light smokers | Heavy smokers |
| Less than 5 minutes | 7 | 27 | 6 | 24 |
| Between 5 – 15 minutes | 11 | 24 | 11 | 26 |
| Between 15 – 30 minutes | 13 | 18 | 16 | 25 |
| Between 30 minutes and 1 hour | 17 | 19 | 24 | 17 |
| Between 1 and 2 hours | 20 | 10 | 16 | 5 |
| Over 2 hours | 33 | 2 | 26 | 3 |
| *Base = 100%* | *275* | *341* | *493* | *330* |

**Table 12.15    Percentage of light and heavy smokers reporting
craving for a smoke if tobacco is not available.
Percentage of smoking category at HALS2**

|  | Males | | Females | |
| --- | --- | --- | --- | --- |
| Craving | Light smokers | Heavy smokers | Light smokers | Heavy smokers |
| Never | 34 | 13 | 30 | 12 |
| Hardly ever | 15 | 8 | 16 | 11 |
| Occasionally | 26 | 23 | 29 | 20 |
| Frequently | 15 | 24 | 13 | 20 |
| Always | 11 | 33 | 12 | 37 |
| *Base = 100%* | *274* | *340* | *491* | *329* |

**Table 12.16** **Young, middle aged and elderly respondents desire to stop smoking as a percentage of current smoking category at HALS2. ('Don't know' omitted)**

| Age at HALS2 | Light cigarette | | | Heavy cigarette | | | Pipe or cigar only | | |
|---|---|---|---|---|---|---|---|---|---|
| | 25-45 | 46-66 | >66 | 25-45 | 46-66 | >66 | 25-45 | 46-66 | >66 |
| **Males** | | | | | | | | | |
| *Desire to stop smoking* | | | | | | | | | |
| None | 25 | 24 | 53 | 14 | 27 | 42 | 50 | 55 | 82 |
| Slight/moderate | 28 | 32 | 19 | 30 | 28 | 29 | 33 | 29 | 13 |
| Strong | 45 | 43 | 28 | 54 | 45 | 29 | 17 | 16 | 5 |
| *Base = 100%* | *127* | *90* | *58* | *168* | *139* | *31* | *36* | *55* | *39* |
| **Females** | | | | | | | | | |
| None | 20 | 23 | 38 | 20 | 21 | (5) | | | |
| Slight/moderate | 38 | 31 | 33 | 33 | 30 | (4) | | | |
| Strong | 43 | 46 | 30 | 47 | 49 | (8) | | | |
| *Base = 100%* | *232* | *168* | *80* | *173* | *138* | *17* | | | |

**Table 12.17** **Regular cigarette smokers' opinions as to whether they were smoking 'more', the 'same' or 'less' than seven years ago, compared to the recorded difference between the number of cigarettes smoked at HALS1 and HALS2. Percentage of opinion group**

| | Respondent's opinion | | | | | | | | |
|---|---|---|---|---|---|---|---|---|---|
| Age at HALS2 | 25-45 | | | 46-66 | | | 67+ | | |
| | Less | Same | More | Less | Same | More | Less | Same | More |
| **Cigarettes HALS1 to HALS2** | | | **Males** | | | | | | |
| Decrease | 50 | 27 | 8 | 52 | 29 | 10 | 88 | 45 | 0 |
| No change | 14 | 32 | 19 | 26 | 41 | 10 | 5 | 32 | 0 |
| Increase | 36 | 41 | 74 | 22 | 30 | 80 | 7 | 23 | (1) |
| *Base = 100%* | *78* | *124* | *53* | *86* | *110* | *20* | *42* | *40* | *1* |
| **Females** | | | | | | | | | |
| Decrease | 58 | 24 | 10 | 67 | 32 | 16 | 73 | 44 | (2) |
| No change | 23 | 35 | 22 | 20 | 37 | 38 | 16 | 40 | (2) |
| Increase | 19 | 42 | 67 | 13 | 32 | 47 | 11 | 16 | (5) |
| *Base = 100%* | *86* | *182* | *86* | *91* | *152* | *45* | *37* | *43* | *9* |

**Table 12.18** **Numbers of respondents who were ex-regular smokers at HALS1 but who claimed always to have been non-smokers at HALS2, by age and socio-economic group**

|  | Males | Females |  | Males | Females |
|---|---|---|---|---|---|
| **Age at HALS1** |  |  | **Socio-economic group** |  |  |
| **18-38** | 5 | 37 |  |  |  |
| **39-59** | 21 | 43 | Non-manual | 18 | 60 |
| **60+** | 9 | 36 | Manual | 17 | 56 |
| **Total** | 35 | 116 |  | 35 | 116 |

# TRENDS IN ALCOHOL CONSUMPTION | 13

## Margaret J Whichelow

Alcohol consumption has been assessed in several different ways: by asking the respondents whether they drank, and if so whether only on special occasions or more regularly; by asking them to define their own drinking as light, moderate or heavy; by enquiry about past drinking; by a seven-day 'drinks diary' taking them through their consumption 'last week'; and by asking questions about dependence — the CAGE questions (Mayfield et al. 1974), see Appendix A. Even if complete honesty on the part of respondents is assumed (and of course it cannot be), none of these provides a reliable categorisation on its own. People's own estimates of what constitutes 'light' or 'heavy' drinking depend on personal norms and reference groups, and one person's 'light' may be equivalent to another's 'heavy'.

Although the 'drinks diary' provides a quantitative estimate of alcohol consumption, it only refers to the week previous to the interview, which may not be typical of any particular person's drinking habits. Furthermore, calculations of the last week's alcohol consumption are made assuming that half a pint of beer, a glass of wine and a pub measure of spirits each contain one unit of alcohol, but beers vary considerably in their alcohol content and drinks taken at home will vary in quantity, where the amount served may well be larger than that bought in a pub (Turner, 1990), so that this measure of alcohol consumption can only be approximate. However, for large groups, as in the two HALS Surveys this method is accepted as giving a guide to consumption levels. The units of alcohol consumed have been categorised as 'prudent', 'unwise' and 'excessive' using currently recommended levels (see Appendix A). The limits for 'prudent' drinking are 1-21 units per week for men and 1-14 units for women, for 'unwise' drinking, 22-50 units for men and 15-35 units for women, and for 'excessive' drinking, over 50 and 35 units respectively for men and women. Lower limits are set for women, as evidence suggests that smaller amounts of alcohol are more hazardous to the health of women (Royal College of Psychiatrists, 1979). Very few women record enough drinks to place them in the 'excessive' category, so for most purposes the 'unwise' and 'excessive' categories have been combined.

## Self assessment of drinking habit

Based on the responses to the first few questions in the drinking section of the questionnaire, the respondents were classified as non-drinkers or very special occasions drinkers, ex-drinkers, occasional drinkers and regular drinkers. It has been suggested that in surveys on alcohol consumption under-reporting may occur, particularly at heavy levels of drinking, and that also the heavier drinkers may be under-represented (Smyth and Browne, 1991). In order to determine whether there had been a differential rate of attrition of groups with different drinking habits between HALS1 and HALS2 the full HALS1 sample is included in Table 13.1 with the HALS2 sub-sample at 1984/5 and 1991/2. There is no consistent difference between the full HALS1 sample and the sub-sample distributions, overall, or at any age. Between HALS1 and HALS2 there has been a small overall increase in the number who report always having been non-drinkers, noticeably women, and an increase in the number of ex-drinkers in both sexes, along with a decrease in occasional, but not regular, drinkers. The fact that some respondents reported at HALS2 always having been non-drinkers, whilst at HALS1 admitting to drinking at some level at that time or previously, is interesting, and may be because of the way people interpret words like 'always', 'ever' and 'never'. The proportion of ex-drinkers rises at all ages in the men, and in all but one age group, 32-38 at HALS1, in the women. Similarly the proportion of occasional drinkers fell in all but one group. As expected, at each age women non-drinkers out-number the non-drinking men, whilst regular drinking was more prominent amongst the men.

Although the proportions in the self-assessed drinking habit groups are similar in HALS1 and HALS2, there has been considerable movement between the groups (Table 13.2). Actual consumption (Table 13.9) shows similar changes from HALS1 to HALS2. With increasing age and in both sexes non-drinkers are more likely to remain non-drinkers, and if they do take up drinking it is on an occasional basis. Amongst the young men 46% of those who were non-drinkers at HALS1 had become occasional drinkers by HALS2, whereas only 22% of the older male non-drinkers at HALS1 had become occasional drinkers. A similar pattern was seen for the women. A large proportion − range 10% to 45% − of those reporting to be ex-drinkers at HALS1, now claim never to have drunk on more than just 'special occasions'. Among those reporting at HALS1 to be occasional drinkers a smaller but significant number are now claiming to be non-drinkers. Most, however, still classify themselves as occasional drinkers, and the majority of regular drinkers at HALS1 still maintain that status.

The findings from HALS1 and HALS2 shown in Table 13.3 are in line with the well-established social class differences in drinking habit (Smyth and Browne, 1991). At both HALS1 and HALS2 there are more non-drinkers in the manual groups, particularly amongst the manual women. The same is true of ex-drinkers, whilst there are more occasional and regular drinkers of both sexes in non-manual groups. There has been a marked increase in the number of professional women who are regular drinkers between HALS1 and HALS2 and a smaller increase in regular drinking in the professional men

and unskilled women.

Sex differences in self-assessment of the level of drinking are apparent for both current drinkers and ex-drinkers, with women being much more likely to report being light drinkers, and most unlikely to admit to previous heavy drinking (Table 13.4). Ex-drinking men are more likely than those currently drinking to admit to heavy drinking, but less likely to report moderate drinking, except in the oldest group. There has been a decrease from HALS1 to HALS2 in the reporting of moderate drinking by men who are current drinkers and ex-drinking women, and in reporting heavy drinking by ex-drinking men. Whilst this may reflect a (small) change in drinking habit, it may also reflect changes in the social acceptability of heavier levels of drinking.

## Alcohol consumption

The results of the more objective (although admittedly flawed) assessment of units of alcohol consumed, show that there has been a small reduction in mean consumption by men and women by HALS2, in both the whole Survey population and the drinkers, although there are no significant changes between HALS1 and HALS2 at any age group. Comparison of the whole HALS1 population with the HALS2 sub-sample in 1984/5 shows that the alcohol consumption levels are very similar and that there has been no selective loss of any level of alcohol consumers (Table 13.5). The results for the drinkers only are shown graphically in Fig. 13.1, where the similarities between HALS1 and HALS2 for both sexes are apparent. For men, there is a steady fall in alcohol consumption from the youngest to the oldest age group, whereas for women who drink there is very little change in consumption with age. At all ages the consumption by women is much less than that by men. Indeed it is noteworthy that in the men under 45 years, the mean consumption is above the 'prudent' level of 21 units, whereas the highest mean consumption in women is only just over half of their 'prudent' level of 15 units.

Despite the small overall change in consumption there has been individual change. The respondents were asked to compare their drinking at HALS2 with that at HALS1 and this comparison was related to the change in units of alcohol consumed (Table 13.6). The majority of respondents, particularly if they reported no change in alcohol consumption, accurately categorized themselves within ±7 units. Those who claimed to be drinking more were more likely to be accurate than those who claimed to be drinking less, which was unexpected, since under-reporting rather than over-reporting is the norm. Similarly the percentage of people claiming to drink the same who actually drink more is no greater than those who actually drink less.

In most regions there has been little change between HALS1 and HALS2 in the amount of alcohol consumed by drinkers or in the number of non-drinkers (Table 13.7). There are, however, a few exceptions, particularly for women in Wales where not only has the proportion of drinkers increased but there has also been a slight increase in the units of alcohol consumed by drinkers. In contrast, fewer women in London and to a lesser extent the South East were drinking in 1991/2 than in 1984/5 and those who drank were drinking less. Male drinkers in London and the South East showed the same decrease in alcohol consumption.

The age trends in alcohol consumption, demonstrated in Fig. 13.1 are also apparent when the amount of alcohol consumed is categorised as 'nil', 'prudent', 'unwise' and 'excessive'. Amongst the men the proportion of 'prudent' drinkers remains fairly constant over the complete age range whilst that of the 'unwise' and 'excessive' drinkers falls steadily

with age (Table 13.8). In the youngest age group about 30% of the men but only 8% of the women consumed alcohol above the 'prudent' level. In the women the percentages of all drinkers fell with advancing age. Between HALS1 and HALS2 there was a small drop in the 'unwise' and 'excessive' male drinkers, which has occurred predominantly in the middle aged group and a small increase in young non-drinkers. There are no appreciable changes between HALS1 and HALS2 in the drinking characteristics of women. The levels of consumption above the prudent level for men are similar to those reported by the GHS, (1991), but in the HALS surveys for women under the age of 65, the proportion of 'unwise' and 'excessive' drinkers is lower. The proportions of non-drinkers in both sexes is considerably higher than those found by the GHS (Smyth and Browne 1991). The difference in methods used to assess drinking may account for the discrepancies, as suggested by Blaxter (1987). Despite the small overall changes in alcohol consumption levels, there were considerable individual changes, as shown in Table 13.9. The 'nil' category is similar to that in Table 13.1, but also includes those who normally drink but did not do so last week. Again, the majority who drank nothing or were prudent drinkers at HALS1 were in the same category at HALS2. Fewer of the 'unwise' or 'excessive' drinkers have remained as such. Many of

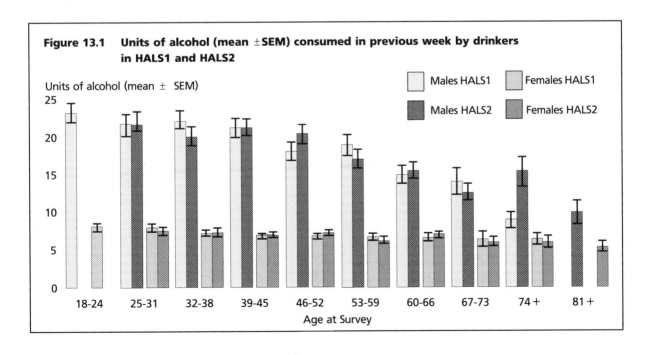

**Figure 13.1   Units of alcohol (mean ±SEM) consumed in previous week by drinkers in HALS1 and HALS2**

the 'unwise' have become 'prudent' drinkers, and only a minority of the HALS1 'excessive' drinkers were drinking excessively in HALS2. However some of the former 'non' and 'prudent' drinkers have now moved into the heavier drinking categories.

The socio-economic group differences noted in Table 13.3 are also apparent when considering alcohol consumption levels (Table 13.10). In both sexes there are more 'prudent' drinkers amongst the non-manual groups, and fewer non-drinkers. In HALS1 there were more 'unwise' and 'excessive' drinkers in the manual men, but by HALS2 this difference had been reduced. Slightly more non-manual than manual women were 'unwise' drinkers, but the largest socio-economic differences, at both HALS1 and HALS2, were in the proportion of non-drinkers. Small regional differences were observed in both surveys for men drinking more than the 'prudent' level of alcohol, with the North having a higher proportion of 'unwise' and 'excessive' drinkers than the South (Table 13.11). There were no North/ South (see Appendix A) differences among the women.

The self-assessed level of drinking in those who drank last week has been related to the category of alcohol consumption in Table 13.12. Almost all those in both sexes claiming to be light drinkers were 'prudent' drinkers, and there was no change between HALS1 and HALS2. For those claiming to be moderate or heavy drinkers there was less consistency. About half of the male and three quarters of the female moderate drinkers were 'prudent' drinkers, and about 10% of the moderately drinking men were 'excessive' drinkers, with over one-third in the 'unwise' category. Men claiming to be heavy drinkers were equally likely to be 'unwise' or 'excessive' drinkers and only a minority were 'prudent' drinkers.

Unreliable reporting of drinking habits was revealed earlier (Table 13.2) and another aspect of this has been found in those claiming to be ex-drinkers. These respondents were asked, along with the current drinkers, if they had any drinks 'last week'. Table 13.13 shows that about 1 in 6 ex-drinkers had drunk 'last week'. Fewer older ex-drinkers had drunk 'last week' in HALS2 than in HALS1 but in the younger age groups the trend was reversed. Otherwise there were no changes between the two

Surveys. As might be expected, almost all those who reported being regular drinkers drank last week, whilst about 80% of the male and just over 70% of female occasional drinkers did so.

## Identification of possible dependent drinkers

The CAGE questions (see Appendix A) have been extensively used and validated as the best instrument for identifying dependent drinkers (Mayfield et al. 1974). These questions were included in both Surveys and the score of positive responses (0 to 4) are presented in Table 13.14 and Table 13.15. Overall, and at any age except for the youngest men, there was little change in the higher scores (indicative of problematic dependent drinking) between HALS1 and HALS2 (Table 13.14). There was a trend, in both sexes, for the percentage with a zero score to increase and for all the higher scores to decrease with advancing age.

In Table 13.15 the changes in CAGE score groups that have taken place between HALS1 and HALS2 are shown. Since all the CAGE questions ask 'Have you ever . . . . . . . . . ?', only the same or a higher score at HALS2 should be possible. However in all groups scoring above zero at HALS1 there are considerable numbers who score less at HALS2 than they did at HALS1. Indeed for those scoring 3 or 4 (the maximum) at HALS1 approximately three quarters are scoring less at HALS2. It can only be speculated as to whether this is mainly due to respondents' amnesia about past drinking problems, or their mis-understanding of the 'ever' part of the questions.

In HALS1 there were slightly more men in the manual than non-manual groups drinking above the 'prudent' level (Table 13.10). However slightly more men in the non-manual groups have a CAGE score of 2 or more at HALS1 (Table 13.16). At HALS2 there is no socio-economic difference for either sex and there are no regional differences at either HALS1 or HALS2 in a CAGE score of 2 or more (Table 13.17). It would be expected that the higher CAGE scores would be found predominantly amongst those who were in the 'unwise' or 'excessive' drinking categories and this is indeed so, as shown in Table 13.18, where the heaviest drinkers are more likely to admit that their drinking causes problems. Very few of the 'prudent' and even fewer of the 'nil' drinkers recorded

CAGE scores above 1. Amongst the men about a quarter of the 'unwise' drinkers and 38% (HALS1) and 47% (HALS2) of the 'excessive' drinkers scored 2 or more. Over 20% of the women who drank more than the 'prudent' level also scored 2 or more. In the respondents who drank heavily there was a reduction in those scoring zero at HALS2 and an increase most noticeably in a score of 2.

## Drinking and smoking

The association between drinking and smoking is well known and was demonstrated in the report of HALS1 (Blaxter, 1987). Table 13.19 shows the changes in smoking habit that have occurred between HALS1 and HALS2 in the different categories of alcohol consumption. In both HALS1 and HALS2 there are more smokers amongst the 'unwise' and 'excessive' drinkers than the 'nil' or 'prudent' drinkers. The 'excessive' drinkers are the most likely to smoke, with 81% of middle aged male 'excessive' drinkers smoking at HALS1. The distribution of smoking categories is similar in the 'nil' and 'prudent' groups, at all ages and in both sexes.

In all groups the proportion of ex-smokers has increased between HALS1 and HALS2 and in most groups the proportion of smokers has declined. However, in the young male 'unwise' and 'excessive' drinking groups and the middle aged females in the heavier drinking category there has been an increase in the proportion of smokers.

## Alcohol consumption & blood pressure

The changes in blood pressure category distribution between HALS1 and HALS2 in the various categories of alcohol con-sumption are given in Table 13.20. The most obvious difference, in the men under 60, is of fewer normoten-sive individuals in the 'unwise' and even fewer in the 'excessive' drinking categories in both HALS1 and HALS2 than in the 'nil' or 'prudent' categories. This is not so for the women, which may be because the amount of alcohol consumed in the 'unwise' and 'excessive' categories is lower than for the men. In the middle aged and elderly respondents, in most drinking groups, there are at HALS2 more treated than untreated hypertensives than there were at HALS1, but

otherwise there have been no obvious changes over seven years. Increasing body mass index is associated with increasing blood pressure, a factor that further discrimination of blood pressure in relation to drinking habits will need to take into account.

## Summary

Overall patterns of alcohol consumption have changed little between HALS1 and HALS2, a result which is in line with the findings of the GHS (1991) between 1984 and 1990, which also observed only small changes. The strength of the HALS longitudinal survey has been that it has been able to reveal considerable changes within groups, demonstrating that whereas questionnaires of the type used here are useful in the description of the characteristics of large groups, they are unreliable for describing individuals. The CAGE questions, although accepted as a reliable way of identifying dependent drinkers, may not be satisfactory for long term studies as many respondents change categories in an illogical fashion. The comparison of smoking habits amongst different levels of drinkers shows that those who drink heavily are also those who smoke heavily, and the least likely to change their addictive behaviours.

### References

Blaxter, M. (1987) 'Alcohol Consumption' in Cox, B.D. et al. 'The Health and Lifestyle Survey', London: Health Promotion Research Trust.

Mayfield, D., McLeod, G. and Hall, P. (1974), 'The CAGE questionnaire: validation of a new alcoholism screening instrument', American Journal of Psychiatry 131, 1121-1123.

Royal College of Psychiatrists (1979), 'Alcohol and Alcoholism', London: Tavistock Publications.

Smyth, M. and Browne, F. (1991), 'General Household Survey 1990', London, HMSO.

Turner, C. (1990), 'How much alcohol is in a standard drink?, An analysis of 125 studies', British Journal of Addiction, 85, 1171-1175.

**Table 13.1** **Self-assessed drinking habit in HALS1 sample and HALS2 sub-sample at HALS1 and HALS2. Percentage of age group**

| | 18-24 | | 25-31 | | 32-38 | | 39-45 | | 46-52 | | 53-59 | | 60-66 | | 67-73 | | 74+ | | All | |
|---|---|---|---|---|---|---|---|---|---|---|---|---|---|---|---|---|---|---|---|---|
| **Age at HALS2** | | 25-31 | | 32-38 | | 39-45 | | 46-52 | | 53-59 | | 60-66 | | 67-73 | | 74-80 | | 81+ | | All |
| **Males** | | | | | | | | | | | | | | | | | | | | |
| **Non-drinker** | | | | | | | | | | | | | | | | | | | | |
| HALS1 sample | 9 | | 10 | | 6 | | 12 | | 12 | | 15 | | 18 | | 22 | | 28 | | 13 | |
| HALS2 sub-sample | 10 | 8 | 10 | 8 | 4 | 5 | 11 | 10 | 13 | 17 | 13 | 15 | 18 | 17 | 21 | 24 | 30 | 29 | 12 | 13 |
| **Ex-drinker** | | | | | | | | | | | | | | | | | | | | |
| HALS1 sample | 3 | | 6 | | 7 | | 7 | | 7 | | 13 | | 6 | | 15 | | 15 | | 8 | |
| HALS2 sub-sample | 3 | 9 | 6 | 11 | 6 | 8 | 7 | 9 | 7 | 10 | 11 | 13 | 5 | 11 | 14 | 20 | 8 | 13 | 7 | 11 |
| **Occasional drinker** | | | | | | | | | | | | | | | | | | | | |
| HALS1 sample | 44 | | 44 | | 45 | | 41 | | 45 | | 43 | | 44 | | 39 | | 38 | | 43 | |
| HALS2 sub-sample | 45 | 47 | 45 | 42 | 44 | 41 | 44 | 39 | 46 | 39 | 45 | 43 | 45 | 45 | 43 | 29 | 43 | 35 | 45 | 41 |
| **Regular drinker** | | | | | | | | | | | | | | | | | | | | |
| HALS1 sample | 43 | | 40 | | 43 | | 41 | | 37 | | 30 | | 33 | | 24 | | 19 | | 36 | |
| HALS2 sub-sample | 42 | 36 | 39 | 39 | 46 | 46 | 39 | 42 | 35 | 35 | 30 | 29 | 32 | 27 | 22 | 27 | 19 | 24 | 36 | 36 |
| **Females** | | | | | | | | | | | | | | | | | | | | |
| **Non-drinker** | | | | | | | | | | | | | | | | | | | | |
| HALS1 sample | 23 | | 22 | | 23 | | 25 | | 33 | | 39 | | 44 | | 59 | | 62 | | 34 | |
| HALS2 sub-sample | 22 | 16 | 23 | 22 | 22 | 24 | 22 | 25 | 31 | 34 | 36 | 42 | 44 | 50 | 58 | 63 | 56 | 54 | 31 | 33 |
| **Ex-drinker** | | | | | | | | | | | | | | | | | | | | |
| HALS1 sample | 7 | | 7 | | 8 | | 6 | | 5 | | 9 | | 8 | | 6 | | 3 | | 7 | |
| HALS2 sub-sample | 6 | 13 | 8 | 12 | 9 | 9 | 6 | 7 | 4 | 9 | 9 | 10 | 8 | 11 | 5 | 6 | 3 | 13 | 7 | 10 |
| **Occasional drinker** | | | | | | | | | | | | | | | | | | | | |
| HALS1 sample | 51 | | 53 | | 50 | | 50 | | 45 | | 38 | | 37 | | 27 | | 24 | | 44 | |
| HALS2 sub-sample | 53 | 51 | 55 | 49 | 51 | 47 | 52 | 43 | 48 | 41 | 37 | 32 | 35 | 28 | 28 | 21 | 26 | 22 | 46 | 40 |
| **Regular drinker** | | | | | | | | | | | | | | | | | | | | |
| HALS1 sample | 19 | | 18 | | 18 | | 19 | | 19 | | 15 | | 11 | | 9 | | 10 | | 16 | |
| HALS2 sub-sample | 20 | 20 | 14 | 17 | 19 | 21 | 20 | 25 | 17 | 16 | 19 | 16 | 13 | 12 | 9 | 10 | 15 | 11 | 17 | 18 |
| *Base = 100%* | *534* | | *487* | | *573* | | *471* | | *419* | | *415* | | *412* | | *314* | | *271* | | *3896* | |
| | *299* | *298* | *239* | *241* | *383* | *383* | *321* | *322* | *280* | *278* | *277* | *277* | *259* | *258* | *148* | *147* | *88* | *87* | *2294* | *2291* |
| | *622* | | *671* | | *762* | | *617* | | *573* | | *483* | | *553* | | *391* | | *407* | | *5079* | |
| | *308* | *308* | *393* | *393* | *542* | *542* | *431* | *430* | *390* | *391* | *314* | *314* | *327* | *324* | *191* | *188* | *144* | *142* | *3040* | *3032* |

**Table 13.2**  **Change in self-assessed drinking habit between HALS1 and HALS2 in those who reported themselves to be 'always non-drinkers', 'ex-drinkers', 'occasional drinkers' or 'regular drinkers' at HALS1. Percentage of HALS1 drinking habit group**

| Age at HALS1 | 18-38 | | | | 39-59 | | | | 60+ | | | |
|---|---|---|---|---|---|---|---|---|---|---|---|---|
| HALS1 drinking habit group | Non-drinker | Ex-drinker | Occ. drinker | Regular drinker | Non-drinker | Ex-drinker | Occ. drinker | Regular drinker | Non-drinker | Ex-drinker | Occ. drinker | Regular drinker |
| **HALS2 category** | | | | | **Males** | | | | | | | |
| Non-drinker | 43 | 10 | 7 | φ | 62 | 29 | 9 | φ | 69 | 23 | 11 | 2 |
| Ex-drinker | 7 | 46 | 10 | 4 | 12 | 40 | 11 | 3 | 8 | 54 | 16 | 3 |
| Occasional drinker | 46 | 42 | 58 | 29 | 25 | 25 | 60 | 22 | 22 | 18 | 56 | 28 |
| Regular drinker | 4 | 2 | 26 | 67 | 2 | 6 | 20 | 75 | 1 | 5 | 17 | 67 |
| | | | | | **Females** | | | | | | | |
| Non-drinker | 60 | 24 | 11 | 3 | 71 | 29 | 22 | 2 | 80 | 45 | 35 | 4 |
| Ex-drinker | 9 | 39 | 10 | 2 | 9 | 31 | 6 | 6 | 6 | 35 | 10 | 10 |
| Occasional drinker | 29 | 35 | 62 | 40 | 19 | 32 | 58 | 29 | 12 | 20 | 43 | 33 |
| Regular drinker | 3 | 3 | 17 | 55 | 1 | 7 | 15 | 63 | 2 | 0 | 11 | 53 |
| *Base = 100%* | *68* | *48* | *409* | *395* | *104* | *72* | *391* | *306* | *101* | *39* | *218* | *134* |
| | *272* | *98* | *651* | *215* | *328* | *68* | *524* | *212* | *331* | *40* | *204* | *77* |

**Table 13.3** **Variations between socio-economic groups' self-assessed drinking habit in HALS1 and HALS2. Percentage of HALS1 socio-economic group**

| HALS | Professional 1 | 2 | Managers Executive 1 | 2 | Other non-manual 1 | 2 | Skilled manual 1 | 2 | Semi-skilled manual 1 | 2 | Unskilled 1 | 2 |
|---|---|---|---|---|---|---|---|---|---|---|---|---|
| **Males** | | | | | | | | | | | | |
| Non-drinker | 7 | 9 | 10 | 11 | 12 | 13 | 12 | 12 | 16 | 14 | 14 | 19 |
| Ex-drinker | 4 | 7 | 5 | 9 | 8 | 9 | 7 | 12 | 10 | 14 | 11 | 11 |
| Occasional drinker | 51 | 42 | 41 | 39 | 40 | 38 | 48 | 43 | 42 | 41 | 46 | 42 |
| Regular drinker | 38 | 42 | 44 | 41 | 40 | 40 | 33 | 33 | 33 | 32 | 29 | 29 |
| **Females** | | | | | | | | | | | | |
| Non-drinker | 15 | 21 | 26 | 29 | 26 | 30 | 36 | 37 | 37 | 36 | 39 | 43 |
| Ex-drinker | 9 | 3 | 4 | 7 | 5 | 9 | 7 | 12 | 10 | 12 | 11 | 12 |
| Occasional drinker | 55 | 45 | 48 | 44 | 51 | 41 | 45 | 38 | 36 | 38 | 37 | 28 |
| Regular drinker | 21 | 31 | 22 | 20 | 19 | 20 | 12 | 14 | 17 | 14 | 14 | 18 |
| *Base = 100%* | *116* | *116* | *437* | *438* | *424* | *425* | *836* | *834* | *342* | *338* | *107* | *108* |
| | *173* | *174* | *545* | *546* | *682* | *681* | *971* | *964* | *495* | *493* | *131* | *131* |

**Table 13.4** **Self-assessed level of present alcohol consumption by drinkers and past level of alcohol consumption by ex-drinkers in HALS1 and HALS2. Percentage of age groups**

| Age at HALS1 HALS | Drinkers 18-38 1 | 2 | 39-59 1 | 2 | 60+ 1 | 2 | Ex-drinkers 18-38 1 | 2 | 39-59 1 | 2 | 60+ 1 | 2 |
|---|---|---|---|---|---|---|---|---|---|---|---|---|
| **Males** | | | | | | | | | | | | |
| Light | 41 | 40 | 48 | 50 | 68 | 70 | 46 | 54 | 52 | 46 | 50 | 51 |
| Moderate | 53 | 52 | 48 | 45 | 31 | 28 | 32 | 30 | 33 | 40 | 32 | 42 |
| Heavy | 6 | 8 | 3 | 5 | 1 | 1 | 22 | 16 | 15 | 14 | 18 | 7 |
| **Females** | | | | | | | | | | | | |
| Light | 59 | 57 | 68 | 64 | 78 | 78 | 72 | 78 | 70 | 80 | 85 | 87 |
| Moderate | 41 | 42 | 32 | 35 | 22 | 22 | 25 | 21 | 26 | 17 | 15 | 13 |
| Heavy | φ | 1 | φ | 2 | 0 | 0 | 3 | 2 | 4 | 3 | 0 | 0 |
| *Base = 100%* | *813* | *774* | *706* | *664* | *360* | *319* | *50* | *83* | *75* | *91* | *38* | *67* |
| | *882* | *842* | *750* | *665* | *298* | *232* | *99* | *129* | *69* | *93* | *40* | *61* |

**Table 13.5** Alcohol consumption in units in the previous week (mean ±SEM) in total HALS1 sample and HALS2 sub-sample in HALS1 and HALS2 for all subjects and drinkers only

| | 18-24 / 25-31 | 25-31 / 32-38 | 32-38 / 39-45 | 39-45 / 46-52 | 46-52 / 53-59 | 53-59 / 60-66 | 60-66 / 67-73 | 67-73 / 74-80 | 74+ / 81+ | Total |
|---|---|---|---|---|---|---|---|---|---|---|
| **All subjects** | | | | | | | | | | |
| **Males** | | | | | | | | | | |
| HALS1 sample | 19.3 ±0.9 | 17.2 ±0.9 | 17.3 ±0.9 | 16.1 ±0.9 | 13.3 ±0.8 | 12.4 ±1.0 | 10.3 ±0.7 | 8.2 ±0.8 | 5.4 ±0.8 | 14.2 ±0.3 |
| HALS2 sub-sample | 18.1 16.5 ±1.2 ±1.2 | 16.5 15.2 ±1.3 ±1.2 | 18.3 17.3 ±1.1 ±1.1 | 15.8 15.4 ±1.1 ±1.1 | 12.1 11.3 ±1.0 ±1.0 | 12.7 10.2 ±1.1 ±0.8 | 10.4 7.8 ±1.0 ±0.8 | 8.5 8.1 ±1.2 ±1.2 | 4.3 5.2 ±0.7 ±1.0 | 14.2 13.0 ±0.4 ±0.4 |
| **Females** | | | | | | | | | | |
| HALS1 sample | 4.5 ±0.3 | 4.3 ±0.3 | 4.0 ±0.3 | 4.1 ±0.2 | 3.7 ±0.2 | 2.9 ±0.2 | 2.4 ±0.2 | 1.7 ±0.2 | 1.7 ±0.2 | 3.4 ±0.1 |
| HALS2 sub-sample | 4.5 4.3 ±0.4 ±0.4 | 3.9 3.8 ±0.4 ±0.3 | 4.0 4.1 ±0.3 ±0.3 | 4.2 4.2 ±0.3 ±0.3 | 3.5 3.0 ±0.3 ±0.3 | 3.2 3.0 ±0.3 ±0.3 | 2.7 2.1 ±0.3 ±0.3 | 1.8 1.4 ±0.4 ±0.3 | 2.0 1.4 ±0.3 ±0.3 | 3.6 3.3 ±0.1 ±0.1 |
| *Base* | 534 | 486 | 573 | 473 | 418 | 415 | 412 | 313 | 271 | 3895 |
| | 299 297 | 239 240 | 383 380 | 323 322 | 279 277 | 277 276 | 259 257 | 148 145 | 88 86 | 2295 2280 |
| | 624 | 672 | 764 | 617 | 574 | 483 | 553 | 391 | 409 | 5087 |
| | 309 306 | 394 387 | 544 539 | 431 429 | 390 390 | 314 314 | 327 323 | 191 188 | 145 141 | 3045 3017 |
| **Drinkers** | | | | | | | | | | |
| **Males** | | | | | | | | | | |
| HALS1 sample | 24.1 ±1.0 | 22.9 ±1.1 | 21.8 ±1.0 | 21.9 ±1.1 | 19.1 ±1.1 | 19.5 ±1.3 | 15.0 ±1.0 | 14.7 ±1.3 | 11.0 ±1.1 | 20.1 ±0.4 |
| HALS2 sub-sample | 23.1 22.1 ±1.3 ±1.4 | 21.7 20.1 ±1.5 ±1.3 | 22.3 21.2 ±1.2 ±1.2 | 21.2 20.4 ±1.3 ±1.3 | 18.1 17.1 ±1.2 ±1.3 | 18.9 15.5 ±1.4 ±1.1 | 15.0 12.6 ±1.2 ±1.1 | 14.1 15.4 ±1.8 ±2.0 | 9.0 9.9 ±1.1 ±1.6 | 19.8 18.5 ±0.5 ±0.5 |
| **Females** | | | | | | | | | | |
| HALS1 sample | 8.1 ±0.4 | 8.1 ±0.5 | 7.5 ±0.4 | 7.0 ±0.3 | 7.3 ±0.4 | 6.7 ±0.4 | 5.9 ±0.4 | 6.0 ±0.7 | 6.4 ±0.5 | 7.2 ±0.2 |
| HALS2 sub-sample | 8.1 7.6 ±0.6 ±0.5 | 8.0 7.4 ±0.6 ±0.6 | 7.3 7.0 ±0.4 ±0.4 | 6.9 7.3 ±0.4 ±0.5 | 6.8 6.2 ±0.4 ±0.5 | 6.7 7.0 ±0.5 ±0.5 | 6.6 6.0 ±0.5 ±0.6 | 6.4 6.0 ±1.1 ±0.8 | 6.4 5.4 ±0.8 ±0.8 | 7.2 6.9 ±0.2 ±0.2 |
| *Base* | 427 | 364 | 453 | 347 | 291 | 264 | 284 | 175 | 133 | 2738 |
| | 235 222 | 181 181 | 314 310 | 241 243 | 187 183 | 186 182 | 180 160 | 89 76 | 42 45 | 1655 1602 |
| | 350 | 356 | 411 | 359 | 287 | 211 | 220 | 109 | 108 | 2411 |
| | 173 172 | 193 198 | 299 315 | 263 249 | 202 187 | 150 133 | 135 113 | 53 45 | 46 37 | 1514 1449 |

**Table 13.6**   Respondents opinions at HALS2 as to whether they were drinking 'more', 'the same' or 'less' than at HALS1, in relation to difference in units of alcohol recorded in HALS1 and HALS2. Percentage of 'less', 'same' and 'more' groups.

| Age at HALS2 | 25-45 | | | 46-66 | | | 67+ | | |
|---|---|---|---|---|---|---|---|---|---|
| | Less | Same | More | Less | Same | More | Less | Same | More |
| **Difference HALS2 minus HALS1 in units of alcohol** | | | | | | | | | |
| | | | | | **Males** | | | | |
| > − 7 | 42 | 20 | 10 | 29 | 18 | 11 | 32 | 13 | (2) |
| − 7 to +7 | 42 | 55 | 37 | 59 | 67 | 48 | 60 | 74 | 0 |
| > +7 | 16 | 26 | 53 | 12 | 15 | 41 | 9 | 13 | (12) |
| | | | | | **Females** | | | | |
| > − 7 | 14 | 5 | 2 | 13 | 4 | 7 | 14 | 6 | 9 |
| − 7 to +7 | 83 | 87 | 67 | 83 | 91 | 75 | 84 | 89 | 73 |
| > +7 | 4 | 7 | 31 | 4 | 5 | 19 | 2 | 5 | 18 |
| Base = 100% | 411 | 308 | 122 | 354 | 312 | 73 | 177 | 187 | 14 |
| | 375 | 409 | 169 | 229 | 429 | 91 | 113 | 149 | 22 |

**Table 13.7  Regional variations in alcohol consumption (mean units ±SEM) in HALS1 and HALS2 in those who drank last week, and percentage of non-drinkers last week in each region**

| HALS | Scotland 1 | Scotland 2 | Wales 1 | Wales 2 | North 1 | North 2 | North West 1 | North West 2 | Yorks/Humber 1 | Yorks/Humber 2 | West Midlands 1 | West Midlands 2 | East Midlands 1 | East Midlands 2 | East Anglia 1 | East Anglia 2 | South West 1 | South West 2 | South East 1 | South East 2 | Greater London 1 | Greater London 2 |
|---|---|---|---|---|---|---|---|---|---|---|---|---|---|---|---|---|---|---|---|---|---|---|
| **Males** | | | | | | | | | | | | | | | | | | | | | | |
| Mean units alcohol | 22.0 | 18.9 | 21.2 | 20.1 | 27.9 | 24.3 | 22.6 | 21.5 | 22.9 | 24.7 | 19.4 | 18.7 | 19.0 | 18.0 | 13.0 | 13.1 | 18.4 | 18.1 | 16.1 | 14.3 | 17.2 | 14.4 |
| ±SEM | ±1.7 | ±1.5 | ±1.9 | ±1.8 | ±2.7 | ±2.5 | ±1.5 | ±1.5 | ±1.7 | ±2.0 | ±1.5 | ±1.8 | ±1.5 | ±1.4 | ±1.4 | ±1.5 | ±1.7 | ±1.7 | ±0.9 | ±0.8 | ±1.4 | ±1.2 |
| n = | (165) | (168) | (93) | (100) | (90) | (92) | (192) | (179) | (164) | (158) | (141) | (138) | (136) | (133) | (63) | (60) | (136) | (134) | (315) | (296) | (160) | (144) |
| Non-drinkers | 33 | 32 | 31 | 25 | 22 | 20 | 23 | 28 | 25 | 26 | 30 | 30 | 29 | 30 | 25 | 29 | 27 | 28 | 30 | 34 | 27 | 34 |
| Base = 100% | 249 | 248 | 136 | 134 | 115 | 115 | 250 | 250 | 219 | 214 | 201 | 197 | 193 | 190 | 84 | 84 | 187 | 186 | 448 | 445 | 218 | 217 |
| **Females** | | | | | | | | | | | | | | | | | | | | | | |
| Mean units alcohol | 6.6 | 6.4 | 6.1 | 6.5 | 7.4 | 7.0 | 7.2 | 8.2 | 7.8 | 6.9 | 6.8 | 7.1 | 7.7 | 7.3 | 6.6 | 6.8 | 7.6 | 6.7 | 6.7 | 6.1 | 8.4 | 7.0 |
| ±SEM | ±0.5 | ±0.5 | ±0.7 | ±0.6 | ±0.6 | ±0.7 | ±0.5 | ±0.6 | ±0.6 | ±0.5 | ±0.6 | ±0.7 | ±0.9 | ±0.8 | ±0.7 | ±0.8 | ±0.6 | ±0.7 | ±0.4 | ±0.3 | ±0.6 | ±0.5 |
| n = | (126) | (125) | (81) | (86) | (106) | (105) | (218) | (213) | (145) | (140) | (119) | (111) | (121) | (115) | (65) | (61) | (113) | (106) | (289) | (272) | (131) | (115) |
| Non-drinkers | 60 | 60 | 51 | 47 | 47 | 47 | 48 | 49 | 47 | 48 | 56 | 59 | 48 | 50 | 50 | 53 | 51 | 54 | 46 | 49 | 50 | 56 |
| Base = 100% | 320 | 316 | 166 | 162 | 199 | 199 | 417 | 414 | 274 | 269 | 275 | 268 | 234 | 231 | 131 | 130 | 233 | 230 | 539 | 535 | 264 | 263 |

**Table 13.8** **Categories of alcohol consumption during the previous week in HALS1 full sample and HALS2 sub-sample at HALS1 and HALS2. Percentage of age group**

| | 18-24 | | 25-31 | | 32-38 | | 39-45 | | 46-52 | | 53-59 | | 60-66 | | 67-73 | | 74+ | | All | |
|---|---|---|---|---|---|---|---|---|---|---|---|---|---|---|---|---|---|---|---|---|
| HALS1 age | | | | | | | | | | | | | | | | | | | | |
| HALS2 age | 25-31 | | 32-38 | | 39-45 | | 46-52 | | 53-59 | | 60-66 | | 67-73 | | 74-80 | | 81+ | | All | |
| **Drinking category** | | | | | | | | | | | | | | | | | | | | |
| **Males** | | | | | | | | | | | | | | | | | | | | |
| **Nil** | | | | | | | | | | | | | | | | | | | | |
| HALS1 sample | 20 | | 25 | | 21 | | 27 | | 30 | | 36 | | 31 | | 44 | | 51 | | 30 | |
| HALS2 sub-sample | 21 | 25 | 24 | 25 | 18 | 18 | 25 | 25 | 33 | 34 | 33 | 34 | 31 | 38 | 40 | 48 | 52 | 48 | 28 | 30 |
| **Prudent** | | | | | | | | | | | | | | | | | | | | |
| HALS1 sample | 45 | | 46 | | 51 | | 45 | | 46 | | 44 | | 54 | | 46 | | 44 | | 47 | |
| HALS2 sub-sample | 46 | 48 | 49 | 48 | 52 | 52 | 45 | 51 | 46 | 48 | 44 | 50 | 55 | 53 | 50 | 43 | 43 | 47 | 48 | 49 |
| **Unwise** | | | | | | | | | | | | | | | | | | | | |
| HALS1 sample | 26 | | 22 | | 21 | | 22 | | 19 | | 16 | | 12 | | 7 | | 4 | | 18 | |
| HALS2 sub-sample | 26 | 21 | 20 | 20 | 21 | 23 | 24 | 18 | 18 | 17 | 19 | 13 | 11 | 7 | 7 | 8 | 5 | 6 | 19 | 16 |
| **Excessive** | | | | | | | | | | | | | | | | | | | | |
| HALS1 sample | 9 | | 7 | | 8 | | 7 | | 5 | | 4 | | 3 | | 3 | | 2 | | 6 | |
| HALS2 sub-sample | 7 | 6 | 7 | 8 | 9 | 6 | 6 | 7 | 3 | 2 | 4 | 3 | 3 | 2 | 3 | 2 | 0 | 0 | 5 | 4 |
| **Females** | | | | | | | | | | | | | | | | | | | | |
| **Nil** | | | | | | | | | | | | | | | | | | | | |
| HALS1 sample | 44 | | 47 | | 46 | | 42 | | 50 | | 56 | | 60 | | 72 | | 74 | | 53 | |
| HALS2 sub-sample | 44 | 44 | 51 | 49 | 45 | 42 | 39 | 42 | 48 | 52 | 52 | 58 | 59 | 65 | 72 | 76 | 68 | 74 | 50 | 52 |
| **Prudent** | | | | | | | | | | | | | | | | | | | | |
| HALS1 sample | 48 | | 45 | | 48 | | 52 | | 45 | | 39 | | 37 | | 25 | | 24 | | 42 | |
| HALS2 sub-sample | 48 | 50 | 42 | 45 | 49 | 52 | 55 | 52 | 47 | 45 | 43 | 39 | 37 | 32 | 25 | 21 | 28 | 25 | 44 | 43 |
| **Unwise/Excessive** | | | | | | | | | | | | | | | | | | | | |
| HALS1 sample | 8 | | 8 | | 6 | | 6 | | 5 | | 5 | | 3 | | 3 | | 3 | | 6 | |
| HALS2 sub-sample | 8 | 6 | 7 | 6 | 6 | 6 | 6 | 6 | 5 | 3 | 5 | 4 | 5 | 3 | 3 | 3 | 3 | 1 | 6 | 5 |
| *Base = 100%* | *534* | | *486* | | *573* | | *473* | | *418* | | *415* | | *412* | | *313* | | *271* | | *3895* | |
| | *297* | *299* | *240* | *239* | *380* | *383* | *323* | *322* | *279* | *277* | *277* | *276* | *259* | *257* | *148* | *145* | *88* | *86* | *2295* | *2280* |
| | *624* | | *672* | | *764* | | *617* | | *574* | | *483* | | *553* | | *391* | | *409* | | *5087* | |
| | *309* | *306* | *394* | *387* | *544* | *539* | *431* | *429* | *390* | *390* | *314* | *314* | *327* | *323* | *191* | *188* | *145* | *141* | *3045* | *3017* |

**Table 13.9  Change in drinking categories from HALS1 to HALS2. Percentage of HALS1 category**

| Age at HALS1 | 18-38 | | | | 39-59 | | | | 60+ | | | |
|---|---|---|---|---|---|---|---|---|---|---|---|---|
| | | | | | HALS1 drinking category | | | | | | | |
| | Nil | Prudent | Unwise | Excessive | Nil | Prudent | Unwise | Excessive | Nil | Prudent | Unwise | Excessive |
| **HALS2 Drinking category** | | | | | **Males** | | | | | | | |
| Nil | 58 | 16 | 8 | 4 | 68 | 19 | 5 | 11 | 78 | 25 | 5 | 0 |
| Prudent | 37 | 64 | 37 | 25 | 30 | 70 | 44 | 8 | 21 | 68 | 65 | (4) |
| Unwise | 3 | 18 | 43 | 38 | 2 | 10 | 43 | 43 | φ | 7 | 28 | (4) |
| Excessive | 2 | 2 | 12 | 32 | 0 | 2 | 8 | 38 | φ | 0 | 2 | (5) |
| | | | | | **Females** | | | | | | | |
| Nil | 65 | 28 | 14 | | 78 | 28 | 8 | | 88 | 40 | 8 | |
| Prudent | 33 | 65 | 53 | | 22 | 67 | 57 | | 12 | 57 | 54 | |
| Unwise/excessive | 2 | 7 | 29 | | φ | 5 | 35 | | φ | 3 | 38 | |
| *Base = 100%* | *190* | *450* | *204* | *71* | *260* | *393* | *182* | *37* | *180* | *252* | *43* | *13* |
| | *575* | *567* | *87* | | *517* | *550* | *63* | | *423* | *204* | *24* | |

**Table 13.10  Non-manual and manual group differences in drinking categories at HALS1 and HALS2. Percentage of HALS1 socio-economic group**

| | Males | | | | Females | | | |
|---|---|---|---|---|---|---|---|---|
| | Non-manual | | Manual | | Non-manual | | Manual | |
| HALS | 1 | 2 | 1 | 2 | 1 | 2 | 1 | 2 |
| **Drinking category** | | | | | | | | |
| Nil | 22 | 25 | 32 | 33 | 42 | 45 | 58 | 58 |
| Prudent | 56 | 55 | 42 | 46 | 51 | 49 | 38 | 38 |
| Unwise | 18 | 17 | 19 | 16 | | | | |
| | | | | | 7 | 6 | 4 | 4 |
| Excessive | 4 | 3 | 7 | 5 | | | | |
| *Base = 100%* | *987* | | *1270* | | *1397* | | *1575* | |

**Table 13.11 Regional ('North'/'South') variations in categories of alcohol consumption. Percentage of regional group**

| | Males | | | | Females | | | |
|---|---|---|---|---|---|---|---|---|
| | HALS1 | | HALS2 | | HALS1 | | HALS2 | |
| | North | South | North | South | North | South | North | South |
| **Drinking category** | | | | | | | | |
| Nil | 28 | 28 | 28 | 32 | 52 | 49 | 52 | 52 |
| Prudent | 44 | 52 | 47 | 52 | 43 | 45 | 43 | 44 |
| Unwise | 21 | 16 | 19 | 14 | 5 | 6 | 5 | 4 |
| Excessive | 7 | 4 | 6 | 3 | | | | |
| Base = 100% | 1167 | 1128 | 1158 | 1122 | 1646 | 1399 | 1628 | 1389 |

**Table 13.12 Self-assessed level of drinking in those who drank 'last week' in comparison to category of alcohol consumption at HALS1 and HALS2. Percentage of self assessed level of drinking group**

| Self-assessed drinking level | Males | | | | | | Females | | | |
|---|---|---|---|---|---|---|---|---|---|---|
| | Light | | Moderate | | Heavy | | Light | | Moderate/Heavy | |
| HALS | 1 | 2 | 1 | 2 | 1 | 2 | 1 | 2 | 1 | 2 |
| **Category of alcohol intake** | | | | | **Age 18-38** | | | | | |
| Prudent | 90 | 90 | 49 | 53 | 13 | 10 | 98 | 98 | 74 | 78 |
| Unwise | 10 | 9 | 38 | 39 | 44 | 43 | 2 | 2 | 26 | 22 |
| Excessive | 0 | φ | 13 | 8 | 42 | 47 | | | | |
| | | | | | **Age 39-59** | | | | | |
| Prudent | 92 | 93 | 45 | 56 | 14 | 15 | 97 | 97 | 76 | 83 |
| Unwise | 8 | 7 | 47 | 37 | 43 | 46 | 3 | 4 | 24 | 17 |
| Excessive | 0 | 0 | 9 | 7 | 43 | 39 | | | | |
| | | | | | **Age 60+** | | | | | |
| Prudent | 95 | 95 | 59 | 66 | (1) | (1) | 97 | 96 | 67 | 80 |
| Unwise | 5 | 5 | 32 | 28 | 0 | (2) | 4 | 4 | 33 | 20 |
| Excessive | 0 | φ | 10 | 6 | (3) | (1) | | | | |
| Base = 100% | 276 | 270 | 409 | 382 | 45 | 58 | 356 | 361 | 308 | 321 |
| | 267 | 291 | 324 | 284 | 21 | 33 | 399 | 343 | 216 | 224 |
| | 203 | 192 | 104 | 85 | 4 | 4 | 173 | 146 | 61 | 49 |

**Table 13.13   Percentage of regular, occasional and ex-drinkers who drank 'last week' in HALS1 and HALS2**

| | Males | | | | | | Females | | | | | |
|---|---|---|---|---|---|---|---|---|---|---|---|---|
| Age at HALS1 | 18-38 | | 39-59 | | 60+ | | 18-38 | | 39-59 | | 60+ | |
| HALS | 1 | 2 | 1 | 2 | 1 | 2 | 1 | 2 | 1 | 2 | 1 | 2 |
| Regular | 98 | 99 | 98 | 99 | 100 | 99 | 95 | 98 | 97 | 98 | 94 | 100 |
| Occasional | 82 | 82 | 78 | 80 | 79 | 78 | 69 | 72 | 77 | 75 | 72 | 71 |
| Ex-drinker | 18 | 20 | 11 | 17 | 18 | 13 | 14 | 17 | 18 | 19 | 30 | 14 |
| *Base = 100%* | *395* | *376* | *306* | *314* | *134* | *130* | *215* | *243* | *212* | *220* | *80* | *71* |
| | *418* | *401* | *403* | *351* | *226* | *190* | *672* | *602* | *538* | *447* | *219* | *164* |
| | *51* | *84* | *75* | *97* | *39* | *68* | *102* | *139* | *72* | *99* | *40* | *65* |

**Table 13.14   CAGE score in HALS1 and HALS2. Percentage of age group**

| Age at HALS1 | 18-24 | | 25-31 | | 32-38 | | 39-45 | | 46-52 | | 53-59 | | 60-66 | | 67-73 | | 74+ | | ALL | |
|---|---|---|---|---|---|---|---|---|---|---|---|---|---|---|---|---|---|---|---|---|
| HALS | 1 | 2 | 1 | 2 | 1 | 2 | 1 | 2 | 1 | 2 | 1 | 2 | 1 | 2 | 1 | 2 | 1 | 2 | 1 | 2 |
| **CAGE score** | | | | | | | | | | | | **Males** | | | | | | | | |
| 0 | 58 | 52 | 52 | 55 | 55 | 59 | 62 | 58 | 70 | 67 | 68 | 74 | 77 | 77 | 78 | 82 | 84 | 92 | 64 | 64 |
| 1 | 26 | 28 | 31 | 25 | 25 | 23 | 23 | 28 | 17 | 19 | 20 | 16 | 18 | 17 | 13 | 15 | 13 | 5 | 22 | 22 |
| 2 | 12 | 13 | 9 | 13 | 13 | 11 | 11 | 12 | 7 | 8 | 8 | 6 | 4 | 5 | 5 | 3 | 2 | 2 | 9 | 9 |
| 3 and 4 | 4 | 8 | 8 | 7 | 7 | 7 | 4 | 3 | 6 | 5 | 4 | 4 | 2 | φ | 4 | 0 | 2 | φ | 5 | 5 |
| | | | | | | | | | | | | **Females** | | | | | | | | |
| 0 | 76 | 74 | 79 | 79 | 79 | 75 | 79 | 74 | 81 | 83 | 80 | 82 | 88 | 86 | 86 | 94 | 95 | 95 | 81 | 79 |
| 1 | 17 | 18 | 14 | 14 | 14 | 16 | 15 | 16 | 12 | 11 | 15 | 12 | 8 | 9 | 13 | 4 | 5 | 5 | 14 | 14 |
| 2 | 6 | 7 | 5 | 6 | 5 | 6 | 5 | 7 | 4 | 4 | 5 | 5 | 3 | 4 | 1 | 2 | 0 | 0 | 5 | 6 |
| 3 and 4 | φ | 1 | 1 | 2 | φ | 2 | 2 | 3 | 3 | 2 | φ | 2 | φ | φ | 0 | 0 | 0 | 0 | 1 | |
| *Base =* | *269* | *269* | *214* | *221* | *363* | *364* | *285* | *287* | *243* | *232* | *239* | *233* | *209* | *212* | *116* | *111* | *62* | *61* | *2000* | *1990* |
| *100%* | *236* | *258* | *301* | *298* | *416* | *407* | *332* | *320* | *263* | *257* | *200* | *183* | *179* | *162* | *79* | *68* | *63* | *63* | *2070* | *2016* |

**Table 13.15    Change in CAGE score from HALS1 to HALS2 in three age groups. Percentage of HALS1 score.**

| Age at HALS1 | 18-39 | | | | 39-59 | | | | 60+ | | | |
|---|---|---|---|---|---|---|---|---|---|---|---|---|
| **HALS1 Score** | **0** | **1** | **2** | **3 & 4** | **0** | **1** | **2** | **3 & 4** | **0** | **1** | **2** | **3 & 4** |
| **HALS2 Score** | | | | | | | **Males** | | | | | |
| 0 | 69 | 45 | 26 | 23 | 78 | 51 | 33 | 11 | 89 | 62 | (4) | (1) |
| 1 | 21 | 32 | 30 | 26 | 17 | 35 | 29 | 25 | 9 | 33 | (6) | (6) |
| 2 | 7 | 17 | 25 | 21 | 5 | 12 | 24 | 31 | 2 | 6 | (4) | (2) |
| 3 and 4 | 3 | 6 | 20 | 30 | 1 | 2 | 14 | 33 | φ | 0 | (1) | (1) |
| | | | | | | | **Females** | | | | | |
| 0 | 82 | 61 | 21 | (4) | 86 | 53 | 38 | (3) | 93 | (14) | (3) | 0 |
| 1 | 14 | 27 | 28 | (1) | 11 | 26 | 31 | (1) | 5 | (3) | (1) | 0 |
| 2 | 3 | 10 | 43 | (2) | 3 | 17 | 19 | (5) | 2 | (1) | (3) | (1) |
| 3 and 4 | φ | 2 | 9 | (3) | 1 | 4 | 13 | (3) | 0 | (1) | 0 | 0 |
| *Base = 100%* | *436* | *221* | *97* | *53* | *455* | *147* | *66* | *36* | *270* | *55* | *15* | *10* |
| | *651* | *130* | *47* | *10* | *513* | *96* | *32* | *12* | *195* | *19* | *7* | *1* |

**Table 13.16    CAGE scores in HALS1 and HALS2 in non-manual and manual groups. Percentage of socio-economic groups**

| | Males | | | | Females | | | |
|---|---|---|---|---|---|---|---|---|
| | Non-manual | | Manual | | Non-manual | | Manual | |
| **HALS** | **1** | **2** | **1** | **2** | **1** | **2** | **1** | **2** |
| **Score** | | | | | | | | |
| 0 | 63 | 63 | 62 | 63 | 79 | 77 | 80 | 79 |
| 1 | 21 | 23 | 24 | 22 | 14 | 14 | 14 | 14 |
| 2 | 10 | 10 | 9 | 10 | 5 | 7 | 5 | 5 |
| 3 and 4 | 6 | 5 | 5 | 5 | 2 | 2 | 1 | 2 |
| *Base = 100%* | *819* | | *1030* | | *879* | | *812* | |

**Table 13.17** **North/South differences in CAGE scores in HALS1 and HALS2**

| | Males | | | | Females | | | |
|---|---|---|---|---|---|---|---|---|
| | North | | South | | North | | South | |
| HALS | 1 | 2 | 1 | 2 | 1 | 2 | 1 | 2 |
| **CAGE score** | | | | | | | | |
| 0 | 61 | 62 | 67 | 66 | 80 | 81 | 81 | 78 |
| 1 | 24 | 23 | 20 | 20 | 14 | 13 | 13 | 14 |
| 2 | 10 | 10 | 9 | 8 | 4 | 5 | 5 | 6 |
| 3 and 4 | 5 | 4 | 5 | 5 | 1 | 1 | 1 | 2 |
| *Base = 100%* | *1022* | *1025* | *978* | *965* | *1089* | *1090* | *981* | *926* |

**Table 13.18** **CAGE scores in HALS1 and HALS2 in regular and occasional drinkers by category of drinking last week. Percentage of drinking category**

| | Males | | | | | | | | Females | | | | | |
|---|---|---|---|---|---|---|---|---|---|---|---|---|---|---|
| | Previous week's drinking category | | | | | | | | | | | | Unwise/ | |
| | Nil | | Prudent | | Unwise | | Excessive | | Nil | | Prudent | | Excessive | |
| HALS | 1 | 2 | 1 | 2 | 1 | 2 | 1 | 2 | 1 | 2 | 1 | 2 | 1 | 2 |
| **CAGE score** | | | | | | | | | | | | | | |
| 0 | 81 | 84 | 73 | 73 | 46 | 45 | 31 | 24 | 90 | 89 | 84 | 82 | 50 | 40 |
| 1 | 13 | 12 | 17 | 18 | 31 | 32 | 31 | 30 | 8 | 7 | 12 | 12 | 28 | 28 |
| 2 | 3 | 3 | 7 | 6 | 14 | 14 | 23 | 35 | 1 | 2 | 4 | 4 | 17 | 27 |
| 3 and 4 | 3 | 2 | 2 | 2 | 9 | 10 | 15 | 12 | 1 | 1 | 1 | 1 | 4 | 5 |
| *Base = 100%* | *223* | *189* | *1095* | *1080* | *426* | *372* | *121* | *101* | *412* | *329* | *1316* | *1242* | *173* | *143* |

**Table 13.19** Smoking habits of 'nil', 'prudent', 'unwise' and 'excessive' drinkers in HALS1 and HALS2. Percentage of category of alcohol consumption

| HALS | Males | | | | | | | | | Females | | | | | |
| | Nil | | Prudent | | Unwise | | Excessive | | | Nil | | Prudent | | Unwise/Excessive | |
| | 1 | 2 | 1 | 2 | 1 | 2 | 1 | 2 | | 1 | 2 | 1 | 2 | 1 | 2 |
|---|---|---|---|---|---|---|---|---|---|---|---|---|---|---|---|
| **HALS1 age 18-38** | | | | | | | | | | | | | | | |
| Non-smokers | 47 | 47 | 45 | 45 | 36 | 31 | 24 | 22 | | 49 | 48 | 48 | 42 | 23 | 2 |
| Occ. smokers | 4 | 1 | 8 | 1 | 7 | 1 | 6 | 0 | | 3 | φ | 3 | 2 | 4 | 1 |
| Ex-smokers | 13 | 18 | 15 | 26 | 15 | 20 | 13 | 15 | | 17 | 20 | 18 | 23 | 16 | 23 |
| Smokers | 37 | 34 | 32 | 28 | 42 | 49 | 58 | 63 | | 31 | 31 | 32 | 32 | 58 | 53 |
| **HALS1 age 39-59** | | | | | | | | | | | | | | | |
| Non-smokers | 28 | 27 | 23 | 24 | 15 | 10 | 8 | 12 | | 47 | 46 | 44 | 40 | 21 | 25 |
| Occ. smokers | 4 | φ | 7 | φ | 7 | φ | 0 | 0 | | 2 | φ | 3 | 1 | 3 | 0 |
| Ex-smokers | 30 | 45 | 37 | 47 | 23 | 43 | 11 | 21 | | 19 | 26 | 23 | 33 | 30 | 27 |
| Smokers | 38 | 28 | 33 | 29 | 56 | 46 | 81 | 68 | | 32 | 27 | 30 | 26 | 46 | 48 |
| **HALS1 age 60+** | | | | | | | | | | | | | | | |
| Non-smokers | 21 | 19 | 18 | 15 | 15 | 6 | 0 | 0 | | 56 | 55 | 46 | 40 | 35 | (6) |
| Occ. smokers | 4 | 1 | 6 | 0 | 7 | 0 | (1) | (1) | | 1 | φ | 3 | 1 | 4 | 0 |
| Ex-smokers | 41 | 51 | 45 | 62 | 44 | 63 | (7) | (4) | | 23 | 29 | 33 | 46 | 38 | (6) |
| Smokers | 33 | 29 | 31 | 23 | 44 | 31 | (5) | (2) | | 19 | 16 | 18 | 13 | 23 | (4) |
| *Base = 100%* | *191* | *204* | *454* | *454* | *205* | *199* | *71* | *60* | | *582* | *547* | *577* | *608* | *88* | *77* |
| | *265* | *267* | *395* | *434* | *182* | *140* | *37* | *34* | | *520* | *564* | *552* | *517* | *63* | *52* |
| | *184* | *207* | *255* | *239* | *43* | *35* | *13* | *7* | | *429* | *457* | *208* | *179* | *26* | *16* |

**Table 13.20  Blood pressure in relation to alcohol consumption in HALS1 and HALS2. Percentage of alcohol consumption category**

| | Males | | | | | | | | Females | | | | | |
| --- | --- | --- | --- | --- | --- | --- | --- | --- | --- | --- | --- | --- | --- | --- |
| | Nil | | Prudent | | Unwise | | Excessive | | Nil | | Prudent | | Unwise/ Excessive | |
| HALS | 1 | 2 | 1 | 2 | 1 | 2 | 1 | 2 | 1 | 2 | 1 | 2 | 1 | 2 |
| **Blood pressure category** | | | | | Age at survey 25-45 | | | | | | | | | |
| Normal | 89 | 91 | 91 | 89 | 82 | 88 | 75 | 86 | 94 | 96 | 95 | 96 | 94 | 97 |
| Borderline | 7 | 2 | 6 | 7 | 10 | 7 | 15 | 4 | 4 | 1 | 3 | 2 | 4 | 2 |
| Untreated hypertensive | 3 | 2 | 4 | 2 | 7 | 4 | 10 | 8 | 1 | 1 | 1 | φ | 1 | 2 |
| Treated hypertensive | φ | 5 | φ | 1 | 1 | 1 | 0 | 2 | 1 | 1 | 1 | 2 | 1 | 0 |
| | | | | | Age at survey 46-66 | | | | | | | | | |
| Normal | 66 | 69 | 63 | 69 | 58 | 58 | 38 | 54 | 65 | 69 | 74 | 77 | 77 | 81 |
| Borderline | 13 | 12 | 18 | 12 | 15 | 17 | 13 | 29 | 13 | 9 | 12 | 7 | 12 | 0 |
| Untreated hypertensive | 13 | 4 | 9 | 7 | 14 | 7 | 29 | 11 | 9 | 4 | 6 | 4 | 5 | 7 |
| Treated hypertensive | 8 | 15 | 11 | 11 | 13 | 19 | 21 | 7 | 13 | 18 | 8 | 12 | 7 | 12 |
| Base = 100% | 179 | 167 | 401 | 378 | 176 | 181 | 61 | 51 | 526 | 444 | 582 | 505 | 80 | 64 |
| | 216 | 219 | 343 | 376 | 118 | 120 | 24 | 20 | 412 | 438 | 351 | 419 | 43 | 43 |

Age at survey 67 +

| | Nil | | Prudent | | Unwise/ Excessive | | | | Nil | | Prudent | | Unwise/ Excessive | |
| --- | --- | --- | --- | --- | --- | --- | --- | --- | --- | --- | --- | --- | --- | --- |
| Normal | 45 | 43 | 53 | 47 | (8) | 38 | | | 38 | 36 | 33 | 47 | (4) | (7) |
| Borderline | 22 | 19 | 20 | 17 | (6) | 24 | | | 21 | 19 | 33 | 17 | (2) | (1) |
| Untreated hypertensive | 17 | 8 | 14 | 9 | (3) | 12 | | | 19 | 8 | 20 | 10 | (2) | (1) |
| Treated hypertensive | 16 | 29 | 13 | 28 | 0 | 26 | | | 23 | 36 | 15 | 26 | (1) | (3) |
| Base = 100% | 182 | 156 | 294 | 187 | 17 | 34 | | | 151 | 299 | 61 | 121 | 9 | 12 |

# CHANGES IN EXERCISE AND LEISURE ACTIVITIES

## 14

Brian D Cox and Margaret J Whichelow

In the report of the first Health and Lifestyle Survey the patterns of active leisure pursuits revealed that the majority of respondents over the age of 40 did not take part in any active (sports) pursuits, that there were socio-economic differences in participation and that women below 40 were less likely than men to take part (Fenner, 1987). Socio-economic, age and sex differences were also found with respect to the less active leisure pursuits. In HALS2 the same questions were posed about sports and other energetic activities, here referred to as 'active leisure pursuits', and other less energetic activities as 'pastimes', with an additional question about long walks. Changes in both types of activity can therefore be examined comparing each cohort at HALS1 and HALS2 and also groups of the same age at the two surveys. Since HALS1, the General Household Survey (GHS) has continued to report on physical and pastime activities (Smyth and Browne, 1992) and a major survey of the energetic non-work activities of British adults has been carried out (Allied Dunbar National Fitness Survey, 1992). The results presented here from HALS1 and HALS2 can be compared with both these studies. Since HALS1, campaigns to encourage the British population to become more active in order to minimise the risk of heart disease and other ailments have continued, and the comparison of HALS1 and HALS2 can be used to assess the success and level of awareness effected by these campaigns. The health benefits for men and women of all ages of taking regular exercise are well established (Royal College of Physicians, 1991) and the physical and psychological effects of exercise have been reviewed in the Allied Dunbar National Fitness Survey (1992).

Controversy has reigned as to whether frequent very intensive exercise is necessary to promote any benefit for cardio-vascular health (Morris et al. 1980) or whether lower levels of exercise can also be associated with good health (Cox, 1989).

## Active Leisure Pursuits

The proportions of men and women taking part in the fortnight prior to interview in the most popular activities are shown in Table 14.1 and Table 14.2. Comparison of the HALS1 full sample with the HALS2 sub-sample at HALS1 shows that the HALS2 sub-sample is representative of the original sample at almost all age groups for all the activities. As shown in the HALS1 report (Fenner, 1987) and by the General Household Survey (1992) there is a marked decrease, with advancing age, in the proportion of respondents taking part in every activity except bowls and golf. It would therefore be expected that, in the seven years between the two Surveys, the proportion of each age group of respondents taking part in each activity would have declined, but this is not always the case. For 'Keep fit, Yoga', particularly in the women, there has been an increase in participation by HALS2 at most ages. The same pattern is seen for cycling, swimming, football (in men under 52), golf for men of all ages and middle aged women and bowls for the middle aged and elderly. In contrast there has been a decline in jogging greater than expected for the youngest age group, and in dancing for all groups.

These patterns are further illustrated in Table 14.3 where a wider range of activities is shown by age at

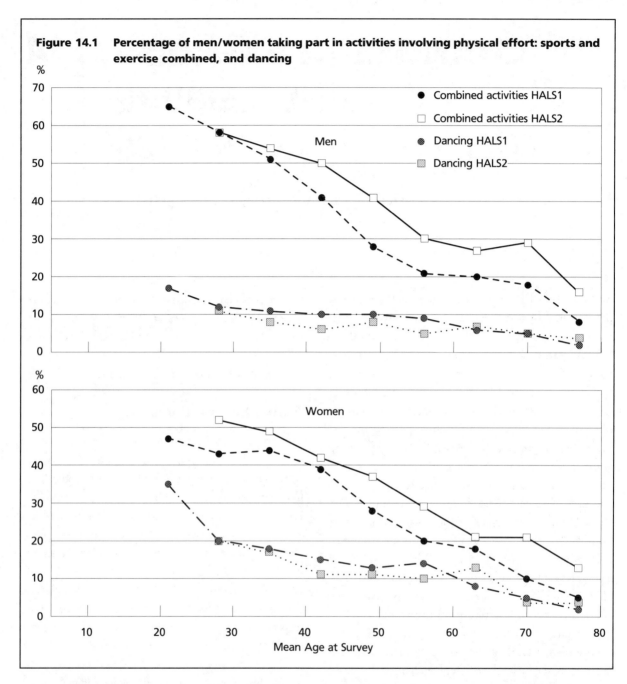

**Figure 14.1** Percentage of men/women taking part in activities involving physical effort: sports and exercise combined, and dancing

Survey. The very small proportion of women, and, except for football in those below 40, of men who play in team or competitive sports is striking.

The trends of increasing participation during the past few years in most activities are also reported by the GHS (Smyth and Browne, 1992) which compared participation in a wide variety of sports, and other energetic activities, in 1987 and 1990. The increase in active leisure pursuit participation since HALS1 is clearly seen at most ages when the activities are grouped as in Table 14.4 and Figure 14.1. These groupings were used when the relationships between various types and levels of exercise and a number of

measures of health were reported for the HALS1 respondents (Cox, 1989). Keep fit, yoga, cycling, jogging, swimming, backpacking, hiking, mountaineering, athletics, rowing/canoeing, skating, skipping and trampolining, which have principally an aerobic component were grouped as 'individual' activities. Team/competitive sports, requiring continuous intense physical effort and which have strong isometric as well as aerobic components, included squash, basketball, badminton, tennis, table tennis, hockey, football, rugby, self-defence, gymnastics, weight/circuit training, fencing and volleyball. Other activities, golf, cricket, sailing, bowls, riding, snow sports, rounders and tug-of-war ( most of which were done by very few people) were grouped as 'recreational' activities. All types of activity, except dancing, had increased to some extent in both sexes in HALS2, when comparison was made with the same age group at HALS1. However, Table 14.5 shows that this increase in participation is not matched by the respondents' opinions at HALS2 of their level of exercise compared to seven years ago. More respondents at almost all ages said that they took less exercise than seven years ago, than reported taking more exercise than seven years ago. As would be expected, this trend was particularly marked in the elderly. In those aged 46 to 66 at HALS2, where the increase in the combined activities (Table 14.4) was most marked, consistently more respondents reported taking less exercise. The possibility that the respondents are less active in other areas of their lives, such as general walking or activities associated with their occupation, may explain these anomalies and cannot therefore be excluded. However the responses may also suggest an increased awareness of exercise as an important feature of lifestyle.

Lower levels of participation in active leisure pursuits by manual groups than by non-manual groups, at all ages and by both men and women were reported in HALS1 (Fenner, 1987) and by the GHS (Smyth and Browne, 1992). This socio-economic difference is apparent for all types of activity undertaken except dancing (Table 14.6). For all three types of activity, 'individual', 'competitive' and 'recreational' there was an increase in participation from HALS1 to HALS2 in both the non-manual and manual groups, so that the socio-economic group difference seen at HALS1 was maintained at HALS2. This is reminiscent of the changes seen in other lifestyle habits, such as diet (Chapter 11) where all groups have reduced their intake of fatty foods, so that although the diet has improved, the manual groups still have poorer diets than the non-manual. Dancing is the one activity where there is no class difference at HALS1 and where there has been a similar marked decrease in participation by both socio-economic groups.

The socio-economic structure of the northern and southern regions (see Appendix A) of the country are different, with a higher proportion of manual workers

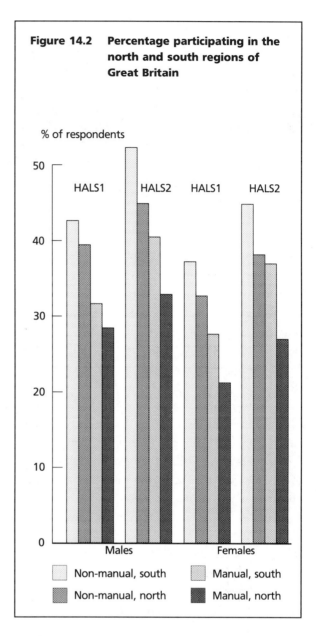

**Figure 14.2    Percentage participating in the north and south regions of Great Britain**

in the northern region, so regional comparison of participation in active leisure pursuits require socio-economic variations to be taken into consideration, as shown in Table 14.7. For each category of activity there are clear regional and socio-economic group differences, as well as changes between HALS1 and HALS2. For the individual activities, at both Surveys, participation is higher in non-manual than manual respondents in both regions, and in the south for both socio-economic groups. Although not quite so consistent, the same trend is seen for the 'competitive' and 'recreational' activities. Thus when the activities are all combined the non-manual/south, non-manual/north, manual/south and manual/north graduation is very clear, for men and women, (Figure 14.2). Dancing, however, shows a different pattern. Similar proportions of non-manual and manual men are dancers in the south, but in the north a higher percentage of non-manual than manual men mention dancing. This difference is preserved from HALS1 to HALS2.

At both Surveys the respondents were asked whether they believed they were more or less active than people of their own age. At HALS2 more respondents than at HALS1 in almost all age groups reported being less active, and conversely fewer reported being more active (Table 14.8). Again this is in conflict with the increase in the numbers taking part in sports and other energetic activities. It is interesting that a higher proportion of men over 60 (HALS1) and 67 (HALS2) and women over 67 (HALS1) and 74 (HALS2) report being more active for their age than do those in the younger age groups.

A further subjective assessment of activity was obtained from the responses to the question 'Do you think you get enough exercise'? Many fewer respondents believed that they got enough exercise at HALS2 than at HALS1, and this was particularly apparent amongst the youngest and oldest men (Table 14.9). The groups of men in the ages 39-59 at HALS1 had not changed their opinions. These groups tended to show larger increases in participation in active leisure pursuits than other groups of men or women, and were likely to report playing sports at HALS1 and HALS2 as being health promoting factors in their lives (Chapter 16).

An assessment of the respondents' subjective view of whether they took enough exercise, in relation to their level of activity, is shown in Table 14.10. This was calculated from participation in activities, the number of occasions on which they were performed and the duration of the activity. The majority of young respondents who did not take part in any active leisure pursuits reported not getting enough exercise, particularly at HALS2. The trend, in both sexes and in both Surveys, is for the proportion believing that they do not get enough exercise to decrease with increasing time spent on activities. Nevertheless, even for the most energetic respondents, particularly the women spending over 16 hours in the previous fortnight on active leisure

pursuits, up to 46% believe they get insufficient exercise. In all categories more respondents report not getting enough exercise at HALS2, suggesting, once again, a much greater awareness of the importance of exercise in 1991/2. However the significant proportion in the 'nil activity' category who believe they do get enough exercise suggests that health campaigns still have a long way to go in this area.

## Walking

Walking is considered separately from other energetic activities as it is part of so many everyday activities and notoriously difficult to assess with precision. Although the questions about walking during weekdays and weekends specifically excluded walking 'at work' and asked about 'walks', walking to and from work, and to and from shopping etc., it was obvious from many replies that walking at work and around the house had been included. At HALS2 a specific question was also included about 'long walks', over two miles, but here again accuracy could not be guaranteed. From the short times recorded for such walks it was evident in a few cases that those respondents must have walked less than 2 miles.

Because of the way it was reported walking at weekends was less likely to be confounded by the inclusion of walking at work, than that reported for weekdays, weekend walking is shown here in Table 14.11. In general more men and women are in the nil walking category at HALS2 than seven years previously, but when comparing like ages there is little overall change. In all age groups there is a reduction over the seven years between the two Surveys in the percentage walking for over one hour a day. Since the prevalence of such walking declines with increasing age this might be expected, but comparison of the respondents at HALS2 with those of the same age at HALS1 shows that, except for the older women, the decline in the proportion going for walks of an hour or more is greater than would be expected for the 7-year age change. In contrast, however, the GHS reports a small increase in the proportion of their respondents going for walks between 1987 and 1990.

The proportion of respondents claiming to go for walks of 2 miles or more does not decline appreciably with age, until age 74 (Table 14.12). Those going for long walks, but who do not take part in any other active leisure pursuits, are also shown in Table 14.12. Here it is evident that, although for half the younger long walking respondents, walks form the only energetic activity recorded, it is the only activity for almost all the older long walking subjects.

It has been suggested by Morris (1987) that a fast pace of walking is protective against coronary heart disease. In HALS2 the respondents were asked to assess their usual pace of walking and the results are shown in Table 14.13 for non-manual and manual socio-economic groups. In non-manual and manual men and women very few young respondents reported walking at a slow pace. With increasing age there was a higher proportion of slow walkers, particularly amongst the manual group. Socio-economic group differences were apparent for brisk walkers, where the non-manual outnumbered the manual, but not amongst the average or fast walkers. There was, not unexpectedly, a lower proportion of brisk walkers amongst the elderly. In middle-age a greater proportion of men and women in the manual than in the non-manual groups report an average or slow pace of walking.

## Pastimes

Although of less importance for cardio-vascular health, participation in non-energetic pursuits (pastimes) can be important from the point of view of social integration and mental stimulation. The same list of activities was used in both Surveys so that the degrees of change in participation in individual pastimes and in the number of pastimes undertaken can be examined.

Table 14.14 shows that the proportion taking part in each pastime is higher in the HALS2 sub-sample at HALS1 than the HALS1 full sample in most age groups. Attrition, between HALS1 and HALS2, is greatest in the non-participants over 60 years of age. Men are more likely than women to go fishing, play darts/snooker, watch sports, do hobbies/crafts, bet, go to the pub and play bingo, whereas knitting/sewing, voluntary work and going to church are more popular for women. There are age trends with the prevalence of most pastimes being lower in the oldest group. Participation in a number of pastimes has increased between HALS1 and HALS2, notably visiting the coast/parks and museums etc., going to the cinema (women), watching sports and betting (women), whilst knitting/sewing has declined markedly in women.

When the number of pastimes engaged in (including in this case gardening and DIY) are considered clear age trends for HALS1 and HALS2 are apparent (Table 14.15). With increasing age there is an increase in the proportion of respondents engaged in very few pastimes and a decrease in the number carrying out many of these activities. Comparison of the HALS1 full sample and HALS2 sub-sample at HALS1 shows that the HALS2 sub-sample is somewhat under-represented by those carrying out few pastimes in the older age groups. By HALS2 in most age groups there has been an increase in the proportion of respondents engaging in five or more pastimes; in the men aged 39 to 73 at HALS2 and the women between 46 and 80 (HALS2) the increase has been greater than expected for the seven year increase in age.

There are also considerable socio-economic group differences in the number of pastimes pursued as shown in Table 14.16, with the manual groups at all ages and in both surveys more likely than the non-manual to report engaging in few pastimes, whilst there is a higher proportion of non-manual respondents reporting five or more at each age.

Gardening, but not DIY, shows some non-manual/manual differences in the proportions carrying out the activity (Table 14.17). Although at most ages fewer manual than non-manual respondents are gardeners, for the men who are gardeners those in manual occupations spend more hours gardening than do those in non-manual occupations. For both groups there is an increase in the number of hours spent gardening at around retirement age; this is not so apparent for the women, who spend fewer hours gardening than do men. Women are much less likely than men to do DIY, and if they do, they spend less time on it.

## Summary

Increases in participation at most ages in a number of active leisure pursuits between HALS1 and HALS2 have been identified. Despite this there has been an increase in the number of respondents reporting that they do not get enough exercise, and more respondents report that they are less active than report that they are more active, than seven years ago. These views may reflect a greater awareness of the importance of exercise for health. There are clear socio-economic and regional differences in participation in active leisure pursuits such that there is a gradient from high to lower participation from non-manual/south, non-manual/north, manual/south to manual/north for both sexes in both Surveys. Overall most of the respondents who did not participate in any active leisure pursuits thought that they were getting enough exercise, but conversely a substantial proportion of the most active, with over 16 hours activity in the previous two weeks also believed that they did not get enough exercise. Participation in non-energetic pastimes has increased between HALS1 and HALS2 at most ages. There are also socio-economic group differences with the manual respondents less likely than the non-manual to engage in many pastimes.

## References

Allied Dunbar National Fitness Survey (1992), 'A report on activity patterns and fitness levels', London, The Sports Council and the Health Education Authority.

Cox, B.D. (1989), 'Association of leisure and sporting activities with health in the Health and Lifestyle Survey',in 'Fit for Life', Cambridge, The Health Promotion Research Trust.

Fenner, N.P. (1987), 'Leisure, Work and Exercise', in Cox et al., 'The Health and Lifestyle Survey: preliminary report of a nationwide survey of the physical and mental health, attitudes and lifestyle of a random sample of British adults', London, The Health Promotion Research Trust.

Morris, J.N., Everitt, M.G., Pollard, R., Chave, S.P.W. and Semmence, A.M. (1980), 'Vigorous exercise in leisure-time: protection against coronary heart disease', Lancet ii, 1207-1210.

Morris, J.N. (1987) 'Exercise and the incidence of coronary heart disease' in 'Exercise – Heart – Health', London, The Coronary Prevention Group.

Royal College of Physicians (1991), 'Medical aspects of exercise: benefits and risks', Journal of the Royal College of Physicians 25, 193-196.

Smyth, M. and Browne, F. (1992), 'General Household Survey 1990', London, HMSO.

**Table 14.1**   **Selected active leisure pursuits in men, in HALS1 full sample, and HALS2 sub-sample at HALS1 and HALS2. Percentage of age group. (φ leass than 1%; number in brackets less than 0.5%)**

| Age at HALS1 | 18-24 | | 25-31 | | 32-38 | | 39-45 | | 46-52 | | 53-59 | | 60-66 | | 67-73 | | >73 | |
| --- | --- | --- | --- | --- | --- | --- | --- | --- | --- | --- | --- | --- | --- | --- | --- | --- | --- | --- |
| Age at HALS2 | | 25-31 | | 32-38 | | 39-45 | | 46-52 | | 53-59 | | 60-66 | | 67-73 | | 74-80 | | >80 |
| **Keep fit, yoga etc.** | | | | | | | | | | | | | | | | | | |
| HALS1 sample | 16 | | 13 | | 12 | | 7 | | 5 | | 4 | | 4 | | 4 | | 2 | |
| HALS2 sub-sample | 19 | 17 | 11 | 11 | 11 | 10 | 7 | 10 | 4 | 4 | 5 | 3 | 6 | 6 | 4 | 3 | 0 | 7 |
| **Cycling** | | | | | | | | | | | | | | | | | | |
| HALS1 sample | 14 | | 12 | | 10 | | 11 | | 6 | | 8 | | 6 | | 7 | | 3 | |
| HALS2 sub-sample | 13 | 14 | 10 | 13 | 9 | 16 | 12 | 11 | 7 | 8 | 9 | 7 | 8 | 8 | 9 | 9 | 5 | 0 |
| **Swimming** | | | | | | | | | | | | | | | | | | |
| HALS1 sample | 14 | | 10 | | 12 | | 8 | | 5 | | 6 | | 4 | | 2 | | 0 | |
| HALS2 sub-sample | 14 | 11 | 11 | 13 | 11 | 15 | 7 | 11 | 5 | 7 | 7 | 7 | 5 | 6 | 2 | 2 | 1 | 1 |
| **Jogging** | | | | | | | | | | | | | | | | | | |
| HALS1 sample | 23 | | 20 | | 13 | | 9 | | 3 | | 1 | | 1 | | 0 | | 0 | |
| HALS2 sub-sample | 24 | 16 | 17 | 14 | 14 | 11 | 10 | 7 | 4 | 2 | 1 | 1 | 2 | 1 | 0 | 0 | 0 | 0 |
| **Football** | | | | | | | | | | | | | | | | | | |
| HALS1 sample | 26 | | 16 | | 8 | | 4 | | 1 | | 0 | | (2) | | 0 | | 0 | |
| HALS2 sub-sample | 26 | 20 | 15 | 10 | 9 | 6 | 3 | 2 | 1 | φ | 0 | φ | (1) | (1) | 0 | 0 | 0 | 0 |
| **Golf** | | | | | | | | | | | | | | | | | | |
| HALS1 sample | 3 | | 5 | | 4 | | 6 | | 5 | | 3 | | 3 | | 3 | | (1) | |
| HALS2 sub-sample | 3 | 7 | 5 | 9 | 4 | 7 | 4 | 7 | 5 | 6 | 4 | 5 | 4 | 5 | 3 | 1 | 0 | 1 |
| **Bowls** | | | | | | | | | | | | | | | | | | |
| HALS1 sample | (1) | | 1 | | (1) | | 1 | | 2 | | 1 | | 2 | | 2 | | 2 | |
| HALS2 sub-sample | 0 | 1 | 1 | 1 | 0 | 1 | 1 | 3 | 1 | 3 | 1 | 5 | 2 | 9 | 2 | 1 | 2 | 2 |
| **Dancing** | | | | | | | | | | | | | | | | | | |
| HALS1 sample | 17 | | 12 | | 11 | | 10 | | 10 | | 9 | | 6 | | 5 | | 2 | |
| HALS2 sub-sample | 16 | 11 | 13 | 8 | 10 | 6 | 9 | 8 | 10 | 5 | 11 | 7 | 9 | 5 | 7 | 4 | 2 | 2 |
| *Base = 100%* | | | | | | | | | | | | | | | | | | |
| *HALS1* | 534 | | 489 | | 573 | | 474 | | 419 | | 417 | | 412 | | 314 | | 273 | |
| *HALS2* | 299 | 299 | 241 | 241 | 383 | 383 | 324 | 324 | 280 | 280 | 278 | 278 | 259 | 259 | 148 | 148 | 88 | 88 |

**Table 14.2** **Selected active leisure pursuits in women, in HALS1 full sample, and HALS2 sub-sample at HALS1 and HALS2. Percentage of age group. ($\phi$ less than 1%; number in brackets less than 0.5%)**

| Age at HALS1 | 18-24 | | 25-31 | | 32-38 | | 39-45 | | 46-52 | | 53-59 | | 60-66 | | 67-73 | | >73 | |
| Age at HALS2 | | 25-31 | | 32-38 | | 39-45 | | 46-52 | | 53-59 | | 60-66 | | 67-73 | | 74-80 | | >80 |
|---|---|---|---|---|---|---|---|---|---|---|---|---|---|---|---|---|---|---|
| **Keep fit, yoga etc.** | | | | | | | | | | | | | | | | | | |
| HALS1 sample | 23 | | 23 | | 21 | | 18 | | 12 | | 9 | | 8 | | 4 | | 2 | |
| HALS2 sub-sample | 24 | 26 | 23 | 24 | 21 | 19 | 19 | 17 | 11 | 14 | 9 | 10 | 10 | 9 | 4 | 8 | 2 | 3 |
| **Cycling** | | | | | | | | | | | | | | | | | | |
| HALS1 sample | 9 | | 9 | | 10 | | 12 | | 7 | | 8 | | 5 | | 3 | | 1 | |
| HALS2 sub-sample | 8 | 12 | 10 | 12 | 10 | 9 | 13 | 11 | 7 | 6 | 8 | 6 | 6 | 5 | 4 | 3 | 2 | 0 |
| **Swimming** | | | | | | | | | | | | | | | | | | |
| HALS1 sample | 14 | | 13 | | 12 | | 9 | | 7 | | 4 | | 4 | | 2 | | 0 | |
| HALS2 sub-sample | 15 | 11 | 13 | 13 | 13 | 15 | 9 | 11 | 7 | 7 | 3 | 7 | 4 | 6 | 3 | 2 | 0 | 1 |
| **Jogging** | | | | | | | | | | | | | | | | | | |
| HALS1 sample | 12 | | 6 | | 5 | | 4 | | 2 | | 2 | | (2) | | 0 | | (1) | |
| HALS2 sub-sample | 14 | 5 | 7 | 5 | 5 | 3 | 5 | 3 | 2 | 2 | 2 | 1 | $\phi$ | $\phi$ | 0 | 0 | $\phi$ | 0 |
| **Golf** | | | | | | | | | | | | | | | | | | |
| HALS1 sample | (3) | | (2) | | $\phi$ | | 1 | | $\phi$ | | (2) | | 1 | | 0 | | 0 | |
| HALS2 sub-sample | 0 | (1) | $\phi$ | (1) | $\phi$ | 1 | 1 | 3 | (1) | 2 | (1) | 1 | 1 | 2 | 0 | 0 | 0 | 0 |
| **Bowls** | | | | | | | | | | | | | | | | | | |
| HALS1 sample | (1) | | 0 | | 1 | | (1) | | $\phi$ | | $\phi$ | | 1 | | 1 | | (2) | |
| HALS2 sub-sample | (1) | (1) | 0 | 1 | 1 | 2 | (1) | 1 | $\phi$ | 2 | 1 | $\phi$ | 2 | 4 | 2 | 0 | 1 | $\phi$ |
| **Dancing** | | | | | | | | | | | | | | | | | | |
| HALS1 sample | 35 | | 20 | | 18 | | 15 | | 13 | | 14 | | 8 | | 5 | | 2 | |
| HALS2 sub-sample | 37 | 20 | 20 | 17 | 18 | 11 | 16 | 11 | 14 | 10 | 16 | 13 | 8 | 4 | 7 | 4 | 3 | 3 |
| *Base = 100%* | | | | | | | | | | | | | | | | | | |
| *HALS1* | *626* | | *672* | | *766* | | *618* | | *576* | | *486* | | *553* | | *391* | | *410* | |
| *HALS2* | *311* | *311* | *394* | *394* | *545* | *545* | *432* | *432* | *391* | *391* | *315* | *315* | *327* | *327* | *191* | *191* | *146* | *146* |

**Table 14.3** **Leisure activities in the two weeks prior to interview analysed by age at Survey: Percentage of age group. (φ less than 1%; number in brackets less than 0.05%)**

| | Males | | | | | | | | | Females | | | | | | | | |
|---|---|---|---|---|---|---|---|---|---|---|---|---|---|---|---|---|---|---|
| Age at Survey | 18-24 | 25-39 | | 40-54 | | 55-69 | | 70+ | | 18-24 | 25-39 | | 40-54 | | 55-69 | | 70+ | |
| HALS | 1 | 1 | 2 | 1 | 2 | 1 | 2 | 1 | 2 | 1 | 1 | 2 | 1 | 2 | 1 | 2 | 1 | 2 |
| Keep fit/yoga | 16 | 12 | 13 | 5 | 10 | 4 | 4 | 3 | 5 | 23 | 22 | 23 | 14 | 16 | 8 | 10 | 3 | 6 |
| Cycling | 14 | 11 | 14 | 9 | 13 | 7 | 8 | 4 | 6 | 9 | 10 | 12 | 9 | 9 | 6 | 6 | 2 | 3 |
| Jogging | 23 | 16 | 14 | 5 | 9 | 1 | 1 | 0 | φ | 12 | 6 | 5 | 3 | 3 | φ | 2 | 0 | 0 |
| Swimming | 14 | 11 | 12 | 6 | 12 | 4 | 7 | 1 | 3 | 14 | 12 | 22 | 7 | 13 | 4 | 9 | φ | 2 |
| Self-defence/martial arts | 3 | 2 | 3 | φ | 1 | 0 | 0 | 0 | 0 | 1 | φ | φ | (1) | (2) | 0 | 0 | 0 | 0 |
| Hiking/backpacking | 2 | 4 | 2 | 2 | 2 | 2 | φ | 1 | (1) | 2 | 2 | 1 | 2 | 1 | 1 | 1 | (2) | (1) |
| Training (weight/circuit) | 6 | 2 | 3 | φ | 1 | 0 | φ | (1) | 0 | φ | φ | φ | (1) | (3) | 0 | 0 | 0 | 0 |
| Football | 26 | 11 | 15 | 2 | 4 | φ | φ | 0 | φ | 1 | φ | φ | φ | (1) | 0 | 0 | 0 | 0 |
| Squash | 7 | 7 | 5 | 2 | 3 | φ | (1) | 0 | (1) | 4 | 2 | 1 | 1 | φ | φ | φ | (1) | 0 |
| Badminton | 6 | 3 | 4 | 2 | 3 | 1 | 1 | 0 | φ | 5 | 4 | 3 | 2 | 3 | φ | φ | 0 | 0 |
| Table tennis | 5 | 4 | 3 | 1 | 1 | φ | φ | φ | φ | 1 | φ | φ | 1 | φ | φ | φ | 0 | 0 |
| Tennis | 2 | 2 | 2 | 1 | 2 | φ | φ | 0 | φ | 1 | 1 | 1 | 1 | 2 | φ | φ | φ | φ |
| Dancing | 17 | 11 | 10 | 10 | 7 | 7 | 6 | 4 | 4 | 35 | 18 | 17 | 14 | 11 | 9 | 10 | 3 | 4 |
| Golf | 3 | 4 | 8 | 5 | 7 | 3 | 6 | 1 | 3 | φ | φ | φ | 1 | 2 | φ | 1 | 0 | φ |
| Bowls | (1) | φ | 1 | 2 | 2 | 2 | 5 | 2 | 4 | (1) | φ | 1 | φ | 2 | 1 | 1 | φ | 2 |
| *Base = 100%* | 534 | 1134 | 583 | 929 | 734 | 853 | 608 | 455 | 375 | 626 | 1525 | 775 | 1248 | 1013 | 1083 | 746 | 616 | 518 |

**Table 14.4** Active leisure pursuits analysed by category and age in HALS1 full sample, and HALS2 sub-sample at HALS1 and HALS2. Percentage of age group. (φ less than 1%; number in brackets less than 0.5%)

| Age at HALS1 | 18-24 | | 25-31 | | 32-38 | | 39-45 | | 46-52 | | 53-59 | | 60-66 | | 67-73 | | >73 | |
|---|---|---|---|---|---|---|---|---|---|---|---|---|---|---|---|---|---|---|
| Age at HALS2 | | 25-31 | | 32-38 | | 39-45 | | 46-52 | | 53-59 | | 60-66 | | 67-73 | | 74-80 | | >80 |
| **Males** | | | | | | | | | | | | | | | | | | |
| **Individual (keep fit, swimming, etc.)** | | | | | | | | | | | | | | | | | | |
| HALS1 sample | 50 | | 43 | | 38 | | 31 | | 17 | | 17 | | 15 | | 13 | | 6 | |
| HALS2 sub-sample | 52 | 42 | 39 | 40 | 37 | 37 | 31 | 30 | 19 | 20 | 21 | 17 | 18 | 12 | 15 | 12 | 9 | 8 |
| **Competitive/team (football, squash, etc.)** | | | | | | | | | | | | | | | | | | |
| HALS1 sample | 38 | | 28 | | 22 | | 12 | | 5 | | 2 | | 3 | | φ | | 0 | |
| HALS2 sub-sample | 38 | 35 | 28 | 22 | 23 | 18 | 10 | 9 | 6 | 5 | 3 | 3 | 3 | 2 | φ | φ | 0 | 0 |
| **Recreational (golf, bowls, sailing, etc.)** | | | | | | | | | | | | | | | | | | |
| HALS1 sample | 7 | | 8 | | 8 | | 9 | | 10 | | 4 | | 6 | | 4 | | 2 | |
| HALS2 sub-sample | 7 | 11 | 7 | 13 | 8 | 11 | 9 | 11 | 8 | 10 | 5 | 12 | 7 | 14 | 4 | 3 | 2 | 3 |
| **Combined activities (excluding dancing and walking)** | | | | | | | | | | | | | | | | | | |
| HALS1 sample | 65 | | 58 | | 51 | | 41 | | 28 | | 21 | | 20 | | 18 | | 8 | |
| HALS2 sub-sample | 68 | 58 | 55 | 54 | 50 | 50 | 41 | 41 | 29 | 30 | 26 | 27 | 24 | 29 | 19 | 16 | 11 | 10 |
| *Base = 100%* | | | | | | | | | | | | | | | | | | |
| HALS1 | 534 | | 489 | | 573 | | 474 | | 419 | | 417 | | 412 | | 314 | | 273 | |
| HALS2 | 299 | 299 | 241 | 241 | 383 | 383 | 324 | 324 | 280 | 280 | 278 | 278 | 259 | 259 | 148 | 148 | 88 | 88 |
| **Females** | | | | | | | | | | | | | | | | | | |
| **Individual (keep fit, swimming, etc.)** | | | | | | | | | | | | | | | | | | |
| HALS1 sample | 42 | | 40 | | 39 | | 35 | | 25 | | 19 | | 16 | | 9 | | 5 | |
| HALS2 sub-sample | 44 | 50 | 42 | 46 | 40 | 36 | 38 | 34 | 24 | 26 | 20 | 19 | 19 | 17 | 12 | 13 | 6 | 3 |
| **Competitive/team (football, squash, etc.)** | | | | | | | | | | | | | | | | | | |
| HALS1 sample | 12 | | 6 | | 8 | | 8 | | 3 | | 1 | | 1 | | φ | | (1) | |
| HALS2 sub-sample | 14 | 7 | 5 | 6 | 7 | 8 | 8 | 6 | 3 | 2 | (1) | 2 | 1 | (1) | φ | 0 | φ | φ |
| **Recreational (golf, bowls, sailing, etc.)** | | | | | | | | | | | | | | | | | | |
| HALS1 sample | 3 | | 2 | | 4 | | 2 | | 3 | | 1 | | 3 | | 1 | | (2) | |
| HALS2 sub-sample | 3 | 3 | 3 | 3 | 5 | 5 | 2 | 5 | 3 | 4 | 1 | 3 | 3 | 5 | 2 | 0 | (1) | 3 |
| **Combined activities (excluding dancing and walking)** | | | | | | | | | | | | | | | | | | |
| HALS1 sample | 47 | | 43 | | 44 | | 39 | | 28 | | 20 | | 18 | | 10 | | 5 | |
| HALS2 sub-sample | 50 | 52 | 45 | 49 | 45 | 42 | 42 | 37 | 28 | 29 | 21 | 21 | 21 | 21 | 14 | 13 | 8 | 5 |
| *Base = 100%* | | | | | | | | | | | | | | | | | | |
| HALS1 | 626 | | 672 | | 766 | | 618 | | 576 | | 486 | | 553 | | 391 | | 410 | |
| HALS2 | 311 | 311 | 394 | 394 | 545 | 545 | 432 | 432 | 391 | 391 | 315 | 315 | 327 | 327 | 191 | 191 | 146 | 146 |

**Table 14.5**   **Respondents opinions at HALS2 as to whether they were taking more, less or the same amount of exercise as seven years previously ('don't know' excluded). Percentage of age group**

| Age at HALS2 | 25-31 | 32-38 | 39-45 | 46-52 | 53-59 | 60-66 | 67-73 | 74-80 | 81+ |
|---|---|---|---|---|---|---|---|---|---|
| **Males** | | | | | | | | | |
| More exercise | 27 | 22 | 20 | 17 | 14 | 20 | 17 | 3 | 2 |
| Same amount of exercise | 28 | 39 | 42 | 55 | 55 | 47 | 51 | 60 | 38 |
| Less exercise | 45 | 40 | 38 | 28 | 32 | 33 | 33 | 37 | 60 |
| **Females** | | | | | | | | | |
| More exercise | 32 | 29 | 26 | 24 | 17 | 19 | 10 | 5 | 2 |
| Same amount of exercise | 30 | 43 | 41 | 46 | 51 | 47 | 56 | 53 | 43 |
| Less exercise | 38 | 28 | 34 | 31 | 32 | 34 | 35 | 42 | 55 |
| *Base = 100%* | *298* | *239* | *380* | *324* | *278* | *280* | *255* | *143* | *87* |
| | *309* | *389* | *544* | *431* | *388* | *316* | *319* | *190* | *137* |

**Table 14.6** **Active leisure pursuits in the two weeks prior to interview in non-manual and manual socio-economic groups and by age at Survey. Percentage of socio-economic group at each age. (φ less than 1%; number in brackets, less than 0.5%)**

| | Males | | | | | | | | | Females | | | | | | | | |
|---|---|---|---|---|---|---|---|---|---|---|---|---|---|---|---|---|---|---|
| Age at Survey | 18-24 | 25-39 | | 40-54 | | 55-69 | | 70+ | | 18-24 | 25-39 | | 40-54 | | 55-69 | | 70+ | |
| HALS | 1 | 1 | 2 | 1 | 2 | 1 | 2 | 1 | 2 | 1 | 1 | 2 | 1 | 2 | 1 | 2 | 1 | 2 |
| **Active leisure pursuits category** | | | | | | | | | | | | | | | | | | |
| **Individual (keep fit, swimming, etc.)** | | | | | | | | | | | | | | | | | | |
| Non-manual | 56 | 43 | 47 | 29 | 40 | 17 | 22 | 8 | 15 | 51 | 48 | 52 | 34 | 38 | 20 | 26 | 8 | 17 |
| Manual | 46 | 35 | 36 | 19 | 27 | 14 | 15 | 10 | 11 | 35 | 34 | 43 | 23 | 29 | 14 | 19 | 4 | 8 |
| **Competitive/team (football, squash, etc.)** | | | | | | | | | | | | | | | | | | |
| Non-manual | 48 | 30 | 34 | 13 | 18 | 4 | 5 | 0 | 2 | 15 | 10 | 10 | 7 | 9 | 1 | 2 | (1) | 1 |
| Manual | 33 | 18 | 26 | 4 | 7 | (1) | 2 | (2) | (1) | 9 | 4 | 5 | 3 | 3 | (2) | 1 | 0 | 0 |
| **Recreational (golf, bowls, sailing, etc.)** | | | | | | | | | | | | | | | | | | |
| Non-manual | 14 | 10 | 15 | 12 | 14 | 7 | 16 | 3 | 7 | 3 | 5 | 4 | 4 | 6 | 3 | 5 | (1) | 3 |
| Manual | 3 | 6 | 10 | 6 | 7 | 4 | 8 | 3 | 7 | 2 | 2 | 3 | 1 | 4 | 1 | 2 | 1 | 2 |
| **Combined activities (excluding dancing and walking)** | | | | | | | | | | | | | | | | | | |
| Non-manual | 75 | 60 | 61 | 44 | 55 | 23 | 36 | 11 | 21 | 56 | 50 | 56 | 39 | 44 | 22 | 30 | 9 | 20 |
| Manual | 61 | 45 | 52 | 26 | 34 | 18 | 23 | 13 | 18 | 38 | 37 | 45 | 24 | 31 | 15 | 21 | 5 | 9 |
| **Dancing** | | | | | | | | | | | | | | | | | | |
| Non-manual | 26 | 21 | 10 | 20 | 7 | 16 | 6 | 12 | 8 | 45 | 27 | 19 | 20 | 9 | 15 | 10 | 11 | 2 |
| Manual | 25 | 18 | 10 | 17 | 7 | 16 | 5 | 12 | 2 | 38 | 25 | 16 | 23 | 13 | 19 | 10 | 12 | 5 |
| *Base = 100%* | 174 | 522 | 218 | 418 | 370 | 322 | 262 | 160 | 145 | 319 | 726 | 337 | 609 | 498 | 437 | 365 | 227 | 210 |
| | 338 | 592 | 351 | 510 | 364 | 527 | 344 | 294 | 228 | 290 | 771 | 426 | 625 | 505 | 629 | 373 | 370 | 300 |

**Table 14.7** **Active leisure pursuits undertaken in the two weeks prior to interview in those aged between 25 and 70 at Survey, analysed by north/south region of residence and by non-manual and manual socio-economic group: Age standardised to 1991 Census. Percentage in regional socio-economic group**

| | Males | | | | Females | | | |
|---|---|---|---|---|---|---|---|---|
| | North | | South | | North | | South | |
| HALS | 1 | 2 | 1 | 2 | 1 | 2 | 1 | 2 |
| **Active leisure pursuits category** | | | | | | | | |
| **Individual (keep fit, swimming, etc.)** | | | | | | | | |
| Non-manual | 26.2 | 33.3 | 31.2 | 36.8 | 29.8 | 34.8 | 33.1 | 39.5 |
| Manual | 20.3 | 22.9 | 26.4 | 28.3 | 19.9 | 25.6 | 25.4 | 33.7 |
| **Competitive/team (football, squash, etc.)** | | | | | | | | |
| Non-manual | 14.6 | 16.3 | 16.5 | 21.6 | 4.0 | 5.1 | 7.0 | 7.3 |
| Manual | 7.8 | 11.9 | 8.1 | 10.9 | 2.3 | 2.2 | 2.7 | 3.9 |
| **Recreational (golf, bowls, sailing, etc.)** | | | | | | | | |
| Non-manual | 9.3 | 12.6 | 9.4 | 16.6 | 3.8 | 3.6 | 3.0 | 5.9 |
| Manual | 5.8 | 7.3 | 4.6 | 10.7 | 1.0 | 1.8 | 1.7 | 4.0 |
| **Combined activities (excluding dancing and walking)** | | | | | | | | |
| Non-manual | 39.5 | 45.0 | 42.6 | 52.4 | 32.7 | 38.3 | 37.3 | 44.9 |
| Manual | 28.5 | 32.9 | 31.8 | 40.5 | 21.3 | 27.0 | 27.7 | 37.0 |
| **Dancing** | | | | | | | | |
| Non-manual | 19.5 | 10.6 | 17.6 | 6.5 | 20.1 | 12.2 | 20.4 | 11.6 |
| Manual | 15.7 | 7.0 | 17.4 | 6.6 | 21.9 | 12.8 | 20.6 | 12.8 |
| *Base* | *589* | *440* | *833* | *555* | *908* | *659* | *1091* | *751* |
| | *1069* | *721* | *854* | *566* | *1418* | *965* | *977* | *639* |

**Table 14.8** **Respondents reporting being 'more active', 'less active' or 'the same' as others of their age in HALS1 full sample and HALS2 sub-sample at HALS1 and HALS2 ('Don't know' omitted). Percentage of age group.**

| Age at HALS1 | 18-24 | | 25-31 | | 32-38 | | 39-45 | | 46-52 | | 53-59 | | 60-66 | | 67-73 | | 74+ | | All | |
| HALS | 1 | 2 | 1 | 2 | 1 | 2 | 1 | 2 | 1 | 2 | 1 | 2 | 1 | 2 | 1 | 2 | 1 | 2 | 1 | 2 |
|---|---|---|---|---|---|---|---|---|---|---|---|---|---|---|---|---|---|---|---|---|
| **Males** | | | | | | | | | | | | | | | | | | | | |
| More active | 28 | 31 | 29 | 27 | 34 | 34 | 38 | 33 | 37 | 38 | 33 | 29 | 39 | 39 | 38 | 39 | 44 | 49 | 35 | 34 |
| Same as others | 63 | 57 | 58 | 59 | 56 | 55 | 57 | 60 | 55 | 49 | 53 | 57 | 53 | 51 | 55 | 41 | 47 | 35 | 56 | 54 |
| Less active | 9 | 11 | 13 | 14 | 9 | 11 | 5 | 7 | 8 | 14 | 14 | 13 | 9 | 10 | 8 | 19 | 9 | 16 | 9 | 12 |
| **Females** | | | | | | | | | | | | | | | | | | | | |
| More active | 15 | 15 | 20 | 24 | 23 | 24 | 27 | 28 | 29 | 28 | 30 | 31 | 29 | 33 | 36 | 36 | 46 | 35 | 26 | 27 |
| Same as others | 75 | 69 | 71 | 64 | 69 | 65 | 66 | 62 | 63 | 59 | 55 | 55 | 62 | 52 | 57 | 49 | 45 | 51 | 65 | 60 |
| Less active | 10 | 17 | 9 | 12 | 9 | 11 | 7 | 9 | 8 | 11 | 14 | 14 | 9 | 16 | 7 | 15 | 9 | 14 | 9 | 13 |
| Base = 100% | 295 | 298 | 238 | 238 | 380 | 376 | 322 | 322 | 272 | 274 | 275 | 272 | 258 | 257 | 143 | 145 | 86 | 81 | 2269 | 2261 |
| | 305 | 309 | 391 | 389 | 541 | 543 | 429 | 432 | 390 | 391 | 313 | 315 | 321 | 326 | 187 | 190 | 141 | 138 | 3021 | 3006 |

**Table 14.9** **Respondents believing they get enough exercise at HALS1 and HALS2. Percentage of age group**

| Age at HALS1 | 18-24 | 25-31 | 32-38 | 39-45 | 46-52 | 53-59 | 60-66 | 67-73 | 74+ | All |
|---|---|---|---|---|---|---|---|---|---|---|
| **Males** | | | | | | | | | | |
| HALS1 | 56 | 48 | 42 | 45 | 49 | 53 | 68 | 73 | 73 | 54 |
| HALS2 | 42 | 35 | 35 | 47 | 51 | 53 | 63 | 66 | 54 | 46 |
| Difference | (− 14) | (− 13) | (− 7) | (+ 2) | (+ 2) | (0) | (− 6) | (− 7) | (− 19) | (− 8) |
| **Females** | | | | | | | | | | |
| HALS1 | 43 | 46 | 43 | 46 | 53 | 59 | 61 | 72 | 70 | 52 |
| HALS2 | 34 | 35 | 35 | 37 | 47 | 50 | 57 | 66 | 59 | 44 |
| Difference | (− 9) | (− 11) | (− 8) | (− 9) | (− 6) | (− 9) | (− 4) | (− 6) | (− 11) | (− 8) |
| Base = 100% | 292 | 238 | 382 | 321 | 277 | 273 | 256 | 147 | 86 | 2272 |
| | 299 | 240 | 382 | 322 | 279 | 275 | 257 | 147 | 85 | 2286 |
| | 308 | 391 | 541 | 429 | 390 | 313 | 321 | 197 | 141 | 3021 |
| | 310 | 393 | 541 | 431 | 389 | 311 | 325 | 188 | 141 | 3029 |

**Table 14.10** Percentage of respondents at HALS1 and HALS2 who said that they were not getting enough exercise analysed by reported time in last two weeks that they were involved in active leisure pursuits including dancing

| | Males | | | | | | | | Females | | | | | | | | | | |
|---|---|---|---|---|---|---|---|---|---|---|---|---|---|---|---|---|---|---|---|
| Age at Survey | 18-24 | 25-39 | | 40-54 | | 55-69 | | 70+ | | 18-24 | 25-39 | | 40-54 | | 55-69 | | 70+ | | |
| HALS | 1 | 1 | 2 | 1 | 2 | 1 | 2 | 1 | 2 | 1 | 1 | 2 | 1 | 2 | 1 | 2 | 1 | 2 | |
| **Hours of activity** | | | | | | | | | | | | | | | | | | | |
| Nil | 55 | 55 | 68 | 47 | 58 | 32 | 43 | 24 | 29 | 62 | 58 | 70 | 46 | 66 | 31 | 44 | 26 | 30 | |
| 0 – 1 hour | 59 | 70 | 79 | 52 | 81 | 50 | 48 | | | 61 | 60 | 77 | 61 | 68 | 41 | 59 | | | |
| 1 – 2 hours | 60 | 67 | 79 | 56 | 58 | 36 | 29 | {23 | 48} | 69 | 58 | 68 | 52 | 65 | 26 | 47 | {13 | 43} | |
| 2 – 4 hours | 47 | 60 | 63 | 55 | 66 | 32 | 43 | | | 70 | 51 | 62 | 51 | 60 | 29 | 49 | | | |
| 4 – 8 hours | 47 | 49 | 58 | 49 | 57 | 35 | 25 | – | – | 44 | 45 | 54 | 33 | 46 | 34 | 29 | – | – | |
| 8 – 16 hours | 35 | 37 | 40 | 47 | 51 | 17 | 21 | – | – | 36 | 38 | 40 | 25 | 37 | 17 | 27 | – | – | |
| over 16 hours | 16 | 20 | 35 | 21 | 22 | 10 | 21 | – | – | 46 | 25 | – | 41 | 35 | 20 | – | – | – | |
| *Base = 100%* | 139 | 433 | 206 | 457 | 309 | 445 | 282 | 277 | 193 | 234 | 666 | 298 | 613 | 461 | 596 | 375 | 409 | 343 | |
| | 39 | 96 | 48 | 56 | 53 | 18 | 25 | | | 71 | 173 | 97 | 88 | 85 | 54 | 37 | | | |
| | 43 | 86 | 33 | 45 | 48 | 28 | 14 | {31 | 33} | 48 | 123 | 85 | 98 | 68 | 38 | 43 | {30 | 46} | |
| | 62 | 119 | 49 | 67 | 56 | 28 | 30 | | | 79 | 183 | 82 | 96 | 99 | 55 | 43 | | | |
| | 89 | 128 | 62 | 73 | 68 | 34 | 28 | – | – | 73 | 133 | 76 | 103 | 89 | 32 | 31 | – | – | |
| | 66 | 104 | 73 | 43 | 55 | 30 | 28 | – | – | 50 | 74 | 48 | 48 | 38 | 23 | 33 | – | – | |
| | 55 | 68 | 43 | 38 | 32 | 19 | 19 | – | – | 28 | 32 | – | 22 | 20 | 15 | – | – | – | |

**Table 14.11   Amount of walking per day at weekends in HALS1 and HALS2. Percentage of age group**

| Age at HALS1 | 18-24 | | 25-31 | | 32-38 | | 39-45 | | 46-52 | | 53-59 | | 60-66 | | 67-73 | | 74+ | | All | |
| --- | --- | --- | --- | --- | --- | --- | --- | --- | --- | --- | --- | --- | --- | --- | --- | --- | --- | --- | --- | --- |
| HALS | 1 | 2 | 1 | 2 | 1 | 2 | 1 | 2 | 1 | 2 | 1 | 2 | 1 | 2 | 1 | 2 | 1 | 2 | 1 | 2 |
| **Males** | | | | | | | | | | | | | | | | | | | | |
| Nil | 9 | 2 | 11 | 9 | 8 | 13 | 10 | 14 | 18 | 14 | 15 | 11 | 8 | 13 | 18 | 20 | 24 | 31 | 12 | 14 |
| $<\frac{1}{2}$ hour | 6 | 7 | 5 | 14 | 7 | 9 | 6 | 7 | 8 | 9 | 6 | 9 | 5 | 8 | 5 | 13 | 5 | 16 | 6 | 9 |
| $\frac{1}{2}$ - 1 hour | 10 | 14 | 15 | 15 | 15 | 19 | 12 | 17 | 8 | 15 | 12 | 16 | 16 | 13 | 16 | 16 | 21 | 16 | 13 | 16 |
| 1-2 hours | 24 | 29 | 25 | 24 | 28 | 23 | 31 | 24 | 23 | 23 | 25 | 24 | 26 | 31 | 29 | 29 | 26 | 19 | 26 | 25 |
| >2 hours | 48 | 36 | 42 | 34 | 41 | 35 | 38 | 36 | 41 | 36 | 40 | 39 | 42 | 32 | 30 | 15 | 22 | 15 | 40 | 33 |
| Don't know | 2 | 3 | 2 | 3 | 2 | 1 | 4 | 3 | 2 | 2 | 3 | 2 | 4 | 3 | 1 | 7 | 3 | 3 | 3 | 3 |
| **Females** | | | | | | | | | | | | | | | | | | | | |
| Nil | 7 | 11 | 7 | 11 | 14 | 13 | 14 | 15 | 12 | 11 | 19 | 15 | 16 | 18 | 20 | 26 | 30 | 41 | 14 | 15 |
| $<\frac{1}{2}$ hour | 4 | 9 | 6 | 7 | 5 | 8 | 5 | 10 | 6 | 9 | 6 | 10 | 6 | 11 | 9 | 13 | 7 | 14 | 6 | 9 |
| $\frac{1}{2}$ - 1 hour | 12 | 14 | 16 | 17 | 15 | 19 | 12 | 16 | 17 | 17 | 16 | 23 | 20 | 19 | 18 | 17 | 23 | 15 | 16 | 17 |
| 1-2 hours | 26 | 27 | 30 | 26 | 27 | 24 | 29 | 27 | 29 | 23 | 24 | 26 | 25 | 26 | 23 | 24 | 17 | 11 | 26 | 25 |
| >2 hours | 49 | 37 | 40 | 37 | 37 | 35 | 37 | 32 | 31 | 35 | 30 | 22 | 29 | 23 | 25 | 13 | 16 | 7 | 34 | 30 |
| Don't know | 3 | 2 | 2 | 3 | 3 | 2 | 3 | 2 | 5 | 5 | 5 | 4 | 4 | 3 | 5 | 8 | 7 | 13 | 4 | 4 |
| *Base = 100%* | 299 | 299 | 241 | 241 | 383 | 383 | 324 | 324 | 280 | 280 | 278 | 278 | 259 | 259 | 148 | 148 | 88 | 88 | 2300 | 2300 |
| | 311 | 311 | 394 | 394 | 545 | 545 | 432 | 432 | 391 | 391 | 315 | 315 | 327 | 326 | 191 | 190 | 146 | 143 | 3052 | 3047 |

**Table 14.12   Percentage of respondents in HALS2 claiming to take walks of 2 miles or more. Percentage of age group**

| Age at HALS2 | 25-31 | 32-38 | 39-45 | 46-52 | 53-59 | 60-66 | 67-73 | 74-80 | 81+ | All |
| --- | --- | --- | --- | --- | --- | --- | --- | --- | --- | --- |
| **All 2 mile walks** | | | | | | | | | | |
| Males | 27 | 31 | 33 | 45 | 33 | 44 | 36 | 25 | 18 | 34 |
| Females | 41 | 36 | 35 | 35 | 31 | 30 | 30 | 25 | 6 | 32 |
| **Only 2 mile walks – no other sports** | | | | | | | | | | |
| Males | 14 | 15 | 19 | 32 | 26 | 35 | 29 | 22 | 16 | 24 |
| Females | 14 | 16 | 17 | 20 | 19 | 18 | 22 | 19 | 6 | 18 |
| *Base = 100%* | 299 | 241 | 383 | 324 | 280 | 278 | 259 | 148 | 88 | 2300 |
| | 311 | 394 | 545 | 432 | 391 | 315 | 327 | 191 | 146 | 3052 |

**Table 14.13**   **Socio-economic group (non-manual (NM) and manual (M)) variations in walking pace at HALS2. Percentage of age group. ($\phi$ less than 1%; number in brackets less than 0.5%)**

| Age at HALS2 | Males | | | | | | | Females | | | | | |
|---|---|---|---|---|---|---|---|---|---|---|---|---|---|
| | 25-45 | | 46-66 | | 67+ | | | 25-45 | | 46-66 | | 67+ | |
| Socio-economic group | NM | M | NM | M | NM | M | | NM | M | NM | M | NM | M |
| **Walking pace** | | | | | | | | | | | | | |
| Slow | 5 | 4 | 5 | 16 | 22 | 33 | | 8 | 10 | 8 | 16 | 26 | 34 |
| Average | 37 | 40 | 46 | 50 | 51 | 45 | | 46 | 47 | 43 | 47 | 45 | 45 |
| Brisk | 46 | 41 | 43 | 27 | 22 | 17 | | 38 | 35 | 41 | 31 | 23 | 16 |
| Fast | 11 | 15 | 6 | 7 | 3 | 2 | | 8 | 8 | 7 | 5 | 3 | 3 |
| Cannot walk | 0 | 0 | $\phi$ | 0 | 1 | 1 | | 0 | 0 | 0 | (1) | 2 | $\phi$ |
| Don't know | $\phi$ | (1) | (1) | $\phi$ | 0 | $\phi$ | | $\phi$ | (1) | $\phi$ | (2) | 2 | 2 |
| *Base = 100%* | *394* | *513* | *405* | *476* | *194* | *294* | | *577* | *657* | *557* | *566* | *273* | *376* |

**Table 14.14  Participation in pastimes in the previous fortnight at HALS1 and HALS2. Percentage of age group. (φ less than 1%; number in brackets less than 0.5%)**

| HALS1 age | Males | | | | | | Females | | | | | |
|---|---|---|---|---|---|---|---|---|---|---|---|---|
| | 18-38 | | 39-59 | | 60+ | | 18-38 | | 39-59 | | 60+ | |
| HALS | 1 | 2 | 1 | 2 | 1 | 2 | 1 | 2 | 1 | 2 | 1 | 2 |
| Fishing | 4 | | 4 | | 2 | | φ | | (8) | | (2) | |
| | 5 | 6 | 3 | 4 | 2 | 3 | φ | φ | φ | φ | (1) | 0 |
| Parties, socials | 34 | | 21 | | 10 | | 35 | | 24 | | 12 | |
| | 33 | 30 | 23 | 21 | 12 | 11 | 35 | 30 | 27 | 24 | 15 | 12 |
| Darts, snooker | 38 | | 21 | | 7 | | 8 | | 4 | | 1 | |
| | 40 | 23 | 22 | 15 | 9 | 6 | 8 | 5 | 4 | 2 | φ | φ |
| Visiting coast etc | 27 | | 25 | | 20 | | 27 | | 25 | | 17 | |
| | 27 | 34 | 26 | 35 | 23 | 26 | 27 | 37 | 26 | 36 | 21 | 24 |
| Visiting museum etc | 9 | | 9 | | 6 | | 8 | | 9 | | 6 | |
| | 9 | 11 | 9 | 12 | 8 | 9 | 8 | 10 | 10 | 16 | 8 | 10 |
| Acting, singing | 5 | | 4 | | 3 | | 3 | | 5 | | 3 | |
| | 6 | 7 | 4 | 4 | 4 | 3 | 4 | 4 | 6 | 5 | 3 | 3 |
| Going to cinema or theatre | 14 | | 8 | | 5 | | 13 | | 9 | | 6 | |
| | 13 | 15 | 9 | 8 | 6 | 5 | 13 | 18 | 10 | 15 | 6 | 8 |
| Watching sports | 19 | | 12 | | 6 | | 9 | | 3 | | 2 | |
| | 19 | 21 | 13 | 14 | 7 | 8 | 7 | 9 | 5 | 6 | 2 | 3 |
| Knitting, sewing | 1 | | 1 | | 2 | | 50 | | 57 | | 51 | |
| | (7) | φ | 1 | φ | 1 | 1 | 52 | 33 | 59 | 48 | 58 | 42 |
| Hobbies, crafts | 18 | | 16 | | 12 | | 11 | | 13 | | 9 | |
| | 19 | 18 | 17 | 19 | 16 | 14 | 11 | 13 | 14 | 16 | 10 | 12 |
| Voluntary work | 5 | | 9 | | 8 | | 9 | | 11 | | 10 | |
| | 6 | 7 | 10 | 10 | 12 | 9 | 11 | 11 | 13 | 15 | 13 | 11 |
| Playing games of skill | 26 | | 19 | | 11 | | 22 | | 15 | | 13 | |
| | 26 | 30 | 20 | 17 | 11 | 11 | 26 | 26 | 16 | 16 | 15 | 16 |
| Betting | 27 | | 31 | | 27 | | 9 | | 11 | | 7 | |
| | 29 | 29 | 31 | 30 | 28 | 24 | 9 | 12 | 12 | 14 | 8 | 7 |
| Going to a pub | 69 | | 50 | | 30 | | 47 | | 29 | | 11 | |
| | 69 | 62 | 49 | 46 | 33 | 27 | 44 | 41 | 29 | 30 | 14 | 10 |
| Bingo | 19 | | 22 | | 20 | | 13 | | 16 | | 18 | |
| | 19 | 16 | 24 | 20 | 22 | 19 | 14 | 12 | 18 | 18 | 19 | 21 |
| Going to church | 12 | | 15 | | 15 | | 17 | | 22 | | 27 | |
| | 12 | 11 | 16 | 18 | 16 | 14 | 18 | 18 | 23 | 24 | 31 | 32 |
| Attending lectures | 8 | | 5 | | 3 | | 8 | | 8 | | 5 | |
| | 8 | 6 | 6 | 5 | 6 | 4 | 8 | 8 | 9 | 9 | 5 | 5 |
| *Base = 100%* | 1596 | | 1310 | | 999 | | 2064 | | 1680 | | 1354 | |
| | 923 | 923 | 882 | 882 | 495 | 495 | 1250 | 1250 | 1138 | 1138 | 664 | 664 |

**Table 14.15 Level of participation in pastimes by HALS1 full sample and HALS2 sub-sample at HALS1 and HALS2. Percentage of age group**

| Age at HALS1 | 18-24 | | 25-31 | | 32-38 | | 39-45 | | 46-52 | | 53-59 | | 60-66 | | 67-73 | | 74+ | | All | |
| Age at HALS2 | | 25-31 | | 32-38 | | 39-45 | | 46-52 | | 53-59 | | 60-66 | | 67-73 | | 74-80 | | 81+ | | All |
|---|---|---|---|---|---|---|---|---|---|---|---|---|---|---|---|---|---|---|---|---|
| **Number of pastimes** | | | | | | | | | **Males** | | | | | | | | | | | |
| 0/1 | 11 | | 11 | | 11 | | 12 | | 14 | | 21 | | 23 | | 35 | | 47 | | 18 | |
| | 12 | 13 | 10 | 12 | 9 | 9 | 12 | 10 | 14 | 17 | 17 | 18 | 21 | 19 | 27 | 32 | 42 | 62 | 15 | 17 |
| 2 | 14 | | 14 | | 12 | | 15 | | 19 | | 21 | | 24 | | 22 | | 22 | | 17 | |
| | 14 | 15 | 10 | 15 | 12 | 12 | 14 | 16 | 15 | 20 | 21 | 17 | 23 | 20 | 22 | 25 | 26 | 14 | 16 | 17 |
| 3 | 15 | | 19 | | 21 | | 18 | | 20 | | 16 | | 16 | | 18 | | 13 | | 17 | |
| | 14 | 16 | 19 | 18 | 19 | 18 | 17 | 20 | 21 | 13 | 14 | 20 | 14 | 20 | 16 | 19 | 13 | 16 | 17 | 18 |
| 4 | 19 | | 19 | | 19 | | 19 | | 19 | | 17 | | 14 | | 12 | | 9 | | 17 | |
| | 16 | 17 | 21 | 18 | 19 | 20 | 20 | 19 | 20 | 19 | 16 | 17 | 14 | 14 | 18 | 10 | 8 | 5 | 18 | 17 |
| 5+ | 41 | | 38 | | 37 | | 36 | | 28 | | 26 | | 25 | | 13 | | 8 | | 30 | |
| | 43 | 39 | 40 | 36 | 40 | 42 | 37 | 34 | 30 | 32 | 31 | 28 | 28 | 27 | 17 | 14 | 11 | 4 | 34 | 32 |
| Base = 100% | 532 | | 489 | | 572 | | 473 | | 418 | | 414 | | 412 | | 313 | | 272 | | 3895 | |
| | 298 | 299 | 241 | 240 | 383 | 383 | 324 | 324 | 279 | 279 | 277 | 277 | 259 | 257 | 147 | 145 | 88 | 86 | 2296 | 2290 |
| | | | | | | | | | **Females** | | | | | | | | | | | |
| 0/1 | 19 | | 22 | | 19 | | 20 | | 21 | | 27 | | 31 | | 40 | | 54 | | 26 | |
| | 19 | 19 | 22 | 19 | 18 | 20 | 17 | 19 | 19 | 23 | 23 | 23 | 26 | 30 | 34 | 33 | 41 | 50 | 22 | 24 |
| 2 | 19 | | 21 | | 18 | | 20 | | 21 | | 27 | | 31 | | 40 | | 54 | | 21 | |
| | 17 | 19 | 20 | 17 | 18 | 18 | 22 | 15 | 21 | 19 | 20 | 17 | 21 | 19 | 27 | 28 | 25 | 25 | 21 | 19 |
| 3 | 24 | | 18 | | 20 | | 19 | | 20 | | 19 | | 18 | | 15 | | 11 | | 19 | |
| | 24 | 21 | 17 | 20 | 22 | 15 | 19 | 18 | 20 | 16 | 18 | 18 | 20 | 18 | 13 | 20 | 12 | 11 | 19 | 18 |
| 4 | 16 | | 17 | | 16 | | 12 | | 13 | | 15 | | 11 | | 9 | | 7 | | 13 | |
| | 17 | 17 | 18 | 17 | 16 | 19 | 12 | 17 | 14 | 15 | 16 | 17 | 12 | 10 | 10 | 9 | 8 | 8 | 14 | 15 |
| 5+ | 23 | | 22 | | 27 | | 27 | | 22 | | 20 | | 17 | | 12 | | 8 | | 21 | |
| | 23 | 23 | 23 | 27 | 26 | 28 | 30 | 32 | 25 | 26 | 24 | 26 | 21 | 23 | 16 | 11 | 14 | 7 | 24 | 25 |
| Base = 100% | 626 | | 671 | | 766 | | 618 | | 576 | | 485 | | 552 | | 391 | | 409 | | 5094 | |
| | 311 | 310 | 394 | 392 | 545 | 545 | 432 | 430 | 391 | 391 | 315 | 315 | 326 | 326 | 191 | 190 | 146 | 143 | 3051 | 3042 |

**Table 14.16  Socio-economic group difference in levels of participation in pastimes at HALS1 and HALS2. Percentage of non-manual and manual groups**

| HALS1 age | 18-38 | | | | 39-59 | | | | 60+ | | | |
|---|---|---|---|---|---|---|---|---|---|---|---|---|
| | Non-Manual | | Manual | | Non-manual | | Manual | | Non-manual | | Manual | |
| **HALS** | **1** | **2** | **1** | **2** | **1** | **2** | **1** | **2** | **1** | **2** | **1** | **2** |
| **Number of pastimes** | | | | | **Males** | | | | | | | |
| 0/1 | 8 | 8 | 13 | 14 | 10 | 11 | 17 | 18 | 20 | 22 | 31 | 37 |
| 2 | 9 | 11 | 15 | 16 | 14 | 16 | 19 | 19 | 20 | 17 | 25 | 22 |
| 3 | 17 | 19 | 19 | 16 | 15 | 15 | 19 | 20 | 13 | 19 | 15 | 19 |
| 4 | 20 | 17 | 17 | 20 | 19 | 20 | 19 | 16 | 14 | 13 | 14 | 10 |
| 5 | 46 | 45 | 37 | 35 | 41 | 38 | 26 | 26 | 33 | 29 | 15 | 12 |
| | | | | | **Females** | | | | | | | |
| 0/1 | 13 | 15 | 25 | 24 | 14 | 15 | 25 | 27 | 26 | 25 | 35 | 42 |
| 2 | 15 | 17 | 22 | 19 | 19 | 16 | 24 | 18 | 19 | 20 | 28 | 25 |
| 3 | 21 | 19 | 21 | 18 | 20 | 15 | 19 | 19 | 17 | 19 | 16 | 15 |
| 4 | 19 | 17 | 15 | 19 | 14 | 17 | 13 | 15 | 12 | 12 | 10 | 7 |
| 5+ | 33 | 32 | 17 | 21 | 34 | 37 | 19 | 21 | 26 | 23 | 12 | 11 |
| *Base = 100%* | 394 | | 514 | | 404 | | 475 | | 195 | | 290 | |
| | 576 | | 655 | | 557 | | 566 | | 274 | | 376 | |

**Table 14.17** **Percentage of respondents in each age group gardening or performing DIY, and mean hours spent in these activities at HALS1 and HALS. Percentage of non-manual and manual groups**

| Age at HALS1 | 18-24 | | 25-31 | | 32-38 | | 39-45 | | 46-52 | | 53-59 | | 60-66 | | 67-73 | | 74+ | | All | |
|---|---|---|---|---|---|---|---|---|---|---|---|---|---|---|---|---|---|---|---|---|
| HALS | 1 | 2 | 1 | 2 | 1 | 2 | 1 | 2 | 1 | 2 | 1 | 2 | 1 | 2 | 1 | 2 | 1 | 2 | 1 | 2 |
| **Gardening** | | | | | | | | | | *Males* | | | | | | | | | | |
| Non-manual | 15 | 24 | 35 | 34 | 41 | 48 | 53 | 51 | 48 | 55 | 44 | 54 | 54 | 59 | 63 | 63 | 46 | 24 | 44 | 47 |
| Hours | 2.6 | 4.8 | 3.9 | 3.6 | 4.3 | 4.3 | 5.8 | 5.8 | 6.9 | 7.4 | 5.6 | 6.3 | 7.8 | 9.1 | 7.2 | 9.4 | 7.1 | 6.5 | 5.8 | 6.3 |
| Manual | 12 | 26 | 29 | 33 | 30 | 36 | 39 | 45 | 46 | 51 | 44 | 40 | 39 | 46 | 45 | 47 | 44 | 24 | 35 | 39 |
| Hours | 1.9 | 3.3 | 5.5 | 4.9 | 4.4 | 5.0 | 6.2 | 5.1 | 6.2 | 9.0 | 6.9 | 9.3 | 7.6 | 11.7 | 7.6 | 7.7 | 8.9 | 11.4 | 6.3 | 7.3 |
| | | | | | | | | | | *Females* | | | | | | | | | | |
| Non-manual | 6 | 22 | 30 | 34 | 38 | 43 | 37 | 44 | 38 | 42 | 46 | 41 | 48 | 43 | 31 | 29 | 32 | 23 | 35 | 38 |
| Hours | 1.8 | 2.3 | 2.5 | 2.8 | 3.8 | 3.9 | 4.0 | 4.5 | 5.7 | 6.4 | 3.2 | 5.1 | 5.3 | 6.1 | 5.0 | 6.2 | 2.8 | 2.4 | 3.5 | 4.2 |
| Manual | 16 | 17 | 26 | 32 | 28 | 34 | 27 | 35 | 30 | 36 | 30 | 34 | 32 | 30 | 26 | 26 | 24 | 18 | 27 | 30 |
| Hours | 1.7 | 2.5 | 3.2 | 3.7 | 2.6 | 2.9 | 3.7 | 4.2 | 4.7 | 4.8 | 3.9 | 5.4 | 3.4 | 4.8 | 6.0 | 6.2 | 2.8 | 2.4 | 3.5 | 4.2 |
| *Base = 100%* | 96 | | 98 | | 200 | | 158 | | 134 | | 112 | | 106 | | 57 | | 32 | | 993 | |
| | 193 | | 139 | | 183 | | 166 | | 145 | | 165 | | 151 | | 90 | | 53 | | 1285 | |
| | 149 | | 157 | | 271 | | 214 | | 205 | | 138 | | 141 | | 80 | | 53 | | 1408 | |
| | 155 | | 234 | | 268 | | 212 | | 182 | | 173 | | 181 | | 108 | | 87 | | 1600 | |
| **DIY** | | | | | | | | | | | | | | | | | | | | |
| Males | 47 | 41 | 54 | 45 | 53 | 49 | 58 | 50 | 52 | 35 | 42 | 38 | 42 | 36 | 34 | 24 | 20 | 12 | 48 | 40 |
| Hours | 6.1 | 7.6 | 9.5 | 7.6 | 8.4 | 7.0 | 7.4 | 7.6 | 6.5 | 6.1 | 7.4 | 7.5 | 8.1 | 10.0 | 6.5 | 7.2 | 7.1 | 3.9 | 7.6 | 7.5 |
| Females | 11 | 18 | 19 | 18 | 13 | 16 | 16 | 12 | 16 | 11 | 11 | 9 | 10 | 7 | 3 | 3 | 4 | 3 | 13 | 12 |
| Hours | 5.1 | 6.3 | 5.2 | 6.7 | 5.0 | 5.9 | 5.7 | 3.4 | 7.0 | 6.4 | 5.6 | 5.2 | 6.7 | 5.6 | 1.7 | 5.4 | 8.6 | 7.0 | 5.7 | 5.8 |
| *Base = 100%* | 299 | | 241 | | 383 | | 322 | | 280 | | 278 | | 258 | | 146 | | 86 | | 2293 | |
| | 311 | | 394 | | 545 | | 429 | | 391 | | 314 | | 326 | | 190 | | 143 | | 3044 | |

# SOCIAL
# FACTORS

# SOCIAL RELATIONSHIPS AND HEALTH | 15

## Virginia J Swain

Social health is more difficult to define than physical and psychological health, which are areas with well-recognised boundaries. It is often described as combining a number of factors, including personality and psychological traits and the ability to function within a social environment and is a vital aspect of health because, as social beings, we live and interact within complex social organisations. Social health, therefore, adds an extra, broader dimension to the concept of health.

Social relationships have long been considered an important aspect of health (Durkheim, 1897), and many people who work within the fields of sociology and psychiatry have continued to establish a connection between dysfunction in social relationships, ill-health, perceived health status and mortality (Cohen and Syme, 1985; Berkman and Breslow, 1983). Some workers emphasise the need to consider the objectively measured effects of social isolation or having few social roles, activities or commitments, whilst others concentrate on a more subjective measure: feelings of not being respected, loved, supported or cared for.

This Chapter approaches the study of social ties by examining both the more objective measure of social contact, albeit based on reported frequency of contact by respondents, and the more subjective assessment of whether individuals believe they can rely on receiving support and encouragement from their family members.

A number of health measures were used for the initial analysis of social relationships, including self-reported health 'compared with someone of own age', self-reported health compared with seven years

ago (the time of the HALS1 Survey), long-standing illness and symptoms of illness and malaise. The malaise score used as a measure of psycho-social health appears to have a strong association with many of the social relationship and social contact variables (see Appendix A for a definition of malaise).

Table 15.1 shows the malaise score in the full HALS1 sample and the HALS2 sub-group at both Surveys. In the youngest age group, for both men and women, there has been some loss in reaching and re-interviewing respondents who had a high malaise score in the HALS2 sub-sample compared to the HALS1 full sample at HALS1. Both men and women who reported a low level of malaise at HALS1 were less likely to be lost from the sample. This is most noticeable in the older men and women.

The reporting of some malaise symptoms has remained quite static, (Table 15.2a – 15.12b), whilst reporting of other symptoms has changed, in some cases upwards and in others downwards. Lower numbers of men, up to age 60, reported being bored, 'some or all of the time' at HALS2, compared both to their own group seven years ago and to the same age group in 1984/5. For men aged 60 or over there has been a consistent loss from the sample between HALS1 and HALS2 for the reporting of each symptom of approximately 2% – 3% except for 'difficulty sleeping', 'always feeling tired' and 'difficulty concentrating': in those aged 74 and over at HALS1, for these three symptoms, the loss has been much greater. The percentage of women reporting boredom also followed a similar, if less consistent, pattern to the men. Although overall a greater percentage of women than men, report higher levels of every malaise symptom they have shown a tendency not to report many of the symptoms than they did seven years ago, whereas men are more likely to have increased their reporting. The only malaise symptom for which reporting has risen consistently across age cohorts for women is 'difficulty in sleeping'; interestingly, this is not reflected in an upward trend in reporting 'always being tired'.

## Contact with relatives and household structure

Household type is determined by the number of individuals living in the house and their relationship to the respondent. The household grid on the questionnaire was divided into six categories: spouse; living as married; children; parents; other relatives and non-relatives. Household groupings have been derived in the same way as in HALS1. A different set of questions were used in the HALS2 Survey to measure quantitatively contact with family outside the household. At HALS1, information was gathered about the two week period leading up to interview and a number of questions were asked to determine how often respondents visited, or were visited by family and friends, or whether they had contact by telephone or letter. At HALS2 questions were asked about the type and number of relatives living 'in the area or within easy reach', (as perceived by the respondent), who the respondent saw most often and how often. Information was only sought about relatives 'seen' and not about contact with friends. It is not possible, therefore, to examine changes over the seven years between type and amount of contact.

Social contacts are an important aspect of perceived health status when consideration is given to the type of contact and level of support that it provides. The significance of household structure, particularly the differentiation between someone living with others or living alone, is unclear, (Hughes and Gove, 1981; Cramer, 1993). In a study in Sweden, Mullins, Sheppard and Andersson (1991) found a complex picture of interaction between an individual's household circumstances and their feelings of loneliness. They determined that emotional isolation was not something exclusively experienced by people living alone and feeling lonely, whether or not an individual lived alone, was significant in its association with self-assessed health. Moreover, individuals who lived with others but who felt lonely, were more likely to have a pessimistic view of their health than those who lived alone and reported loneliness.

Table 15.3 and Table 15.4 compare the respondent's reported frequency of seeing any relatives by type of household lived in; they show the effects on malaise and illness scores analysed by changing household structure since 1984/5. In Table 15.3 it is evident that more than half of all respondents see relatives weekly or more often and couples with dependent children, in the middle age group, are most likely to have less frequent contact. High malaise is reported by more men and women in all age groups, if they live alone or if they are lone parents, especially for men seeing relatives less than weekly (Table 15.4). Even though they report higher rates of malaise overall, compared with couples, lone women between 24 and 45 at HALS2 do not show any substantial rise in malaise if they do not see relatives weekly or more often and older women show a reverse trend. Men aged 46 and over, who have partners and see other relatives frequently report more malaise symptoms. A similar pattern is evident in females but the gap is smaller. Although we did not find any great differences in frequency of family contact between those who reported suffering from long-standing illness and those who did not, the nature and quality of the contact cannot be established from the information available and must, therefore, be interpreted with caution. We cannot know whether the contact is purely social or part of a responsibility to care for another's well-being. What may be a source of happiness and fulfilment for one individual may be a chore or burden for another.

Table 15.5 compares the change from low levels of malaise and illness for respondents who have become parents since 1984/5 with those who had dependents at both Surveys. The number of individuals changing their status is quite small, nonetheless a difference is obvious for women who have become parents since HALS1. This group of women are more likely to have moved from 'low' to 'average' malaise, but more women who had children at both Surveys shifted into the high illness category at HALS2. A change in parental status does not appear to be associated with increased malaise in men but is so for illness.

## Social Integration

The 'roles and available attachments index' (see Appendix A) has been derived in the same way as at HALS1. It is based on whether an individual is married; living with partner or family; with living children and/or parents; in employment; living in an area for some years and feeling part of the community; and involved in community affairs or visits to a place of worship. A high scoring individual would have many roles, living in a familiar community, with living family, in employment and with an active social life. Many studies have examined the possible ill-effects on men and women of insufficient, or too many or conflicting roles, with employment and parity being popular routes to investigating multiplicity of roles, (Nathanson, 1980; Bartley, Popay and Plewis, 1992).

Table 15.6 shows that the youngest group of respondents are less likely to have a high social integration score; the highest score for level of integration peaks between the ages of 32 and 45 and then gradually falls away. At all ages, except for men aged 74 and over and women between 60 and 66, a smaller proportion of subjects who reported low levels of integration at HALS1 were re-interviewed at HALS2. This is also the case with some of the middle age groups for men and women who scored 'average' in 1984/5. Interestingly, respondents with high scores were more likely to be seen at HALS2, demonstrating perhaps that this group is easier to trace, (maybe the respondents were living at or close to the address where they were originally interviewed). It is also possible that they were more willing to be re-interviewed.

In HALS1 it was found that respondents with low levels of social integration had a greater likelihood of higher rates of illness and malaise, and an extra dimension has been added at HALS2 because when changes in levels of integration between Survey 1 and 2 are examined, the association with malaise, though not illness, (not shown) is very apparent (Table 15.7). Individuals who had moved from 'average or high' to 'low' scores on the roles and available attachment index were much more likely to report 'high' malaise than their counterparts who had moved from 'low' to 'average or high'. This was most pronounced in men aged 39 and over and for women in the oldest age group. However, when self-assessed health 'compared with someone of same age' was examined (Table 15.8), the association was not clear for men until the age of 60 was reached, when there was a contrast between those who changed integration scores. A smaller percentage of men in this age group who moved from 'average or high' to 'low' reported 'excellent or good' health whilst those moving upwards in their score were more likely to report 'excellent or good' health. Men over 60 years who scored 'low' on both occasions reported a greater 'decline' in self-assessed health than did any other group. For women, a low level of social integration is associated with a greater likelihood of reporting their health as 'fair or poor'.

## Perceived social support

The Health and Lifestyle Survey (1987) and Blaxter (1990) illustrated a relationship between levels of perceived support and psycho-social health and illness. Table 15.9 to Table 15.17 evaluate a number of variables including illness, malaise, self-assessed health and life events to assess possible changes between the two Surveys in particular groups.

Levels of perceived social support have remained fairly stable between HALS1 and HALS2 with slightly more respondents having no lack of social support at HALS2 (Table 15.9, Table 15.10). Over 70% of both men and women reported still having no perceived lack of support, and less than one third of the respondents who felt most deprived at HALS1, remained so. Comparison of the HALS1 full sample and the HALS2 sub-sample at HALS1 shows that for both men and women the greatest loss occurred amongst those who had a severe lack of perceived support in 1984/5, (Table 15.11).

Self-assessed health does not show a strong or clear association with perceived support (Table 15.12). A higher percentage of the youngest group of men with 'moderate or severe lack' of support on both occasions report a greater 'improvement' in health when compared with all other groups but the percentage reporting 'excellent or good' health at HALS1 was much lower. This might indicate that although there has been a greater loss of respondents who reported some lack of social support at HALS1, those who report some lack of support and who assess their health to be 'excellent or good', are more likely to be represented at the second Survey. In the middle years a more 'expected' pattern is evident in those who change categories but not in those who remain in the same one: more men in the 35-59 age group who have moved from 'moderate or severe lack' of support to 'no lack' are reporting 'excellent or good' health compared with those moving in the opposite direction. However, middle aged men who have no apparent lack of support at either Survey are no more likely to report 'excellent or good' health at HALS2 than those who felt a lack of support at HALS1 and HALS2. Similarly more women in the younger age groups in all categories are reporting 'excellent or good' health at HALS2. One striking feature of using perceived health status as a dependent variable measured against social support is that, in most cases, respondents who believed they were supported by family or friends on both occasions were more likely to have a positive view of their health and less likely to identify their health as being only 'fair or poor' when compared to all other groups, including the group whose perceived level of support had improved since HALS1. Women at all ages and men between 18 and 38, who consistently report 'no lack' of perceived support, show similar responses to malaise and self-assessed health. A smaller percentage of respondents who had 'no lack' at HALS1 and HALS2 reported high malaise at each Survey compared to the group who felt 'no lack' at HALS1 and who subsequently perceived a drop in support at HALS2, suggesting a difference between the consistent group and those whose levels of support have changed between Surveys.

In HALS1 an association was noted between low support and high malaise and illness levels for men in manual socio-economic groups. This has been re-examined in Table 15.14, using HALS1 socio-economic groups, for respondents who have changed support category between HALS1 and HALS2. It is not obvious from this table that an improvement in perceived social support leads to a clear reduction in reporting of illness or malaise symptoms, but men at all ages in the manual group, and in the non-manual group over 60 years of age, show increasing likelihood of high malaise when deprived of social support, to a degree similar, or even higher than for the group who felt a lack of support at both Surveys. A stronger association is evident in women, particularly for the oldest age group, in reporting symptoms of malaise. In line with HALS1 findings, high support is favourable for women in non-manual families.

Table 15.15 to Table 15.17 examine the relationship between perceived social support as reported in HALS1 and life events involving family and friends which occurred in the intervening seven years (Chapter 10 examines life-events further). Table 15.15 shows a strong association between perceived support in 1984/5 and stressful life events reported at HALS2 as having occurred within the last twelve months. Women of all ages were more likely to report disagreements with family, difficulty with children or loss of contact with family or friends in the previous year if they suffered from lack of support at HALS1. The association is also present for men reporting loss of contact with friends or relatives, for all except the two youngest age groups. Table 15.16 shows that this also holds true for reported divorce or separation during the last seven years (numbers reporting separation or divorce during the last year were too small). Greater caution is needed in interpretation of this association, however, because 'living apart' may not necessarily mean the break-down of a relationship. If we suppose that this is generally the implication and, of course, it is obviously so with divorce, the quality of the relationship may already have been impaired or breaking down at the time of the first Survey, so that feelings of lack of support, low self-esteem and pessimism may have been more pronounced at that time.

At the close of the interview, respondents were asked to recall if 'anything good had happened to them during the last year or 7 years'. Table 15.17 shows that women between the ages of 39 and 59 and men over 60 were more likely to report ongoing satisfaction with their family and life in general if they felt their family to be supportive.

# Summary

The continuing importance of social relationships and social ties, particularly for psycho-social health, has been demonstrated in this chapter. Nearly three quarters of respondents continue to report 'no lack' in perceived social support. Although there are only small numbers reporting change in levels of support, a decline in perceived support appears to have a pronounced effect on psycho-social health in some groups of individuals. Younger men and women appear to be less affected by changing circumstances, maybe because they have a wider circle of people outside the family to whom they can turn. Older respondents seem to be more affected, especially when perceived social support drops. Differences are also apparent between socio-economic groups for malaise but less so for reported illness. A 'deterioration' in amount of support is more likely to be reflected in a higher malaise score for men in manual occupations, in all age groups, whereas only the oldest group of non-manual men is similarly affected. Whichever groups are examined, women who feel an 'ongoing' lack of social support are affected most profoundly. They are more likely to report a high number of illness and malaise symptoms and a greater proportion assess their health as only fair or poor compared with those who report a change from 'no lack' to 'moderate or severe lack' of support.

It is evident that living alone and seeing relatives less than weekly is more likely to be associated with poor psycho-social health for men than for women. A strong relationship has been demonstrated between reported malaise and the amount of social integration. Men are more likely than women to have a high score on the roles and available attachments index, as are subjects in early middle age, but individuals in all age groups who have increased their level of integration between the Surveys consistently show lower reporting of malaise symptoms. This seems to support studies which advocate the beneficial effects of a multiplicity of roles on psycho-social health.

Further analysis is necessary before many of the complexities of social relationships and their change over time can be investigated in relation to health and ill-health in the HALS population.

## References

Bartley M, Popay J, and Plewis I. (1992), Domestic conditions, paid employment and women's experience of health. Sociology of Health and Illness, 14, No.3: 313-343.

Berkman LF, and Breslow L. (1983) Health and Ways of Living, Oxford: Oxford University Press.

Blaxter M. (1990) Health and Lifestyles, London/New York: Routledge.

Cohen S, and Syme L, (Eds) (1985), Social Support and Health. New York: Academic Press.

Cox BD, et al. (1987) Health and Lifestyle Survey, Cambridge: Health Promotion Research Trust.

Cramer D. (1993), Living Alone, Marital Status, Gender and Health. Journal of Community and Applied Social Psychology, 3, 1-15.

Durkheim E. (1897), Le Suicide, Paris.

Hughes M, and Gove WR, (1981), Living alone, social integration and mental health. American Journal of Sociology, 87, pp 48-74.

Mullins LC, Sheppard HL, Andersson L. (1991), Loneliness and Social Isolation in Sweden:Differences in Age, Sex, Labor Force Status, Self-Rated Health, and Income Adequacy. Journal of Applied Gerontology, 10, No. 4: 455-468.

Nathanson CA. (1980), Social Roles and Health Status Among Women: The Significance of Employment. Social Science and Medicine, 14A, 463-471.

**Table 15.1  Change in malaise scores using full HALS1 sample and HALS2 sub-sample at HALS1 and HALS2. Percentage of age group**

| HALS1 age | 18-24 | | 25-31 | | 32-38 | | 39-45 | | 46-52 | | 53-59 | | 60-66 | | 67-73 | | 74+ | | Total | |
| HALS2 age | | 25-31 | | 32-38 | | 39-45 | | 46-52 | | 53-59 | | 60-66 | | 67-73 | | 74-80 | | 81+ | | Total |
|---|---|---|---|---|---|---|---|---|---|---|---|---|---|---|---|---|---|---|---|---|
| **Malaise score** | | | | | | | | | | **Males** | | | | | | | | | | |
| **Low** | | | | | | | | | | | | | | | | | | | | |
| HALS1 sample | 35 | | 37 | | 38 | | 47 | | 47 | | 43 | | 53 | | 55 | | 51 | | 44 | |
| HALS2 sub-sample | 35 | 36 | 39 | 42 | 39 | 44 | 47 | 43 | 47 | 51 | 44 | 50 | 55 | 57 | 62 | 58 | 61 | 43 | 45 | 47 |
| **Average** | | | | | | | | | | | | | | | | | | | | |
| HALS1 sample | 39 | | 40 | | 39 | | 34 | | 34 | | 31 | | 31 | | 27 | | 24 | | 34 | |
| HALS2 sub-sample | 41 | 41 | 38 | 34 | 39 | 38 | 36 | 36 | 34 | 29 | 31 | 30 | 32 | 25 | 26 | 26 | 22 | 31 | 35 | 33 |
| **High** | | | | | | | | | | | | | | | | | | | | |
| HALS1 sample | 26 | | 23 | | 22 | | 19 | | 20 | | 26 | | 17 | | 19 | | 26 | | 22 | |
| HALS2 sub-sample | 24 | 23 | 23 | 25 | 22 | 18 | 18 | 21 | 19 | 20 | 25 | 21 | 14 | 18 | 12 | 16 | 17 | 26 | 20 | 20 |
| *Base = 100%* | *534* | | *489* | | *573* | | *474* | | *419* | | *417* | | *412* | | *314* | | *273* | | *3905* | |
| | *299* | *299* | *241* | *241* | *383* | *383* | *324* | *324* | *280* | *280* | *278* | *278* | *259* | *259* | *148* | *148* | *88* | *88* | *2300* | *2300* |
| | | | | | | | | | | **Females** | | | | | | | | | | |
| **Low** | | | | | | | | | | | | | | | | | | | | |
| HALS1 sample | 25 | | 26 | | 31 | | 31 | | 30 | | 31 | | 33 | | 37 | | 37 | | 31 | |
| HALS2 sub-sample | 27 | 28 | 27 | 31 | 32 | 37 | 34 | 32 | 30 | 31 | 30 | 39 | 35 | 38 | 40 | 33 | 43 | 40 | 32 | 34 |
| **Average** | | | | | | | | | | | | | | | | | | | | |
| HALS1 sample | 38 | | 39 | | 38 | | 34 | | 35 | | 33 | | 32 | | 29 | | 29 | | 35 | |
| HALS2 sub-sample | 38 | 40 | 40 | 36 | 38 | 32 | 33 | 37 | 37 | 35 | 35 | 31 | 31 | 31 | 29 | 29 | 33 | 31 | 36 | 34 |
| **High** | | | | | | | | | | | | | | | | | | | | |
| HALS1 sample | 37 | | 34 | | 31 | | 36 | | 35 | | 35 | | 35 | | 35 | | 34 | | 35 | |
| HALS2 sub-sample | 35 | 32 | 34 | 33 | 30 | 31 | 33 | 31 | 33 | 34 | 35 | 30 | 34 | 32 | 31 | 38 | 24 | 30 | 33 | 32 |
| *Base = 100%* | *626* | | *672* | | *766* | | *618* | | *576* | | *468* | | *553* | | *391* | | *410* | | *5098* | |
| | *311* | *311* | *394* | *394* | *545* | *545* | *432* | *432* | *391* | *391* | *315* | *315* | *327* | *327* | *191* | *191* | *146* | *146* | *3052* | *3052* |

**Table 15.2a** **Change in reporting of specific symptoms of malaise 'during the last month' by men including complete HALS1 sample and HALS2 sub-sample at HALS1 and HALS2. Percentage of age group**

| | 18-24 | | 25-31 | | 32-38 | | 39-45 | | 46-52 | | 53-59 | | 60-66 | | 67-73 | | 74+ | | Total | |
| --- | --- | --- | --- | --- | --- | --- | --- | --- | --- | --- | --- | --- | --- | --- | --- | --- | --- | --- | --- | --- |
| **HALS1 age** | | | | | | | | | | | | | | | | | | | | |
| **HALS2 age** | | 25-31 | | 32-38 | | 39-45 | | 46-52 | | 53-59 | | 60-66 | | 67-73 | | 74-80 | | 81+ | | Total |
| **Malaise symptoms** | | | | | | | | | | | | | | | | | | | | |
| **Difficulty sleeping** | | | | | | | | | | | | | | | | | | | | |
| HALS1 sample | 19 | | 19 | | 21 | | 17 | | 20 | | 23 | | 20 | | 21 | | 27 | | 20 | |
| HALS2 sub-sample | 14 | 21 | 21 | 27 | 23 | 19 | 17 | 26 | 20 | 25 | 21 | 23 | 19 | 23 | 18 | 18 | 19 | 27 | 19 | 23 |
| **Nerves** | | | | | | | | | | | | | | | | | | | | |
| HALS1 sample | 6 | | 5 | | 5 | | 6 | | 6 | | 8 | | 7 | | 7 | | 7 | | 6 | |
| HALS2 sub-sample | 5 | 5 | 5 | 7 | 5 | 5 | 6 | 7 | 6 | 4 | 7 | 6 | 5 | 6 | 5 | 4 | 3 | 6 | 5 | 5 |
| **Always tired** | | | | | | | | | | | | | | | | | | | | |
| HALS1 sample | 22 | | 20 | | 19 | | 18 | | 18 | | 20 | | 16 | | 14 | | 23 | | 19 | |
| HALS2 sub-sample | 23 | 23 | 22 | 23 | 19 | 13 | 17 | 20 | 20 | 20 | 19 | 17 | 14 | 16 | 11 | 20 | 15 | 24 | 18 | 19 |
| **Difficulty concentrating** | | | | | | | | | | | | | | | | | | | | |
| HALS1 sample | 13 | | 11 | | 9 | | 9 | | 10 | | 12 | | 9 | | 11 | | 14 | | 10 | |
| HALS2 sub-sample | 11 | 10 | 11 | 12 | 9 | 11 | 9 | 12 | 11 | 13 | 9 | 12 | 7 | 9 | 9 | 16 | 8 | 20 | 9 | 12 |
| **Worrying over everything** | | | | | | | | | | | | | | | | | | | | |
| HALS1 sample | 14 | | 12 | | 13 | | 12 | | 13 | | 18 | | 14 | | 8 | | 16 | | 13 | |
| HALS2 sub-sample | 14 | 13 | 12 | 14 | 11 | 12 | 11 | 19 | 11 | 12 | 18 | 14 | 12 | 14 | 6 | 11 | 14 | 9 | 12 | 13 |
| **Under strain** | | | | | | | | | | | | | | | | | | | | |
| HALS1 sample | 3 | | 5 | | 8 | | 8 | | 7 | | 10 | | 5 | | 3 | | 4 | | 6 | |
| HALS2 sub-sample | 3 | 5 | 6 | 10 | 9 | 8 | 9 | 7 | 8 | 6 | 10 | 5 | 3 | 3 | 1 | 3 | 1 | 3 | 6 | 6 |
| **Bored** | | | | | | | | | | | | | | | | | | | | |
| HALS1 sample | 16 | | 13 | | 8 | | 8 | | 8 | | 14 | | 9 | | 9 | | 15 | | 11 | |
| HALS2 sub-sample | 16 | 11 | 14 | 8 | 5 | 4 | 8 | 6 | 7 | 6 | 12 | 9 | 6 | 8 | 5 | 10 | 16 | 5 | 9 | 8 |
| **Lonely** | | | | | | | | | | | | | | | | | | | | |
| HALS1 sample | 3 | | 3 | | 2 | | 3 | | 3 | | 5 | | 6 | | 8 | | 14 | | 5 | |
| HALS2 sub-sample | 3 | 2 | 2 | 4 | 1 | 3 | 2 | 1 | 3 | 3 | 4 | 6 | 5 | 3 | 5 | 8 | 11 | 11 | 3 | 4 |
| *Base = 100%* | 534 | | 489 | | 573 | | 474 | | 419 | | 417 | | 412 | | 314 | | 273 | | 3905 | |
| | 299 | 299 | 241 | 241 | 383 | 383 | 324 | 324 | 280 | 280 | 278 | 278 | 259 | 259 | 148 | 148 | 88 | 88 | 2300 | 2300 |

**Table 15.2b** **Change in reporting of specific symptoms of malaise 'during the last month' by women including complete HALS1 sample and HALS2 sub-sample at HALS1 and HALS2. Percentage of age group**

| | 18-24 | | 25-31 | | 32-38 | | 39-45 | | 46-52 | | 53-59 | | 60-66 | | 67-73 | | 74+ | | Total | |
|---|---|---|---|---|---|---|---|---|---|---|---|---|---|---|---|---|---|---|---|---|
| HALS2 age | | 25-31 | | 32-38 | | 39-45 | | 46-52 | | 53-59 | | 60-66 | | 67-73 | | 74-80 | | 81+ | | Total |
| **Malaise symptoms** | | | | | | | | | | | | | | | | | | | | |
| **Difficulty sleeping** | | | | | | | | | | | | | | | | | | | | |
| HALS1 sample | 23 | | 24 | | 21 | | 28 | | 38 | | 36 | | 40 | | 42 | | 40 | | 31 | |
| HALS2 sub-sample | 23 | 26 | 22 | 25 | 19 | 30 | 27 | 36 | 39 | 44 | 39 | 39 | 39 | 43 | 44 | 48 | 40 | 40 | 30 | 36 |
| **Nerves** | | | | | | | | | | | | | | | | | | | | |
| HALS1 sample | 12 | | 10 | | 9 | | 14 | | 16 | | 17 | | 19 | | 14 | | 16 | | 14 | |
| HALS2 sub-sample | 11 | 11 | 10 | 9 | 10 | 10 | 13 | 10 | 13 | 13 | 15 | 15 | 20 | 13 | 12 | 16 | 14 | 10 | 13 | 11 |
| **Always tired** | | | | | | | | | | | | | | | | | | | | |
| HALS1 sample | 35 | | 33 | | 31 | | 33 | | 30 | | 27 | | 22 | | 26 | | 28 | | 30 | |
| HALS2 sub-sample | 34 | 33 | 32 | 30 | 31 | 28 | 32 | 34 | 29 | 27 | 26 | 23 | 22 | 21 | 25 | 27 | 23 | 26 | 29 | 28 |
| **Difficulty concentrating** | | | | | | | | | | | | | | | | | | | | |
| HALS1 sample | 14 | | 11 | | 11 | | 17 | | 17 | | 17 | | 17 | | 17 | | 17 | | 15 | |
| HALS2 sub-sample | 10 | 11 | 10 | 12 | 12 | 17 | 16 | 20 | 16 | 16 | 16 | 15 | 17 | 18 | 15 | 23 | 14 | 16 | 14 | 16 |
| **Worrying over everything** | | | | | | | | | | | | | | | | | | | | |
| HALS1 sample | 26 | | 24 | | 24 | | 26 | | 32 | | 30 | | 31 | | 29 | | 26 | | 27 | |
| HALS2 sub-sample | 27 | 22 | 25 | 23 | 23 | 22 | 24 | 24 | 29 | 27 | 29 | 26 | 31 | 26 | 30 | 29 | 21 | 25 | 26 | 24 |
| **Under strain** | | | | | | | | | | | | | | | | | | | | |
| HALS1 sample | 5 | | 6 | | 6 | | 10 | | 7 | | 8 | | 6 | | 6 | | 5 | | 7 | |
| HALS2 sub-sample | 4 | 5 | 6 | 8 | 6 | 9 | 10 | 7 | 7 | 7 | 9 | 6 | 8 | 4 | 4 | 7 | 3 | 3 | 7 | 7 |
| **Bored** | | | | | | | | | | | | | | | | | | | | |
| HALS1 sample | 19 | | 14 | | 10 | | 7 | | 10 | | 9 | | 10 | | 12 | | 15 | | 12 | |
| HALS2 sub-sample | 19 | 11 | 14 | 9 | 8 | 8 | 6 | 5 | 8 | 9 | 8 | 6 | 8 | 10 | 11 | 13 | 11 | 10 | 10 | 9 |
| **Lonely** | | | | | | | | | | | | | | | | | | | | |
| HALS1 sample | 9 | | 7 | | 8 | | 7 | | 8 | | 8 | | 9 | | 12 | | 17 | | 9 | |
| HALS2 sub-sample | 7 | 5 | 9 | 5 | 8 | 4 | 5 | 4 | 6 | 7 | 8 | 8 | 8 | 9 | 9 | 18 | 10 | 12 | 7 | 7 |
| *Base = 100%* | 626 | | 672 | | 766 | | 618 | | 576 | | 486 | | 553 | | 391 | | 410 | | 5898 | |
| | 311 | 311 | 394 | 394 | 545 | 545 | 432 | 432 | 391 | 391 | 315 | 315 | 327 | 327 | 191 | 191 | 146 | 146 | 3052 | 3052 |

**Table 15.3    Frequency of reporting seeing relative/s by household type at HALS2. Percentage of household type**

| | | Males | | | | Females | | |
|---|---|---|---|---|---|---|---|---|
| | Daily | Weekly | < weekly | Base = 100% | Daily | Weekly | < weekly | Base = 100% |
| **Household type** | | | | | | | | |
| **Age at HALS2 25-45** | | | | | | | | |
| Alone | 15 | 57 | 29 | *69* | 24 | 49 | 27 | *41* |
| Alone with depend. children | – | – | – | *–* | 33 | 45 | 22 | *95* |
| Couple | 16 | 58 | 26 | *134* | 22 | 52 | 26 | *152* |
| Couple with depend. children | 16 | 50 | 34 | *482* | 25 | 50 | 25 | *665* |
| Couple with adult children | 17 | 51 | 32 | *59* | 25 | 53 | 22 | *137* |
| **Age at HALS2 46-66** | | | | | | | | |
| Alone | 20 | 44 | 36 | *61* | 23 | 54 | 23 | *146* |
| Alone with adult children | 23 | 55 | 23 | *22* | 29 | 54 | 16 | *68* |
| Couple | 20 | 54 | 26 | *375* | 28 | 50 | 22 | *496* |
| Couple with depend. children | 12 | 43 | 45 | *108* | 16 | 40 | 44 | *82* |
| Couple with adult children | 13 | 50 | 38 | *254* | 22 | 53 | 25 | *287* |
| **Age at HALS2 67+** | | | | | | | | |
| Alone | 24 | 52 | 24 | *105* | 20 | 54 | 27 | *312* |
| Alone with adult children | – | – | – | *–* | 21 | 43 | 36 | *42* |
| Couple | 16 | 54 | 31 | *303* | 16 | 53 | 31 | *239* |
| Couple with adult children | 11 | 64 | 25 | *28* | 29 | 38 | 33 | *21* |

Alone includes single, separated, divorced or widowed. Couple includes married and cohabiting.

**Table 15.4**  **Percentage reporting high malaise by household type and frequency of seeing relatives at HALS2**

| | Males | | | Females | | |
|---|---|---|---|---|---|---|
| | Daily | Weekly | < weekly | Daily | Weekly | < weekly |
| **Household type** | | | | | | |
| **Age at HALS2 25-45** | | | | | | |
| Alone or lone parents | (2) | 31 | 42 | 47 | 51 | 50 |
| Couple or couple with children | 14 | 17 | 19 | 29 | 25 | 30 |
| *Base = 100%* | *11* | *45* | *24* | *45* | *74* | *42* |
| | *108* | *349* | *218* | *234* | *483* | *237* |
| **Age at HALS2 46-66** | | | | | | |
| Alone | (8) | 44 | 46 | 53 | 41 | 41 |
| Couple | 27 | 16 | 14 | 33 | 27 | 29 |
| *Base = 100%* | *19* | *39* | *28* | *55* | *116* | *49* |
| | *121* | *374* | *242* | *215* | *433* | *217* |
| **Age at HALS2 67+** | | | | | | |
| Alone | 23 | 33 | 34 | 37 | 46 | 27 |
| Couple | 22 | 17 | 9 | 29 | 29 | 26 |
| *Base = 100%* | *26* | *63* | *32* | *70* | *175* | *93* |
| | *50* | *180* | *101* | *42* | *135* | *81* |

**Table 15.5** **Malaise and illness at HALS2 in respondents with low malaise and illness at HALS1. Effect of change in household structure for couples aged 18-38 at HALS1. Percentage of household type**

| | Low malaise at HALS1 | | | |
| | **Males** | | **Females** | |
| | **No dependents HALS1 Dependents at HALS2** | **Dependents at HALS1 and HALS2** | **No dependents HALS1 Dependents at HALS2** | **Dependents at HALS1 and HALS2** |
|---|---|---|---|---|
| **Malaise at HALS2** | | | | |
| Low | 70 | 66 | 46 | 65 |
| Average | 23 | 28 | 41 | 26 |
| High | 7 | 6 | 14 | 10 |
| *Base = 100%* | *30* | *133* | *22* | *158* |

| | Low illness at HALS1 | | | |
|---|---|---|---|---|
| **Illness at HALS2** | | | | |
| Low | 46 | 65 | 58 | 57 |
| Average | 42 | 29 | 39 | 30 |
| High | 12 | 6 | 3 | 13 |
| *Base = 100%* | *41* | *158* | *36* | *196* |

**Table 15.6**  **Change in roles and available attachments index score (RAAI) including full HALS1 sample and HALS2 sub-group at HALS1 and HALS2. Percentage of age group**

| HALS1 age | 18-24 | | 25-31 | | 32-38 | | 39-45 | | 46-52 | | 53-59 | | 60-66 | | 67-73 | | 74+ | | Total | |
|---|---|---|---|---|---|---|---|---|---|---|---|---|---|---|---|---|---|---|---|---|
| HALS2 age | | 25-31 | | 32-38 | | 39-45 | | 46-52 | | 53-59 | | 60-66 | | 67-73 | | 74-80 | | 81+ | | Total |
| **RAAI score** | | | | | | | | | | **Males** | | | | | | | | | | |
| **Low** | | | | | | | | | | | | | | | | | | | | |
| HALS1 sample | 21 | | 20 | | 11 | | 13 | | 12 | | 21 | | 32 | | 46 | | 57 | | 23 | |
| HALS2 sub-sample | 13 | 17 | 15 | 9 | 9 | 10 | 8 | 8 | 10 | 15 | 18 | 26 | 27 | 35 | 43 | 52 | 67 | 78 | 18 | 21 |
| **Average** | | | | | | | | | | | | | | | | | | | | |
| HALS1 sample | 64 | | 36 | | 35 | | 35 | | 44 | | 50 | | 54 | | 52 | | 43 | | 46 | |
| HALS2 sub-sample | 73 | 41 | 31 | 31 | 32 | 26 | 33 | 34 | 43 | 50 | 49 | 61 | 57 | 62 | 55 | 47 | 33 | 22 | 45 | 42 |
| **High** | | | | | | | | | | | | | | | | | | | | |
| HALS1 sample | 15 | | 43 | | 53 | | 52 | | 44 | | 29 | | 14 | | 2 | | 0 | | 31 | |
| HALS2 sub-sample | 14 | 41 | 54 | 60 | 59 | 63 | 59 | 58 | 47 | 35 | 33 | 14 | 15 | 3 | 2 | 1 | 0 | 0 | 37 | 37 |
| *Base = 100%* | *534* | | *489* | | *573* | | *474* | | *419* | | *417* | | *412* | | *314* | | *273* | | *3905* | |
| | *299* | *293* | *241* | *236* | *383* | *380* | *324* | *317* | *280* | *274* | *278* | *275* | *259* | *255* | *148* | *145* | *88* | *87* | *2300* | *2262* |
| | | | | | | | | | | **Females** | | | | | | | | | | |
| **Low** | | | | | | | | | | | | | | | | | | | | |
| HALS1 sample | 25 | | 19 | | 15 | | 17 | | 24 | | 31 | | 54 | | 64 | | 80 | | 33 | |
| HALS2 sub-sample | 16 | 16 | 17 | 13 | 13 | 10 | 14 | 15 | 22 | 25 | 27 | 40 | 54 | 57 | 61 | 73 | 73 | 88 | 27 | 29 |
| **Average** | | | | | | | | | | | | | | | | | | | | |
| HALS1 sample | 59 | | 54 | | 51 | | 49 | | 50 | | 56 | | 43 | | 36 | | 20 | | 48 | |
| HALS2 sub-sample | 65 | 48 | 51 | 40 | 48 | 39 | 48 | 49 | 51 | 54 | 57 | 56 | 43 | 41 | 39 | 28 | 26 | 11 | 50 | 43 |
| **High** | | | | | | | | | | | | | | | | | | | | |
| HALS1 sample | 15 | | 27 | | 34 | | 34 | | 26 | | 13 | | 3 | | 0 | | (1) | | 19 | |
| HALS2 sub-sample | 19 | 36 | 32 | 48 | 39 | 51 | 38 | 36 | 28 | 21 | 16 | 4 | 3 | 2 | 0 | 0 | (1) | (1) | 24 | 28 |
| *Base = 100%* | *626* | | *672* | | *766* | | *618* | | *576* | | *486* | | *553* | | *391* | | *410* | | *5098* | |
| | *311* | *304* | *394* | *390* | *545* | *538* | *432* | *423* | *391* | *385* | *315* | *313* | *327* | *313* | *191* | *189* | *146* | *137* | *3052* | *2992* |

**Table 15.7    Malaise score at HALS1 and HALS2 in relation to change in roles and available attachments index score (RAAI) at HALS1 and HALS2. Percentage of RAAI group**

| Age at HALS1 | 18-38 | | | | 39-59 | | | | 60+ | | | |
|---|---|---|---|---|---|---|---|---|---|---|---|---|
| RAAI | Aver/ high | Low | Low | Aver/ high | Aver/ high | Low | Low | Aver/ high | Aver/ high | Low | Low | Aver/ high |
| HALS | 1 | 2 | 1 | 2 | 1 | 2 | 1 | 2 | 1 | 2 | 1 | 2 |
| **Malaise** | | | | | **Males** | | | | | | | |
| Low | 31 | 25 | 29 | 32 | 46 | 34 | 35 | 38 | 62 | 39 | 57 | 65 |
| Average | 43 | 49 | 35 | 40 | 40 | 32 | 29 | 38 | 26 | 33 | 28 | 22 |
| High | 26 | 26 | 36 | 28 | 15 | 34 | 35 | 24 | 12 | 28 | 15 | 13 |
| | | | | | **Females** | | | | | | | |
| Low | 20 | 17 | 17 | 33 | 25 | 27 | 25 | 35 | 40 | 28 | 28 | 31 |
| Average | 38 | 38 | 36 | 31 | 42 | 36 | 30 | 35 | 33 | 31 | 33 | 39 |
| High | 42 | 46 | 47 | 36 | 33 | 37 | 46 | 30 | 27 | 41 | 39 | 29 |
| *Base = 100%* | 77 | | 75 | | 68 | | 34 | | 87 | | 46 | |
| | 85 | | 118 | | 139 | | 77 | | 104 | | 51 | |

**Table 15.8    Self-assessed health at HALS1 and HALS2 in relation to change in roles and available attachment index scores (RAAI). Percentage of RAAI group**

| | Males | | | | | | | | Females | | | | | | | |
|---|---|---|---|---|---|---|---|---|---|---|---|---|---|---|---|---|
| **RAAI** | Aver/high | Low | Low | Aver/high | Low | Low | Aver/high | Aver/high | Aver/high | Low | Low | Aver/high | Low | Low | Aver/high | Aver/high |
| **HALS** | 1 | 2 | 1 | 2 | 1 | 2 | 1 | 2 | 1 | 2 | 1 | 2 | 1 | 2 | 1 | 2 |

**Age at HALS1 18-38**

**Self-assessed health**

| | | | | | | | | | | | | | | | | |
|---|---|---|---|---|---|---|---|---|---|---|---|---|---|---|---|---|
| Excellent/good | 70 | 80 | 69 | 76 | 62 | 71 | 76 | 82 | 72 | 72 | 73 | 81 | 66 | 69 | 78 | 83 |
| Difference | (+10) | | (+7) | | (+9) | | (+6) | | (0) | | (+8) | | (+3) | | (+5) | |
| Fair/poor | 30 | 20 | 31 | 24 | 38 | 29 | 24 | 18 | 28 | 28 | 27 | 19 | 34 | 31 | 22 | 17 |
| *Base = 100%* | 76 | | 75 | | 34 | | 723 | | 85 | | 118 | | 64 | | 960 | |

**Age at HALS1 39-59**

**Self-assessed health**

| | | | | | | | | | | | | | | | | |
|---|---|---|---|---|---|---|---|---|---|---|---|---|---|---|---|---|
| Excellent/good | 74 | 59 | 62 | 50 | 64 | 53 | 76 | 75 | 71 | 67 | 73 | 77 | 55 | 61 | 77 | 77 |
| Difference | (-15) | | (-12) | | (-11) | | (-1) | | (-4) | | (+4) | | (+6) | | (0) | |
| Fair/poor | 27 | 41 | 38 | 50 | 36 | 47 | 24 | 25 | 30 | 33 | 27 | 23 | 45 | 39 | 23 | 23 |
| *Base = 100%* | 68 | | 34 | | 66 | | 696 | | 139 | | 77 | | 146 | | 752 | |

**Age at HALS1 60+**

**Self-assessed health**

| | | | | | | | | | | | | | | | | |
|---|---|---|---|---|---|---|---|---|---|---|---|---|---|---|---|---|
| Excellent/good | 72 | 64 | 67 | 71 | 75 | 57 | 76 | 71 | 71 | 68 | 60 | 66 | 71 | 68 | 79 | 70 |
| Difference | (-8) | | (+4) | | (-18) | | (-5) | | (-3) | | (+6) | | (-3) | | (-9) | |
| Fair/poor | 28 | 36 | 33 | 29 | 25 | 43 | 24 | 29 | 29 | 32 | 40 | 34 | 29 | 32 | 20 | 30 |
| *Base = 100%* | 87 | | 45 | | 146 | | 207 | | 104 | | 50 | | 327 | | 152 | |

**Table 15.9    Percentage change in perceived social support between HALS1 and HALS2 by age group.**

| Perceived social support HALS1 | Males | | | Females | | |
|---|---|---|---|---|---|---|
| | Severe lack | Moderate lack | No lack | Severe lack | Moderate lack | No lack |
| **HALS2** | | | **HALS1 age 18-38** | | | |
| Severe lack | 23 | 10 | 4 | 30 | 11 | 4 |
| Moderate lack | 46 | 37 | 25 | 37 | 32 | 17 |
| No lack | 31 | 53 | 72 | 33 | 56 | 79 |
| *Base = 100%* | *106* | *285* | *525* | *103* | *342* | *795* |
| | | | **HALS1 age 39-59** | | | |
| Severe lack | 29 | 9 | 5 | 32 | 10 | 3 |
| Moderate lack | 37 | 39 | 18 | 36 | 32 | 15 |
| No lack | 34 | 52 | 77 | 32 | 58 | 82 |
| *Base = 100%* | *93* | *274* | *506* | *72* | *315* | *742* |
| | | | **HALS1 age 60+** | | | |
| Severe lack | 34 | 13 | 6 | 23 | 10 | 4 |
| Moderate lack | 36 | 30 | 20 | 40 | 35 | 15 |
| No lack | 30 | 57 | 74 | 37 | 55 | 80 |
| *Base = 100%* | *53* | *132* | *302* | *65* | *138* | *441* |

**Table 15.10    Percentage in perceived social support groups at HALS1 compared with HALS2 by age group**

| HALS1 age | Males | | | | | | Females | | | | | |
|---|---|---|---|---|---|---|---|---|---|---|---|---|
| | 18-38 | | 39-59 | | 60+ | | 18-38 | | 39-59 | | 60+ | |
| HALS | 1 | 2 | 1 | 2 | 1 | 2 | 1 | 2 | 1 | 2 | 1 | 2 |
| **Perceived social support** | | | | | | | | | | | | |
| Severe lack | 12 | 8 | 11 | 9 | 11 | 11 | 8 | 8 | 6 | 7 | 10 | 8 |
| Moderate lack | 31 | 31 | 31 | 27 | 27 | 24 | 28 | 23 | 28 | 21 | 22 | 22 |
| No lack | 57 | 61 | 58 | 65 | 62 | 65 | 64 | 69 | 66 | 72 | 69 | 71 |
| *Base = 100%* | *916* | | *873* | | *487* | | *1240* | | *1129* | | *644* | |

**Table 15.11** **Change in level of perceived social support including complete HALS1 sample and HALS2 sub-sample at HALS1 and HALS2. Percentage of age group**

| | 18-24 | | 25-31 | | 32-38 | | 39-45 | | 46-52 | | 53-59 | | 60-66 | | 67-73 | | 74+ | | Total | |
| --- | --- | --- | --- | --- | --- | --- | --- | --- | --- | --- | --- | --- | --- | --- | --- | --- | --- | --- | --- | --- |
| HALS2 age | | 25-31 | | 32-38 | | 39-45 | | 46-52 | | 53-59 | | 60-66 | | 67-73 | | 74-80 | | 81+ | | Total |
| **Perceived social support** | | | | | | | | **Males** | | | | | | | | | | | | | |
| **Severe lack** | | | | | | | | | | | | | | | | | | | | | |
| HALS1 sample | 16 | | 13 | | 11 | | 11 | | 11 | | 13 | | 13 | | 12 | | 13 | | 12 | |
| HALS2 sub-sample | 13 | 7 | 12 | 8 | 10 | 8 | 10 | 9 | 11 | 10 | 11 | 8 | 10 | 11 | 11 | 12 | 17 | 12 | 11 | 9 |
| **Moderate lack** | | | | | | | | | | | | | | | | | | | | | |
| HALS1 sample | 37 | | 35 | | 28 | | 33 | | 33 | | 26 | | 26 | | 23 | | 25 | | 30 | |
| HALS2 sub-sample | 34 | 32 | 34 | 36 | 27 | 28 | 34 | 30 | 31 | 24 | 28 | 26 | 27 | 24 | 28 | 26 | 24 | 22 | 30 | 28 |
| **No lack** | | | | | | | | | | | | | | | | | | | | | |
| HALS1 sample | 48 | | 52 | | 61 | | 56 | | 56 | | 61 | | 61 | | 65 | | 61 | | 57 | |
| HALS2 sub-sample | 53 | 61 | 53 | 57 | 63 | 64 | 56 | 62 | 58 | 67 | 60 | 66 | 63 | 65 | 61 | 63 | 58 | 66 | 58 | 63 |
| *Base = 100%* | *534* | | *488* | | *572* | | *473* | | *417* | | *415* | | *411* | | *313* | | *270* | | *3893* | |
| | *299* | *298* | *240* | *239* | *382* | *381* | *323* | *323* | *280* | *277* | *277* | *275* | *259* | *256* | *148* | *147* | *87* | *85* | *2295* | *2281* |
| | | | | | | | | **Females** | | | | | | | | | | | | | |
| **Severe lack** | | | | | | | | | | | | | | | | | | | | | |
| HALS1 sample | 10 | | 8 | | 7 | | 6 | | 10 | | 9 | | 11 | | 12 | | 15 | | 9 | |
| HALS2 sub-sample | 8 | 7 | 10 | 11 | 7 | 7 | 5 | 8 | 7 | 8 | 8 | 5 | 11 | 5 | 9 | 7 | 12 | 13 | 8 | 8 |
| **Moderate lack** | | | | | | | | | | | | | | | | | | | | | |
| HALS1 sample | 32 | | 26 | | 29 | | 29 | | 30 | | 25 | | 23 | | 17 | | 22 | | 26 | |
| HALS2 sub-sample | 33 | 22 | 26 | 24 | 26 | 22 | 28 | 22 | 32 | 22 | 23 | 19 | 22 | 22 | 23 | 22 | 21 | 22 | 26 | 22 |
| **No lack** | | | | | | | | | | | | | | | | | | | | | |
| HALS1 sample | 59 | | 66 | | 64 | | 65 | | 60 | | 66 | | 66 | | 70 | | 63 | | 64 | |
| HALS2 sub-sample | 59 | 71 | 64 | 66 | 67 | 70 | 67 | 71 | 61 | 71 | 70 | 76 | 67 | 72 | 68 | 72 | 67 | 65 | 65 | 70 |
| *Base = 100%* | *626* | | *668* | | *765* | | *617* | | *574* | | *485* | | *553* | | *390* | | *410* | | *5087* | |
| | *311* | *309* | *392* | *391* | *544* | *543* | *432* | *430* | *390* | *388* | *315* | *312* | *327* | *319* | *191* | *184* | *145* | *142* | *3047* | *3018* |

**Table 15.12**  Self-assessed health at HALS1 and HALS2 in relation to perceived social support. Percentage of perceived social support group. (M/s, moderate, severe)

| | Males | | | | | | | | Females | | | | | | | |
|---|---|---|---|---|---|---|---|---|---|---|---|---|---|---|---|---|
| **Perceived social support** | No lack | M/s lack | M/s lack | No lack | M/s lack 1 & 2 | | No lack 1 & 2 | | No lack | M/s lack | M/s lack | No lack | M/s lack 1 & 2 | | No lack 1 & 2 | |
| **HALS** | 1 | 2 | 1 | 2 | 1 | 2 | 1 | 2 | 1 | 2 | 1 | 2 | 1 | 2 | 1 | 2 |
| **Age at HALS1 18-38** | | | | | | | | | | | | | | | | |
| **Self-assessed health** | | | | | | | | | | | | | | | | |
| Excellent/good | 75 | 77 | 71 | 78 | 57 | 73 | 84 | 87 | 74 | 78 | 71 | 80 | 65 | 75 | 82 | 84 |
| Difference | (+2) | | (+7) | | (+16) | | (+3) | | (+4) | | (+9) | | (+10) | | (+2) | |
| Fair/poor | 25 | 23 | 29 | 22 | 44 | 26 | 16 | 13 | 26 | 22 | 29 | 20 | 35 | 25 | 18 | 16 |
| *Base = 100%* | 148 | | 183 | | 207 | | 377 | | 167 | | 225 | | 217 | | 626 | |
| **Age at HALS1 39-59** | | | | | | | | | | | | | | | | |
| **Self-assessed health** | | | | | | | | | | | | | | | | |
| Excellent/good | 77 | 69 | 67 | 72 | 72 | 70 | 78 | 71 | 69 | 71 | 67 | 70 | 64 | 66 | 79 | 77 |
| Difference | (−8) | | (+5) | | (−2) | | (−7) | | (+2) | | (+3) | | (+2) | | (−2) | |
| Fair/poor | 23 | 31 | 33 | 28 | 28 | 30 | 22 | 29 | 31 | 29 | 33 | 30 | 36 | 34 | 21 | 23 |
| *Base = 100%* | 116 | | 174 | | 191 | | 390 | | 133 | | 206 | | 179 | | 605 | |
| **Age at HALS1 60+** | | | | | | | | | | | | | | | | |
| **Self-assessed health** | | | | | | | | | | | | | | | | |
| Excellent/good | 71 | 62 | 73 | 66 | 67 | 52 | 78 | 73 | 64 | 63 | 67 | 74 | 67 | 59 | 77 | 70 |
| Difference | (−9) | | (−7) | | (−15) | | (−5) | | (−1) | | (+7) | | (−8) | | (−7) | |
| Fair/poor | 29 | 38 | 27 | 34 | 33 | 48 | 22 | 27 | 36 | 37 | 33 | 26 | 33 | 41 | 23 | 30 |
| *Base = 100%* | 77 | | 90 | | 93 | | 224 | | 87 | | 99 | | 102 | | 350 | |

**Table 15.13  High malaise score in respondents with different levels of perceived social support (PSS) at HALS1 and HALS2. Percentage of PSS group and age group with high malaise**

| Age at HALS1 | Males | | | | | | Females | | | | | |
|---|---|---|---|---|---|---|---|---|---|---|---|---|
| | 18-38 | | 39-59 | | 60+ | | 18-38 | | 39-59 | | 60+ | |
| HALS | 1 | 2 | 1 | 2 | 1 | 2 | 1 | 2 | 1 | 2 | 1 | 2 |
| **Perceived social support** | | | | | | | | | | | | |
| No lack at HALS1 and HALS2 | 17 | 18 | 17 | 15 | 8 | 16 | 24 | 24 | 25 | 23 | 25 | 26 |
| No lack at HALS1 but mod/severe lack at HALS2 | 21 | 26 | 16 | 22 | 12 | 37 | 31 | 37 | 38 | 40 | 36 | 47 |
| Moderate/severe lack at HALS1 and HALS2 | 28 | 26 | 23 | 22 | 26 | 22 | 56 | 49 | 53 | 45 | 62 | 48 |
| *Base = 100%* | 308 | | 390 | | 224 | | 628 | | 606 | | 354 | |
| | 148 | | 116 | | 78 | | 167 | | 136 | | 87 | |
| | 208 | | 193 | | 94 | | 218 | | 181 | | 103 | |

**Table 15.14a High illness and high malaise reported by men in relation to change in perceived social support (PSS) and HALS1 socio-economic group. Percentage of PSS and HALS1 socio-economic group.**

| Age at HALS1 | 18-38 | | | | 35-59 | | | | 60+ | | | |
|---|---|---|---|---|---|---|---|---|---|---|---|---|
| Socio-economic group | Non-manual | | Manual | | Non-manual | | Manual | | Non-manual | | Manual | |
| HALS | 1 | 2 | 1 | 2 | 1 | 2 | 1 | 2 | 1 | 2 | 1 | 2 |
| **Perceived social support** | | | | | **High illness** | | | | | | | |
| No lack HALS1 but some lack HALS2 | 13 | 11 | 14 | 13 | 14 | 9 | 18 | 32 | 15 | 21 | 23 | 38 |
| Some lack HALS1 but no lack HALS2 | 9 | 15 | 15 | 15 | 11 | 19 | 26 | 34 | 29 | 37 | 32 | 27 |
| Some lack HALS1 and HALS2 | 12 | 14 | 12 | 20 | 11 | 26 | 27 | 28 | 16 | 28 | 30 | 38 |
| No lack HALS1 and HALS2 | 11 | 15 | 11 | 13 | 11 | 16 | 16 | 24 | 19 | 24 | 19 | 23 |
| | | | | | **High Malaise** | | | | | | | |
| No lack HALS1 but some lack HALS2 | 24 | 22 | 18 | 29 | 20 | 20 | 12 | 23 | 5 | 21 | 18 | 28 |
| Some lack HALS1 but no lack HALS2 | 33 | 26 | 29 | 14 | 20 | 27 | 34 | 35 | 14 | 20 | 18 | 16 |
| Some lack HALS1 and HALS2 | 27 | 21 | 27 | 27 | 21 | 19 | 24 | 24 | 16 | 15 | 31 | 25 |
| No lack HALS1 and HALS2 | 16 | 18 | 18 | 19 | 16 | 13 | 18 | 18 | 8 | 13 | 7 | 18 |
| *Base = 100%* | 63 | | 80 | | 51 | | 65 | | 39 | | 39 | |
| | 66 | | 116 | | 83 | | 91 | | 35 | | 56 | |
| | 73 | | 131 | | 81 | | 112 | | 32 | | 61 | |
| | 188 | | 185 | | 184 | | 205 | | 85 | | 137 | |

**Table 15.14b** **High illness and high malaise reported by women at HALS2 in relation to change in perceived social support (PSS) and HALS1 socio-economic group. Percentage of PSS and HALS1 socio-economic group**

| Age at HALS1 | 18-38 | | | | 35-59 | | | | 60+ | | | |
|---|---|---|---|---|---|---|---|---|---|---|---|---|
| Socio-economic group | Non-manual | | Manual | | Non-manual | | Manual | | Non-manual | | Manual | |
| HALS | 1 | 2 | 1 | 2 | 1 | 2 | 1 | 2 | 1 | 2 | 1 | 2 |
| **Perceived social support** | | | | | **High illness** | | | | | | | |
| No lack HALS1 but some lack HALS2 | 19 | 22 | 27 | 28 | 26 | 26 | 54 | 45 | 24 | 37 | 40 | 57 |
| Some lack HALS1 but no lack HALS2 | 19 | 23 | 27 | 19 | 18 | 26 | 29 | 35 | 20 | 34 | 46 | 53 |
| Some lack HALS1 and HALS2 | 33 | 30 | 34 | 33 | 32 | 37 | 36 | 52 | 42 | 60 | 39 | 57 |
| No lack HALS1 and HALS2 | 17 | 15 | 19 | 19 | 23 | 23 | 31 | 34 | 26 | 32 | 34 | 38 |
| | | | | | **High Malaise** | | | | | | | |
| No lack HALS1 but some lack HALS2 | 18 | 34 | 40 | 38 | 32 | 28 | 42 | 51 | 24 | 39 | 47 | 57 |
| Some lack HALS1 but no lack HALS2 | 31 | 33 | 37 | 34 | 34 | 36 | 47 | 41 | 27 | 16 | 42 | 42 |
| Some lack HALS1 and HALS2 | 53 | 55 | 58 | 45 | 43 | 38 | 51 | 53 | 24 | 44 | 50 | 51 |
| No lack HALS1 and HALS2 | 24 | 21 | 24 | 28 | 19 | 19 | 33 | 29 | 23 | 20 | 27 | 30 |
| *Base = 100%* | 72 | | 94 | | 65 | | 71 | | 41 | | 44 | |
| | 109 | | 113 | | 87 | | 115 | | 44 | | 55 | |
| | 78 | | 137 | | 84 | | 94 | | 50 | | 51 | |
| | 314 | | 307 | | 318 | | 382 | | 132 | | 216 | |

**Table 15.15** Relationship between reporting a life event at HALS2 as having occurred in the past year and perceived social support (PSS) at HALS1. Percentage of PSS and age group.

| Perceived social support at HALS1 | Severe lack | Moder. lack | No lack | Severe lack | Moder. lack | No lack | Severe lack | Moder. lack | No lack |
|---|---|---|---|---|---|---|---|---|---|
| Age at HALS1 | | 18-38 | | | 39-59 | | | 60+ | |
| **Males** | | | | | | | | | |
| Disagreement with friend/relative/s | 13 | 13 | 10 | 9 | 8 | 5 | 4 | 3 | 2 |
| Disagreement with partner/spouse | 11 | 9 | 7 | 3 | 4 | 2 | 9 | 1 | 0 |
| Lost contact with friend/relative/s | 12 | 13 | 11 | 6 | 6 | 6 | 11 | 5 | 5 |
| Any difficulty with children | 22 | 20 | 15 | 20 | 19 | 13 | 22 | 9 | 6 |
| *Base = 100%* | *106* | *228* | *527* | *94* | *276* | *510* | *57* | *133* | *304* |
| | *76* | *207* | *415* | *67* | *234* | *460* | *22* | *96* | *229* |
| | *106* | *228* | *527* | *94* | *276* | *510* | *57* | *133* | *304* |
| | *65* | *195* | *385* | *74* | *248* | *440* | *36* | *102* | *257* |
| **Females** | | | | | | | | | |
| Disagreement with friend/relative/s | 28 | 18 | 12 | 8 | 10 | 7 | 6 | 3 | 2 |
| Disagreement with partner/spouse | 19 | 12 | 7 | 13 | 6 | 5 | 5 | 2 | 2 |
| Lost contact with friend/relative/s | 17 | 11 | 10 | 9 | 9 | 5 | 7 | 6 | 3 |
| Any difficulty with children | 29 | 28 | 24 | 25 | 23 | 21 | 16 | 9 | 9 |
| *Base = 100%* | *103* | *343* | *801* | *74* | *318* | *745* | *71* | *145* | *447* |
| | *70* | *261* | *665* | *45* | *240* | *607* | *20* | *44* | *206* |
| | *103* | *343* | *801* | *74* | *318* | *745* | *71* | *145* | *447* |
| | *82* | *262* | *664* | *61* | *283* | *683* | *38* | *107* | *387* |

**Table 15.16** Percentage at HALS2 reporting divorce or living apart during last seven years by perceived social support at HALS1

| | Males | | Females | | | Base = 100% | | |
|---|---|---|---|---|---|---|---|---|
| Age at HALS1 | 18-38 | 39-59 | 18-38 | 39-59 | | | | |
| **Perceived social support at HALS1** | | | | | | | | |
| Severe lack | 18 | 7 | 26 | 8 | *83* | *74* | *86* | *49* |
| Moderate lack | 18 | 5 | 18 | 6 | *230* | *250* | *293* | *270* |
| No lack | 10 | 3 | 12 | 4 | *444* | *480* | *730* | *665* |

**Table 15.17    Percentage at HALS2 reporting ongoing general satisfaction with family and/or 'life' by perceived social support at HALS1**

| Age at HALS1 | 18-38 | | 39-59 | | 60+ | | Base = 100% | | | | | |
|---|---|---|---|---|---|---|---|---|---|---|---|---|
| | Males | Females | Males | Females | Males | Females | | | | | | |
| **Perceived social support at HALS1** | | | | | | | | | | | | |
| Severe lack | 16 | 16 | 7 | 5 | 5 | 14 | 106 | 103 | 94 | 74 | 57 | 71 |
| Moderate lack | 14 | 13 | 9 | 13 | 8 | 8 | 288 | 343 | 276 | 318 | 133 | 145 |
| No lack | 12 | 12 | 9 | 16 | 12 | 12 | 527 | 801 | 510 | 745 | 304 | 447 |

# CHANGING VIEWS ON HEALTH AND ILL-HEALTH | 16

## Virginia J Swain

This chapter deals specifically with the changing views about health and ill-health of the respondents who took part in the first Health and Lifestyle Survey in 1984/5 and the second Survey conducted during 1991/2. It is concerned primarily with describing the change which has occurred between HALS1 and HALS2 in reported health related lifestyle or circumstances and respondents' ideas about disease aetiology. The tables focus on a selection of activities which subjects reported doing or which they would like to do to maintain good health, whether or not they consider their life to be more healthy than seven years ago, (as distinct from their health actually being better or worse, which is discussed in Chapter 4) and changing beliefs about the principal causes of specific diseases.

Understanding how attitudes and beliefs about health, ill-health and disease processes are formed, and their subsequent transfer into 'healthy' or 'unhealthy' behaviour, is an important concern for health promotion workers and the implementation of health education and effective programmes of preventive medicine. The interaction between these different factors in people's lives is sometimes neither obvious nor straight forward. For the purposes of this chapter therefore, the main variables against which the measures of 'attitude' and 'belief' are set are demographic and thus act as a source of initial information and a basis for future study.

## Changing Behaviour

The respondents were asked at HALS2 whether they did anything to keep healthy or to improve their health. The format of the question was the same for HALS2 as it was for HALS1, and it was asked early in the interview to avoid influence from later, more specific questions about the respondents' dietary, exercise, drinking or smoking habits.

Table 16.1 shows the percentage of respondents in the full HALS1 sample who reported not doing anything to improve their health or to keep healthy and those who reported between one and three activities. The values for the HALS2 sub-sample, (respondents who were subsequently re-interviewed at HALS2), at HALS1, are shown alongside their HALS2 values. Overall there has been a slight loss from the sample between HALS1 and HALS2 of those subjects who reported not doing anything or only doing one thing to improve health, so that slightly more respondents who claimed to do two or three things were interviewed at HALS2. In almost all age groups there has been an increase from HALS1 to HALS2 in the percentages reporting two or three activities to keep healthy or to improve their health, particularly marked in the older age groups, and therefore a decrease in those who report doing nothing or only one activity.

Although some respondents reported a change in their socio-economic status between HALS1 and HALS2 (Chapter 2), as in the rest of the book, socio-economic status at HALS1 has been employed (except for Table 16.6), for simplicity. Overall, fewer men and women in the manual socio-economic group reported doing two or more items both at HALS1 and HALS2 compared with the non-manual group (Table 16.2). There has been an increase, among young men in the non-manual group, in the proportions claiming to do three things to improve health. Young men in manual occupations, on the other hand, have not increased their health promoting activities over the seven years. However, among the oldest men in the manual group, there was an 8% increase in the proportions reporting three health-promoting activities compared to a 1% drop in those who were in the non-manual occupations. In contrast to the young men, women aged 18 to 59 and in the manual group at HALS1, have shown a larger percentage rise in claiming to do three activities to keep healthy than their non-manual counterparts.

There has been some change between HALS1 and HALS2 in the type of behaviours respondents report to maintain or improve health (Table 16.3). The most notable changes have occurred in diet for men, and physical activities for both sexes. Physical activity was the most favoured answer for men at HALS1 and HALS2 but more men at all ages, except between 67 and 73, now mention diet as a means of keeping healthy. Women show no clear overall increase; the biggest rise in claiming diet to be important has occurred for women between the ages of 39 and 45 and between 53 and 59. However, women are still more likely than men to mention diet. The changes which have occurred in the reporting of different types of physical activities, notably walking, sport and general exercise, include an 8% overall increase in the numbers of men and women mentioning walking. Using HALS1 ages, women reported walking more frequently at HALS2 for all ages up to 66 years and men between the ages of 25 and 73 were more likely to report it. A similar rise in reporting is also evident for general exercise but the percentage reporting taking part in sport has dropped for men between the ages of 18 and 38 whilst remaining fairly constant in other age groups for men and most age groups for women. 'Job or work' was reported less frequently by all men as a means of promoting health except for those aged between 25 and 31 at HALS1 but was mentioned more often by all women up to retirement age.

Table 16.4 demonstrates both the difference

between the non-manual and manual socio-economic groups and the change in the items of health promoting behaviour mentioned from HALS1 to HALS2. At HALS1, most items were more likely to be mentioned by men and women in the non-manual than in the manual group, with 'walking' showing the greatest similarity in reporting between socio-economic groups for all but the oldest subjects. The only exception to this at HALS1 was for reporting of 'job or work' which was claimed to be health promoting by twice as many men in manual occupations, aged 39 and above, than in the equivalent non-manual group. The change in reporting between HALS1 and HALS2 has tended to follow the same pattern for both socio-economic groups with a slightly higher proportion of men who were in the non-manual group, in the two youngest age bands, reporting general exercise, walking and diet to promote health and a bigger fall being evident for the men who were in the manual group, and over 39 years of age, saying their job or work kept them healthy. A slightly different pattern is apparent for women. Women aged between 18 and 59 and in the manual group at HALS1, showed a bigger increase in reporting general exercise by HALS2 compared with the women who were in the non-manual group, similarly, a higher proportion of the youngest women who were in the manual group reported taking part in sporting activity at HALS2 whereas a smaller percentage of women who were in the non-manual group did so.

Respondents were asked if there were 'things you would like to do to keep or improve health – but don't do'. Table 16.5 shows that a high percentage of respondents at HALS1 and HALS2 felt they would like to do more sport or exercise; a slightly higher percentage of women, between the ages of 25 and 59 at HALS1, reported sport or exercise at HALS2 but only the youngest group of men mentioned it more often at HALS2 than at HALS1. For both men and women in the younger groups a slightly higher percentage reported a desire to improve their diet or lose weight and a higher proportion of women, up to the age of 45, expressed a desire to give up smoking or reduce the amount of cigarettes they smoked.

Figure 16.1 shows the overlap between the respondents' claims to do things to keep healthy and their desire (or otherwise) to do other things at

**Figure 16.1    Proportion of men and women at HALS1 and HALS2 claiming to do and/or wanting to do things to keep healthy in HALS1 non-manual and manual socio-economic groups**

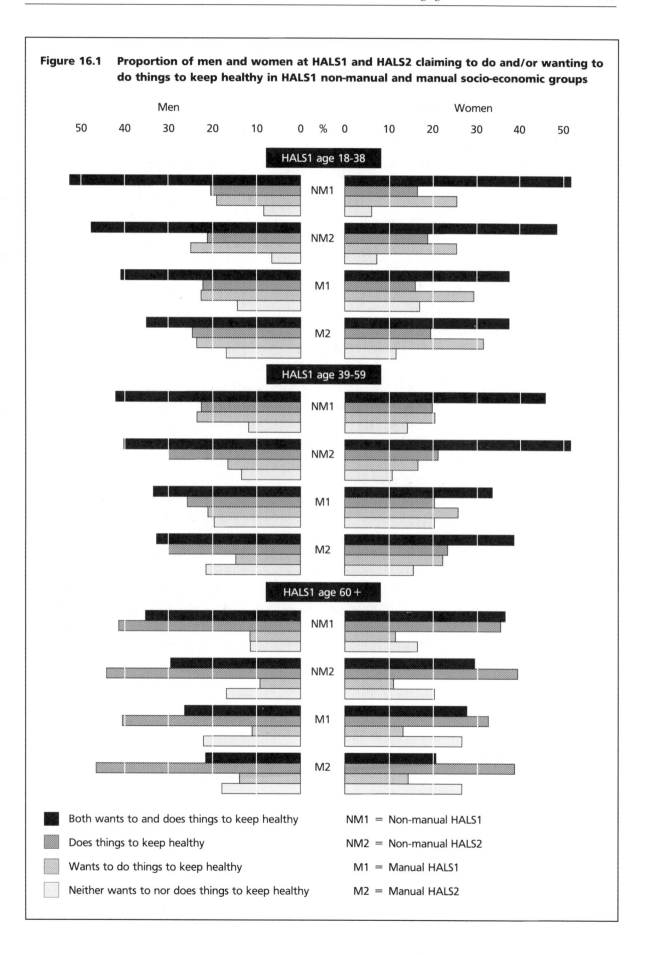

Men                                                                                          Women

50    40    30    20    10    0    %    0    10    20    30    40    50

HALS1 age 18-38

HALS1 age 39-59

HALS1 age 60 +

NM1
NM2
M1
M2

■  Both wants to and does things to keep healthy        NM1 = Non-manual HALS1

▨  Does things to keep healthy                          NM2 = Non-manual HALS2

▨  Wants to do things to keep healthy                    M1 = Manual HALS1

□  Neither wants to nor does things to keep healthy      M2 = Manual HALS2

HALS1 and HALS2. At one extreme there are respondents who neither do, nor wish to do, anything and at the other, individuals who both claim to do things to maintain health and mention other things they would like to do – but do not do. Non-manual respondents at both Surveys are more likely to say they do some things and would like to do others, and the proportion of these groups are smaller in the oldest respondents. A higher proportion of older than younger respondents and manual than non-manual respondents neither 'do nor want to do things to keep them healthy'.

Two separate questions in the schedule asked respondents, 'is there is any way in which your life has become more healthy/less healthy in the last seven years'? If they answered 'yes' to either question they were asked to explain fully, this was recorded verbatim by the interviewer and coded in-house. Table 16.6 to Table 16.9 consider the respondents' own views about whether they believe their life has become more healthy or less healthy during the last seven years, and the ways in which this has occurred. Only respondents who identified change are included, subjects who did not consider their life to be any more healthy or less healthy are omitted from the tables.

Of the men, only those in the youngest age group were more likely to say that their life was more healthy compared to seven years ago than to say it was less healthy. From the HALS2 age of 32 onwards a greater proportion reported life to be less healthy. Women show three upward 'steps' in the percentage reporting life to be less healthy, the first occurring in the age band 39 to 45 the next at 53 to 59 and the last one occurring at 74 to 80. Men show a greater consistency in reporting life to be less healthy between the ages of 25 and 59, with only two main changes occurring at the later ages of 60 to 66 and at 81 and over. Both men and women show a sudden large fall in the percentage reporting life to be more healthy, in men from the HALS2 age of 74 onwards and for women at the earlier age of 67. A larger percentage of women in the two youngest age groups claimed their life to be more healthy rather than less healthy, but from the age of 74 a much greater proportion of women identify their life as less healthy when compared to men. Using HALS2 socio-economic groups, men and women in non-manual

groups were more likely to report life as being more healthy than were individuals in manual groups, yet a higher proportion of the youngest group of men and women in non-manual classes also reported their life as less healthy.

It is well recognised that there is a relationship between poverty and ill-health (Quick and Wilkinson 1991). Blaxter (1990) also analysed the association between household income and self-assessed health, attitudes, behaviour and beliefs about causes of specific diseases using the HALS1 data. Table 16.7 shows respondents' claims that their life has become more healthy or less healthy in the last seven years against monthly household income as reported at HALS2 (see Appendix A for a description of household income). In the youngest age group household income and reporting life to be more healthy are positively associated for both men and women. Other age groups show less clear trends.

At HALS1 and HALS2 respondents were asked whether they were currently suffering with any long-standing illness, disability or infirmity. Verbatim answers were coded in-house about the type of condition or disease suffered (see Chapter 4). Table 16.8 compares disease status groups at HALS1 and HALS2 against their likelihood of reporting life to be more healthy or less healthy. There does not appear to be any clear trend in reporting life to be more healthy according to disease status at HALS1 or HALS2. This may indicate that an individual's assessment of their life as being more healthy than seven years ago is not necessarily dependent on having a long-standing illness or developing a disease within the seven year time-span, but, as is demonstrated further on in the chapter, many respondents, particularly older subjects, do associate the improvement of a condition with their life being more healthy. Differences are more evident, however, in those who reported life to be less healthy. It is perhaps not surprising that men and women aged between 18 and 59 at HALS1, who have developed a chronic illness since the first Survey, at HALS1, are more likely to report life to be less healthy than those who were suffering with chronic ill-health on both occasions. For the oldest subjects, a greater percentage of those with continuing ill-health were most likely to report their life as less healthy.

Having considered differences between age, sex,

socio-economic group, household income and disease status in respondents who reported their life to be more or less healthy in the last seven years, Table 16.9 shows some of the reasons given by subjects in explaining why their lives have become more, or less, healthy. Women in all age groups were more likely than men to mention the improvement of a condition or improved dietary habits as being beneficial. In the youngest age group a higher percentage of women reported taking more exercise. Men, however, were more likely to report cutting down or stopping smoking and also, in the 25-45 age group at HALS2, were more likely to report starting to smoke or increasing the number of cigarettes smoked as a reason why their life was less healthy. 40% of men and 45% of women, aged over 67 at HALS2, mentioned the improvement of a condition as being a beneficial influence on their life since 1984/5, but even more mention the worsening of a condition as a reason for their life being less healthy. Nearly a third of men aged 46 to 66, and 28% of men aged 67 and over said that changing their job or retiring had made their life more healthy.

## Causes of Diseases

Respondents were asked to identify possible causes for a number of conditions or diseases, with known lifestyle or behavioural components in their aetiology, at HALS1 and HALS2. The format of the questions was open-ended so that individual views could be recorded without prompted causes being offered by the interviewer. Answers were coded by the interviewer into a coding scheme in the questionnaire (see Appendix C), 'other' answers were recorded verbatim and coded in-house.

Table 16.10 illustrates some of the changes which have occurred in the most frequently suggested causes associated with age, sex and socio-economic classification for all eleven conditions asked about in the schedule. Overall at HALS2, fewer subjects answered 'don't know' when asked about the cause of specified diseases, except for those respondents, aged over 60 at HALS1, who were still more likely to be unable to suggest a cause of a disease. Many more respondents are now identifying diet as a cause of many of the diseases and are more aware of the relationship between aspects of the diet and particular conditions. For example; although 'other bad diet'

was reported more frequently by all groups of subjects, more respondents in all age groups and both socio-economic groups, except the oldest men in the non-manual group, also mentioned a diet low in fibre or roughage as a cause of haemorrhoids at HALS2. When asked about the causes of obesity, overeating, per se, became a less popular answer by men in non-manual groups and by some women in both socio-economic groups, with greater emphasis being placed at HALS2 than HALS1, by both occupational groups, on eating 'wrong' foods. Heredity or family has been offered more frequently at HALS2 than it was at HALS1 as a cause for many diseases. An increased percentage of men and women below HALS1 age 60 attributed worry, tension or stress as a cause of stomach ulcers at HALS2, but in addition, more subjects identified dietary habits, alcohol and smoking as possible causes. Other beliefs which were reported by only a few respondents at the first Survey but which have become more prominent at HALS2 are infection or virus as a cause of liver trouble and passive smoking as a cause of lung cancer.

Table 16.11 lists the most popular ideas offered at HALS2 about the causes of heart problems in relation to whether or not the respondent reported ever having suffered with angina or a heart attack. As has been found in other studies (Cox et al. 1987), individuals who reported having suffered from heart trouble at some time in the past were often less likely to offer possible relevant causes which have a behavioural component such as smoking, diet or lack of exercise, and were more likely to attribute more external causes such as overwork or worry, tension and stress. Moreover, men in both age groups and women in the youngest group who reported having suffered with heart problems were more likely to say they did not know what caused heart trouble.

## Summary

Differences are still obvious between the sexes and between socio-economic groups in many areas of health behaviour, attitudes and beliefs. Women place a greater emphasis than men on social, environmental and dietary factors as influences on health, although a higher proportion of men appear to be aware of the beneficial effects of diet at HALS2 when compared to

HALS1. Although an increased proportion of men and women in both socio-economic groups are reporting taking part in more health promoting activity, respondents who were in non-manual groups at HALS1 still tend to report doing more to maintain their health at both Surveys than their counterparts in manual groups.

It is evident that respondents at HALS2 have assimilated many of the health messages which have been most actively disseminated during the last seven years. More individuals tend to report doing more exercise or changing their diet, implying that they recognise the potential beneficial effects in maintaining good health. Dietary habits have featured strongly both in actual changes which have occurred (Chapter 11) and in an increasing recognition of their role in the aetiology of disease.

### References

Blaxter M. (1990), Health and Lifestyles, London/New York: Routledge.

Cox BD et al. (1987), Health and Lifestyle Survey, Cambridge: Health Promotion Research Trust.

Quick A, and Wilkinson RG. (1991), Income and Health, London: Socialist Health Association.

**Table 16.1    Change in number of activities undertaken to maintain or improve health by men in full HALS1 sample and HALS2 sub-sample at HALS1 and HALS2. Percentage of age group**

| HALS1 age → / HALS2 age → | 18-24 / 25-31 | 25-31 / 32-38 | 32-38 / 39-45 | 39-45 / 46-52 | 46-52 / 53-59 | 53-59 / 60-66 | 60-66 / 67-73 | 67-73 / 73-80 | 74+ / 81+ | All / All |
|---|---|---|---|---|---|---|---|---|---|---|
| **Number of things done to keep healthy** | | | | | | | | | | |
| **Men** | | | | | | | | | | |
| **None** | | | | | | | | | | |
| HALS1 | 34 | 31 | 36 | 38 | 41 | 40 | 32 | 28 | 32 | 35 |
| HALS2 sub-sample | 33 33 | 33 39 | 33 38 | 37 36 | 39 36 | 39 29 | 31 23 | 26 34 | 28 42 | 34 34 |
| **One** | | | | | | | | | | |
| HALS1 | 31 | 31 | 29 | 27 | 28 | 24 | 25 | 26 | 27 | 28 |
| HALS2 sub-sample | 30 29 | 30 25 | 32 24 | 27 21 | 26 19 | 22 20 | 23 17 | 23 16 | 26 18 | 27 22 |
| **Two** | | | | | | | | | | |
| HALS1 | 23 | 24 | 19 | 22 | 22 | 17 | 20 | 28 | 22 | 22 |
| HALS2 sub-sample | 25 25 | 25 21 | 20 19 | 23 22 | 23 24 | 18 23 | 22 31 | 31 23 | 23 19 | 23 23 |
| **Three (maximum)** | | | | | | | | | | |
| HALS1 | 12 | 15 | 16 | 14 | 10 | 20 | 23 | 18 | 20 | 16 |
| HALS2 sub-sample | 12 13 | 13 15 | 15 19 | 13 22 | 12 22 | 22 27 | 24 30 | 20 28 | 23 21 | 16 22 |
| *Base = 100%* | *534* | *489* | *572* | *474* | *419* | *417* | *411* | *314* | *273* | *3903* |
| | *299 299* | *241 241* | *382 382* | *324 324* | *280 280* | *278 278* | *259 259* | *148 148* | *88 88* | *2299 2299* |
| **Women** | | | | | | | | | | |
| **None** | | | | | | | | | | |
| HALS1 | 42 | 41 | 39 | 41 | 41 | 42 | 35 | 39 | 45 | 41 |
| HALS2 sub-sample | 41 39 | 39 37 | 40 39 | 39 32 | 41 33 | 40 33 | 30 30 | 36 38 | 43 51 | 39 36 |
| **One** | | | | | | | | | | |
| HALS1 | 24 | 23 | 25 | 21 | 22 | 25 | 23 | 24 | 26 | 24 |
| HALS2 sub-sample | 26 25 | 25 20 | 24 19 | 22 19 | 21 18 | 27 18 | 23 21 | 22 16 | 22 19 | 24 20 |
| **Two** | | | | | | | | | | |
| HALS1 | 21 | 22 | 20 | 20 | 21 | 19 | 22 | 18 | 16 | 20 |
| HALS2 sub-sample | 22 22 | 23 26 | 19 22 | 21 25 | 22 21 | 18 25 | 24 26 | 21 23 | 19 19 | 21 23 |
| **Three (maximum)** | | | | | | | | | | |
| HALS1 | 13 | 14 | 16 | 18 | 17 | 14 | 19 | 19 | 13 | 16 |
| HALS2 sub-sample | 11 15 | 13 18 | 17 20 | 19 24 | 17 29 | 14 24 | 24 23 | 22 23 | 16 11 | 17 21 |
| *Base = 100%* | *626* | *672* | *766* | *618* | *576* | *486* | *553* | *390* | *408* | *5095* |
| | *311 311* | *394 394* | *545 545* | *432 432* | *391 390* | *315 315* | *327 327* | *190 190* | *144 144* | *3049 3048* |

**Table 16.2**  **Socio-economic variations in number of activities undertaken to maintain or improve health reported at HALS1 and HALS2. Percentage of non-manual and manual groups**

| HALS1 age and SEG | 18-38 | | | | 39-59 | | | | 60+ | | | |
| | Non-manual | | Manual | | Non-manual | | Manual | | Non-manual | | Manual | |
| HALS | 1 | 2 | 1 | 2 | 1 | 2 | 1 | 2 | 1 | 2 | 1 | 2 |
|---|---|---|---|---|---|---|---|---|---|---|---|---|
| **Number of things done to keep healthy** | | | | | | **Males** | | | | | | |
| None | 28 | 31 | 37 | 40 | 35 | 29 | 41 | 37 | 24 | 26 | 33 | 31 |
| One | 29 | 24 | 32 | 27 | 22 | 20 | 28 | 20 | 21 | 13 | 25 | 19 |
| Two | 25 | 21 | 20 | 21 | 25 | 23 | 18 | 23 | 27 | 33 | 23 | 22 |
| Three (maximum) | 18 | 24 | 11 | 11 | 18 | 28 | 13 | 20 | 29 | 28 | 19 | 27 |
| | | | | | | **Females** | | | | | | |
| None | 32 | 33 | 46 | 43 | 34 | 27 | 46 | 37 | 28 | 31 | 40 | 41 |
| One | 25 | 21 | 25 | 20 | 23 | 18 | 23 | 19 | 25 | 15 | 21 | 22 |
| Two | 24 | 25 | 18 | 22 | 21 | 26 | 20 | 21 | 20 | 27 | 22 | 21 |
| Three (maximum) | 20 | 21 | 10 | 15 | 22 | 29 | 11 | 22 | 27 | 27 | 17 | 16 |
| *Base = 100%* | 379 | | 515 | | 405 | | 476 | | 196 | | 296 | |
| | 572 | | 657 | | 558 | | 567 | | 274 | | 378 | |

**Table 16.3** **Items volunteered as 'the most important things you do to keep or improve health' at HALS1 and HALS2 (up to 3 items allowed per respondent). Percentage of age group**

| Age at HALS1 | 18-24 | | 25-31 | | 32-38 | | 39-45 | | 46-52 | | 53-59 | | 60-66 | | 67-73 | | 74+ | | All | |
| HALS | 1 | 2 | 1 | 2 | 1 | 2 | 1 | 2 | 1 | 2 | 1 | 2 | 1 | 2 | 1 | 2 | 1 | 2 | 1 | 2 |
|---|---|---|---|---|---|---|---|---|---|---|---|---|---|---|---|---|---|---|---|---|
| **Things done to keep healthy** | | | | | | | **Males** | | | | | | | | | | | | | |
| Dietary habits | 8 | 17 | 20 | 17 | 20 | 22 | 16 | 23 | 15 | 23 | 20 | 19 | 15 | 17 | 16 | 16 | 11 | 14 | 16 | 20 |
| Stopped/ reduced smoking | 3 | 4 | 5 | 3 | 5 | 5 | 4 | 2 | 3 | 6 | 9 | 4 | 5 | 5 | 6 | 3 | 1 | 3 | 5 | 4 |
| Walking | 10 | 10 | 12 | 15 | 11 | 20 | 20 | 28 | 19 | 30 | 23 | 44 | 34 | 43 | 28 | 35 | 36 | 27 | 19 | 27 |
| Sport | 41 | 36 | 36 | 27 | 32 | 20 | 20 | 21 | 18 | 19 | 11 | 11 | 11 | 16 | 6 | 5 | 5 | 3 | 23 | 20 |
| General exercise | 32 | 31 | 23 | 27 | 24 | 31 | 20 | 25 | 16 | 17 | 14 | 23 | 19 | 24 | 13 | 18 | 11 | 14 | 20 | 25 |
| Job/work | 12 | 11 | 9 | 12 | 11 | 8 | 12 | 10 | 13 | 8 | 13 | 8 | 10 | 9 | 9 | 2 | 6 | 0 | 11 | 9 |
| Take medicine | (1) | 0 | 2 | (1) | 0 | (1) | 0 | (3) | 2 | 3 | 1 | 4 | 3 | 2 | 2 | 2 | 2 | 6 | 1 | 2 |
| | | | | | | | **Females** | | | | | | | | | | | | | |
| Dietary habits | 25 | 29 | 34 | 34 | 32 | 31 | 34 | 40 | 34 | 36 | 25 | 30 | 30 | 28 | 23 | 26 | 19 | 14 | 30 | 31 |
| Stopped/ reduced smoking | 2 | 2 | 3 | 3 | 2 | 3 | 4 | 2 | 4 | 3 | 2 | 3 | 5 | 1 | 1 | 1 | 1 | 0 | 3 | 2 |
| Walking | 11 | 18 | 15 | 24 | 16 | 22 | 19 | 29 | 21 | 32 | 22 | 32 | 31 | 36 | 29 | 29 | 18 | 15 | 19 | 27 |
| Sport | 21 | 20 | 15 | 15 | 15 | 16 | 11 | 13 | 7 | 9 | 6 | 10 | 7 | 7 | 8 | 2 | 2 | 2 | 11 | 12 |
| General exercise | 29 | 32 | 25 | 33 | 27 | 28 | 24 | 30 | 16 | 22 | 13 | 21 | 13 | 17 | 12 | 14 | 10 | 7 | 21 | 25 |
| Job/work | 3 | 4 | 4 | 5 | 3 | 5 | 5 | 7 | 6 | 10 | 9 | 6 | 6 | 4 | 3 | 3 | 2 | 1 | 5 | 6 |
| Take medicine | 2 | (1) | 1 | (3) | 1 | (3) | 1 | 1 | 2 | 4 | 4 | 5 | 4 | 5 | 4 | 7 | 3 | 6 | 2 | 3 |
| Base = 100% | 299 | | 241 | | 382 | | 324 | | 280 | | 278 | | 259 | | 148 | | 88 | | 2299 | |
| | 311 | | 394 | | 545 | | 432 | | 391 | | 315 | | 327 | | 190 | | 144 | | 3049 | |

**Table 16.4** **Percentage volunteering activities undertaken to maintain or improve health at HALS1 and HALS2 by HALS1 socio-economic groups (SEG)**

| HALS1 age | 18-38 | | | | 39-59 | | | | 60+ | | | |
| HALS1 SEG | Non-manual | | Manual | | Non-manual | | Manual | | Non-manual | | Manual | |
| HALS | 1 | 2 | 1 | 2 | 1 | 2 | 1 | 2 | 1 | 2 | 1 | 2 |
|---|---|---|---|---|---|---|---|---|---|---|---|---|
| **Things done to keep healthy** | | | | | **Males** | | | | | | | |
| Dietary habits | 23 | 29 | 11 | 13 | 21 | 28 | 13 | 17 | 19 | 19 | 11 | 14 |
| Walking | 11 | 17 | 12 | 15 | 20 | 35 | 21 | 33 | 39 | 41 | 28 | 36 |
| Sport | 42 | 32 | 32 | 24 | 23 | 24 | 10 | 12 | 12 | 13 | 6 | 9 |
| General exercise | 29 | 36 | 23 | 26 | 19 | 27 | 15 | 18 | 21 | 26 | 12 | 17 |
| Job/work | 9 | 7 | 13 | 12 | 8 | 7 | 16 | 11 | 5 | 4 | 12 | 6 |
| Reduced/stopped smoking | 5 | 5 | 4 | 3 | 5 | 4 | 5 | 4 | 5 | 6 | 4 | 3 |
| | | | | | **Females** | | | | | | | |
| Dietary habits | 36 | 37 | 27 | 26 | 37 | 38 | 26 | 33 | 32 | 28 | 20 | 21 |
| Walking | 15 | 24 | 14 | 20 | 21 | 34 | 20 | 29 | 31 | 35 | 25 | 26 |
| Sport | 23 | 19 | 11 | 14 | 11 | 15 | 7 | 7 | 8 | 7 | 3 | 3 |
| General exercise | 33 | 33 | 22 | 29 | 23 | 29 | 13 | 21 | 13 | 17 | 12 | 12 |
| Job/work | 4 | 4 | 2 | 5 | 7 | 9 | 6 | 7 | 4 | 4 | 5 | 2 |
| Reduced/stopped smoking | 3 | 3 | 2 | 3 | 4 | 2 | 2 | 3 | 2 | 1 | 3 | 1 |
| *Base = 100%* | 379 | | 515 | | 405 | | 476 | | 196 | | 296 | |
| | 572 | | 657 | | 558 | | 567 | | 274 | | 378 | |

**Table 16.5** **Respondents reporting 'things would like to do to improve health – but don't do' at HALS1 and HALS2. Percentage of age group**

| HALS1 age | 18-24 | | 25-31 | | 32-38 | | 39-45 | | 46-52 | | 53-59 | | 60-66 | | 67-73 | | 74+ | | All | |
|---|---|---|---|---|---|---|---|---|---|---|---|---|---|---|---|---|---|---|---|---|
| HALS | 1 | 2 | 1 | 2 | 1 | 2 | 1 | 2 | 1 | 2 | 1 | 2 | 1 | 2 | 1 | 2 | 1 | 2 | 1 | 2 |
| **Things would like to do** | | | | | | | | | | | **Males** | | | | | | | | | |
| More sport/ exercise | 52 | 54 | 56 | 56 | 54 | 51 | 52 | 45 | 40 | 40 | 37 | 32 | 29 | 27 | 26 | 23 | 22 | 21 | 44 | 42 |
| Improve diet | 4 | 7 | 4 | 7 | 7 | 6 | 5 | 4 | 4 | 1 | 3 | 2 | 2 | (1) | 0 | 1 | 0 | 0 | 4 | 4 |
| Lose weight | 1 | 2 | 2 | 2 | 4 | 6 | 2 | 4 | 3 | 3 | 2 | 3 | 2 | 1 | 0 | 1 | 0 | 0 | 2 | 3 |
| Reduce/give up smoking | 7 | 5 | 9 | 8 | 8 | 9 | 5 | 6 | 8 | 7 | 7 | 5 | 4 | 4 | 1 | 5 | 5 | 2 | 6 | 6 |
| | | | | | | | | | | | **Females** | | | | | | | | | |
| More sport/ exercise | 62 | 58 | 53 | 54 | 59 | 60 | 48 | 55 | 43 | 51 | 40 | 42 | 35 | 28 | 26 | 28 | 16 | 16 | 46 | 48 |
| Improve diet | 10 | 11 | 6 | 7 | 6 | 10 | 7 | 5 | 6 | 3 | 5 | 3 | 2 | 2 | 3 | 2 | 1 | 1 | 6 | 6 |
| Lose weight | 4 | 6 | 5 | 7 | 7 | 7 | 6 | 8 | 7 | 7 | 6 | 4 | 4 | 3 | 2 | 1 | 2 | 0 | 5 | 6 |
| Reduce/give up smoking | 5 | 8 | 8 | 9 | 8 | 11 | 7 | 9 | 6 | 6 | 4 | 4 | 2 | 2 | 1 | 0 | 0 | 0 | 5 | 7 |
| *Base = 100%* | *291* | | *241* | | *383* | | *324* | | *280* | | *278* | | *259* | | *148* | | *88* | | *2300* | |
| | *311* | | *394* | | *545* | | *432* | | *391* | | *315* | | *327* | | *191* | | *146* | | *3052* | |

**Table 16.6** **Age and socio-economic group (SEG) variations in respondents claiming their life to be more healthy or less healthy than 7 years ago ('unchanged' omitted)**

| HALS2 age | 25-31 | 32-38 | 39-45 | 46-52 | 53-59 | 60-66 | 67-73 | 74-80 | 81+ | All |
|---|---|---|---|---|---|---|---|---|---|---|
| | | | | | Percentage of age group | | | | | |
| | | | | | **Males** | | | | | |
| More healthy | 40 | 37 | 37 | 31 | 28 | 34 | 28 | 10 | 11 | 31 |
| Less healthy | 38 | 39 | 40 | 37 | 38 | 46 | 45 | 47 | 55 | 41 |
| *Base = 100%* | *299* | *241* | *383* | *324* | *279* | *278* | *259* | *148* | *88* | *2299* |
| | | | | | **Females** | | | | | |
| More healthy | 43 | 39 | 36 | 35 | 28 | 32 | 18 | 13 | 5 | 31 |
| Less healthy | 33 | 28 | 38 | 37 | 45 | 45 | 46 | 62 | 65 | 41 |
| *Base = 100%* | *310* | *393* | *545* | *432* | *391* | *315* | *326* | *190* | *143* | *3045* |

| | Percentage of non-manual (NM) and manual (M) group | | | | | | | | | | | |
|---|---|---|---|---|---|---|---|---|---|---|---|---|
| | Males | | | | | | Females | | | | | |
| HALS2 age | 25-45 | | 46-66 | | 67+ | | 25-45 | | 46-66 | | 67+ | |
| HALS2 SEG | NM | M | NM | M | NM | M | NM | M | NM | M | NM | M |
| More healthy | 40 | 36 | 36 | 26 | 26 | 15 | 42 | 35 | 34 | 30 | 14 | 13 |
| Less healthy | 48 | 30 | 39 | 42 | 47 | 48 | 38 | 29 | 41 | 43 | 52 | 57 |
| *Base = 100%* | *451* | *466* | *397* | *485* | *194* | *298* | *604* | *638* | *579* | *553* | *289* | *365* |

**Table 16.7** **Respondents claiming their life to be more healthy or less healthy than 7 years ago. Percentage of HALS2 household income group**

| Household income £/month | Males ≤320 | Males 321-860 | Males 861-1500 | Males 1501+ | Females ≤320 | Females 320-860 | Females 861-1500 | Females 1501+ |
|---|---|---|---|---|---|---|---|---|
| **HALS2 age 25-45** | | | | | | | | |
| Life more healthy | (5) | 29 | 37 | 45 | 33 | 36 | 38 | 44 |
| Life less healthy | (10) | 40 | 36 | 42 | 31 | 30 | 29 | 40 |
| **HALS2 age 46-66** | | | | | | | | |
| Life more healthy | 21 | 30 | 34 | 32 | 28 | 33 | 29 | 40 |
| Life less healthy | 41 | 51 | 36 | 36 | 50 | 45 | 44 | 34 |
| **HALS2 age 67+** | | | | | | | | |
| Life more healthy | 9 | 19 | 32 | 27 | 14 | 13 | 7 | 35 |
| Life less healthy | 56 | 46 | 45 | 33 | 57 | 57 | 56 | 30 |
| *Base = 100%* | *15* | *133* | *325* | *324* | *52* | *269* | *374* | *359* |
| | *33* | *226* | *267* | *236* | *76* | *363* | *214* | *219* |
| | *64* | *244* | *69* | *33* | *171* | *267* | *43* | *20* |

**Table 16.8** **Respondents claiming their life to be more healthy or less healthy than 7 years ago tabulated by disease status at HALS1 and HALS2. Percentage of disease status group.**

| HALS2 age | Reporting life more healthy 25-45 Males | Females | 46-66 Males | Females | 67+ Males | Females | Reporting life less healthy 25-45 Males | Females | 46-66 Males | Females | 67+ Males | Females |
|---|---|---|---|---|---|---|---|---|---|---|---|---|
| **Disease status** | | | | | | | | | | | | |
| No disease HALS1 Disease HALS2 | 41 | 39 | 31 | 29 | 15 | 15 | 53 | 53 | 58 | 59 | 51 | 64 |
| No disease HALS1/2 | 37 | 38 | 31 | 31 | 18 | 11 | 35 | 30 | 29 | 32 | 32 | 42 |
| Disease HALS1/2 | 40 | 38 | 29 | 36 | 23 | 18 | 48 | 45 | 53 | 54 | 65 | 66 |
| Disease HALS1 No disease HALS2 | 40 | 47 | 32 | 36 | 23 | 10 | 35 | 24 | 38 | 44 | 47 | 49 |
| *Base = 100%* | *118* | *121* | *159* | *190* | *75* | *139* | *118* | *121* | *158* | *190* | *75* | *140* |
| | *603* | *898* | *430* | *604* | *200* | *251* | *603* | *897* | *430* | *604* | *200* | *251* |
| | *120* | *133* | *211* | *236* | *167* | *188* | *120* | *133* | *211* | *236* | *167* | *188* |
| | *82* | *97* | *82* | *108* | *53* | *78* | *82* | *97* | *82* | *108* | *53* | *78* |

**Table 16.9** **Reasons given by respondents for life becoming more healthy or less healthy in the last 7 years (multiple answers possible). Percentage of those who reported improvement or deterioration.**

| HALS2 age | 25-45 | | 46-66 | | 67+ | |
|---|---|---|---|---|---|---|
| | Males | Females | Males | Females | Males | Females |
| **Life more healthy** | | | | | | |
| Better social/ family/environment | 6 | 8 | 4 | 14 | 6 | 9 |
| Improved diet | 39 | 46 | 26 | 34 | 7 | 15 |
| Reduced/stopped smoking | 20 | 10 | 21 | 10 | 13 | 2 |
| More exercise | 26 | 30 | 16 | 15 | 16 | 12 |
| Job change/retirement | 16 | 11 | 31 | 15 | 28 | 11 |
| Less stress | 12 | 9 | 27 | 29 | 24 | 21 |
| Improved condition | 7 | 11 | 13 | 23 | 40 | 45 |
| *Base = 100%* | *352* | *482* | *271* | *365* | *97* | *91* |
| **Life less healthy** | | | | | | |
| Worse social/ family/environment | 6 | 11 | 4 | 10 | 4 | 4 |
| Poor diet | 6 | 7 | 2 | 2 | 1 | 1 |
| Increased/started smoking | 12 | 7 | 1 | 2 | 0 | (1) |
| Less exercise | 28 | 26 | 15 | 10 | 8 | 5 |
| Work problems | 29 | 17 | 14 | 9 | 1 | (1) |
| Increased stress | 23 | 17 | 12 | 15 | 2 | 5 |
| Det. of condition | 23 | 33 | 64 | 67 | 77 | 77 |
| Ageing | 2 | 2 | 8 | 6 | 12 | 13 |
| Less mobility | 1 | 1 | 5 | 4 | 14 | 17 |
| *Base = 100%* | *360* | *419* | *357* | *478* | *235* | *361* |

**Table 16.10    Changes in beliefs from HALS1 to HALS2 about causes of diseases with known environmental components in their aetiology by non-manual (NM) and manual (Man) socio-economic groups in HALS1**

| Age at HALS1 | | Percentage of age and socio-economic group ('–' not mentioned or less than 1%) | | | | | | | | | | | |
|---|---|---|---|---|---|---|---|---|---|---|---|---|---|
| | | 18-38 | | 39-59 | | 60+ | | 18-38 | | 39-59 | | 60+ | |
| HALS | | 1 | 2 | 1 | 2 | 1 | 2 | 1 | 2 | 1 | 2 | 1 | 2 |
| **Stomach ulcers** | | | | | *Males* | | | | | | *Females* | | |
| Worry/tension/ | NM | 65 | 76 | 71 | 76 | 65 | 55 | 64 | 77 | 75 | 76 | 64 | 56 |
| stress | Man | 43 | 58 | 57 | 59 | 45 | 43 | 46 | 62 | 56 | 60 | 45 | 43 |
| Alcohol | NM | 14 | 22 | 6 | 15 | 9 | 17 | 9 | 17 | 5 | 11 | 5 | 7 |
| | Man | 18 | 29 | 13 | 18 | 12 | 13 | 12 | 19 | 8 | 15 | 6 | 8 |
| Bad diet | NM | 34 | 55 | 32 | 45 | 38 | 46 | 33 | 47 | 34 | 47 | 35 | 49 |
| | Man | 26 | 37 | 27 | 36 | 32 | 36 | 26 | 39 | 28 | 41 | 32 | 41 |
| Fried/fatty | NM | 8 | 8 | 7 | 10 | 5 | 5 | 12 | 12 | 7 | 12 | 8 | 8 |
| foods | Man | 18 | 17 | 14 | 17 | 11 | 12 | 24 | 26 | 18 | 19 | 11 | 14 |
| 'Acid' foods | NM | 6 | 8 | 3 | 6 | 3 | 4 | 7 | 8 | 4 | 8 | 4 | 7 |
| | Man | 6 | 8 | 4 | 7 | 5 | 11 | 6 | 8 | 4 | 8 | 3 | 6 |
| Irregular meals/ | NM | 7 | 6 | 5 | 7 | 4 | 4 | 5 | 5 | 6 | 8 | 6 | 7 |
| shift work | Man | 5 | 5 | 8 | 6 | 5 | 7 | 3 | 3 | 6 | 6 | 7 | 5 |
| Heredity/family | NM | 1 | 3 | 2 | 5 | 3 | 3 | 1 | 3 | 1 | 4 | 3 | 4 |
| | Man | 2 | 1 | – | 1 | 1 | 1 | – | 2 | 1 | 2 | 1 | 2 |
| Smoking | NM | 2 | 5 | 2 | 5 | 3 | 5 | 3 | 6 | 3 | 7 | 2 | 3 |
| | Man | 3 | 5 | 3 | 6 | 3 | 8 | 1 | 6 | 2 | 8 | 3 | 3 |
| Don't know | NM | 4 | 4 | 6 | 4 | 9 | 13 | 5 | 3 | 4 | 4 | 7 | 10 |
| | Man | 12 | 7 | 7 | 7 | 10 | 16 | 11 | 6 | 7 | 7 | 16 | 17 |
| **Chronic bronchitis** | | | | | | | | | | | | | |
| Smoking | NM | 59 | 68 | 59 | 63 | 48 | 51 | 61 | 74 | 62 | 70 | 45 | 48 |
| | Man | 53 | 68 | 50 | 55 | 37 | 44 | 57 | 69 | 60 | 70 | 40 | 46 |
| Heredity/family | NM | 7 | 11 | 12 | 13 | 15 | 16 | 7 | 10 | 16 | 18 | 22 | 20 |
| | Man | 5 | 7 | 8 | 7 | 12 | 9 | 5 | 8 | 9 | 13 | 13 | 13 |
| Damp – weather | NM | 14 | 15 | 15 | 12 | 18 | 15 | 16 | 15 | 14 | 13 | 11 | 14 |
| or clothes | Man | 15 | 12 | 19 | 17 | 21 | 20 | 13 | 15 | 15 | 15 | 18 | 14 |
| Weak chest/lungs | NM | 5 | 6 | 5 | 9 | 6 | 10 | 10 | 15 | 9 | 14 | 12 | 15 |
| | Man | 3 | 6 | 4 | 5 | 7 | 6 | 9 | 12 | 7 | 10 | 11 | 12 |
| Air pollution | NM | 18 | 28 | 23 | 33 | 19 | 29 | 10 | 21 | 17 | 27 | 12 | 18 |
| | Man | 10 | 23 | 14 | 27 | 16 | 23 | 8 | 18 | 9 | 19 | 11 | 14 |
| Working | NM | 12 | 20 | 12 | 15 | 13 | 10 | 6 | 13 | 7 | 12 | 6 | 6 |
| conditions | Man | 11 | 16 | 12 | 13 | 11 | 9 | 5 | 9 | 4 | 8 | 5 | 6 |
| Don't know | NM | 15 | 8 | 11 | 9 | 12 | 12 | 11 | 6 | 9 | 7 | 16 | 14 |
| | Man | 21 | 14 | 14 | 15 | 14 | 17 | 17 | 10 | 11 | 6 | 16 | 15 |
| *Base = 100%* | NM | 393 | | 405 | | 196 | | 577 | | 558 | | 275 | |
| | Man | 514 | | 476 | | 296 | | 657 | | 567 | | 380 | |

**Table 16.10    Changes in beliefs about causes of diseases (cont.)**

| Age at HALS1 | | 18-38 | | 39-59 | | 60+ | | 18-38 | | 39-59 | | 60+ | |
|---|---|---|---|---|---|---|---|---|---|---|---|---|---|
| HALS | | 1 | 2 | 1 | 2 | 1 | 2 | 1 | 2 | 1 | 2 | 1 | 2 |
| **High blood pressure** | | | | | **Males** | | | | | | | **Females** | | |
| Smoking | NM | 12 | 21 | 8 | 17 | 5 | 9 | 9 | 18 | 7 | 13 | 4 | 6 |
| | Man | 7 | 18 | 7 | 12 | 2 | 5 | 6 | 16 | 6 | 13 | 4 | 5 |
| Alcohol | NM | 5 | 12 | 9 | 11 | 10 | 11 | 4 | 9 | 4 | 7 | 6 | 7 |
| | Man | 6 | 14 | 12 | 14 | 6 | 9 | 4 | 10 | 5 | 7 | 6 | 6 |
| Type of diet | NM | 18 | 31 | 20 | 32 | 17 | 21 | 14 | 28 | 11 | 23 | 15 | 18 |
| | Man | 11 | 25 | 11 | 18 | 10 | 11 | 6 | 19 | 9 | 16 | 12 | 9 |
| Salt | NM | 4 | 5 | 3 | 3 | 4 | 2 | 6 | 6 | 3 | 4 | 3 | 2 |
| | Man | 4 | 5 | 3 | 3 | 1 | 2 | 6 | 5 | 3 | 3 | 1 | 1 |
| Obesity/ overweight | NM | 17 | 19 | 19 | 14 | 7 | 10 | 18 | 28 | 20 | 25 | 8 | 10 |
| | Man | 10 | 15 | 11 | 13 | 5 | 5 | 18 | 27 | 16 | 19 | 6 | 5 |
| Lack of exercise | NM | 5 | 8 | 6 | 8 | 4 | 6 | 2 | 8 | 2 | 4 | 2 | 2 |
| | Man | 4 | 8 | 3 | 6 | 3 | 3 | 1 | 4 | 1 | 3 | 1 | 1 |
| Heredity/family | NM | 5 | 15 | 10 | 12 | 9 | 12 | 8 | 15 | 12 | 20 | 10 | 11 |
| | Man | 3 | 6 | 3 | 6 | 4 | 4 | 3 | 7 | 5 | 9 | 5 | 4 |
| Old age | NM | 1 | 3 | 2 | 3 | 5 | 1 | 3 | 3 | 2 | 3 | 4 | 3 |
| | Man | 1 | 3 | 2 | 1 | 2 | 4 | 2 | 1 | 1 | 1 | 3 | 1 |
| Overwork | NM | 3 | 1 | 2 | 2 | 3 | 1 | 3 | 3 | 2 | 1 | 1 | 2 |
| | Man | 3 | 2 | 1 | 3 | 1 | 4 | 4 | 3 | 3 | 3 | 1 | 2 |
| Don't know | NM | 12 | 5 | 11 | 8 | 14 | 14 | 12 | 4 | 13 | 9 | 22 | 22 |
| | Man | 16 | 9 | 19 | 15 | 33 | 33 | 19 | 9 | 20 | 16 | 32 | 32 |
| **Obesity** | | | | | | | | | | | | | |
| Worry/tension/ stress | NM | 8 | 9 | 12 | 8 | 4 | 3 | 15 | 11 | 14 | 11 | 10 | 2 |
| | Man | 7 | 7 | 4 | 5 | 2 | 1 | 13 | 11 | 13 | 7 | 4 | 1 |
| Alcohol | NM | 7 | 10 | 8 | 12 | 11 | 14 | 2 | 5 | 2 | 4 | 4 | 4 |
| | Man | 9 | 10 | 8 | 12 | 10 | 14 | 2 | 4 | 2 | 5 | 1 | 3 |
| Overeating | NM | 67 | 64 | 71 | 69 | 71 | 75 | 72 | 69 | 67 | 74 | 74 | 73 |
| | Man | 61 | 64 | 66 | 68 | 66 | 68 | 70 | 68 | 67 | 70 | 73 | 74 |
| Eating 'wrong' foods | NM | 29 | 42 | 24 | 36 | 22 | 32 | 27 | 37 | 24 | 33 | 20 | 28 |
| | Man | 18 | 31 | 21 | 30 | 19 | 25 | 26 | 31 | 24 | 31 | 23 | 28 |
| Lack of exercise | NM | 26 | 37 | 25 | 36 | 32 | 33 | 16 | 30 | 15 | 25 | 15 | 26 |
| | Man | 29 | 38 | 26 | 31 | 30 | 36 | 14 | 23 | 12 | 20 | 18 | 21 |
| Heredity/family | NM | 15 | 25 | 11 | 19 | 15 | 16 | 8 | 16 | 12 | 19 | 10 | 15 |
| | Man | 5 | 11 | 8 | 11 | 7 | 7 | 4 | 9 | 6 | 12 | 6 | 9 |
| 'Glands' or hormones | NM | 20 | 26 | 17 | 18 | 12 | 8 | 21 | 29 | 22 | 26 | 19 | 13 |
| | Man | 13 | 17 | 11 | 12 | 8 | 7 | 17 | 25 | 15 | 20 | 13 | 7 |
| Don't know | NM | 1 | – | 1 | 1 | 1 | – | 1 | – | 2 | 1 | 3 | 1 |
| | Man | 4 | 3 | 3 | 3 | 4 | 5 | 3 | 3 | 2 | 2 | 3 | 4 |
| *Base = 100%* | NM | | 393 | | 405 | | 196 | | 577 | | 558 | | 275 |
| | Man | | 514 | | 476 | | 296 | | 657 | | 567 | | 380 |

**Table 16.10    Changes in beliefs about causes of diseases (cont.)**

| Age at HALS1 | | 18-38 | | 39-59 | | 60+ | | 18-38 | | 39-59 | | 60+ | |
|---|---|---|---|---|---|---|---|---|---|---|---|---|---|
| HALS | | 1 | 2 | 1 | 2 | 1 | 2 | 1 | 2 | 1 | 2 | 1 | 2 |
| **Stroke** | | | | | **Males** | | | | | | **Females** | | |
| Worry/tension/ | NM | 33 | 40 | 34 | 39 | 34 | 36 | 32 | 38 | 31 | 37 | 35 | 41 |
| stress | Man | 34 | 38 | 34 | 41 | 25 | 35 | 30 | 36 | 31 | 38 | 30 | 32 |
| Alcohol | NM | 3 | 8 | 3 | 7 | 1 | 4 | 2 | 3 | 1 | 2 | 1 | – |
| | Man | 2 | 10 | 2 | 4 | – | 3 | 2 | 4 | – | 3 | – | 1 |
| Diet | NM | 14 | 26 | 11 | 19 | 7 | 7 | 10 | 18 | 7 | 9 | 3 | 4 |
| | Man | 6 | 18 | 6 | 7 | 2 | 3 | 4 | 14 | 2 | 7 | 1 | 4 |
| Obesity/ | NM | 7 | 11 | 7 | 10 | 4 | 4 | 6 | 10 | 6 | 11 | 3 | 4 |
| overweight | Man | 8 | 11 | 8 | 11 | 3 | 3 | 7 | 9 | 5 | 9 | 2 | 1 |
| Lack of exercise | NM | 9 | 13 | 6 | 10 | 3 | 6 | 3 | 7 | 3 | 6 | 2 | 2 |
| | Man | 6 | 11 | 4 | 6 | 2 | 4 | 2 | 6 | 2 | 3 | 1 | 1 |
| Heredity/family | NM | 3 | 11 | 4 | 11 | 7 | 4 | 4 | 7 | 5 | 9 | 5 | 6 |
| | Man | 2 | 4 | 3 | 2 | 2 | 4 | 1 | 5 | 2 | 4 | 1 | 2 |
| Old age | NM | 9 | 10 | 8 | 8 | 10 | 8 | 11 | 10 | 11 | 10 | 5 | 7 |
| | Man | 10 | 8 | 6 | 4 | 5 | 7 | 7 | 6 | 6 | 5 | 3 | 6 |
| High blood | NM | 10 | 15 | 14 | 24 | 26 | 25 | 13 | 25 | 23 | 37 | 28 | 36 |
| pressure | Man | 7 | 14 | 14 | 20 | 17 | 18 | 10 | 19 | 21 | 29 | 24 | 22 |
| Sudden/over | NM | 4 | 4 | 6 | 5 | 7 | 6 | 6 | 3 | 3 | 4 | 4 | 4 |
| exertion | Man | 10 | 7 | 8 | 5 | 5 | 4 | 5 | 4 | 4 | 4 | 5 | 3 |
| Smoking | NM | 7 | 14 | 3 | 10 | 2 | 6 | 5 | 10 | 3 | 6 | – | 1 |
| | Man | 3 | 12 | 4 | 7 | 1 | 1 | 3 | 9 | 3 | 5 | – | 1 |
| Don't know | NM | 23 | 16 | 20 | 13 | 18 | 19 | 28 | 19 | 23 | 14 | 26 | 21 |
| | Man | 24 | 19 | 23 | 17 | 36 | 31 | 36 | 25 | 28 | 20 | 36 | 40 |
| **Liver trouble** | | | | | | | | | | | | | |
| Alcohol | NM | 79 | 89 | 77 | 83 | 67 | 67 | 73 | 85 | 73 | 82 | 55 | 55 |
| | Man | 74 | 86 | 71 | 75 | 61 | 59 | 66 | 79 | 68 | 76 | 46 | 49 |
| Diet | NM | 11 | 18 | 8 | 16 | 15 | 15 | 9 | 14 | 9 | 12 | 14 | 19 |
| | Man | 5 | 11 | 8 | 11 | 6 | 11 | 6 | 10 | 6 | 8 | 9 | 10 |
| Heredity/family | NM | 1 | 4 | 2 | 4 | 4 | 2 | 3 | 5 | 3 | 4 | 3 | 3 |
| | Man | 1 | 2 | 2 | 1 | 1 | 1 | 1 | 3 | 1 | 2 | 1 | 1 |
| Infection/virus | NM | – | 6 | – | 6 | – | 5 | – | 6 | – | 8 | – | 3 |
| | Man | – | 2 | – | 3 | – | 1 | – | 5 | – | 3 | – | 2 |
| Don't know | NM | 14 | 9 | 18 | 11 | 21 | 25 | 18 | 10 | 20 | 12 | 31 | 30 |
| | Man | 21 | 10 | 21 | 19 | 31 | 32 | 29 | 16 | 26 | 19 | 44 | 39 |
| *Base = 100%* | NM | | 393 | | 405 | | 196 | | 577 | | 558 | | 275 |
| | *Man* | | 514 | | 476 | | 296 | | 657 | | 567 | | 380 |

Percentage of age and socio-economic group ('–' not mentioned or less than 1%)

## Table 16.10 Changes in beliefs about causes of diseases (cont.)

| Age at HALS1 | | 18-38 | | 39-59 | | 60+ | | 18-38 | | 39-59 | | 60+ | |
|---|---|---|---|---|---|---|---|---|---|---|---|---|---|
| HALS | | 1 | 2 | 1 | 2 | 1 | 2 | 1 | 2 | 1 | 2 | 1 | 2 |
| **Heart trouble** | | | | | **Males** | | | | | | **Females** | | |
| Smoking | NM | 37 | 50 | 28 | 42 | 19 | 21 | 34 | 43 | 29 | 41 | 15 | 19 |
| | Man | 35 | 47 | 26 | 34 | 15 | 19 | 33 | 46 | 28 | 39 | 12 | 15 |
| Worry/tension/ | NM | 37 | 41 | 34 | 39 | 33 | 39 | 29 | 40 | 40 | 43 | 33 | 39 |
| stress | Man | 20 | 29 | 27 | 36 | 28 | 31 | 27 | 32 | 27 | 34 | 34 | 33 |
| Alcohol | NM | 9 | 21 | 6 | 9 | 5 | 5 | 8 | 11 | 3 | 6 | 1 | 5 |
| | Man | 8 | 17 | 4 | 9 | 3 | 4 | 6 | 11 | 6 | 7 | 3 | 2 |
| Wrong diet | NM | 33 | 55 | 28 | 37 | 10 | 19 | 30 | 46 | 21 | 31 | 9 | 11 |
| | Man | 20 | 39 | 13 | 21 | 6 | 9 | 17 | 38 | 8 | 21 | 3 | 8 |
| Fatty foods | NM | 14 | 19 | 9 | 13 | 4 | 6 | 12 | 17 | 9 | 11 | 5 | 8 |
| | Man | 11 | 17 | 7 | 14 | 3 | 9 | 8 | 15 | 7 | 15 | 4 | 7 |
| Over-eating | NM | 9 | 9 | 8 | 9 | 5 | 7 | 7 | 10 | 7 | 7 | 3 | 6 |
| | Man | 9 | 9 | 7 | 9 | 5 | 6 | 6 | 10 | 7 | 7 | 2 | 4 |
| Obesity/ | NM | 18 | 23 | 21 | 21 | 14 | 13 | 26 | 27 | 22 | 27 | 14 | 13 |
| overweight | Man | 18 | 19 | 18 | 20 | 12 | 12 | 22 | 24 | 24 | 25 | 14 | 13 |
| Lack of exercise | NM | 21 | 37 | 17 | 27 | 10 | 14 | 14 | 27 | 12 | 18 | 6 | 6 |
| | Man | 16 | 34 | 11 | 18 | 7 | 9 | 7 | 18 | 6 | 12 | 3 | 4 |
| Sudden/over- | NM | 4 | 3 | 7 | 5 | 13 | 7 | 3 | 4 | 5 | 4 | 11 | 11 |
| exertion | Man | 8 | 5 | 10 | 6 | 11 | 14 | 5 | 2 | 5 | 5 | 11 | 10 |
| Heredity/family | NM | 15 | 26 | 17 | 25 | 20 | 20 | 15 | 28 | 24 | 34 | 23 | 28 |
| | Man | 9 | 12 | 12 | 16 | 12 | 11 | 8 | 17 | 13 | 22 | 12 | 17 |
| Overwork | NM | 5 | 3 | 4 | 3 | 7 | 7 | 5 | 4 | 7 | 6 | 10 | 7 |
| | Man | 4 | 3 | 7 | 6 | 10 | 10 | 6 | 3 | 8 | 4 | 10 | 10 |
| Don't know | NM | 4 | 2 | 7 | 4 | 15 | 12 | 10 | 3 | 9 | 5 | 18 | 13 |
| | Man | 11 | 6 | 13 | 7 | 19 | 21 | 17 | 8 | 13 | 6 | 24 | 21 |
| **Migraine** | | | | | | | | | | | | | |
| Worry/tension/ | NM | 49 | 56 | 45 | 44 | 38 | 37 | 57 | 64 | 58 | 60 | 44 | 46 |
| stress | Man | 45 | 48 | 41 | 44 | 36 | 35 | 51 | 59 | 49 | 53 | 41 | 40 |
| Foods/food | NM | 18 | 30 | 22 | 30 | 14 | 15 | 37 | 55 | 45 | 51 | 24 | 23 |
| allergy | Man | 12 | 20 | 13 | 22 | 5 | 8 | 29 | 52 | 31 | 43 | 17 | 17 |
| Heredity/family | NM | 7 | 12 | 8 | 13 | 10 | 16 | 7 | 11 | 6 | 14 | 11 | 14 |
| | Man | 4 | 7 | 5 | 5 | 7 | 6 | 3 | 5 | 4 | 5 | 5 | 6 |
| Eye strain/TV | NM | 5 | 7 | 3 | 6 | 3 | 4 | 4 | 9 | 4 | 5 | 3 | 3 |
| | Man | 5 | 8 | 5 | 7 | 4 | 6 | 5 | 6 | 3 | 3 | 3 | 4 |
| Don't know | NM | 30 | 24 | 29 | 27 | 40 | 40 | 18 | 10 | 14 | 15 | 34 | 31 |
| | Man | 33 | 29 | 32 | 28 | 45 | 48 | 24 | 13 | 22 | 20 | 35 | 38 |
| Base = 100% | NM | | 393 | | 405 | | 196 | | 577 | | 558 | | 275 |
| | Man | | 514 | | 476 | | 296 | | 657 | | 567 | | 380 |

**Table 16.10    Changes in beliefs about causes of diseases (cont.)**

| | | | | | | | | | | | | | |
|---|---|---|---|---|---|---|---|---|---|---|---|---|---|
| | | Percentage of age and socio-economic group ('–' not mentioned or less than 1%) | | | | | | | | | | | |
| Age at HALS1 | | 18-38 | | 39-59 | | 60+ | | 18-38 | | 39-59 | | 60+ | |
| HALS | | 1 | 2 | 1 | 2 | 1 | 2 | 1 | 2 | 1 | 2 | 1 | 2 |
| **Lung cancer** | | | | | Males | | | | | Females | | | |
| Smoking | NM | 94 | 99 | 86 | 93 | 84 | 87 | 92 | 98 | 88 | 94 | 82 | 85 |
| | Man | 90 | 95 | 83 | 90 | 72 | 77 | 89 | 93 | 84 | 92 | 75 | 81 |
| Heredity/family | NM | 4 | 8 | 8 | 8 | 4 | 10 | 4 | 9 | 4 | 9 | 3 | 8 |
| | Man | 2 | 4 | 3 | 5 | 4 | 5 | 2 | 4 | 2 | 6 | 2 | 4 |
| Air pollution | NM | 14 | 24 | 21 | 29 | 20 | 20 | 7 | 15 | 13 | 20 | 9 | 14 |
| | Man | 10 | 18 | 15 | 24 | 17 | 20 | 6 | 14 | 7 | 13 | 9 | 10 |
| Other pollution/ | NM | 8 | 16 | 13 | 19 | 11 | 6 | 7 | 10 | 7 | 12 | 9 | 3 |
| chemicals | Man | 5 | 10 | 10 | 14 | 7 | 9 | 4 | 8 | 5 | 9 | 6 | 6 |
| Living environ- | NM | 6 | 9 | 4 | 9 | 3 | 4 | 2 | 6 | 2 | 5 | 3 | 3 |
| ment housing etc. | Man | 2 | 6 | 4 | 8 | 3 | 5 | 1 | 4 | 2 | 3 | 1 | 2 |
| Passive smoking | NM | – | 4 | – | 3 | – | 1 | – | 3 | – | 3 | – | – |
| | Man | – | 3 | – | 2 | – | 1 | – | 3 | – | 3 | – | 1 |
| Don't know | NM | 4 | 1 | 6 | 3 | 8 | 9 | 5 | 1 | 6 | 3 | 13 | 11 |
| | Man | 6 | 2 | 8 | 3 | 14 | 13 | 8 | 5 | 11 | 6 | 17 | 12 |
| **Piles or haemorrhoids** | | | | | | | | | | | | | |
| Constipation | NM | 9 | 14 | 19 | 18 | 26 | 27 | 21 | 33 | 37 | 46 | 49 | 50 |
| | Man | 7 | 13 | 22 | 20 | 28 | 32 | 23 | 32 | 43 | 46 | 47 | 49 |
| Low fibre/ | NM | 7 | 16 | 12 | 14 | 11 | 8 | 11 | 22 | 14 | 17 | 5 | 10 |
| roughage diet | Man | 4 | 8 | 5 | 9 | 4 | 6 | 9 | 16 | 6 | 14 | 4 | 8 |
| Other bad diet | NM | 17 | 20 | 18 | 25 | 19 | 22 | 19 | 31 | 20 | 25 | 13 | 14 |
| | Man | 8 | 19 | 11 | 15 | 9 | 10 | 12 | 20 | 12 | 20 | 12 | 14 |
| Pregnancy | NM | 3 | 4 | 2 | 3 | 3 | – | 16 | 24 | 13 | 18 | 8 | 9 |
| | Man | 3 | 4 | 1 | 2 | – | – | 18 | 26 | 11 | 12 | 6 | 5 |
| Sitting on wet/ | NM | 14 | 15 | 7 | 10 | 5 | 8 | 11 | 7 | 4 | 5 | 2 | 6 |
| cold surfaces | Man | 22 | 22 | 16 | 17 | 9 | 9 | 10 | 10 | 5 | 5 | 4 | 2 |
| Sitting | NM | 8 | 5 | 9 | 10 | 9 | 9 | 6 | 5 | 8 | 7 | 6 | 4 |
| | Man | 9 | 8 | 11 | 13 | 9 | 12 | 4 | 5 | 4 | 5 | 6 | 3 |
| Don't know | NM | 44 | 35 | 37 | 34 | 33 | 32 | 30 | 19 | 19 | 16 | 27 | 27 |
| | Man | 50 | 41 | 36 | 35 | 41 | 41 | 36 | 26 | 27 | 22 | 27 | 29 |
| *Base = 100%* | NM | | *393* | | *405* | | *196* | | *577* | | *558* | | *275* |
| | Man | | *514* | | *476* | | *296* | | *657* | | *567* | | *380* |

**Table 16.10   Changes in beliefs about causes of diseases (cont.)**

| | | Percentage of age and socio-economic group ('–' not mentioned or less than 1%) | | | | | | | | | | | |
|---|---|---|---|---|---|---|---|---|---|---|---|---|---|
| Age at HALS1 | | 18-38 | | 39-59 | | 60+ | | 18-38 | | 39-59 | | 60+ | |
| HALS | | 1 | 2 | 1 | 2 | 1 | 2 | 1 | 2 | 1 | 2 | 1 | 2 |
| **Severe depression** | | | | | Males | | | | | | Females | | |
| Worry/tension/ | NM | 44 | 44 | 47 | 48 | 46 | 41 | 42 | 47 | 42 | 46 | 41 | 38 |
| stress | Man | 40 | 45 | 51 | 54 | 50 | 46 | 45 | 43 | 48 | 52 | 50 | 48 |
| Loneliness | NM | 10 | 12 | 7 | 10 | 12 | 8 | 15 | 15 | 17 | 20 | 18 | 24 |
| | Man | 7 | 11 | 8 | 7 | 12 | 12 | 12 | 11 | 16 | 18 | 23 | 22 |
| Financial | NM | 18 | 23 | 21 | 30 | 19 | 20 | 18 | 27 | 15 | 23 | 11 | 18 |
| problems | Man | 22 | 29 | 20 | 22 | 14 | 15 | 17 | 25 | 15 | 21 | 11 | 14 |
| Attitude to life – | NM | 15 | 14 | 17 | 17 | 19 | 18 | 15 | 18 | 16 | 20 | 22 | 24 |
| give in to things | Man | 12 | 12 | 10 | 10 | 13 | 14 | 13 | 13 | 12 | 12 | 17 | 13 |
| Unemployment | NM | 12 | 12 | 11 | 9 | 5 | 8 | 8 | 11 | 7 | 8 | 3 | 5 |
| | Man | 16 | 14 | 12 | 11 | 6 | 4 | 9 | 9 | 4 | 6 | 4 | 3 |
| Bereavement | NM | 9 | 18 | 9 | 13 | 7 | 14 | 12 | 21 | 16 | 23 | 12 | 16 |
| | Man | 6 | 10 | 6 | 9 | 7 | 11 | 7 | 12 | 7 | 14 | 12 | 11 |
| Heredity/family | NM | 5 | 11 | 4 | 9 | 5 | 11 | 5 | 9 | 6 | 12 | 6 | 9 |
| | Man | 1 | 3 | 2 | 3 | 2 | 5 | 2 | 8 | 4 | 4 | 2 | 2 |
| Marital problems/ | NM | 5 | 13 | 10 | 15 | 7 | 8 | 11 | 17 | 13 | 17 | 6 | 4 |
| divorce/separation | Man | 6 | 12 | 6 | 5 | 2 | 5 | 9 | 11 | 5 | 9 | 2 | 4 |
| Family | NM | 9 | 18 | 11 | 17 | 14 | 11 | 14 | 19 | 13 | 17 | 8 | 9 |
| relationships | Man | 8 | 11 | 8 | 12 | 4 | 7 | 12 | 19 | 9 | 18 | 10 | 10 |
| Childbirth | NM | 2 | 2 | 1 | 1 | 1 | – | 9 | 11 | 6 | 7 | 2 | 3 |
| | Man | 1 | – | 1 | – | – | – | 8 | 9 | 4 | 4 | 2 | 1 |
| Medical problems | NM | 6 | 12 | 8 | 10 | 5 | 9 | 6 | 13 | 9 | 11 | 5 | 8 |
| | Man | 2 | 5 | 4 | 6 | 5 | 4 | 5 | 9 | 6 | 8 | 4 | 5 |
| Don't know | NM | 13 | 12 | 11 | 10 | 13 | 14 | 10 | 8 | 10 | 7 | 10 | 10 |
| | Man | 16 | 14 | 9 | 12 | 12 | 21 | 15 | 11 | 6 | 8 | 6 | 11 |
| *Base = 100%* | NM | | 393 | | 405 | | 196 | | 577 | | 558 | | 275 |
| | Man | | 514 | | 476 | | 296 | | 657 | | 567 | | 380 |

**Table 16.11  Professed beliefs at HALS2 about heart problems in relation to whether or not the respondent reported they had angina or heart attack**

| | | Percentage of group giving cause | | | |
|---|---|---|---|---|---|
| Age at HALS2 | | 45-66 | 66+ | 45-66 | 66+ |
| | | Males | | Females | |
| Cause | Heart trouble | | | | |
| Smoking | Yes | 34 | 22 | 39 | 19 |
| | No | 38 | 20 | 40 | 16 |
| Worry/tension/ | Yes | 41 | 39 | 42 | 43 |
| stress | No | 37 | 34 | 37 | 34 |
| Alcohol | Yes | 9 | 7 | 4 | 2 |
| | No | 10 | 4 | 7 | 4 |
| Wrong diet | Yes | 23 | 11 | 15 | 8 |
| | No | 29 | 13 | 26 | 9 |
| Fatty foods | Yes | 17 | 6 | 9 | 5 |
| | No | 13 | 8 | 16 | 9 |
| Over-eating | Yes | 5 | 8 | 4 | 5 |
| | No | 10 | 6 | 7 | 5 |
| Obesity/overweight | Yes | 18 | 8 | 22 | 7 |
| | No | 21 | 14 | 27 | 15 |
| Lack of exercise | Yes | 12 | 8 | 5 | 2 |
| | No | 23 | 11 | 16 | 6 |
| Sudden/over- | Yes | 2 | 12 | 7 | 13 |
| exertion | No | 6 | 11 | 5 | 10 |
| Heredity/family | Yes | 22 | 10 | 28 | 19 |
| | No | 20 | 15 | 27 | 22 |
| Overwork | Yes | 7 | 14 | 11 | 18 |
| | No | 4 | 7 | 4 | 7 |
| High blood pressure | Yes | 6 | 2 | 4 | 1 |
| | No | 2 | 3 | 3 | 2 |
| High cholesterol | Yes | 2 | 2 | 4 | 0 |
| | No | 2 | 1 | 3 | 0 |
| Lifestyle | Yes | 1 | 1 | 0 | 0 |
| | No | 2 | 1 | 1 | 1 |
| Don't know | Yes | 8 | 19 | 9 | 11 |
| | No | 5 | 18 | 6 | 19 |
| *Base = 100%* | *Yes* | *89* | *107* | *76* | *88* |
| | *No* | *759* | *361* | *1021* | *531* |

# SUMMARY

# IMPLICATIONS FOR HEALTH POLICY | 17

**Mildred Blaxter**

In 1992, the White Paper 'The Health of the Nation' noted that:

*The need for monitoring and research is especially important in tackling the variation in health between different groups in the population... Effective strategies, whether national or local, will need to be sensitive to these variations, and focus on the settings in which they are most evident.*

In recognition of this need, surveys of health and health behaviour have proliferated since the first Health and Lifestyle Survey in 1984/5, at both the national level (with, for instance, the Health Survey for England 1991 (1993) and the Allied Dunbar National Fitness Survey (1992)) and at local levels where health regions and districts have been very active in attempting to measure the health needs of their areas.

However, almost all are snapshots at one time, or have geographically restricted samples. HALS1 provided a great deal of evidence about the 'variation in health' of which the White Paper speaks. The repetition of this Survey, seven years later, offers to those interested in health policy some information about general stability and change. Even more importantly, it presents a view of health events and life events in individuals over time – albeit over a relatively short period. Thus, speculation about cause and effect can be much more firmly grounded.

Comparisons between HALS1 and HALS2 may take several forms, though they are not always easy to isolate. The preceding chapters demonstrate them all. Firstly, general temporal change or stability in the health, the social circumstances, or the behaviour of the population can be examined.

Examples are seen in Chapter 2, the main purpose of which is to test the make-up of the HALS2 sample, and examine the extent to which it has become selected. However, it is also a very clear demonstration of the fluidity of society, and the way in which surveys at any one point of time may give an apparent solidity to demographic characteristics which they rarely merit. Remembering that the most socially unstable individuals were more likely to be lost from the sample, it is notable that within seven years 10% of those aged 18-45 in 1984/5 who were married became divorced or separated. Among the divorced at HALS1, 40% had remarried by HALS2. Nearly half of the mothers living alone with children were in other types of household – 37% of them in couple households – seven years later, though age-for-age the rate of single parenthood had not greatly changed. Of the men who were unemployed at HALS1, 60% of those aged 18-38 were employed at HALS2, though again the overall rate of unemployment was little different. Only 35% of women under 60 whose occupation was household duties at HALS1 were similarly occupied at HALS2.

Other examples of the individual change concealed by apparent overall stability are noted later: for instance, overall rates of alcohol consumption are very similar at the two dates, but there is a great deal of change in individuals' behaviour.

On the other hand, many general societal changes over the seven years can be identified, where differences between the two Surveys cannot be explained simply by seven years of ageing in the Survey population. These are, for the most part, already known, but the amount of detail available about each individual may assist in understanding how they have come about. Dietary changes, discussed later, are one example. A considerable increase in the use of medication among all age and social groups and in all areas is another (Chapter 7). The general increase in the prevalence of overweight is another (Chapter 6). There are also suggestions of an increased prevalence of certain medical conditions – asthma, diabetes among men, migraine in younger women, heart problems at older ages (Chapter 4). Whether these self-reported prevalences represent true rises (as in some cases they are thought to be) or whether they are diagnostic and identification changes, can be ascertained only where there is other evidence within the Survey. Such evidence exists, for instance, in the case of hypertension, discussed later.

Secondly, individual change can be identified. By comparison with the distribution of characteristics by age seven years ago, some attempt can be made to show whether this change is a simple ageing effect. If change is not general, but is confined to certain groups, some cause other than ageing can be sought.

It is also possible to examine characteristics of the individual which may be expected to be relatively stable over time, such as attitudes, personality factors or cognitive functioning (or, perhaps, examine the reliability of the measuring instruments used). These issues have great practical as well as methodological importance, and though many remain to be addressed in detail, Chapters 8 and 9 report very interesting findings. For instance, longitudinal changes in the measures of mental state and personality suggest that 'Type A' behaviour is, at least in part, under the influence of environmental factors, and not completely intrinsic to the individual. Neuroticism – at least as measured on the scale used – was shown to be affected by present emotional state, and is not necessarily an enduring trait. There was considerable consistency over time in the measures of cognitive functioning, though an unexpected improvement between cohorts on all measures. The scores in a reasoning test, however, thought to be an intellectual ability likely to be retained over time, showed a marked impairment over the seven years among older individuals.

Most of the health-related lifestyle factors discussed below show the anticipated changes characteristic of people now seven years older, but many also show distinctive changes among particular groups, where causal factors may be sought in individual circumstances. Where these result in 'healthier' or 'unhealthier' behaviour, there are obvious policy implications.

## Risk factors and health-related behaviour

'The Health of the Nation' (1992) noted that:

*Many people die prematurely or suffer debilitating ill-health from conditions which are to a large extent preventible. The way in which people live and the lifestyles they adopt can have profound effects on subsequent health...over the next decade, gains in health will increasingly depend on effective preventive interventions.*

The Health Survey for England 1991 (1993) did in fact suggest that, by some indicators, people are becoming more health-conscious. At most ages, rather high proportions of respondents to HALS2 said that they thought their life was unhealthier than seven years previously (Chapter 16). However, this is not necessarily to be taken at face value: it may in fact represent a greater emphasis on the importance of healthy behaviour. Although younger men were not likely to report being more active in 'health promoting activities' than the equivalent age group seven years before, from about age 45 on both men and women were significantly more likely to report 'doing things to improve their health'. More exercise was reported, and there was a greater emphasis on diet.

The health promotion programme outlined by 'The Health of the Nation' (1992) identified five key priority areas:
– Coronary heart disease and stroke
– Cancers
– Mental illness
– HIV/AIDS and sexual health
– Accidents

and offered targets for each: for instance, to reduce the death rate under age 65 from CHD and stroke by at least 40% by the year 2000, and to reduce the rate for lung cancer under age 75 by at least 30% in men and 15% in women by the year 2010. The findings from HALS are extremely relevant to the first of the above priority areas, risk factors for CHD and stroke, although they cannot contribute to the last two.

There is also information relevant to the aim of reducing lung cancer, and perhaps also relevant to a better understanding of the determinants of mental health.

CHD and stroke were selected as a priority area because of their major contribution to mortality, and also because, it was suggested, behavioural risk factors are especially implicated. Although the death rate from CHD has been declining since the late 1970s, it remains in Britain one of the highest in the world, and accounted for 26% of deaths in England in 1991. Stroke accounted for 12% of deaths. The main risk factors, the White Paper suggested, are
– cigarette smoking (also, of course, a crucial factor in the incidence of lung cancer)
– raised blood cholesterol, to which obesity and the dietary intake of saturated fatty acids contribute
– raised blood pressure, to which obesity and excessive alcohol consumption contribute
– lack of physical activity, which in turn contributes to obesity.

The Health Survey for England 1991 (1993) examined these four risk factors and concluded that only 12% of men and 11% of women were free of all of them (though it must be noted that this includes the categorisation of over two-thirds of the population as having cholesterol levels above that approved, a level which is the subject of some dispute (Consensus Conference, 1989).

HALS cannot exactly replicate the Health Survey for England 1991 (1993), since there are no data on blood cholesterol. Evidence can, however, be offered on the other risk factors and their correlates, considering not only the population prevalences found but also individual, cohort and societal changes over seven years.

*Cigarette smoking*: The specific target set by the White Paper is to reduce the prevalence of cigarette smoking to no more than 20% in the population by the year 2000 in both men and women, with consequent reduction in death rates from lung cancer. It may be noted that the target of a 30% reduction in male mortality from lung cancer is in line with current trends, since mortality from this cause is showing a regular decline. The target for women may be more difficult to achieve, as rates are currently level or rising.

Between the HALS Surveys, the continuing decrease in regular smokers is demonstrated in both men and women (Chapter 12). Among men, 41% described themselves as regular smokers at HALS1, and 33% at HALS2. The reduction among women was smaller, from 31% to 27%. The most notable reduction in the proportion of regular smokers was among men aged 46 + at HALS2, rather than among young men. The implication may be that while the White Paper targets for reduction in lung cancer may continue to be approached, as currently middle-aged men give up smoking, there cannot necessarily be optimistic predictions about men at present young, or about women.

HALS1 and HALS2 together offer the opportunity to consider the dynamic processes over time which produce these smoking prevalences. It is notable that it is the occasional smokers who were likely to give up smoking (for instance, 60% of male occasional smokers aged 39-59 in 1984/5). Among young women, however, 41% of those who were occasional smokers at HALS1 had become regular smokers seven years later. Heavy smokers, particularly among the younger men and women, were very much less likely to give up. One positive finding, among all groups, was the general change to lower-tar cigarettes.

Some evidence can also be offered about the health effects of smoking. Lung function measurements (Chapter 5) show the clear deterioration over seven years for those who continue to smoke, and the improvement on giving up. There is some indication of the continuation of the differential effects according to social class which were noted in the analysis of HALS1. Though the well-known social class difference in smoking prevalence remains, there is no indication that it is now those in higher occupational classes who are disproportionately likely to give up smoking. However, there is a suggestion that giving up may improve lung function more in men and women in non-manual than in manual groups – that is, where environmental factors may be presumed to be more favourable.

Interesting differences in the general trend towards less smoking are noted in different areas of the country: for instance, there appears to be little change in Wales, the North, or the W. Midlands. All these, and many similar issues which await more detailed analysis, should offer important information for health education policy.

*Diet*: Similarly, on the topic of diet (Chapter 11), the general changes in dietary habits which are well-known — the reduction in the consumption of saturated fats, cheese, chips, eggs, meats, cooked breakfasts, and the increase in pasta, poultry, wholemeal/brown bread — can be considered as individual, or as cohort, changes.

The specific 'risk factor' target of the White Paper is to reduce the percentage of food energy derived by the population from saturated fatty acids by at least 35% by the year 2005 to no more than 11% of food energy, and to reduce total fat by at least 12%. In relation to cancer, it is noted that there is 'mounting, though as yet inconclusive' evidence that diets low in meat and fat, and high in vegetables, starchy foods, cereals and fruits, may be associated with a lower incidence of some cancers. The general dietary changes confirmed in HALS2 are, therefore, progress towards the White Paper's targets, though in this survey rather little change was found in the consumption of fruit and vegetables.

Over half of the younger people, aged 25-45 in 1991, said that they had changed their diet. It is notable, however, that only 17% of these said that it was in response to health campaigns (and another 10% to lose weight). This has policy implications for the determinants of change, and the extent to which they are specifically health-related choices. The data have great potential for the investigation of change at the individual level, including such issues as the diets associated with smoking on which important findings have been reported from the earlier survey.

*Alcohol consumption*: The Health of the Nation's target for this risk factor is to reduce by 30% the proportion of men who drink more than 21 units a week, and of women who drink more than 14 units, to 18% and 7% of the adult population respectively. HALS2 reports (Chapter 13) little overall change in the levels of drinking or the amount consumed since 1984/5, and thus suggests little progress towards this target. It does, however, show considerable change in individuals. For instance, fewer than half of those males categorised as 'heavy' drinkers at HALS1 were still 'excessive' drinkers seven years later. On the other hand, among young men, nearly half of those

who were non-drinkers at HALS1 had become occasional drinkers at HALS2. These longitudinal data show that, for a high proportion of the population, drinking habits are not a stable personal characteristic but change with life circumstances. For health promotion, this suggests a rather different model from that which sees behaviour as essentially a characteristic of the individual.

*Exercise*: The Health Survey for England 1991 (1993) reported that only 20% of men and 12% of women exercised at the level recommended as protective against CHD. HALS does not offer comparable data about the intensity of exercise, but does in fact show that exercise levels in the population are improving. Although approximately one-third of respondents (if the very oldest are excluded) said that they took less exercise than they had when seven years younger, and between a third and a half believed their exercise was inadequate, the levels reported for almost all age groups were higher than those at the equivalent ages seven years before (Chapter 14). For the individual, strenuous activity, of course, declines with age. The decline was less than would be predicted from HALS1 data, however, and for some age groups exercise levels even increased. Thus, comparing cohorts, among those aged 46-52 30% of men and 41% of women engaged in individual exercise activities (keep-fit, etc.) compared with 17% and 28% respectively of the same age group in 1984/5. A higher proportion of young men aged 25-31 engaged in competitive team sports than seven years before. There may have been some general reduction in the time spent walking, but in general this 'risk factor' of inadequate exercise seems to have improved. Certainly, more awareness of the importance of exercise was expressed (Chapters 14 and 16).

*Overweight*: Nevertheless, the survey confirmed an increase in the prevalence of overweight (Chapter 6). The Health Survey for England 1991 (1993) similarly noted a sharp rise, with almost a doubling in the population of men rated as obese between 1986/7 and 1991. 'The Health of the Nation' pointed out that 24% of women and 37% of men were overweight in 1986/7, and 12% of women and 8% of men were obese.

Comparing age cohorts, the Health Survey of 1991 noted an average increase in height of 0.8 cm for men and 1.0 cm for women between 1980 and 1991. Increases of the same order were found between HALS1 and HALS2.

Mean increases in weight were, however, greater than would be predicted from this height increase and from the expected age-associated gain in weight. For instance, 18% of women aged 32-38 were obese, twice the proportion in the same age group at HALS1, and 51% of men aged 32-38 were overweight or obese, compared with 41% of the age group at the first Survey. 'The Health of the Nation' (1992) offered the target of reducing the proportion of men and women aged 16-64 who are obese by at least 25% and 33% respectively by the year 2005, to no more than 6% of men and 8% of women. The evidence here should raise concern about the probability of reaching this target. Those individuals who were overweight or obese in 1984/5, especially those under 60 years of age, were very unlikely to have achieved an acceptable weight seven years later.

*Blood pressure*: Obesity, diet, excessive alcohol and exercise may all, of course, be associated with raised blood pressure and one of The Health of the Nation targets is to reduce mean systolic blood pressure in the adult population by at least 5 mm Hg by the year 2005. The Health Survey for England identified 16% of men and 17% of women with raised blood pressure.

A notable finding of HALS2 (Chapter 5) is in fact a general reduction in blood pressure, despite the rise in obesity. In Western industrialised populations blood pressure can be expected to rise with age, and this effect is shown in most age groups (an exception being young women). The rise is less than would be predicted from measures at the relevant ages in HALS1, however, with the result that, comparing like ages, mean rates are lower at HALS2, and greater proportions of each age up to 60 for men and 80 for women are normotensive. Artefactual explanations – the deaths of those who already had disease at HALS1, or the identification at that Survey and consequent treatment of previously undiagnosed hypertension – can have made only a small contribution to this. A greater contribution is obviously made by the fact that a much larger proportion of the population was being treated for hypertension at HALS2, especially at older ages. For

instance, within an age-cohort, the percentage of men aged 53-59 treated for hypertension at HALS1 was 12%; seven years later 23% of the same group were receiving treatment. Across cohorts, this 23% compares with 16% of the relevant group aged 60-66 at HALS1. High proportions were also receiving drugs with anti-hypertensive effects, for conditions other than raised blood pressure. The implication of this evidence is that action by the Health Service in monitoring, diagnosing and treating raised blood pressure may well be the most important factor for the achievement of this 'risk factor' target.

## The effect of the social environment upon health

'The Health of the Nation' (1992) acknowledges that, of course, not all ill-health, potentially preventible, is associated with behaviour which is within the individual's control. Health hazards imposed by the environment, poverty, poor housing, unemployment, working situations, and social marginalisation or isolation also have policy implications. For many of these, HALS now offers the opportunity to add to the evidence which is merely associative by demonstrating any effect of change in the individual's circumstances.

Seven years is, of course, a rather short period for clear effects upon health to be demonstrated. However, many preliminary findings reported in this volume go some way towards the identification of causal mechanisms. For instance, the effect of health status upon employment status can be explored, if tentatively: a surprising finding is that as many as 53% of those who at HALS1 had a chronic disease or handicap and were unemployed were in employment seven years later – an only slightly smaller proportion than among the unemployed without any chronic health problem (Chapter 4). There are suggestions (though numbers are small) that becoming unemployed has a clearly harmful effect upon the mental health of men in middle age, though not the young, and becoming employed after unemployment has a clear beneficial effect (Chapter 8).

It was demonstrated in HALS1 that the gap between social classes in various measures of health, including people's own assessments, widens as age increases. A further example of the value of the repeated study is that this can now be shown to be probably a true ageing effect rather than a historical difference between cohorts (Chapter 4). Those in manual occupational classes at HALS1 were more likely than those in non-manual classes to say that their health had worsened over the seven years, after middle age but not before.

Marriage or the breaking of relationships can also be shown to have a probable 'effect' on health, especially psychosocial health (Chapters 4 and 8). Those who were married in 1984/5 and separated/divorced in 1991 were particularly likely to have high 'malaise' scores. The very interesting data of Chapter 10 on 'life events' also considers the effect of changes in life circumstances. Getting married is associated with better mental health: divorce with worse, though for men rather than women. Widowhood, and living alone, are associated with a marked deterioration in mental health (Chapters 8 and 10). There is also a clear demonstration of the harmful effect on psychosocial health of a decline in perceived social support (Chapter 15).

Though some of these findings do not have policy implications which are as immediate or straightforward as the findings on personal behaviour, nevertheless they promise to add to our understanding of the determinants of health: on the one hand, they identify the vulnerable; on the other, they begin to illustrate how general social and economic changes in society can affect the nation's health.

### References

The Health of the Nation: A Strategy for Health in England (1992) London: HMSO.

Health Survey for England 1991 (1993) London: HMSO.

Allied Dunbar National Fitness Survey (1992): 'A Report on activity patterns and fitness levels' London: The Sports Council and the Health Education Authority.

Consensus Conference (1989): Blood Cholesterol Measurement in the Prevention of Coronary Heart Disease, London: King Edward's Hospital Fund for London.

# APPENDICES

# MEASURES AND DEFINITIONS OF TERMS

The interview questionnaire, which was very similar to that used in the first Survey, was piloted in a separate field study. The measurements schedule was almost identical to the previous one and the self-completion questionnaire was the same in the two Surveys (see Appendix C for interview schedule).

This Appendix contains notes on the derivation of the measures, and discusses their reliability and validity where appropriate. Further information will be found in the Users' Manuals which accompany the datasets and which will be available from the ESRC Data Archive at the University of Essex from January 1994.

## Active leisure pursuits

The same list of sports and other energetic activities was used in HALS1 and HALS2, except that in HALS2 'yoga' was separated from 'keep fit' and a question was asked about long walks (over two miles). The frequency of participation in each activity and average duration per session during the previous fortnight was recorded. The additional physical activities recorded at Q88 were recoded, into activities in Q87 or into additional codes such as snow sports, hockey, tug-of-war, trampolining, etc. as appropriate. The grouped activities 'individual', 'team, competitive' and 'other' included all the activities recorded in Q87 and Q88, except for dancing and walking, as described in Chapter 14.

## Alcohol consumption

The questions asking respondents to describe their drinking behaviour were tested in the pilot studies in the first Survey and found to cover the variety of possible responses. The questions on cutting down and giving up drinking alcohol are similar to those used in the national surveys of drinking habits (Wilson, 1980, Dight, 1976), with which the results can be compared.

It is generally agreed that the 'diary' method, taking the respondent back through one week, is the most reliable way of estimating alcohol intake (see e.g. Pernanen, 1974). This is the method used in the national surveys, and comparison is again possible.

The usual categories used in the tables to describe alcohol consumption are:

- *Non-drinker or very occasional drinker:* Always been a non-drinker or only drinks 'on very special occasions'.
- *Ex-drinker:* Not currently a regular drinker, but used to be more than a very occasional drinker.
- *Regular drinker:* Describes self as 'an occasional drinker' or a 'regular drinker'.

Based on the diary, respondents are further categorised as:

- Regular or ex-drinker who drank nothing 'last week'.
- Regular or ex-drinker, prudent 'last week'.
- Regular or ex-drinker, unwise 'last week'.
- Regular or ex-drinker, excessive drinker 'last week'.

In some tables, non-drinkers, 'special occasions drinkers' and those who drank nothing 'last week' are combined as 'non or only occasional drinkers'.

## Levels of consumption

In the first survey the reported number of units of alcohol consumed were based on Imperial measures served in pubs in England. Since then there has been an increasing tendency to employ metric measures and millilitres (ml) of pure alcohol as recommended by Turner (1990) and Miller et al. (1991). The present Survey recorded half pints of beer (approximately 290ml), glasses of wine (average 115ml), small glasses of fortified wine (56ml) and pub measures of spirits (28ml), each taken as equivalent to one unit (10ml) of pure alcohol. Since the assessment of alcohol consumption is not precise, with beers varying in their alcohol content, and with the amounts of spirits and wine served in the home often larger, but by an unknown amount, than standard pub measures, for most purposes consumption per week has been categorised as 'prudent', 'unwise', and 'excessive'. Since the 1984/5 Survey the banding of these categories has changed (Smyth and Browne, 1992). In this report the 1990 categories will be used. They are shown below with those used in the 1984/5 survey for comparison.

|  | *New Categories* | *Units* | *Old Categories* | *Units* |
|---|---|---|---|---|
| *Males* | Prudent | 1-21 | Light | 1-10 |
|  | Unwise | 22-50 | Moderate | 11-50 |
|  | Excessive | >50 | High | >50 |
| *Females* | Prudent | 1-14 | Light | 1-5 |
|  | Unwise | 15-35 | Moderate | 6-35 |
|  | Excessive | >35 | High | >35 |

## Problem drinkers

In order to identify the group who may be described as 'problem drinkers' (who are probably, but not necessarily, heavy drinkers) a simple instrument of four questions is used – Q65a, Q66a, b and c – known as the CAGE questionnaire. This cannot be presumed to identify 'alcoholics' reliably, but a full screening questionnaire for alcoholism was inappropriate. The brief instrument is derived from the Michigan Alcohol Screening Test and has been validated in a clinical setting (Mayfield et al. 1974). It has been found to correlate well with biochemical measures (Saunders and Kershaw, 1980).

## Area of residence

The five categories used, based on the interviewer's judgement, are:
- *High rise:* high rise development.
- *Built up:* built up area with no open space adjacent.
- *Built up with open space:* built up area with adjacent open space or large garden.
- *Rural:* in a country district.
- *Other.*

## Attitudinal and belief measures

The majority of the questions on attitudes and beliefs are, as in HALS1, based on issues and concepts developed in more intensive studies (e.g. D'Houtard and Field, 1984; Pill and Stott, 1985; Herzlich, 1973; Blaxter and Paterson, 1982) though some of the questions have been used before e.g. on health behaviour and on the causes of illness (Harris and Guten, 1979; Pill and Stott, 1982; Blaxter, 1984). Many of these questions were designed not only, or principally, to give individual items of information, but were used as part of complex indices summarising attitudinal 'sets' or orientations.

## Block counting test

This test has been used by psychologists for many years as a simple measure of visuospatial reasoning ability. Subjects are shown drawings representing three-dimensional piles of square blocks, and are asked to say how many blocks are contained in each pile. To obtain the correct answer, they must count the blocks which are hidden from view as well as the ones that are visible. This requires subjects to make inferences about the three-dimensional structure of simple shapes. The six drawings used in the survey were shown at the end of the nurse's visit. Subjects were asked to write down their responses, taking as much time as they needed.

## Blood pressure

For this Survey the WHO criteria of hypertension have been adopted (WHO, 1978) defined by the following values:
- Normal blood pressure is a systolic pressure of 140 mm Hg or less and a diastolic of 90mm Hg or less.

- Borderline hypertension is defined as the blood pressure being between 141-159 mm Hg systolic and 91-94 mm Hg diastolic.
- Hypertension in adults is regarded as a systolic pressure equal to or greater than 160 mm Hg and diastolic pressure of 95 mm Hg or above.
- Treated hypertensives are those being actively treated by drug therapy for hypertension. Blood pressure measurement may be normal depending on the effectiveness of therapy.

## Body Mass Index

Body Mass Index or Quetelet's Index is calculated by the formula WEIGHT (in kilos) over HEIGHT (in metres) squared ($WT/HT^2$).

Body Mass Index Categories: The categories recommended by the Fogarty Conference, USA (Bray, 1979) and Royal College of Physicians (1983), for Body Mass Index values are as follows:

|  | *Male* | *Female* |
|---|---|---|
| Underweight | Up to 20.0 | Up to 18.6 |
| Acceptable/Normal | 20.1 – 25.0 | 18.7 – 23.8 |
| Overweight | 25.1 – 29.9 | 23.9 – 28.5 |
| Obese | 30.0 and over | 28.6 and over |

## Breakfast: see Food

## Children

'Dependent' children are defined as those under 16 years.

## Choice reaction time: see Reaction time

## Dental roll

Respondents who took part in the measurements section of the Survey were asked to place a dental roll in their mouths, and keep it there until it was well soaked with saliva. The roll was then placed in a specimen tube and sent by first class post to Dr M. Jarvis at the Addiction Research Unit, Maudesley Hospital, London SE. The amount of salivary cotinine

was determined to obtain an indication of active and passive smoking levels. These results will be available at a later date.

## Disease prevalence: see Health, self-declared

## Education

Various ways of defining education are available in the data at HALS1. At HALS2 information was collected on 'highest educational qualification obtained'. The next question asked whether the qualification had been achieved in the past seven years. In Chapter 2 (Demographic Changes) HALS1 and HALS2 values have been compared but elsewhere HALS1 values have usually been used.

The categories used are:

- *No educational qualifications:* Work-related certificates which do not represent any academic qualifications are included.
- *'O'level, etc.:* CSE, GCE 'O'level, GCSE School Certificate, Scottish School Leaving Certificate (SLC) lower, Scottish SCE/SUPE lower, City and Guilds Craft/Ordinary/Intermediate/Part 1.
- *'A'level, etc.:* GCE 'A'/'S' level, Higher School Certificate, Matriculation, Scottish SCE/SLC/SUPE higher, ONC/OND/City and Guilds Advanced Level/Final level/Part 11 or 111, HNC/HND, City and Guilds Advanced/Full Technological Certificate, RSA/other clerical and commercial.
- *Semi-professional/professional:* Nursing qualifications, teaching qualifications, membership of professional institute.
- *Degree:* First or higher degree.

In some tables "A' level and above' refers to the last three of these categories. Those with overseas qualifications are usually omitted from tables where education is a variable.

## Employment status

Rigorous cross-checks were performed within the data, and all anomalous or difficult cases examined individually, in order to provide the relatively simple classification which is used in the tables:

- *Employed:* includes those temporarily sick, and (unless otherwise stated) both full time and part time employed. Full-time work is defined as 30 hours/week and over. This category includes those in temporary or casual work, and those waiting to start a job already obtained.
- *Unemployed:* includes all those technically unemployed, i.e. in the labour market but not employed. They may or may not describe themselves as currently 'actively looking for work'.
- *Permanently sick:* defined as out of the labour market (below retirement age) because of permanent illness.
- *Household duties (sometimes called housewife):* all those women and a few men, below retirement age, who so described themselves and were not in the labour market.
- *Retired:* all of retirement age (65+ males, 60+ females) who are not employed, together with those below retirement age who so described themselves, are not in the labour market, and are not engaged in household duties. The decision to categorise women over 60, not in the labour market, as 'retired' rather than 'household duties' (even if they described themselves as 'housewife') was taken in order to ensure uniformity: the women themselves might use either description. It should be noted that 'housewife' refers only to those under 60, and a woman over 60 described as 'retired' has not necessarily worked outside the home.

## Ethnic group

Assumed ethnic group is based on the interviewer's assessment:

| | |
|---|---|
| Indian (incl. E African) Pakistani, Bangladeshi, Black, African, West Indian, Other non-white | *Non-white* |
| White, European | *White* |

## Eysenck Personality Inventory (EPI)

This is a self-completion questionnaire devised by Eysenck and Eysenck, (1964). It contains 57 questions about behaviour, each requiring a yes/no response. 24 of the items comprise the Extraversion scale (see Extraversion), another 24 comprise the Neuroticism scale (see Neuroticism) and 9 items comprise the Lie scale, an index of the extent to which people give socially desirable responses.

## Extraversion

This is a personality trait which refers to the way in which people habitually behave, especially in social situations. One extreme is extraversion; the other is introversion. Extraverts are sociable, need people to talk to, crave excitement and act impulsively. Introverts are quiet, retiring, introspective and cautious. The Extraversion scale of the Eysenck Personality Inventory comprises 24 questions about such behaviours, which require yes/no answers. The score is summed and the higher the score the more extraverted the individual. Subjects with more than two missing responses are not included in the tables.

## Family contact: see Social support

## Food

The questions were selected, after the three pilot studies prior to the first Survey, to be readily understood by all types of respondents. The first two questions in the section, about special diets, had been used in the MRC National Survey of Health and Development (Wadsworth, 1980) and also checked against self-reported diseases (Chapter 4). Additional questions in this Survey about change in eating habits were based on those used in the West of Scotland Twenty-07 study.

The questions regarding meal and eating patterns were similar to those used by the British Nutrition Foundation (1985). In pilot surveys the respondents were asked when and where they ate their breakfast, midday and evening meals. However, that format proved unsatisfactory in pilot studies in the north where the number of shift workers was high. The questions used in both Surveys allowed for subjects with irregular eating habits and for the different terminology used in different parts of the country.

Meals and eating patterns were defined as follows:

- *Breakfast:* Food eaten within two hours of rising.
- *Light breakfast:* Toast/bread/breakfast cereal/porridge, fruit etc.
- *Cooked breakfast:* Eggs/bacon/sausage etc.
- *Main meals:* A main dish, usually cooked, with one or more vegetables.
- *Light meals:* Respondent's own definition of a meal lying between a main meal and a snack.
- *Snacks:* Something eaten between meals.
- *Meals away from home:* Includes food (e.g. sandwiches) taken to eat away from home, particularly at work.
- *Regular eaters:* Respondents who reported usually eating the same number of meals each day, at the same time each day.

Questions were designed to determine the frequency with which the majority of foods were eaten, and in some cases (e.g. bread) the amount. Food frequency assessment is probably the most suitable approach for assessing the quality of the diet in large-scale surveys (Willet and MacMahon, 1984). The questions on the frequency of food consumption are similar to those used in other surveys (Yarnell et al. 1983; Bull, 1985). The six categories of frequency of consumption of foods were:

- *Never:* never, or on very rare occasions.
- *Rarely:* sometimes, but less than once or twice a week.
- *Once or twice a week.*
- *Most days:* 3-6 days a week.
- *Daily.*
- *More than once a day.*

No attempt was made to assess the total energy intake, as in a pilot study detailed dietary recall using food models to determine energy intake showed little relationship to assessments from the subjects' reports on usual eating.

Other definitions:

- *Brown Bread:* Includes wholemeal, brown and granary bread.
- *Slices of bread per day:* Slices of bread plus rolls, converted to slices, assuming one roll is equivalent to one and a half slices.
- *Breakfast cereal:* Includes porridge.
- *Salad:* Includes raw vegetables.

- *Red Meat:* Beef/lamb/pork/gammon/ham/veal.
- *Processed meats:* Sausages, meat pies and pasties, bought cooked meats, burgers etc.
- *Margarine:* Hard and soft margarine, excluding polyunsaturated margarine and low fat spread.

# Gardening and DIY (Do-it-yourself)

The time spent on gardening and on DIY was assessed over the seven days before interview. DIY includes car maintenance.

# General Health Questionnaire (GHQ)

This self-completion questionnaire was developed by Goldberg (1972) as a screening instrument for psychiatric disorder. The 30-item version (GHQ-30) which comprises 30 questions about a range of psychiatric symptoms was used. Respondents are required to tick one of four categories according to the degree to which they have recently experienced the particular symptom. The categories are 'Not at all', 'No more than usual', 'Rather more than usual' and 'Much more than usual'. Responses were dichotomised so that the first two categories received a score of 0 (symptom absent), and the second two a score of 1 (symptom present). This is the scoring method recommended by Goldberg, and yields a total score out of 30. Subjects who had more than two missing responses are not included in the tables.

The validity of the GHQ has been investigated in a two-stage design, where the GHQ has been followed by a clinical interview to confirm the presence of psychiatric disorder (Tarnopolsky, et al. 1979). It has been found that a cut-point between 4 and 5 is useful for most purposes. People scoring 5 or more are more likely to be clinically confirmed cases of psychiatric disorder than those obtaining lower scores, although a high percentage of those scoring 5 + turn out to be 'non-cases'. The GHQ can also be used as a continuous variable, corresponding to the number of psychiatric symptoms (mostly minor ones) which the person has experienced recently.

# Handicap: see Health, self-declared

# Health (Self-declared)

## Disease prevalence

The wording of the question, (Q28) ascertaining current self-declared disease is that which is regularly used in the General Household Survey and is common in other health surveys. The validity of the answers is discussed briefly in Chapter 2 of the report of the first HALS Survey (Blaxter, 1987).

Diseases were coded by ICD Chapter (International Classification of Diseases, 1977), with the most common conditions within a Chapter selected for individual coding.

'Past' diseases, in reply to the question 'Have you ever had...?' (Q30) were selected to include those which might have some lifestyle component in their aetiology, although in fact the list covers most of the common or more serious diseases. Myalgic Encephalomyelitis (ME) or Post-Viral Fatigue Syndrome was asked about for the first time in HALS2. The question about heart problems was separated from the others in the HALS2 schedule. A subsequent question asked about types of heart problems to separate congenital problems from other types of heart trouble.

In the tables, 'has' a given disease condition is defined by the answer to Q.28.

'Ever had' a given disease condition is defined by the answer to Q.30.

## Disability or handicap

Q.28c and 29a-g are designed as a 'screen' which enables the respondents to be categorised as having 'limiting' or 'non-limiting' disease, so that comparison can be made with the General Household Survey, and also as mildly, moderately or severely handicapped in accordance with the definitions of the National Survey of the Handicapped and Impaired (Harris, 1971). The categories used are:

- *None:* chronic disease or impairment exists, but is stated to have no effect upon daily life.
- *Mild:* chronic disease or impairment is said to limit the subject's activities 'compared with people of your own age', but not to the extent of limiting work or social activities.
- *Moderate:* Subject is limited 'in the amount of work, or the kind of work, you can do, or in your social life' and/or cannot climb stairs.

- *Severe handicap, unable to work:* Subject cannot work (or do housework) though not housebound.
- *Severe handicap, housebound:* Subject cannot walk outside the house without aids, though not bed/chairfast.
- *Severe handicap, bed/chairfast:* Subject cannot walk inside the house and requires help with activities of daily living.

The last three categories are often combined as 'severe handicap'.

## Illness

The symptom list chosen to measure this dimension of health represents those complaints which are most common in adults, as recorded in consultation rates (Royal College of General Practitioners, 1982) and in smaller surveys in the community (e.g. Hannay, 1978; Blaxter, 1985).

The categories of high, average and low illness are based on a simple additive score of the number of symptoms declared 'within the last month' from the following list: headache, hay fever, constipation, trouble with eyes, a bad back, colds and flu, trouble with feet, kidney or bladder trouble, painful joints, palpitations or breathlessness, trouble with ears, indigestion or other stomach trouble, sinus trouble or catarrh, persistent cough, faints or dizziness, and (women only) trouble with periods or the menopause.

The arbitrary categories derived from the distributions found in the data, which are used in the tables are:

- *High illness:* 4 + symptoms.
- *Average illness:* 2/3 symptoms.
- *Low illness:* 0/1 symptoms.

## Malaise

This dimension of health (which is not presented as a psychological instrument, but simply as a measure of self-perceived psycho-social well-being) is based, in a similar way to the illness score, on the 'symptoms': difficulty sleeping, always feeling tired, difficulty concentrating, worrying 'over every little thing', 'nerves', feeling bored, feeling lonely, feeling 'under so much strain that your health is likely to suffer' (with extra weight given to 'always' experiencing the last three).

The categories used in the tables are:

- *High malaise:* 4 + symptoms.
- *Average malaise:* 2/3 symptoms.
- *Low malaise:* 0/1 symptoms.

## Household structure

Various categories and combined categories of household are used in the tables and are defined in the headings. Couples can be either married or cohabiting.

## Hypertension: see Blood pressure.

## 'Illness' score: see Health, self-declared

## Income, household

Net household income, is quoted in the tables in £/month. For single-person households, this is of course the respondent's income. It should be noted that this information is not available at HALS2 for approximately 18% of the sample. Analysis of HALS1 values of those with household income 'refused' or 'not known' at HALS2 suggests that men were slightly more likely to be in a medium-to-low income group, but women to have been in the lowest or highest income groups at HALS1.

## Life events

Life event questions were not asked in HALS1. The 26 life events questions used in HALS2 were developed by Huppert and colleagues for the Healthy Ageing Study (Economic and Social Research Council). They were devised for HALS2 from two scales, the West of Scotland Twenty-07 Study of Health in the Community and the National Survey of Health and Development, (Rodgers, 1991), both funded by the Medical Research Council.

For each event, the West of Scotland Twenty-07 Study used a series of seven supplementary questions, whereas the National Survey of Health and Development and HALS2 ask two: how much the event disrupted or changed the respondent's life and how much it caused them worry or stress (each on a 3 point scale: 'not at all', 'somewhat', 'a great deal').

In addition to the previous scales which only use a one-year time frame, questions were also asked about the past 7 years, in order to cover the follow-up period from HALS1. Since reports over seven

years are less reliable than over one year, a question about the past seven years was asked only if the respondent did not report the particular event in the past year, and then only for selected events (16 of the original 26). 25 of the events were 'adverse' (i.e. usually rated as such by independent judges) and the last one was an open-ended question about the occurrence of positive events, and the nature of such events.

## Lung function: see Respiratory Function

## 'Malaise' score: see Health, self-declared

## Marital status

'Marital status' normally refers to legal status, i.e. those who are cohabiting are not defined as married. 'Couple', as a household description, refers to those who are cohabiting as well as the married.

'Separated', however, is not necessarily a legal status but refers to all those who are permanently (as far as can be ascertained) living apart from a spouse.

## Memory

The memory test involved recall of items from a list of 10 common foods, read aloud to respondents a few minutes earlier. Respondents were required to make a decision about each food (whether or not it contained dietary fibre) at the time the list was presented. Recall was tested without prior warning ('incidental memory') following a distracting task. The measure is the total number of foods recalled.

## Neuroticism

The term refers generally to emotional instability. The Neuroticism scale of the Eysenck Personality Inventory (see above) makes the assumption that individuals have a characteristic way of responding emotionally (stable or unstable) and the scale is intended to measure this personality trait. The Neuroticism scale comprises twenty four questions about emotional responses, to which the subject is required to give a yes/no answer. The questions are concerned primarily with anxiety, depression and irritability. The scores are added; high scores correspond to emotional instability, low scores to emotional stability. Subjects who had more than two missing responses are not included in the tables.

# Occupational group: see Socio-economic group or social class

# Obesity and overweight: see Body Mass Index

# Pastimes

Participation in leisure activities, which do not require physical effort, were also enquired about in both Surveys, as they can form an important part of the respondent's social and non-working life.

# Reaction time (RT)

RT is the time taken for a person to respond as quickly as possible to the appearance of a target stimulus. In the survey, RT was measured using a specially designed portable machine (Bartram Associates, Cambridge). Numerals were displayed on a small screen at the top of the unit. Below were five keys, the central one labelled '0' and the remainder labelled (from left to right) 1,2,3 and 4. Subjects were asked to rest the appropriate finger(s) on the key(s) and, when a numeral appeared on the screen, to press as quickly as possible the key corresponding to that numeral. Only one numeral appeared at a time. There were two test conditions, simple RT and choice RT.

## Simple reaction time

Simple RT is the time taken to respond to a single, known target. In this case, only the digit '0' appeared and subjects were required to press the centre key labelled '0'. The second finger of the preferred hand rested on the centre key in readiness for responding. There were eight practice trials and twenty test trials. The time between a response and the next appearance of the digit was randomly varied between one and three seconds. The mean RT in milliseconds (msec) and the standard deviation were recorded for the twenty test trials.

## Choice reaction time

Choice RT is the time taken to respond when the target is not known in advance and the subject must choose the appropriate response. In this case, the digit 1,2,3 or 4 could appear and the subject was required to press the corresponding key. The second and third fingers of each hand rested on the appropriate keys in readiness for responding. There were eight practice trials and forty test trials (ten each of the four digits in random order). The time between a response and the next appearance of a digit was the same as for simple RT. The mean and the standard deviation of the reaction time on test trials were recorded separately for correct and incorrect responses. The number of errors was also recorded.

# Reasoning: see Block counting test

# Region

The units used are the Standard Regions of the Registrar General, with Scotland and Wales regarded as single regions. In most tables the regions are grouped into 'North': Scotland, Wales, North, North West, Yorkshire/Humberside and West Midlands and 'South': East Midlands, East Anglia, South West, South East and Greater London.

# Respiratory function

Respiratory function was measured using a portable electronic spirometer. The respondent was instructed to take a deep breath, and blow into the spirometer as hard, and as fast and for as long as he or she could. After a practice attempt, three measurements of lung function were then recorded by the spirometer:

1. $FEV_1$ (Forced Expiratory Volume in one second) which is the volume of air in litres expelled in the first second by the respondent.
2. PEF (Peak Expiratory Flow) which is the fastest rate of exhalation in litres per minute recorded during the measurement.
3. FVC (Forced Vital Capacity) which is the total amount of air in litres exhaled by the respondent. This is a reflection of functional lung capacity.

# The Choice Reaction time

## Respiratory Function Categories

In HALS1 these categories were derived using simple regression equations which did not take into account the fact that respiratory function does not peak until about age 25. Thus the equations used in HALS1 over-estimated the predicted values for those under 25 years of age. In HALS2 the polynomial regression equations for lung function derived by Strachan et al. (1991) were used. These were derived from over 1500 of the HALS1 subjects who were lifetime non-smokers with no history of respiratory problems.

For simplicity in analysing the data obtained, the respondents have been grouped into four categories. The first category (Excellent) is composed of those whose performance with the spirometer was equal to or in excess of predicted values for their age, sex and height. The second category (Good) comprises those in whom the values obtained were up to 2.0 standard deviations below the predicted value. In the third category (Fair to Poor) are those whose performance was between 2.0 and 4.0 standard deviations below the predicted value. Those respondents whose performance fell more than 4.0 standard deviations below the predicted value were regarded as having grossly impaired respiratory function (Very poor) and included in this category are those individuals who were unable to carry out the measurements because they suffered from chronic respiratory problems. Excluded from the analyses were respondents with transitory acute respiratory problems, such as a cold or 'flu.

# Roles and available attachments

This index was formed by scoring various demographic and lifestyle characteristics: e.g. marital status, living children, living parents, household structure, employment, whether born in area, whether lived in area for seven years or more, says 'feels part of community', been to place of worship in last two weeks, been involved in community work in past two weeks. These items (weighted) gave a range of scores of 0-18. The categories used in the tables are:

- Low 0-7
- Medium 8-10
- High 11 +

# Simple reaction time: see Reaction time

# Snacks: see Food

# Smoking

The order and phrasing of some of the questions in this section have been changed in HALS2, since the complex routing in HALS1 resulted in questions being missed on some occasions. The layout of questions used in the current Survey, designed to elicit the same information as before, has been used successfully in a national survey (Allied Dunbar National Fitness Survey, 1992) and a local survey currently being carried out by the Department of Community Medicine, University of Cambridge (The Ely Diabetes Project). The 1984/5 and 1991/2 smoking questions were compared in a pilot survey and shown to categorise respondents' smoking habits in exactly the same way.

Questions were designed to enable the categorisation of the respondents by their cigarette smoking habits, and consumption of all forms of smoked tobacco. Cigarette smoking was by far the most usual form of tobacco usage by men, and the only form of tobacco smoked by women.

Respondents are categorised as:
- *Current regular smoker:* Currently smokes at least one cigarette and/or pipe and/or cigar per day on average.
- *Current occasional smoker:* Currently smokes, but less than one cigarette and/or pipe and/or cigar per day on average.
- *Ex-(regular) smoker:* Does not now smoke but used to smoke at least one cigarette and/or pipe and/or cigar per day.
- *Never smoked:* Does not now smoke, and has never smoked as much as one cigarette and/or pipe and/or cigar per day.

Cigarette smokers are categorised as:
- *Current regular cigarette smoker:* Currently smokes at least one cigarette per day.
- *Light cigarette smoker:* smokes 1-15 cigarettes per day.
- *Heavy cigarette smoker:* smokes more than 15 cigarettes per day.

- *Occasional cigarette smoker:* Currently smokes cigarettes but less than one per day on average.
- *Ex-(regular) cigarette smoker:* Does not now smoke cigarettes but used to smoke at least one per day for a period of at least six months.

Tar levels of cigarettes were recorded as Low, Low middle, Middle, Middle high or High in both surveys. During the present Survey, in accordance with EC legislation, mg tar started to be recorded on cigarette packages, and some respondents reported these, which were converted to tar level categories:

- *Low tar:* 0-9.9mg
- *Low-middle tar:* 10-14.99mg
- *Middle tar:* 15-17.99mg
- *High tar:* over 18mg

## Social support

The questions designed to measure social support or social networks were derived largely from work in the United States (House et al. 1982; Berkman and Syme, 1979; Blazer and Kaplan, 1983) though similar methods have been used in smaller studies in Britain (Pill and Stott, 1980). The questions were tested in the pilot studies for acceptability.

### Index of Perceived Social Support

This index was formed from Q.13, with a range of 7-21. The responses were heavily skewed, with 60% of the population obtaining the maximum score, i.e. no lack of perceived support.

| The categories used in the tables: | Score |
|---|---|
| • Severe lack of perceived social support | 7-17 |
| • Moderate lack of perceived social support | 18-20 |
| • No lack of perceived social support | 21 |

### Indices of Family Contact

Derived from Q10 of the schedule. The categories used in the tables for the frequency of seeing relatives are:

- *Daily:* includes most days
- *Weekly:* At least weekly, 2 or 3 times a week.
- *Less than weekly:* At least monthly, more than once a year, less than once a year.

## Socio-economic group or social class

Because of the importance of this descriptive variable, many cross-checks were performed within the data to ensure that it is as accurate as possible.

The basic classification used in the tables is the Office of Population Censuses and Surveys (1980) socio-economic grouping, S.E.G. S.E.G. was chosen in preference to Social Class in most tables as being the better system for the examination of lifestyles. However, the Registrar General's Social Class (RGSC), usually grouped as non-manual and manual, is used in some tables. The majority of tables use a condensed version of S.E.G.:

1. *Professional:* S.E.G. 3,4. Employed and self-employed professional.
2. *Employers/managers:* S.E.G. 1,2,13. Employers and managers, large and small, including farmers.
3. *Other non-manual:* S.E.G. 5,6. Intermediate and junior non-manual.
4. *Skilled manual/own account:* S.E.G. 8,9,12.14. Foremen, supervisors, skilled manual workers, own-account manual workers, own-account farmers.
5. *Semi-skilled manual:* S.E.G. 7,10,15. Semi-skilled manual workers, personal service workers, general agricultural workers.
6. *Unskilled manual:* S.E.G. 11. Unskilled manual workers.

This condensed classification omits Armed Services, those who have never had an occupation, and those for whom occupational information is missing. Those without a past or present occupational group include students, young people who have never been employed, those who have never been able to work because of disability, and women who have never had an occupation outside the home.

### Collapsed S.E.G.

The above six categories are commonly collapsed to form a manual/non-manual distinction:

- *Non-manual:* Groups 1, 2, 3
- *Manual:* Groups 4, 5, 6

### Extended S.E.G.

The six categories are derived from seventeen in the basic classification. For particular purposes, other or more detailed combinations may be used.

## Household socio-economic group

This classification uses the condensed SEG groups 1-6, based on the current occupation of the 'head of household', or the past or 'usual' occupation of the retired, unemployed, etc. This is equivalent to the respondent's own occupation for almost all men, and for single and divorced women. Married women and widows are categorised by their husband's or ex-husband's occupation in the standard manner. In a few cases where a husband is not in the labour market, household S.E.G. can be based on a wife's occupation. The advantage of the use of household S.E.G. is that comparatively few people remain unclassified.

## Sport: see Active leisure pursuits

## Type A behaviour pattern

This term refers to a pattern of behaviour which has been associated with a raised incidence of heart disease (Jenkins et al. 1974) and is sometimes described as coronary-prone behaviour. Its characteristics are being hard-driving, competitive and pressed for time. It can be measured clinically (Friedman and Rosenman, 1959) or by questionnaire (Jenkins et al. 1967). In the present survey we used nine of the ten items of the Framingham Type A scale (Haynes et al. 1978). Respondents are required to indicate, in a self-completion questionnaire, how well the list of behaviours characterises them.

A description which fitted the subject well was scored 1, and a description which did not fit at all was scored 0. Intermediate categories received intermediate scores in accordance with the Framingham coding. The scores were summed and converted to a ratio of the maximum possible Type A behaviour which was a value of 1.00 multiplied by 100. Subjects who failed to answer more than one of the 9 questions are not included in the tables.

## Walking

Respondents were asked how much time per weekday and weekend day they spent walking when not at work – going to work, shopping, walking the dog, for pleasure etc. Walking, reported in this way, is difficult to quantify accurately, as recall can be unreliable (Allied Dunbar National Fitness Survey, 1992). Broad bands of time spent walking per weekend day, with those who cannot walk included in the nil walking category, have been used to indicate walking activity. In HALS2 an additional question about walks of over 2 miles was included, as used by the General Household Survey (Smyth and Browne, 1992) and the Allied Dunbar National Fitness Survey (1992).

## Working status: see Employment status

### References

Allied Dunbar National Fitness Survey (1992), 'A report on activity patterns and fitness levels', London: The Sports Council and the Health Education Authority.

Berkman, L.F. and Syme, L. (1979), 'Social networks, host resistance and mortality: a nine-year follow up study of Alameda County residents', American Journal Epidemiology, 109, 186-204.

Blazer, D.G. and Kaplan, B.H. (1983), 'The assessment of social support in an elderly community population', American Journal of Social Psychiatry, 3, 29-36.

Blaxter, M. (1984), 'Causes of disease: women talking', Social Science and Medicine, 17, 59-69.

Blaxter, M. (1985), 'Self-definition of health status and consulting rates in primary care', Quarterly Journal of Social Affairs, 1, 131-171.

Blaxter, M. (1987), in Cox B.D. et al. 'The Health and Lifestyle Survey: preliminary report of a nationwide survey of the physical and mental health, attitudes and lifestyle of a random sample of 9003 British adults', London: The Health Promotion Research Trust.

Blaxter, M. and Paterson, E. (1982), 'Mothers and Daughters: Health Attitudes and Behaviour in Two Generations', London: Heinmann Educational Books.

Bray, G.A. ed. (1979), 'Obesity in America', Proceedings of the 2nd Fogarty International Centre Conference on Obesity, No.79, Washington: US: DHEW.

British Nutrition Foundation (1985), 'Eating in the early 1980s. Attitudes and behaviour: main findings', London: The British Nutrition Foundation.

Bull, N.L. (1985), 'Dietary habits of 15 to 25 year olds', Human Nutrition: Applied Nutrition, 38A, 1-68.

d'Houtard, A. and Field, M.G. (1984), 'The image of health: variations in perceptions by social class in a French population', Sociology of Health and Illness, 6, 30-60.

Dight, S. (1976), 'Scottish Drinking Habits, Edinburgh: HMSO.

Eysenck, H.J. and Eysenck, B.G. (1964), 'Manual of the Eysenck Personality Inventory', London: Hodder and Stoughton.

Friedman, M. and Rosenman, R.H. (1959), 'Association of specific overt behaviour pattern with blood and cardiovascular findings', Journal of the American Medical Association', 169, 1286-1296.

Goldberg, D.P. (1972), 'The Detection of Psychiatric Illness by Questionnaire', London: Oxford University Press.

Hannay, D.R. (1978), 'Symptom prevalence in the community', Journal of the Royal College General Practitioners, 28, 492-499.

Harris, A. (1971), 'National Survey of the Handicapped and Impaired', London: HMSO.

Harris, D.M. and Guten, S. (1979) 'Health protective behaviour', Journal of Health and Social Behaviour, 20, 17-29.

Haynes, S.G., Frienleib, M., Levine, S., Scotch, N. and Kannel, W.B. (1978), 'The relationship of psychosocial factors to coronary heart disease in The Framingham Study. 11: Prevalence of coronary heart disease', American Journal of Epidemiology, 107, 362-383.

Herzlich, C. (1973), 'Health and Illness: a social psychological analysis', London: Academic Press.

House, J.S., Robbins, C. and Metzner, H.L. (1982), 'The associations of social relationships and activities mortality: Prospective evidence from the Tecumseh Community Health Study', American Journal of Epidemiology, 109, 186-204.

International Classification of Diseases (1977), 'Manual of the International Classification of Diseases, Injuries and Causes of Death', London: HMSO and Geneva: WHO.

Jenkins, C.D., Rosenman, R.H. and Friedman, M. (1967), 'Development of an objective psychological test for the determination of the coronary prone behaviour in employed men', Journal of Chronic Diseases, 20, 371-379.

Jenkins, C.D., Rosenman, R.M. and Zyzanski, S.J. (1974), 'Prediction of clinical coronary heart disease by a test of the coronary-prone behaviour', New England Journal of Medicine, 290, 1271-1275.

Mayfield, D., McCleod, G. and Hall, P. (1974), 'The CAGE questionnaire: validation of a new alcoholism screening instrument', American Journal of Psychiatry, 131, 1121-1123.

Miller, W.R., Heather, N. and Hall, W. (1991), 'Calculating standard drink units: international comparisons', British Journal of Addiction, 86, 43-47.

Office of Population Censuses and Surveys (1980), 'Classification of occupations and coding index', London: HMSO.

Pernanen, K. (1974), 'Validity of survey data on alcohol use', Research Advances in Alcohol and Drug Problems, Chichester: Wiley.

Pill, R. and Stott, N.C.H. (1980), 'A study of health beliefs, attitudes and behaviour among working class mothers (Report)', Department of General Practice, Welsh National School of Medicine.

Pill, R. and Stott, N.C.H. (1982), 'Concept of illness causation and responsibility: some preliminary data from a sample of working class mothers', Social Science and Medicine, 16, 43-52.

Pill, R. and Stott, N.C.H. (1985) 'Choice or chance, further ideas of illness and responsibility for health', Social Science and Medicine, 21, 975.

Rodgers, B. (1991), 'Models of Stress, vulnerability and affective disorder', Journal of Affective Disorders, 21, 1-13.

Royal College of General Practitioners (1982), 'Morbidity Statistics from General Practice 1970-1971', Studies on Medical and Population subjects No.46, London: HMSO.

Royal College of Physicians (1983), 'Obesity Report', Journal of The Royal College of Physicians, 17, 5-65.

Saunders, W.M. and Kershaw, P.W. (1980), 'Screening tests for alcoholism – findings from a community study', British Journal of Addiction, 75, 37.

Smyth, M. and Browne, F. (1992), 'General Household Survey 1990', London: HMSO.

Strachan, D.P., Cox, B.D., Erzinclioglu, S.W., Walters, D.E. and Whichelow, M.J. (1991), 'Ventilatory function and winter fresh fruit consumption in a random sample of British adults', Thorax, 46, 624-629.

Tarnopolsky, A., Hand, D.J., McLean, E.,K., Roberts, H. and Wiggins, R.,D. (1979), 'Validity and use of a screening questionnaire (GHQ) in the community', British Journal of Psychiatry, 134, 508-515.

Turner, C. (1990), 'How much alcohol is in a 'standard drink'? An analysis of 125 studies'. British Journal of Addiction, 85, 1171-1175.

Wadsworth M.E.J. (1980), Personal communication.

WHO (1978), 'Arterial Hypertension', Geneva: World Health Organisation.

Willet, W.C. and MacMahon, B. (1984), 'Diet and Cancer – an overview', New England Journal of Medicine, 310, 633-638.

Wilson, P. (1980), 'Drinking in England and Wales', London: HMSO.

Yarnell, J.W.G., Fehily, A.M., Millbank, J.E., Sweetman, P.M., and Walker, C.L. (1983), 'A short dietary questionnaire for use in an epidemiological survey: comparison with weighed dietary records', Human Nutrition: Applied Nutrition, 37A, 103-111.

# APPENDIX | B

## INSTRUMENTATION, VALIDATION

## AND CALIBRATION

All equipment was evaluated and assessed by 'in house' trials and by three major feasibility and pilot studies prior to the first survey in the field, involving over 300 respondents. The spirometers, stadiometers, blood pressure machines and reaction timers were those used in the 1984/5 survey.

## Training and instruction

All nurses attended a one day training and briefing session. Most of the nurses had previous experience in field studies, usually with the MRC study of hypertension, the MRC Survey of Health and Development or the previous Health and Lifestyle Survey. Detailed instruction was given in the use of the equipment at these training sessions. During the fieldwork the progress of the nurses was monitored both by the research team at Cambridge and by the supervisors from Social and Community Planning Research.

## Electronic scales

The electronic scales (Salter) displayed values digitally to the nearest 0.2kg. Respondents were weighed without shoes, and allowances were made of 0.9kg and 0.6kg for men and women respectively in light clothing, and 1.5kg and 0.9kg for heavier clothing. Providing the scales were set on a firm, level surface the pilot studies had showed that there was no significant problem of measurement variability. The calibration of the scales was checked at the beginning and end of each wave of data collection and the nurses were asked to check the scales daily by using themselves as a reference weight.

## Stadiometer

The stadiometer used for the survey had been previously evaluated and assessed for use before the first Survey in the MRC Survey of Health and Development in a study of over 3,000 individuals (Bradden, et al. 1986). The stadiometer incorporated a spirit level to ensure that the top plate was resting horizontally on the respondent's head and the scale was read to the nearest 0.1cm. Assessment of observer variability indicated that although there was some variation between observers, as in the OPCS study of heights and weights (Knight, 1984), the large number of field workers (over 120) ensured that a small bias on the part of any one interviewer would not have a significant effect on the overall results. The results from the first survey gave an average height of 173.5cm for men aged 18-93 compared to the OPCS values of 173.9cm for men aged 16-64. The difference is probably due to the inclusion of the older men in the Health and Lifestyle Survey.

## Girth (waist) and hip measurements

Girth (waist) was measured at the narrowest point or, if that could not be ascertained, midway between the iliac crest and the bottom rib, using a good quality dressmaker's measuring tape.

Hip circumference was measured, in cm, at the widest point below the iliac crest with the same tape.

## Spirometer

An electronic spirometer (Micro Medical Ltd.) chosen for its portability and simplicity in operation was used for the respiratory function measurements. It was developed in the Department of Clinical Physics and Bioengineering, Guy's Hospital and had been evaluated before the first Survey by the Department of Community Medicine at St. Thomas's Hospital who subsequently published their findings (Gunawardena, Houston and Smith, 1987), and the Health and Safety Executive (personal communication). The spirometer was found to give satisfactorily reproducible results with coefficients of variation of ± 2.2% for Forced Expiratory Volume in one second and ± 2.5% for Forced Vital Capacity (Melia et al. 1985). The device was assessed as having a comparable accuracy to the Vitalograph spirometer against which it was calibrated (Chowiencyzk and Lawson (1982).

The pocket spirometers were calibrated at the start of each wave of data collection and rechecked at the end. In the few instances where significant changes had occurred between calibrations the values obtained by the nurse were discarded. The nurses were encouraged to check the device by using the instrument on themselves as a rough calibration guide before each series of measurements, so that any major fault could be detected and the instrument replaced.

## Dental roll

Dental rolls were used to collect saliva for cotinine measurements, which can be used to assess passive as well as active smoking. Each respondent was asked to place a dental roll in his/her mouth and move it around within the mouth for 3-5 minutes until it was well saturated with saliva. The roll was then placed in a small specimen tube and dispatched by first class post in a padded envelope to Dr Martin Jarvis in London for cotinine assay. If samples were not to be mailed immediately they were kept in a domestic freezer. Cotinine results are not reported in this document, but will be available at a later date.

## Blood-pressure machine

The blood-pressure instrument chosen, after evaluation against many others, was an Accutorr (Datascope Ltd.). The machine was assessed in the Physiological Measurement Laboratory at Addenbrookes Hospital Cambridge by comparison with intra-arterial catheterisation in the same arm, and with other automated blood-pressure instruments. The advantages of having a robust reliable instrument with a detection system, not subject to background noise interference which had been reported by many nurses who had used other instruments in previous field trials, outweighed the disadvantages of a requirement for a power supply, and the instrument's weight (Bruner et al. 1981).

## GP referrals

If the nurse discovered that the respondent's blood pressure was elevated, particularly if he/she was not already being treated for hypertension, she would advise the respondent to visit his/her General Practitioner, and request permission for the blood-pressure readings to be forwarded to the GP. If consent was given the nurse entered the blood-pressure readings, the respondent's name and address and that of the GP onto a form, which was then sent to the survey director, Dr Cox, who wrote to the GP.

## Reaction timer

The reaction timer used for the Survey was purpose designed and built (Batvale Ltd.). Each timer measured 18 x 12 x 4cm depth. It housed a 5 x 2cm screen on which 1cm high digits were presented, and 5 response keys each 1.5cm square. Preprogrammed random time sequences were incorporated into the instruments so that each respondent was faced with the same apparently randomly generated numbers to react to. Each instrument was checked against another instrument by operating both simultaneously. The electronically generated sequences were identical in respect of time course, each digit appearing between 1 and 3 seconds after the response to the previous digit.

Simple reaction time was the time for the subject to press the central key (marked '0') as quickly as possible when the digit '0' appeared on the screen.

The mean response time and standard deviation appeared on the screen recorded in seconds and milliseconds.

Choice reaction time was the time taken to press as quickly and accurately as possible, one of four keys marked '1' to '4' when the corresponding digit appeared on the screen. The mean reaction time and standard deviation appeared on the screen separately for correct and incorrect responses. The number of incorrect responses also appeared.

## References

Bradden, F.E.M. Rodgers, B., Wadsworth, M.E.J. and Davies, J.M.C. (1986), 'Onset of obesity in a 36 year birth cohort study', British Medical Journal, 293, 299-303.

Bruner, J.M.R. Krenis, L.J., Kurisman, J.M. and Sherman, A.P. (1981), 'Comparison of direct and indirect methods of measuring arterial blood pressure'. Medical Instrumentation, 15, 11-21, 97-101.

Chowiencyzk, P.J., and Lawson, C.P., (1982), 'Pocket-sized device for measuring forced expiratory volume in one second and forced vital capacity', British Medical Journal, 285, 15-17.

Gunawardena, K.A., Houston, K., and Smith, A.P., (1987), 'Evaluation of the turbine pocket spirometer', Thorax, 42, 689-693.

Knight, I. (1984), 'The heights and weights of adults in Great Britain', OPCS, HMSO.

Melia, R.J.W. Swan, A.V., Clarke, G., du Ve Florey, C. and Nelson, A.M. (1985), 'Suitability of new turbine spirometer for epidemiological surveys in children', Bulletin of European Physiopathology and Respiration, 21, 43-47.

# APPENDIX | C

## SCHEDULES

SCPR
SOCIAL & COMMUNITY
PLANNING RESEARCH

*Head Office: 35 NORTHAMPTON SQUARE,*
*LONDON EC1V 0AX. Telephone 071-250 1866*

*Field and DP Office: BRENTWOOD, ESSEX*
*Northern Field Office: DARLINGTON, CO. DURHAM*

P.1178

## HEALTH AND LIFESTYLE SURVEY

1991/2

SERIAL NUMBER:

CARD NUMBER: 02

WARD:

1984/85 NURSE OUTCOME:     Measured      1

Not measured   2

INTRODUCTION: I work for SCPR, an independent research institute, and we are carrying out a large-scale national survey about people's attitudes towards health, and about the way they live. You were interviewed seven years ago (in 1985) and this survey is a follow-up to see how your health, attitudes and lifestyle may have changed since then.

TIME AT START OF INTERVIEW:

BATCH

e. HOUSEHOLD CONTINUATION GRID. COMPLETE IF NECESSARY.

| RELATIONSHIP TO RESPONDENT | | | | | | SEX | | AGE LAST BIRTHDAY |
|---|---|---|---|---|---|---|---|---|
| Spouse | Living as Married | Son/ daughter (incl. adopted & steps) | Parent (incl. in-laws) | Other relatives (incl. other in-laws, grand-children & grandparents) | Non-relative (incl. fosters) | M | F | (IN YEARS) |
| 1 | 2 | 3 | 4 | 5 | 6 | 1 | 2 | |
| 1 | 2 | 3 | 4 | 5 | 6 | 1 | 2 | |
| 1 | 2 | 3 | 4 | 5 | 6 | 1 | 2 | |
| 1 | 2 | 3 | 4 | 5 | 6 | 1 | 2 | |
| 1 | 2 | 3 | 4 | 5 | 6 | 1 | 2 | |
| 1 | 2 | 3 | 4 | 5 | 6 | 1 | 2 | |
| 1 | 2 | 3 | 4 | 5 | 6 | 1 | 2 | |
| 1 | 2 | 3 | 4 | 5 | 6 | 1 | 2 | |
| 1 | 2 | 3 | 4 | 5 | 6 | 1 | 2 | |
| 1 | 2 | 3 | 4 | 5 | 6 | 1 | 2 | |
| 1 | 2 | 3 | 4 | 5 | 6 | 1 | 2 | |

HOUSEHOLD

1. I would like to start by collecting some brief information about you and your household.

a. First, what is your date of birth?   DAY [ ]  MONTH [ ]  YEAR [ ]

b. So can I check, on your last birthday you were aged ...?   AGE: [ ]

c. RECORD RESPONDENT'S SEX:   Male 1   Female 2

d. In addition to you how many other people live in this household?

   NUMBER OF OTHER PEOPLE: [ ]

   Lives on own   00   GO TO Q2

   [ ]   ASK e.

e. IF OTHER PEOPLE IN HOUSEHOLD AT d.

   Who lives in the household with you?

   RECORD BELOW DETAILS OF ALL IN HOUSEHOLD APART FROM RESPONDENT

| RELATIONSHIP TO RESPONDENT | | | | | | SEX | | AGE LAST BIRTHDAY |
|---|---|---|---|---|---|---|---|---|
| Spouse | Living as Married | Son/ daughter (incl. adopted & steps) | Parent (incl. in-laws) | Other relatives (incl. other in-laws, grand-children & grandparents) | Non-relative (incl. fosters) | M | F | (IN YEARS) |
| 1 | 2 | 3 | 4 | 5 | 6 | 1 | 2 | |
| 1 | 2 | 3 | 4 | 5 | 6 | 1 | 2 | |
| 1 | 2 | 3 | 4 | 5 | 6 | 1 | 2 | |
| 1 | 2 | 3 | 4 | 5 | 6 | 1 | 2 | |
| 1 | 2 | 3 | 4 | 5 | 6 | 1 | 2 | |
| 1 | 2 | 3 | 4 | 5 | 6 | 1 | 2 | |
| 1 | 2 | 3 | 4 | 5 | 6 | 1 | 2 | |
| 1 | 2 | 3 | 4 | 5 | 6 | 1 | 2 | |
| 1 | 2 | 3 | 4 | 5 | 6 | 1 | 2 | |
| 1 | 2 | 3 | 4 | 5 | 6 | 1 | 2 | |
| 1 | 2 | 3 | 4 | 5 | 6 | 1 | 2 | |
| 1 | 2 | 3 | 4 | 5 | 6 | 1 | 2 | |

f. CHECK NUMBER OF ROWS COMPLETED IN GRID = ENTRY AT d. OR IF MORE THAN 12, CONTINUE OPPOSITE.

2a. Do you have any (other) children of your own who are not living with you?

(CHILDREN OF ANY AGE)

| | | |
|---|---|---|
| Yes | 1 | ASK b. |
| No | 2 | GO TO Q3 |

b. IF YES (CODE 1 AT a.)

How many (other) children do you have?

NUMBER OF (OTHER) CHILDREN: [ ]

---

### HEALTH ATTITUDES AND BELIEFS

**ALL**

3a. I am now going to ask you some general questions about health and your opinions about it. There are no right and wrong answers. We just want to know what you think.

Would you say that for someone of your age, your own health is generally ... READ OUT ...

CODE ONE ONLY

| | |
|---|---|
| ... excellent, | 1 |
| good, | 2 |
| fair, | 3 |
| or poor? | 4 |
| Don't know | 8 |

b. Do you do anything at the moment to keep yourself healthy or improve your health?

| | | |
|---|---|---|
| Yes | 1 | ASK Q4 |
| No | 2 | GO TO Q5 |

---

IF YES (CODE 1 AT Q3b)

4. What are the three most important things you do to keep or improve your health?

DO NOT PROMPT.
CODE 3 ITEMS BELOW ONLY.
(ACCEPT ONE OR TWO IF NO MORE OFFERED).

| | | |
|---|---|---|
| DIET: | Keep to a medical/slimming diet | 01 |
| | Other dietary habits | 02 |
| DRINKING: | Stopped or reduced drinking | 03 |
| SMOKING: | Stopped or reduced smoking | 04 |
| MEDICINES: | Take medicines | 05 |
| PHYSICAL ACTIVITIES: | Housework | 06 |
| | Gardening | 07 |
| | Walking | 08 |
| | Play particular sport(s) | 09 |
| | Physical leisure activities generally | 10 |
| JOB: | Job/work keeps healthy | 11 |
| SLEEP: | Type of sleeping habits | 12 |
| SOCIAL: | Type of social activities | 13 |
| MENTAL STATE: | Mental attitude, lack of stress | 14 |
| | Use special techniques - yoga/meditation etc. | 15 |
| HOUSING/AREA: | Housing/area conditions | 16 |
| FRESH AIR: | Get (more) fresh air | 17 |
| OTHER (SPECIFY): | | |
| 1. _____ | | 18 |
| 2. _____ | | 19 |
| 3. _____ | | 20 |

**ALL**

5a. Are there any things you would like to do
to keep yourself healthy but don't do?

Yes | 1 | ASK b.
No | 2 | GO TO Q6

IF YES (CODE 1 AT a.)

b. What would you like to do?
CODE UP TO THREE THINGS

| | |
|---|---|
| Sport/exercise | 01 |
| Diet/nutrition generally | 02 |
| Lose weight | 03 |
| Cut down or give up smoking | 04 |
| Cut down or give up alcohol | 05 |
| Pursue hobbies | 06 |
| Change/get job | 07 |
| Change social life | 08 |
| | 09 |
| | 10 |
| | 11 |
| Don't know | 98 |

Other (SPECIFY)  1. _____
2. _____
3. _____

**ALL**

6a. Is there any way in which your life is
healthier now than it was seven years ago?

Yes | 1 | ASK b.
No | 2 | ASK Q7

IF YES (CODE 1 AT a.)

b. In what ways has it become more healthy?
PROBE FULLY. RECORD VERBATIM

**ALL**

7a. Is there any way in which your life has become
less healthy in the last seven years?

Yes | 1 | ASK b.
No | 2 | GO TO Q8

IF YES (CODE 1 AT a.)

b. In what ways has it become less healthy?
PROBE FULLY. RECORD VERBATIM

**ALL**

8a. How long have you lived in this area?

CODE ONE ONLY

| | |
|---|---|
| Less than 1 year | 1 |
| 1 year, less than 2 years | 2 |
| 2 years, less than 7 years | 3 |
| 7 years or more | 4 |
| Can't say | 8 |

b. Were you born in this area?

| | |
|---|---|
| Yes | 1 |
| No | 2 |
| Don't know/Can't remember | 8 |

c. Do you feel part of the community?

| | |
|---|---|
| Yes | 1 |
| No | 2 |
| Don't know | 8 |

d. And do you have any friends in this community?

| | |
|---|---|
| Yes | 1 |
| No | 2 |
| No friends at all | 7 |
| Don't know | 8 |

**9a.** ALL

(Apart from those who live with you,) do any of your (children or other) relatives live in the area or within easy reach?

| | | |
|---|---|---|
| Yes | 1 | ASK b. |
| No | 2 | GO TO Q10 |
| No relatives | 3 | GO TO Q.12 |

**b.** IF YES (CODE 1 AT a.)

How many of each of these relatives live in the area or within easy reach of the area? Starting with...

READ OUT...

INSERT NUMBER FOR EACH CATEGORY OR CODE "00" FOR NONE OR "98" FOR UNKNOWN

... Children?
... Grandchildren?
... Parents?
... Brothers/sisters?
... Other relatives?

**10.** IF HAS RELATIVES (CODES 1 OR 2 AT Q9a.) ASK AS APPROPRIATE

Thinking of all your relatives, (apart from those who live with you), how often do you see any of your (children or other) relatives to speak to?

PROMPT IF NECESSARY

> IF SEES DIFFERENT RELATIVE EVERY DAY, CODE AS "DAILY"

CODE ONE ONLY

| | |
|---|---|
| Never | 0 |
| Daily | 1 |
| 2 or 3 times a week | 2 |
| At least weekly | 3 |
| At least monthly | 4 |
| More than once a year | 5 |
| Less than once a year | 6 |
| Don't know | 8 |

**11a.** IF HAS RELATIVE(S) (CODES 1 OR 2 AT Q9a.)

(Apart from those who live with you,) which one of your relatives do you have the most contact with?

> IF CLAIM TO CONTACT TWO OR MORE RELATIVES EQUALLY, PROMPT TO ESTABLISH WHICH ONE THEY HAVE MOST CONTACT WITH. IF CANNOT SPECIFY ONE PERSON THEN MULTI-CODE.

> CODE STEP-RELATIVES IN "OTHER CATEGORIES"

| | | |
|---|---|---|
| No contact | 00 | GO TO Q12 |
| Daughter | 01 | |
| Daughter-in-law | 02 | |
| Son | 03 | |
| Son-in-law | 04 | ASK b. |
| Mother | 05 | |
| Father | 06 | |
| Sister/brother | 07 | |
| Granddaughter/grandson | 08 | |
| Other female relative | 09 | |
| Other male relative | 10 | |
| Don't know | 98 | |

**b.** IF HAS CONTACT WITH RELATIVE(S)

How often do you see him/her/them to talk to?

PROMPT IF NECESSARY

CODE ONE ONLY

| | |
|---|---|
| Daily | 1 |
| 2 or 3 times a week | 2 |
| At least weekly | 3 |
| At least monthly | 4 |
| More than once a year | 5 |
| Less than once a year | 6 |
| Don't know | 8 |

**12.** ALL

How often do you see any of your neighbours to have a chat, or to do something with?

PROMPT IF NECESSARY

CODE ONE ONLY

| | |
|---|---|
| Never | 0 |
| Daily | 1 |
| 2 or 3 times a week | 2 |
| At least weekly | 3 |
| At least monthly | 4 |
| More than once a year | 5 |
| Less than once a year | 6 |
| Don't know | 8 |

ALL

14. SHOW CARD B. On this card are things people have said about health. I'd like you to say how far you agree with each statement. The answers you can give are shown on top of the card.
READ OUT EACH ITEM AND CODE

| STATEMENT | Strongly Agree | Agree | All depends (Don't know) | Disagree | Strongly disagree |
|---|---|---|---|---|---|
| a. It's sensible to do exactly what the doctors say | 1 | 2 | 3 | 4 | 5 |
| b. To have good health is the most important thing in life | 1 | 2 | 3 | 4 | 5 |
| c. Generally health is a matter of luck | 1 | 2 | 3 | 4 | 5 |
| d. If you think too much about your health, you are more likely to be ill | 1 | 2 | 3 | 4 | 5 |
| e. Suffering sometimes has a divine purpose | 1 | 2 | 3 | 4 | 5 |
| f. I have to be very ill before I'll go to the doctor | 1 | 2 | 3 | 4 | 5 |
| g. People like me don't really have time to think about their health | 1 | 2 | 3 | 4 | 5 |
| h. The most important thing is the constitution (the health) you are born with. | 1 | 2 | 3 | 4 | 5 |

15. I'm now going to read out some different kinds of disease and ask you what in your opinion causes them.

What do you believe causes stomach ulcers?

DO NOT PROMPT
CODE ALL THAT APPLY

| | |
|---|---|
| Worry/Tension/Stress | 01 |
| Alcohol | 02 |
| Bad diet | 03 |
| Fried/Fatty foods | 04 |
| "Acid" foods | 05 |
| Irregular meals/Shift work | 06 |
| Lack of exercise | 07 |
| Family or heredity | 08 |
| Other (SPECIFY) i) | 09 |
| ii) | 10 |
| Don't know | 98 |

---

13. SHOW CARD A. I would now like you to think about your family. By family I mean those you live with as well as those elsewhere. Here are some comments people have made about their family. I'd like you to say how far each statement is true for you. Use this card to give your reply. CODE ONE ONLY FOR EACH QUESTION.

a. There are members of my family (friends) who make me feel loved. Is this... READ OUT
not true, 1
partly true, 2
or, certainly true? 3

b. Do things to make me feel happy.
Not true, 1
partly true, 2
or, certainly true. 3

c. There are members of my family (friends) who can be relied on no matter what happens.
Not true, 1
partly true, 2
or, certainly true. 3

d. Would see that I am taken care of if I needed to be.
Not true, 1
partly true, 2
or, certainly true. 3

e. There are members of my family (friends) who accept me just as I am.
Not true, 1
partly true, 2
or, certainly true. 3

f. Make me feel an important part of their lives.
Not true 1
partly true, 2
or, certainly true. 3

g. Give me support and encouragement.
Not true, 1
partly true, 2
or, certainly true. 3

16a. What do you believe causes <u>chronic bronchitis</u>?

DO NOT PROMPT

CODE ALL THAT APPLY

| | |
|---|---|
| Smoking | 01 |
| Overweight | 02 |
| Family or heredity | 03 |
| Damp weather or clothes | 04 |
| Weak chest/lungs | 05 |
| Air pollution | 06 |
| Working conditions | 07 |
| | 08 |
| | 09 |
| Don't know | 98 |

Other (SPECIFY) i) _____

ii) _____

b. What do you believe causes <u>high blood pressure</u>?

DO NOT PROMPT

CODE ALL THAT APPLY

| | |
|---|---|
| Smoking | 01 |
| Worry/Tension/Stress | 02 |
| Alcohol | 03 |
| Type of diet | 04 |
| Salt | 05 |
| Overweight | 06 |
| Lack of exercise | 07 |
| Family or heredity | 08 |
| Age | 09 |
| | 10 |
| | 11 |
| Don't know | 98 |

Other (SPECIFY) i) _____

ii) _____

c. What do you believe causes <u>obesity or being overweight</u>?

DO NOT PROMPT

CODE ALL THAT APPLY

| | |
|---|---|
| Worry/Tension/Stress | 01 |
| Alcohol | 02 |
| Overeating | 03 |
| Eating wrong foods | 04 |
| Lack of exercise | 05 |
| Family or heredity | 06 |
| 'Glands' or hormones | 07 |
| | 08 |
| | 09 |
| Don't know | 98 |

Other (SPECIFY) i) _____

ii) _____

17a. What do you believe causes <u>migraine</u>?

DO NOT PROMPT

CODE ALL THAT APPLY

| | |
|---|---|
| Worry/Tension/Stress | 01 |
| Alcohol | 02 |
| Foods, food allergy | 03 |
| Family or heredity | 04 |
| Pollution | 05 |
| Environment (housing/local conditions) | 06 |
| | 07 |
| | 08 |
| Don't know | 98 |

Other (SPECIFY) i) _____

ii) _____

b. What do you believe causes <u>liver trouble</u>?

DO NOT PROMPT

CODE ALL THAT APPLY

| | |
|---|---|
| Worry/Tension/Stress | 01 |
| Alcohol | 02 |
| Diet | 03 |
| Overweight | 04 |
| Family or heredity | 05 |
| Pollution | 06 |
| | 07 |
| | 08 |
| Don't know | 98 |

Other (SPECIFY) i) _____

ii) _____

c. What do you believe causes <u>a stroke</u>?

DO NOT PROMPT

CODE ALL THAT APPLY

| | |
|---|---|
| Worry/Tension/Stress | 01 |
| Alcohol | 02 |
| Diet | 03 |
| Overweight | 04 |
| Lack of exercise | 05 |
| Family or heredity | 06 |
| Environment (housing/local conditions) | 07 |
| Old age | 08 |
| High blood pressure | 09 |
| Sudden/over exercise | 10 |
| | 11 |
| | 12 |
| Don't know | 98 |

Other (SPECIFY) i) _____

ii) _____

18. What do you believe causes <u>lung cancer</u>?

    **DO NOT PROMPT**
    **CODE ALL THAT APPLY**

    | | |
    |---|---|
    | Smoking | 01 |
    | Alcohol | 02 |
    | Diet | 03 |
    | Overweight | 04 |
    | Lack of exercise | 05 |
    | Family or heredity | 06 |
    | Air pollution | 07 |
    | Other pollution/chemicals | 08 |
    | Environment (housing/local conditions) | 09 |
    | Other (SPECIFY) i) _____ | 10 |
    | ii) _____ | 11 |
    | Don't know | 98 |

19. What do you believe causes <u>heart trouble</u>?

    **DO NOT PROMPT**
    **CODE ALL THAT APPLY**

    | | |
    |---|---|
    | Smoking | 01 |
    | Worry/Tension/Stress | 02 |
    | Alcohol | 03 |
    | Wrong diet | 04 |
    | Fatty foods | 05 |
    | Overeating | 06 |
    | Obesity/Overweight | 07 |
    | Lack of exercise | 08 |
    | Over-exertion/sudden exercise | 09 |
    | Family or heredity | 10 |
    | Overworking | 11 |
    | Other (SPECIFY) i) _____ | 12 |
    | ii) _____ | 13 |
    | Don't know | 98 |

20a. What do you think causes <u>severe depression</u>?

    **DO NOT PROMPT**
    **CODE ALL THAT APPLY**

    | | |
    |---|---|
    | Worry/Tension/Stress | 01 |
    | Family or heredity | 02 |
    | Loneliness | 03 |
    | Financial problems | 04 |
    | Attitude/Give in to things | 05 |
    | Bereavement | 06 |
    | Marital problems/Divorce/Separation | 07 |
    | Family relationships | 08 |
    | Menopause | 09 |
    | Childbirth | 10 |
    | Unemployment | 11 |
    | Other (SPECIFY) i) _____ | 12 |
    | ii) _____ | 13 |
    | Don't know | 98 |

b. What do you think causes <u>piles and haemorrhoids</u>?

    **DO NOT PROMPT**
    **CODE ALL THAT APPLY**

    | | |
    |---|---|
    | Constipation | 01 |
    | Diet-low fibre/roughage | 02 |
    | Other bad diet | 03 |
    | Pregnancy | 04 |
    | Sitting on cold surfaces | 05 |
    | Sitting on wet surfaces | 06 |
    | Other (SPECIFY) i) _____ | 07 |
    | ii) _____ | 08 |
    | Don't know | 98 |

---

| HEALTH |
|---|

**ALL**

Now I would like to ask you about your health.

21. Are there any things about your life now that have a <u>good</u> effect on your health?

    | | | |
    |---|---|---|
    | Yes | 1 | ASK Q22 |
    | No | 2 | GO TO Q23 |
    | Don't know | 8 | |

22. **IF YES (CODE 1 AT Q21)**
What are they?
**CODE ALL THAT APPLY**

| | |
|---|---|
| Able to get about | 01 |
| Environment/housing | 02 |
| Work | 03 |
| Financial/Standard of living/Income | 04 |
| Family/Marital relationships | 05 |
| Friends/Neighbours/Social activity | 06 |
| Behaviour (smoking, drinking, exercise, etc) | 07 |
| Contentment | 08 |
| Other (SPECIFY) _____ | 09 |
| Don't know | 98 |

23a. **ALL**
Are there any things about your life now that have a **bad** effect on your health?

| | | |
|---|---|---|
| Yes | 1 | ASK b. |
| No | 2 | GO TO Q24 |
| Don't know | 8 | |

b. **IF YES (CODE 1 AT a.)**
What are they?
**CODE ALL THAT APPLY**

| | |
|---|---|
| Unable to get about | 01 |
| Environment/housing | 02 |
| Work | 03 |
| Financial/Standard of living/Income | 04 |
| Family or marital problems/relationships | 05 |
| Friends/Neighbours/Social activity | 06 |
| Behaviour (smoking/drinking/exercise, etc) | 07 |
| Stress and worry | 08 |
| Other (SPECIFY) _____ | 09 |
| Don't know | 98 |

24. **ALL**
Do you feel that you lead ... **READ OUT** ...
**CODE ONE ONLY**

| | |
|---|---|
| ... a very healthy life, | 1 |
| a fairly healthy life, | 2 |
| a not very healthy life, | 3 |
| or, an unhealthy life? | 4 |
| Don't know | 8 |

25a. **ALL**
Do you think that compared to seven years ago your health is generally ... ?

| | | |
|---|---|---|
| ... Better, | 1 | ASK b. |
| worse, | 2 | ASK c. |
| or about the same? | 3 | GO TO Q26 |
| Can't say | 8 | |

b. **IF BETTER (CODE 1 AT a.)**
Do you think it is ... **READ OUT** ...

| | |
|---|---|
| ... a bit better | 1 |
| or a lot better? | 2 |
| Can't say | 8 |

c. **IF WORSE (CODE 2 AT a.)**
Do you think it is ... **READ OUT** ...

| | |
|---|---|
| ... a bit worse | 1 |
| or a lot worse? | 2 |
| Can't say | 8 |

26a. **ALL**
At the <u>moment</u> do you have anything on prescription. (IF FEMALE UNDER 50: Other than the oral contraceptive)?

| | |
|---|---|
| Yes | 1 |
| No | 2 |

b. At the <u>moment</u> do you take any tonics, vitamin pills or anything similar?

| | |
|---|---|
| Yes | 1 |
| No | 2 |

c. **INTERVIEWER: RECORD SEX**

| | | |
|---|---|---|
| Female | A | ASK d. |
| Male | B | GO TO Q28 |

d. **IF FEMALE**
Have you had a cervical smear test in the past 3 years?

| | |
|---|---|
| Yes | 1 |
| No | 2 |
| Don't know | 8 |

**27a.** IF FEMALE
INTERVIEWER CHECK AGE AT Q1b. AND RECORD:

| | | |
|---|---|---|
| Aged 49 or less | 1 | **ASK b.** |
| Aged 50 or more | 2 | **GO TO Q28** |

**b.** IF FEMALE AGED 49 OR LESS (CODE 1 AT a.)
Do you <u>usually</u> take an oral contraceptive?

Yes 1
No 2

> IF 'JUST STOPPED', CODE 'YES'

**c.** Are you pregnant at the moment?

| | | |
|---|---|---|
| Yes | 1 | **ASK d.** |
| No | 2 | **GO TO Q28** |

**d.** IF PREGNANT (CODE 1 AT c.)
How many months pregnant are you?
**NUMBER OF MONTHS (TO NEAREST MONTHS):** [ ]

**28a.** ALL
Do you have any long-standing illness, disability or infirmity?

| | | |
|---|---|---|
| Yes | 1 | **ASK b.** |
| No | 2 | **GO TO Q30** |

**b.** IF HAS LONG-STANDING ILLNESS (CODE 1 AT a.)
What is the matter with you?
**RECORD IN FULL**

**c.** Does it limit your activities in any way compared with other people of your own age?

| | | |
|---|---|---|
| Yes | 1 | **ASK Q29** |
| No | 2 | **GO TO Q30** |

**29a.** IF LIMITS ACTIVITIES (CODE 1 AT Q28c.)
How does it affect you, do you have to take special care some of the time?

Yes 1
No 2

**b.** Are you limited in the amount of work, or the kind of work you can do, or in your social life?

Yes 1
No 2

**c.** Are you unable to work (or do housework)?

Yes 1
No 2

**d.** Can you climb stairs?

Yes 1
No 2

**e.** Can you walk around outside without help or aids?

| | | |
|---|---|---|
| Yes | 1 | **GO TO Q30** |
| No | 2 | **ASK f.** |

**f.** IF NO (CODE 2 AT e.)
Can you walk around the house (flat) without help or aids?

Yes 1
No 2

**g.** Do you have to have help with things like dressing or feeding?

Yes 1
No 2

**ALL**

30a. Have you ever had asthma?

b. IF YES, PROBE: Has it ever been treated by a doctor or at hospital?
REPEAT a. AND b. FOR EACH OTHER ITEM LISTED BELOW.

| | a. No | a. Yes, treated | b. Yes, not treated |
|---|---|---|---|
| Asthma | 1 | 2 | 3 |
| Chronic Bronchitis | 1 | 2 | 3 |
| Other chest trouble | 1 | 2 | 3 |
| Diabetes | 1 | 2 | 3 |
| Stomach or other digestive disorder | 1 | 2 | 3 |
| Piles or haemorrhoids | 1 | 2 | 3 |
| Liver trouble | 1 | 2 | 3 |
| Rheumatic disorder or arthritis | 1 | 2 | 3 |
| Lung cancer | 1 | 2 | 3 |
| Other cancer | 1 | 2 | 3 |
| Severe depression or other nervous illness | 1 | 2 | 3 |
| Varicose veins | 1 | 2 | 3 |
| High blood pressure | 1 | 2 | 3 |
| Stroke | 1 | 2 | 3 |
| Migraine | 1 | 2 | 3 |
| Back trouble | 1 | 2 | 3 |
| Epilepsy/fits | 1 | 2 | 3 |
| ME or Post Viral Fatigue Syndrome or Chronic Fatigue Syndrome | 1 | 2 | 3 |

**ALL**

31a. Have you ever had any heart problems?

Yes 1 ASK b.
No 2 GO TO Q33

b. IF HAS HAD HEART PROBLEMS (CODE 1 AT a.)
Have you ever had ... READ OUT AND CODE YES OR NO FOR EACH ...

| | Yes | No |
|---|---|---|
| ... a heart attack? | 1 | 2 |
| ... angina? | 1 | 2 |
| ... valve disease? | 1 | 2 |
| ... hole in the heart? | 1 | 2 |
| ... rheumatic heart disease? | 1 | 2 |
| ... any other heart problem? (SPECIFY) _____ | 1 | 2 |

32a. INTERVIEWER CHECK Q31b. AND RECORD:

Respondent has had a heart attack or angina 1 ASK b.
Respondent has not had a heart attack or angina 2 GO TO Q33

b. IF HAD HEART ATTACK/ANGINA (CODE 1 AT a.)
How old were you when you first experienced a heart attack/angina?

AGE IN YEARS: [  ]

**ALL**

33. Have either of your parents ever had a heart attack or angina?

Yes 1
No 2
Don't know 8

IF QUERIED TAKE NATURAL PARENTS

**All**

34. Within the last month have you suffered from any problems with ... READ OUT AND CODE YES OR NO FOR EACH ...

| | Yes | No |
|---|---|---|
| ... Headaches? | 1 | 2 |
| ... Hay fever? | 1 | 2 |
| ... Difficulty sleeping? | 1 | 2 |
| ... Constipation? | 1 | 2 |
| ... Trouble with eyes? | 1 | 2 |

35a. Within the last month have you suffered from any problems with ...

| | Yes | No |
|---|---|---|
| ... A bad back? | 1 | 2 |
| ... Nerves? | 1 | 2 |
| ... Colds and flu? | 1 | 2 |
| ... Trouble with feet? (CORNS, BUNIONS, ATHLETE'S FOOT, ETC.) | 1 | 2 |
| ... Always feeling tired? | 1 | 2 |

b. Within the last month have you suffered from any problems with ....

| | Yes | No |
|---|---|---|
| ... Kidney or bladder trouble? | 1 | 2 |
| ... Painful joints? | 1 | 2 |
| ... Difficulty concentrating? | 1 | 2 |
| ... Palpitations or breathlessness? | 1 | 2 |
| ... Trouble with ears? | 1 | 2 |

36a. And within the <u>last month</u> have you suffered from any problems with ...

| | Yes | No |
|---|---|---|
| ... Worrying over every little thing? | 1 | 2 |
| ...Indigestion or other stomach trouble? | 1 | 2 |
| ... Sinus trouble or catarrh? | 1 | 2 |
| ... Persistent cough? | 1 | 2 |
| ... Faints or dizziness? | 1 | 2 |

b. ALL

INTERVIEWER CHECK SEX:

| | | |
|---|---|---|
| Female | A | GO TO c. |
| Male | B | GO TO Q37 |

c. INTERVIEWER CHECK AGE:

| | | |
|---|---|---|
| Aged less than 60 | A | ASK d. |
| Aged 60 or more | B | GO TO Q37 |

d. IF FEMALE UNDER 60 (CODE B AT c.)

Within the last month have you suffered from any trouble with periods or the menopause?

| | |
|---|---|
| Yes | 1 |
| No | 2 |

37a. ALL

How often do you feel that you are under so much strain that your health is likely to suffer ... READ OUT ...

CODE ONE ONLY

| | |
|---|---|
| ... always, | 1 |
| often, | 2 |
| sometimes, | 3 |
| or never? | 4 |

b. How often do you feel bored ... READ OUT ...

CODE ONE ONLY

| | |
|---|---|
| ... always, | 1 |
| often, | 2 |
| sometimes, | 3 |
| or never? | 4 |

c. How often do you feel lonely ... READ OUT ...

CODE ONE ONLY

| | |
|---|---|
| ... always, | 1 |
| often, | 2 |
| sometimes, | 3 |
| or never? | 4 |

38. ALL

How much in the past month have your activities been limited by your health ... READ OUT ...

| | |
|---|---|
| ... not at all, | 1 |
| a little, | 2 |
| quite a lot, | 3 |
| or a great deal? | 4 |
| Can't say | 8 |

39a. Have you visited or been seen by your Doctor (GP) in the past month because of illness or a possible health problem?

| | | |
|---|---|---|
| Yes | 1 | ASK b. |
| No | 2 | GO TO Q40 |

b. IF SEEN DOCTOR IN PAST MONTH (CODE 1 AT a.)

How many times in the past month have you been seen?

NUMBER OF TIMES: [ ]

40a. ALL

Have you been seen at a Hospital Outpatients clinic in the past month?

| | |
|---|---|
| Yes | 1 |
| No | 2 |

b. And have you been in hospital, either overnight or as a day patient, in the past month?

| | |
|---|---|
| Yes | 1 |
| No | 2 |

41. About how many hours of sleep do you usually get?

CODE ONE ONLY

| | |
|---|---|
| Less than 6 hours | 1 |
| 6 hours, less than 7 hours | 2 |
| 7 hours, less than 8 hours | 3 |
| 8 hours, less than 9 hours | 4 |
| 9 hours, less than 10 hours | 5 |
| 10 hours | 6 |
| More than 10 hours | 7 |
| Don't know | 8 |

**ALL**

42a. How tall are you?  **ROUND DOWN TO NEAREST ½"**

IF GIVEN IN CENTIMETRES,
RECORD HERE:

HEIGHT:  FEET  INCHES

Don't know  998

b. How much do you weigh?

IF GIVEN IN KILOS,
RECORD HERE:

WEIGHT:  STONES  POUNDS

Don't know  9998

c. Would you say that for your height
you are ... **READ OUT** ...

**CODE ONE ONLY**

... about the right weight,  1
too heavy,  2
or too light?  3
Don't know  8

43a. Compared to seven years ago, do you
now weigh ... **READ OUT** ...

... more,  1  ASK b.
less,  2  ASK c.
or about the same?  3  GO TO Q44
Can't say  8

**IF MORE (CODE 1 AT a.)**

b. Overall, how much more do you weigh now
than you did seven years ago?

IF GIVEN IN KILOS,
RECORD HERE:

GAINED:  stones  lbs

Don't know  9998

**NOW GO TO Q44**

**IF LESS (CODE 2 AT a.)**

c. Overall, how much less do you weigh now,
than you did seven years ago?

IF GIVEN IN KILOS,
RECORD HERE:

LOST:  stones  lbs

Don't know  9998

---

FOOD AND DRINK

**ALL**

Now I would like to ask about what you eat.

44a. Are you on a special diet of any sort for
health reasons?

Yes  1  ASK b.
No  2  GO TO Q45

**IF ON SPECIAL DIET (CODE 1 AT a.)**

b. What is this diet for?

**CODE ALL THAT APPLY**

Obesity/to lose weight  01
High blood pressure/heart disease  02
Ulcers, (gastric, peptic, stomach, duodenal)  03
Gall stones  04
Kidney failure  05
Diabetes  06
Food allergy  07
Osteoporosis  08
Coeliac disease  09

Other (SPECIFY) _____  10

c. What sort of diet is it?
RECORD VERBATIM.  PROBE FOR CLARIFICATION.

d. CODE BELOW ANSWERS RECORDED AT c.  USE
'OTHER' IF DOES NOT FIT A PRECODE

**CODE ALL THAT APPLY**

Low calorie  01
Low carbohydrate  02
Low fat  03
Low salt  04
High fibre  05
Low protein  06
Gluten free  07
Avoid dairy products  08
High calcium (including dairy products)  09
Other  10

**ALL**

45a. Would you say that you usually eat the right amount of food for you?

Yes   1   GO TO Q46
No   2   ASK b.
Can't say   8   GO TO Q46

IF NO AT a.

b. Do you eat too much or too little?

Too much   1
Too little   2
Can't say   8

**ALL**

46a. On weekdays (workdays), how soon after you get up do you usually have something to eat?

NOTE: This meal would normally be breakfast but count first food eaten.

If breakfast in bed, count this.

Less than ½ hour   1
1/2 hour, but less than 1 hour   2
1 hour, but less than 2 hours   3
2 hours, but less than 3 hours   4
3 hours, but less than 4 hours   5
4 hours or more   6

b. How often do you have a cooked breakfast? (First meal after getting up)

CODE ONE ONLY

Every day   1
Most days (3-6)   2
Once or twice a week   3
Less than once a week   4
Never   5

47. Apart from breakfast, how many main or cooked meals, that is a meal that has a main course with one or more vegetables, do you usually have during the day?

NUMBER: [ ]

NOTE: FOR SHIFT WORKERS AND OTHERS WITH ERRATIC LIVES, ASK FOR MEALS EATEN IN PREVIOUS WEEK

**ALL**

48a. Apart from breakfast, how many other lighter meals do you usually have during the day?

NUMBER OF LIGHT MEALS PER DAY: [ ]

NOTE: FOR SHIFT WORKERS AND OTHERS WITH ERRATIC LIVES, ASK FOR MEALS EATEN IN PREVIOUS WEEK

b. (Including meals taken to work) how often do you have a meal away from home?

CODE ONE ONLY

More than once a day   1
Once a day   2
Most days (3-6)   3
Once or twice a week   4
Less than once a week   5
Never   6

49a. How many times a day do you have a snack or something to eat between meals or before going to bed?

CODE ONE ONLY

Once or twice   1
Three or four   2
More than four   3
Occasionally or never   4

b. Do you eat regularly, that is have the same number of meals and snacks at roughly the same time each day?

Yes   1
No   2
Varies   3

ALL

50. How often do you eat fried food, don't count chips?

CODE ONE ONLY

| | |
|---|---|
| More than once a day | 1 |
| Once a day | 2 |
| Most days (3-6) | 3 |
| Once or twice a week | 4 |
| Less than once a week | 5 |
| Never | 6 |

51a. What sort of bread do you eat? That includes rolls, baps and anything else made from bread.

IF RESPONDENT MENTIONS MORE THAN ONE SORT, RING "1" FOR SORT EATEN MOST OFTEN, THEN "2" AND "3" FOR OTHERS AS APPROPRIATE. IF OVER 3 TYPES, USE CODE 3 FOR REMAINDERS.

| | 1st | 2nd | 3rd | |
|---|---|---|---|---|
| White | 1 | 2 | 3 | |
| Granary/Wheatmeal/Brown | 1 | 2 | 3 | IF ANY BREAD CODED ASK b. |
| Wholemeal | 1 | 2 | 3 | |
| Crispbreads | 1 | 2 | 3 | |
| Pitta - white | 1 | 2 | 3 | |
| Pitta - wholemeal | 1 | 2 | 3 | |
| Nan, chapatis | 1 | 2 | 3 | |
| Other (SPECIFY) _____ | 1 | 2 | 3 | |
| Does not eat any bread | 0 | | | GO TO Q54 |

IF EATS BREAD

b. I am going to ask you how much bread you usually eat in a day.

First, how many slices of bread or crispbread do you usually eat each day, including toast or sandwiches?

| | |
|---|---|
| None | 00 |
| Less than one slice a day | 90 |
| NUMBER OF SLICES: [ ] | |
| Don't know | 98 |

IF EATS BREAD

52a. In addition, how many rolls, baps or similar types of bread do you usually eat each day?

(IF SOMETIMES EAT ROLLS AND SOMETIMES BREAD SLICES, RECORD AT Q51b. ONLY)

| | |
|---|---|
| None | 00 |
| Less than one a day | 90 |
| NUMBER OF ROLLS: [ ] | |
| Don't know | 98 |

b. What do you usually spread on bread?
IF SOFT MARGERINE ASK: What brand?

CODE ONE ONLY

| | | |
|---|---|---|
| Butter | 01 | |
| Hard margarine | 02 | |
| Polyunsaturated margarine | 03 | |
| Low fat spread | 04 | ASK c. |
| Low fat, polyunsaturated margarine | 05 | |
| Soft margarine (BRAND) _____ | 06 | |
| Other (SPECIFY) _____ | 07 | |
| Nothing | 08 | GO TO Q53 |

IF SPREADS SOMETHING ON BREAD (CODES 01-07 AT b.)

c. Do you spread this ... READ OUT ...

CODE ONE ONLY

| | |
|---|---|
| ... thick, | 1 |
| medium | 2 |
| thin, | 3 |
| or just a scrape? | 4 |

IF EATS BREAD

53. On weekdays (workdays), how often do you have sandwiches or similarly filled types of bread or rolls?

CODE ONE ONLY

| | |
|---|---|
| More than once a day | 1 |
| Every (working) day | 2 |
| Most days (three or four days a week) | 3 |
| Once or twice a week | 4 |
| Less than once a week | 5 |
| Never | 6 |

ALL

54. How many cups of tea do you usually drink in a day? READ OUT ...

CODE ONE ONLY

| | | |
|---|---|---|
| ... one or two | 1 | |
| three or four | 2 | ASK Q55 |
| five or six | 3 | |
| more than six | 4 | |
| or none? | 5 | GO TO Q56 |

**ALL**

**58.** **SHOW CARD C.** I am going to read out a list of foods. Using this card, please tell me how often you eat each of them. **READ OUT EACH FOOD IN TURN AND CODE IN GRID.**

| | MORE THAN ONCE A DAY | ONCE A DAY | MOST DAYS (3-6) | ONCE OR TWICE A WEEK | LESS THAN ONCE A WEEK | NEVER |
|---|---|---|---|---|---|---|
| Fresh fruit in summer | 5 | 4 | 3 | 2 | 1 | 6 |
| Fresh fruit in winter | 5 | 4 | 3 | 2 | 1 | 6 |
| Salads or raw veg. in summer | 5 | 4 | 3 | 2 | 1 | 6 |
| Salads or raw veg. in winter | 5 | 4 | 3 | 2 | 1 | 6 |
| Tinned fruit | 5 | 4 | 3 | 2 | 1 | 6 |
| Chips | 5 | 4 | 3 | 2 | 1 | 6 |
| Potatoes (NOT CHIPS) | 5 | 4 | 3 | 2 | 1 | 6 |
| Root vegetables like carrots, turnips and parsnips | 5 | 4 | 3 | 2 | 1 | 6 |
| Peas and beans (ALL KINDS; INC. BAKED BEANS, LENTILS) | 5 | 4 | 3 | 2 | 1 | 6 |
| Green vegetables | 5 | 4 | 3 | 2 | 1 | 6 |
| Other cooked vegetables, inc. onions & mushrooms | 5 | 4 | 3 | 2 | 1 | 6 |
| Nuts | 5 | 4 | 3 | 2 | 1 | 6 |
| Potato crisps or similar snacks | 5 | 4 | 3 | 2 | 1 | 6 |
| Sweets, chocolates | 5 | 4 | 3 | 2 | 1 | 6 |
| Pasta (spaghetti, noodles), or rice | 5 | 4 | 3 | 2 | 1 | 6 |
| Breakfast cereal (inc. porridge) | 5 | 4 | 3 | 2 | 1 | 6 |
| Biscuits | 5 | 4 | 3 | 2 | 1 | 6 |
| Cakes of all kinds | 5 | 4 | 3 | 2 | 1 | 6 |
| Sweets or puddings, fruit pies and flans and tarts | 5 | 4 | 3 | 2 | 1 | 6 |
| Ice cream, mousse, yoghurt, milk puddings | 5 | 4 | 3 | 2 | 1 | 6 |

---

**55.** **IF DRINKS TEA (CODES 1-4 AT Q54)**

How much sugar do you usually have in tea?

**CODE ONE ONLY**

| | |
|---|---|
| 1 or less teaspoons | 1 |
| Over 1, to 2 teaspoons | 2 |
| More than 2 teaspoons | 3 |
| None | 4 |

**56a.** **ALL**

How many cups of coffee do you usually drink in a day? **READ OUT** ...

| | | |
|---|---|---|
| ... one or two | 1 | |
| three or four | 2 | ASK b. |
| five or six | 3 | |
| more than six | 4 | |
| or none? | 5 | GO TO Q57 |

**b.** **IF 'DRINKS COFFEE' (CODES 1-4 AT a.)**

How much sugar do you usually have in coffee?

**CODE ONE ONLY**

| | |
|---|---|
| 1 or less teaspoons | 1 |
| Over 1, to 2 teaspoons | 2 |
| More than 2 teaspoons | 3 |
| None | 4 |

**57a.** **ALL**

How much milk do you usually have each day? Please include milk used in drinks, on cereal and in cooking (eg. custard, milk puddings)?

**CODE ONE ONLY**

| | | |
|---|---|---|
| None | 1 | GO TO Q58 |
| Less than 1/2 pint | 2 | |
| 1/2-1 pint | 3 | |
| Over 1, to 2 pints | 4 | ASK b. |
| More than 2 pints | 5 | |
| Don't know | 8 | |

**b.** **IF HAS MILK (CODES 2 TO 5/8 AT a.)**

What sort of milk do you usually use?

**IF 'DON'T KNOW', CODE AS SILVERTOP (CODE 1)**

**CODE ALL THAT APPLY**

| | |
|---|---|
| Silver Top/Sterilised/Pasteurised/Homogenised (full cream) | 1 |
| Gold Top | 2 |
| Skimmed or semi-skimmed milk | 3 |
| Evaporated milk | 4 |
| Powdered milk (SPECIFY) _____ | 5 |
| Other (SPECIFY) _____ | 6 |

**59. SHOW CARD C.** And how often do you eat these foods ... **READ OUT** ...

| | MORE THAN ONCE A DAY | ONCE A DAY | MOST DAYS (3-6) | ONCE OR TWICE A WEEK | LESS THAN ONCE A WEEK | NEVER |
|---|---|---|---|---|---|---|
| Soft drinks like squash or cola | 5 | 4 | 3 | 2 | 1 | 6 |
| Pure fruit juice | 5 | 4 | 3 | 2 | 1 | 6 |
| Jam/marmalade/golden syrup/ honey | 5 | 4 | 3 | 2 | 1 | 6 |
| Cheese | 5 | 4 | 3 | 2 | 1 | 6 |
| Eggs | 5 | 4 | 3 | 2 | 1 | 6 |
| Cream | 5 | 4 | 3 | 2 | 1 | 6 |
| Fish | 5 | 4 | 3 | 2 | 1 | 6 |
| Shellfish (Seafood) | 5 | 4 | 3 | 2 | 1 | 6 |
| Poultry | 5 | 4 | 3 | 2 | 1 | 6 |
| Sausages/tinned meat/pate/meat pies/pasties/burgers etc. | 5 | 4 | 3 | 2 | 1 | 6 |
| Beef/lamb/pork/ham/bacon | 5 | 4 | 3 | 2 | 1 | 6 |
| Chinese meals/dishes | 5 | 4 | 3 | 2 | 1 | 6 |
| Indian meals/dishes | 5 | 4 | 3 | 2 | 1 | 6 |
| Pizzas | 5 | 4 | 3 | 2 | 1 | 6 |
| Soup | 5 | 4 | 3 | 2 | 1 | 6 |

Can you think of any other sorts of food which you eat regularly? (SPECIFY)

| | | | | | | |
|---|---|---|---|---|---|---|
| 1. _____ | 5 | 4 | 3 | 2 | 1 | 6 |
| 2. _____ | 5 | 4 | 3 | 2 | 1 | 6 |
| 3. _____ | 5 | 4 | 3 | 2 | 1 | 6 |
| 4. _____ | 5 | 4 | 3 | 2 | 1 | 6 |

---

**60a.** Overall do you think you are eating differently compared to 7 years ago?

| | | |
|---|---|---|
| Yes | 1 | ASK b. |
| No | 2 | GO TO Q61 |
| Don't know | 8 | |

**IF EATING DIFFERENTLY (CODE 1 AT a.)**

b. Do you think you are eating ... **READ OUT** ...

| | |
|---|---|
| ... a bit differently, | 1 |
| or a lot differently? | 2 |
| Don't know | 8 |

> DIFFERENTLY = AMOUNT OR TYPE OF FOODS

c. What were your reasons for changing?

**DO NOT PROMPT**
**CODE ALL THAT APPLY**

| | |
|---|---|
| To improve appearance/change weight | 01 |
| Because of health problem | 02 |
| Because of health campaigns | 03 |
| Change in income | 04 |
| Food availability | 05 |
| Convenience | 06 |
| Change in taste preference | 07 |
| To suit others in the household | 08 |
| Other (SPECIFY) _____ | 09 |
| Don't know | 98 |

**ALL**

**61.** Thinking overall about the things you eat, would you say that your diet is ... **READ OUT** ...

| | |
|---|---|
| ... as healthy as it could be, | 1 |
| quite good but could improve, | 2 |
| or not very healthy? | 3 |
| Don't know | 8 |

DRINKING

ALL

62a. Now I would like to ask you about alcoholic drinks.
Would you say that you now are ... **READ OUT** ...

CODE <u>ONE</u> ONLY

| | | |
|---|---|---|
| ... a non drinker, | 1 | ASK b. |
| a very special occasions drinker, | 2 | |
| an occasional drinker, | 3 | GO TO Q63 |
| or a regular drinker? | 4 | |

IF NON OR SPECIAL OCCASIONS DRINKER (CODE 1 OR 2 AT a.)

b. Have you always been a non (special occasions) drinker?

| | | |
|---|---|---|
| Yes | 1 | GO TO Q70 |
| No | 2 | ASK c. |

IF NOT ALWAYS NON/SPECIAL OCCASIONS DRINKER (CODE 2 AT b.)

c. How old were you when you gave up more regular drinking?

AGE GAVE UP [ ] YEARS

Don't know 98

IF OCCASIONAL/REGULAR DRINKER (CODE 3 OR 4 AT Q 62a.) OR PREVIOUS REGULAR DRINKER (CODE 2 AT Q62b.)

63a. Would you say that you are (were) ... **READ OUT** ...

| | |
|---|---|
| ... a light drinker, | 1 |
| a moderate drinker, | 2 |
| or a heavy drinker? | 3 |
| Don't know | 8 |

b. Has a doctor or anyone else ever suggested that you should cut down on drinking?

| | | |
|---|---|---|
| No | 1 | GO TO Q65 |

**IF YES PROBE:** Who suggested it?
CODE ONE ONLY. GIVE PRIORITY TO HIGHEST IN LIST

| | | |
|---|---|---|
| Yes, doctor | 2 | ASK Q64 |
| Yes, relative/spouse | 3 | |
| Yes, workmate/friend | 4 | |
| Yes, other | 5 | |

IF SOMEONE SUGGESTED CUTTING DOWN (CODES 2-5 AT Q63b.)

64. Why did they suggest that you cut down?
CODE ONE ONLY
(TAKE MOST IMPORTANT)

| | |
|---|---|
| Health reasons | 1 |
| Driving | 2 |
| Other (SPECIFY) _____ | 3 |
| Don't know | 8 |

ALL OCCASIONAL/REGULAR DRINKERS OR PREVIOUS REGULAR DRINKERS

65a. Have you ever felt you ought to cut down on your drinking?

| | | |
|---|---|---|
| Yes | 1 | ASK b. |
| No | 2 | GO TO Q66 |

IF HAS EVER WANTED TO CUT DOWN (CODE 1 AT a.)

b. Have you ever succeeded in cutting down for at least a month?

| | |
|---|---|
| Yes | 1 |
| No | 2 |

c. Why did you decide (you ought) to cut down on your drinking?
CODE ALL THAT APPLY

| | | |
|---|---|---|
| Health reasons | 1 | ASK d. |
| Driving | 2 | |
| Other (SPECIFY) _____ | 3 | GO TO Q66 |
| Don't know | 8 | |

IF HEALTH REASONS (CODE 1 AT c.)

d. What were the health reasons?
PROBE FULLY. RECORD VERBATIM.

**66a. IF OCCASIONAL/REGULAR DRINKER (CODES 3 OR 4 AT Q62a.) OR PREVIOUS REGULAR DRINKER (CODE 2 AT Q62b.)**

Have (Did) people ever annoy(ed) you by criticising your drinking?

| | |
|---|---|
| Yes | 1 |
| No | 2 |

b. Have (Did) you ever felt (feel) bad or guilty about your drinking?

| | |
|---|---|
| Yes | 1 |
| No | 2 |

c. Have you ever had a drink first thing in the morning to steady your nerves or get rid of a hangover?

| | |
|---|---|
| Yes | 1 |
| No | 2 |

d. Have you had any alcoholic drinks during the past week?

| | | |
|---|---|---|
| Yes | 1 | ASK Q67 |
| No | 2 | GO TO Q69 |

**67a. IF HAD DRINKS IN PAST WEEK (CODE 1 AT Q66d.)**

I would now like to learn what you had to drink last week. Let's start with yesterday and work backwards.

Yesterday was _____ (NAME DAY OF WEEK AND CODE).

| | |
|---|---|
| Monday | 1 |
| Tuesday | 2 |
| Wednesday | 3 |
| Thursday | 4 |
| Friday | 5 |
| Saturday | 6 |
| Sunday | 7 |

b. COMPLETE DRINK DIARY ON OPPOSITE PAGE. START WITH RELEVANT DAY OF WEEK (YESTERDAY) AND WORK BACKWARDS THROUGH PAST WEEK.

FIRST ASK ABOUT DRINK CONSUMED IN DAYTIME AND THEN IN EVENING. PROBE: Anything else?

FOR EACH TYPE OF DRINK CONSUMED, RECORD AMOUNT DRUNK. ASK FOR AMOUNTS IN PUB MEASURES (P = pints, M = measures, G = glasses). RING P, G or M TO SHOW MEASURE USED.

IF OTHER/MIXED, INCLUDES LOW ALCOHOL WINES ENTER AMOUNT. RING G OR M. SPECIFY UNDERNEATH TYPE OF DRINK.

IF ESTIMATE, INDICATE BY 'E'.

IF 'NIP', 'SPOONFUL', WRITE IN.

---

DRINK DIARY

| DAY | None/Low Alcohol at that time | Beer Cider Lager Shandy Stout | Sherry Vermth | Wines | Spirits e.g. Whisky, Gin, Rum, Vodka | Liquers e.g. Brandy, TiaMaria etc. | Other/Mixed (Specify type as well as amount) |
|---|---|---|---|---|---|---|---|
| MONDAY — Amount | 0 | P | G | G | G / M | G / M | Amount ........ Type ........ G / M |
| MONDAY — Amount | 0 | P | G | G | G / M | G / M | Amount ........ Type ........ G / M |
| TUESDAY — Amount | 0 | P | G | G | G / M | G / M | Amount ........ Type ........ G / M |
| TUESDAY — Amount | 0 | P | G | G | G / M | G / M | Amount ........ Type ........ G / M |
| WEDS — Amount | 0 | P | G | G | G / M | G / M | Amount ........ Type ........ G / M |
| WEDS — Amount | 0 | P | G | G | G / M | G / M | Amount ........ Type ........ G / M |
| THURS — Amount | 0 | P | G | G | G / M | G / M | Amount ........ Type ........ G / M |
| THURS — Amount | 0 | P | G | G | G / M | G / M | Amount ........ Type ........ G / M |
| FRIDAY — Amount | 0 | P | G | G | G / M | G / M | Amount ........ Type ........ G / M |
| FRIDAY — Amount | 0 | P | G | G | G / M | G / M | Amount ........ Type ........ G / M |
| SATE — Amount | 0 | P | G | G | G / M | G / M | Amount ........ Type ........ G / M |
| SATE — Amount | 0 | P | G | G | G / M | G / M | Amount ........ Type ........ G / M |
| SUN DE — Amount | 0 | P | G | G | G / M | G / M | Amount ........ Type ........ G / M |
| SUN DE — Amount | 0 | P | G | G | G / M | G / M | Amount ........ Type ........ G / M |

68. **IF COMPLETED DIARY**

Was this last week's drinking ... READ OUT ...

CODE ONE ONLY

| | |
|---|---|
| ... reasonably typical of your usual pattern, | 1 |
| rather less than usual, | 2 |
| or rather more than usual? | 3 |

69. **IF OCCASIONAL/REGULAR DRINKER OR PREVIOUS REGULAR DRINKER**

Do you think that compared with seven years ago you drink ... READ OUT .

| | |
|---|---|
| ... less, | 1 |
| about the same, | 2 |
| or more? | 3 |
| Don't know | 8 |

---

**SMOKING**

**ALL**

70. Now I would like to ask you some questions about smoking.

Have you ever smoked a cigarette or cigar or pipe, more than just a few times as an experiment?

| | | |
|---|---|---|
| Yes | 1 | ASK Q71 |
| No | 2 | GO TO Q81 |

71a. **IF EVER SMOKED**

Do you smoke cigarettes at all nowadays?

| | | |
|---|---|---|
| Yes | 1 | ASK b. |
| No | 2 | GO TO Q75 |

b. **CURRENT SMOKERS**

How many cigarettes do you generally smoke in a day?

IF RANGE GIVEN, ESTABLISH AVERAGE NO. PER DAY

| | | |
|---|---|---|
| Less than 1 per day | 00 | GO TO Q73 |
| More than 1 per day - give number | [ ] | ASK c. |

c. What is the maximum number of cigarettes you have regularly smoked in a day?

| | |
|---|---|
| Number per day | [ ] |
| 97 or more | 97 |

d. Nowadays, do you mainly smoke ... READ OUT ...

CODE ONE ONLY

| | | |
|---|---|---|
| ... filter tipped cigarettes, | 1 | ASK Q72 |
| plain or untipped cigarettes, | 2 | GO TO Q74 |
| or hand rolled cigarettes? | 3 | GO TO Q74 |

72. **CURRENT REGULAR (NON-HANDROLLED) CIGARETTE SMOKERS**

What is the tar level of the cigarettes you usually smoke?

CODE ONE ONLY

| | | |
|---|---|---|
| High | 1 | |
| Middle to high | 2 | |
| Middle | 3 | GO TO Q74 |
| Low to middle | 4 | |
| Low | 5 | |
| Don't know | 6 | |

73a. **CURRENT OCCASIONAL SMOKERS (CODE 00 AT Q71b.)**

Were you ever a regular smoker, that is smoking at least one cigarette a day for 6 months or more?

| | | |
|---|---|---|
| Yes | 1 | ASK b. |
| No | 2 | GO TO Q74 |

b. IF YES AT a. (CODE 1)

How many cigarettes did you generally smoke in a day? (WHEN A REGULAR SMOKER)

IF VARIED, PROBE FOR AVERAGE

| | |
|---|---|
| Number per day | [ ] |
| 97 or more | 97 |

c. How long ago did you stop being a regular cigarette smoker?

ROUND UP TO NEAREST MONTH/YEAR

| | |
|---|---|
| IF LESS THAN 1 YEAR ENTER NO. OF MONTHS: | [ ] |
| IF 1 YEAR OR MORE ENTER NO. OF YEARS: | [ ] |

74. **ALL CURRENT SMOKERS**

Compared with seven years ago, do you nowadays ... READ OUT ...

| | | |
|---|---|---|
| ... smoke less, | 1 | GO TO Q76 |
| smoke more, | 2 | |
| or about the same? | 3 | |
| Don't know | 8 | |

**EX-SMOKERS (CODE 2 AT Q71a.)**

75a. Were you ever a regular cigarette smoker, that is smoking at least one cigarette a day for 6 months or more?

Yes   1   ASK b.
No   2   GO TO Q77

b. IF YES AT a. (CODE 1)
How long ago did you completely stop smoking cigarettes?

ROUND UP TO NEAREST MONTH/YEAR

IF LESS THAN 1 YEAR ENTER NO. OF MONTHS:

IF 1 YEAR OR MORE ENTER NO. OF YEARS:

c. So can I just check - how old were you when you stopped smoking cigarettes?

AGE:

d. Over the period you were a smoker, roughly how many cigarettes did you generally smoke in a day?

Number smoked per day

(IF RANGE GIVEN, ESTABLISH AVERAGE)

97 or more   97

e. What reasons made you decide to give up smoking cigarettes?

CODE ALL THAT APPLY

Ill health at time of giving up   1   ASK f.
Expense   2
Fear of ill health in future   3
Social pressure/to please someone else   4   GO TO Q76
Pregnancy   5
Just wanted to give up   6
Other reasons (SPECIFY)   7

_____

f. What was wrong with you when you gave up smoking cigarettes? PROBE FULLY. RECORD VERBATIM.

---

76. **IF CURRENT SMOKER (CODE 1 AT Q71a.) OR HAS SMOKED REGULARLY IN PAST (CODE 1 AT Q73a. OR CODE 1 AT Q75a.)**
How old were you when you started to smoke cigarettes?

AGE IN YEARS:

77a. **ALL WHO HAVE EVER SMOKED (CODE 1 AT Q70a.)**
Have you ever smoked cigars regularly - that is at least one cigar a day?

Yes   1   ASK b.
No   2   GO TO Q78

b. IF YES AT a.
How old were you when you first started to smoke cigars regularly?

AGE IN YEARS:

c. Do you smoke cigars at present?

Yes   1   ASK e.
No   2   ASK d.

d. IF DO NOT CURRENTLY SMOKE CIGARS (CODE 2 AT c.)
How long ago did you stop smoking cigars regularly?

Less than 1 year   00

No. of years

e. **ALL WHO HAVE SMOKED CIGARS (CODE 1 AT a.)**
How many cigars do (did) you regularly smoke in a week?

No. per week

f. Compared to seven years ago, do you think that you now smoke more or fewer cigars?

Smokes fewer   1
The same   2
Smokes more   3
Don't know   8

CODE 'THE SAME' IF HAS BEEN AN EX-CIGAR SMOKER FOR MORE THAN SEVEN YEARS

**ALL CURRENT SMOKERS**

80a. How soon after waking do you have your first smoke of the day?

CODE <u>ONE</u> ONLY

| | |
|---|---|
| Less than 5 minutes | 1 |
| 5, less than 15 minutes | 2 |
| 15, less than 30 minutes | 3 |
| 30 minutes, less than 1 hour | 4 |
| 1 hour, less than 2 hours | 5 |
| 2 hours or longer | 6 |
| Don't know | 8 |

b. On occasions when you can't smoke or you haven't got any cigarettes, cigars or a pipe on you, do you feel a craving for one?

PROMPT IF NECESSARY

CODE <u>ONE</u> ONLY

| | |
|---|---|
| Never | 1 |
| Hardly ever | 2 |
| Occasionally | 3 |
| Frequently | 4 |
| Always | 5 |

c. Do you ever feel that you want to give up smoking altogether?

| | | |
|---|---|---|
| Yes | 1 | ASK d. |
| No | 2 | ASK e. |
| Can't say | 8 | |

d. IF YES AT c.

How much? Would you say ... READ OUT ...

| | |
|---|---|
| ... slightly, | 1 |
| moderately, | 2 |
| quite strongly, | 4 |
| or very strongly? | 5 |
| Don't know | 8 |

e. ALL CURRENT SMOKERS

Would you give up smoking altogether if you could do so easily?

PROMPT IF NECESSARY

| | |
|---|---|
| Yes, definitely | 1 |
| Yes, probably | 2 |
| No | 3 |
| Don't know | 8 |

---

78a. **ALL WHO HAVE EVER SMOKED (CODE 1 AT Q70a.)**

Have you ever smoked a pipe regularly - that is at least one bowl of tobacco a day?

| | | |
|---|---|---|
| Yes | 1 | ASK b. |
| No | 2 | GO TO Q79 |

b. How old were you when you first started to smoke a pipe?

AGE IN YEARS: [ ]

c. Do you smoke a pipe at present?

| | | |
|---|---|---|
| Yes | 1 | ASK e. |
| No | 2 | ASK d. |

d. IF DO NOT CURRENTLY SMOKE PIPE (CODE 2 AT c.)

How long ago did you stop smoking a pipe?

LESS THAN 1 YEAR: 00

NO. OF YEARS: [ ]

e. **ALL WHO HAVE EVER SMOKED PIPE (CODE 1 AT a.)**

How many ounces of pipe tobacco do (did) you regularly smoke in a week?

OUNCES PER WEEK: [ ]

Don't know 98

f. Compared to seven years ago, do you think that you are now smoking more or less pipe tobacco?

CODE 'THE SAME' IF IT HAS BEEN AN EX-SMOKER FOR MORE THAN SEVEN YEARS

| | |
|---|---|
| Smokes less | 1 |
| The same | 2 |
| Smokes more | 3 |
| Don't know | 8 |

79. **ALL WHO HAVE EVER SMOKED (CODE 1 AT Q70a.)**

INTERVIEWER CHECK Q71a., Q77a. AND Q78a. AND RECORD <u>ALL</u> THAT APPLY

| | | |
|---|---|---|
| Current cigarette smoker | 1 | ASK Q80 |
| Current cigar smoker | 2 | |
| Current pipe smoker | 3 | |
| Does not currently smoke anything | 4 | GO TO Q81 |

**ALL**

81a. (Apart from you), does anyone else in this household smoke regularly?

Yes 1 ASK b.
No 2
Lives on own 3 GO TO Q82

b. Do they/any of them smoke in the house, or only away from home or outside?

Yes - smokes in the house 1
No - they all smoke away from the house 2

---

**EXERCISE AND LEISURE**

**ALL**

82a. Now let's talk about exercise, and leisure activities. Overall, do you think that you get enough exercise?

Yes 1
No 2
Don't know 8

b. In general, compared with men/women (AS APPROPRIATE) of your own age, are you physically ... **READ OUT** ...

... more active, 1
less active, 2
or, about average? 3
Don't know 8

83a. On weekdays (working days) when not at work, how much time on average per day do you spend walking – getting to work, shopping, walking the dog, for pleasure and so on?

TIME PER DAY: [ ] [ ] HOURS [ ] [ ] MINS
Don't know 9998

b. At weekends (rest days) how much time on average per day do you spend walking?

TIME PER DAY: [ ] [ ] HOURS [ ] [ ] MINS
Don't know 9998

---

**ALL**

84. Compared to people of your own age, which of the following best describes your usual walking pace? ... **READ OUT** ...

... slow, 1
average, 2
fairly brisk, 3
or fast? 4
It depends/Don't know 8

85a. In the last 7 days, have you done any gardening (outside of work - IF APPLICABLE)?

Yes 1 ASK b.
No 2 GO TO Q86

b. How much time, overall, did you spend gardening in the last 7 days?

TOTAL TIME IN LAST 7 DAYS: [ ] [ ] HOURS [ ] [ ] MINS
Don't know 9998

c. Would you describe any of the gardening as 'heavy'?

Yes 1
No 2
Don't know 8

86a. In the last 7 days, have you done any DIY (outside of work - IF APPLICABLE): by DIY, I mean house and car maintenance, building, carpentry, etc.?

Yes 1 ASK b.
No 2 GO TO Q87

b. How much time, overall, did you spend on DIY in the last 7 days?

TOTAL TIME IN LAST 7 DAYS: [ ] [ ] HOURS [ ] [ ] MINS
Don't know 9998

c. Would you describe any of this work as 'heavy'?

Yes 1
No 2
Don't know 8

**ALL**

**87a.** **SHOW CARD D.** In the last fortnight have you done any of the activities on this card? (outside of work - IF APPLICABLE)

|  |  |
|---|---|
| Yes | 1 ASK b. |
| No | 2 GO TO Q88 |

b. Which of these activities have you done in the last fortnight? **RING CODE 1 IN COLUMN b. OF GRID FOR EACH ONE**

**FOR EACH DONE AT b. ASK c. and d.**

c. How many times have you done ... (ACTIVITY) ... in the last fortnight? **ENTER NUMBER IN COLUMN c. OF GRID**

d. On average, how long did you spend doing it each time? **IF ACTIVITY DONE FOR DIFFERENT LENGTHS OF TIMES, GET ESTIMATED AVERAGE TIME. ENTER IN COLUMN d. OF GRID**

|  | b. DONE | c. NO. OF TIMES IN FORTNIGHT | d. AVERAGE TIME EACH TIME DONE Hours Minutes |
|---|---|---|---|
| Keep fit, aerobics etc. | 1 | ☐☐ | ☐☐ ☐☐ |
| Yoga | 1 | ☐☐ | ☐☐ ☐☐ |
| Cycling | 1 | ☐☐ | ☐☐ ☐☐ |
| Golf | 1 | ☐☐ | ☐☐ ☐☐ |
| Jogging, Running | 1 | ☐☐ | ☐☐ ☐☐ |
| Swimming | 1 | ☐☐ | ☐☐ ☐☐ |
| Table tennis | 1 | ☐☐ | ☐☐ ☐☐ |
| Basketball | 1 | ☐☐ | ☐☐ ☐☐ |
| Football | 1 | ☐☐ | ☐☐ ☐☐ |
| Rugby | 1 | ☐☐ | ☐☐ ☐☐ |
| Badminton | 1 | ☐☐ | ☐☐ ☐☐ |
| Tennis | 1 | ☐☐ | ☐☐ ☐☐ |
| Squash, Fives, Rackets | 1 | ☐☐ | ☐☐ ☐☐ |
| Cricket | 1 | ☐☐ | ☐☐ ☐☐ |
| Windsurfing, Sailing | 1 | ☐☐ | ☐☐ ☐☐ |
| Self defence, Boxing, Wrestling | 1 | ☐☐ | ☐☐ ☐☐ |
| Back-packing, Hiking, etc. | 1 | ☐☐ | ☐☐ ☐☐ |
| Walks of 2 miles or more | 1 | ☐☐ | ☐☐ ☐☐ |
| Dancing | 1 | ☐☐ | ☐☐ ☐☐ |

**ALL**

**88a.** Have you done any other physical activities in the last fortnight?

|  |  |
|---|---|
| Yes | 1 ASK b. |
| No | 2 GO TO Q89 |

b. What did you do? **RECORD EACH BELOW AND ASK FOR EACH:**

c. How many times have you ... (ACTIVITY) in the last fortnight? **ENTER NUMBER IN COLUMN c. OF GRID**

d. On average, how long did you spend doing it each time? **IF ACTIVITY DONE FOR DIFFERENT LENGTHS OF TIME, GET ESTIMATED AVERAGE TIME. ENTER IN COLUMN d. OF GRID.**

| OTHER ACTIVITIES: | c. NO. OF TIMES IN FORTNIGHT | d. AVERAGE TIME EACH TIME DONE Hours Minutes |
|---|---|---|
| 1. _____ | ☐☐ | ☐☐ ☐☐ |
| 2. _____ | ☐☐ | ☐☐ ☐☐ |
| 3. _____ | ☐☐ | ☐☐ ☐☐ |
| 4. _____ | ☐☐ | ☐☐ ☐☐ |

**ALL**

**89a.** Compared with 7 years ago, do you nowadays spend more, less or about the same amount of time on sport and physical activities?

**CODE ONE ONLY**

|  |  |
|---|---|
| Now spend more time | 1 ASK b. |
| Now spend less time | 2 GO TO Q91 |
| About the same time | 3 GO TO Q92 |
| Don't know | 8 |

**IF MORE TIME (CODE 1 AT a.)**

b. Would you say that you now spend ... **READ OUT** ...

|  |  |
|---|---|
| ... a bit more time, | 1 |
| or a lot more time? | 2 |
| Can't say | 8 |

90. **IF MORE TIME (CODE 1 AT Q89a.)**
Why do you now spend more time than seven years ago on sport or physical activities?

**DO NOT PROMPT**
**CODE ALL THAT APPLY**

| | |
|---|---|
| Will power/to get or keep fit | 01 |
| More leisure time | 02 |
| To take part with family | 03 |
| More money | 04 GO TO Q92 |
| Better facilities | 05 |
| Better health | 06 |
| Other (DESCRIBE) _____ | 07 |
| Can't say | 98 |

91a. **IF LESS TIME (CODE 2 AT Q89a.)**
Would you say that you now spend ... READ OUT ...

| | |
|---|---|
| ... a bit less time, | 1 |
| or a lot less time? | 2 |
| Can't say | 8 |

b. Why do you spend less time on sport or physical activities than seven years ago?

**DO NOT PROMPT**
**CODE ALL THAT APPLY**

| | |
|---|---|
| Less leisure time | 01 |
| Family ties | 02 |
| Companions not available | 03 |
| Less money | 04 |
| Less facilities | 05 |
| Poor health/injuries | 06 |
| Other (DESCRIBE) _____ | 07 |
| Can't say | 98 |

92. **ALL**
**SHOW CARD E.** In the past fortnight have you done any of the activities on this card (outside of work - IF APPLICABLE)?

| | | |
|---|---|---|
| Yes | 1 | ASK Q93 |
| No | 2 | GO TO Q94 |
| Don't know | 8 | |

93. **IF YES (CODE 1 AT Q92)**
**CONTINUE WITH SHOWCARD E.** Which of these have you done in the last fortnight?
**RING CODE FOR EACH ACTIVITY DONE.**

| | |
|---|---|
| Fishing | 01 |
| Parties, dances, socials | 02 |
| Darts, billiards, snooker | 03 |
| Visited coast, rivers, parks, countryside, (other than fishing) | 04 |
| Visited historic buildings, museum, exhibitions or zoos | 05 |
| Amateur music, acting or singing | 06 |
| Gone to cinema, theatre, concert | 07 |
| Gone to watch a sports event | 08 |
| Knitting or sewing | 09 |
| Hobbies, crafts, creative arts or collecting things | 10 |
| Community, social or voluntary work | 11 |
| Played games of skill (computer games, chess, cards, scrabble etc.) | 12 |
| Betting, football pools, other gambling | 13 |
| Been to a pub | 14 |
| Been to a social club or bingo | 15 |
| Been to church or other place of worship | 16 |
| Been to a class or lecture (other than to do with work, school or college) | 17 |

94a. **ALL**
Compared to 7 years ago, do you think that you have more or less time for leisure activities?

| | |
|---|---|
| More time | 1 |
| About the same | 2 |
| Less time | 3 |
| Can't say/Don't know | 8 |

b. In general, do you get out and about as much as you would like to?

| | |
|---|---|
| Yes | 1 |
| No | 2 |
| Can't say | 8 |

**BACKGROUND INFORMATION**

95a. Now I would like to ask you some questions about what you are currently doing.

At the present time are you in paid work, a full-time student or doing something else?

PROBE TO DETERMINE CURRENT STATUS

NOTE: 1) FULL-TIME STUDENT (CODE 09) HAS PRIORITY OVER WORKING.
2) IN WORK (CODES 01 & 02) INCLUDES WORK THROUGH A GOVT. SCHEME

| | | |
|---|---|---|
| Work full-time (30+ hrs) | 01 | ASK b. |
| Work part-time (less than 30 hrs) | 02 | |
| Waiting to start a job already obtained | 03 | |
| Unemployed and <u>actively</u> looking for work | 04 | GO TO Q99 |
| Unemployed, wanting work but <u>not</u> actively looking | 05 | |
| Out of work as temporarily sick | 06 | |
| Permanently sick or disabled | 07 | |
| Wholly retired from work | 08 | |
| In full-time education | 09 | GO TO Q98 |
| Looking after home or family | 10 | |
| Other (SPECIFY) | 11 | |

CODE <u>ONE</u> ONLY

b. IF CURRENTLY IN WORK (CODE 01 OR 02 AT a.)
How many hours do you normally work in a week?
ROUND UP TO NEAREST HOUR
HOURS A WEEK: [ ]

c. Do you do shift work?
Yes 1
No 2

d. How much physical effort is involved in your job, is there ... READ OUT ...
... none, 1
a little, 2
some, 3
or a lot? 4
Don't know 8
CODE ONE ONLY

---

IF <u>CURRENTLY IN WORK</u> (CODE 01 OR 02 AT Q95a.)

96a. How long have you been in this job?

ROUND UP TO NEAREST MONTH/ YEAR

IF <u>LESS THAN ONE YEAR</u> WRITE IN NO. OF <u>MONTHS</u>: [ ] ASK b.
IF <u>ONE TO SIX YEARS</u> WRITE IN NO. OF YEARS: [ ]
IF <u>SEVEN YEARS OR MORE</u>, WRITE IN NO. OF YEARS: [ ] GO TO Q100

b. IF IN JOB LESS THAN SIX YEARS
Since 1985 (seven years ago), have you had any <u>other</u> full or part-time jobs?
Yes 1 ASK c.
No 2 GO TO Q97

c. IF HAD OTHER JOBS (CODE 1 AT b.)
How many other jobs have you had in the past seven years? ... READ OUT ...
One, 1
two, 2
three, 3
or four or more? 4
Can't remember/Don't know 8
CODE <u>ONE</u> ONLY

97a. IF CURRENTLY IN WORK OR IN JOB LESS THAN SIX YEARS
In the past 7 years, how long have you been in paid work altogether?
ROUND UP TO NEAREST MONTH/ YEAR
IF <u>LESS THAN ONE YEAR</u> WRITE IN NO. OF <u>MONTHS</u>: [ ]
IF <u>ONE YEAR OR MORE</u> WRITE IN NO. OF YEARS: [ ]

b. Since 1985 (seven years ago) have you been unemployed and available for work for at least a month?
Yes 1 ASK c.
No 2 GO TO Q100

c. IF HAS BEEN UNEMPLOYED SINCE 1985
In total, how long have you been unemployed and available for work since 1985?
ROUND UP TO NEAREST MONTH/ YEAR
IF <u>LESS THAN ONE YEAR</u> WRITE IN NO. OF <u>MONTHS</u>: [ ]
IF <u>ONE YEAR OR MORE</u> WRITE IN NO. OF YEARS: [ ] GO TO Q100

**IF RETIRED/STUDENT/PERMANENTLY SICK/LOOKING AFTER HOME/OTHER (CODES 07-11 AT Q95a.)**

98. Have you been ... (CURRENT STATUS) ... for the whole of the last 7 years?

| | | |
|---|---|---|
| Yes | 1 | GO TO Q102 |
| No | 2 | ASK Q99 |

ASK 'DISABLED', 'RETIRED' ETC APPROPRIATE

99a. **IF CODES 03-08 AT Q95a. OR CODE 2 AT Q98**

How long is it since you were last in paid work?

IF NECESSARY, PROBE FOR ESTIMATE

CODE ONE ONLY

| | | |
|---|---|---|
| Never in paid work | 01 | GO TO Q102 |
| Under 3 months | 02 | |
| 3, less than 6 months | 03 | |
| 6 months, less than a year | 04 | |
| 1 year, less than 2 years | 05 | ASK b. |
| 2 years, less than 4 years | 06 | |
| 4 years, less than 7 years | 07 | |
| 7 years or more | 08 | GO TO Q102 |
| Can't say | 98 | |

b. **IF IN PAID WORK DURING LAST 7 YEARS AGO (CODES 02-07 AT a.)**

How many full or part-time jobs have you had in the past 7 years? ... READ OUT ...

CODE ONE ONLY

| | |
|---|---|
| One, | 1 |
| two, | 2 |
| three, | 3 |
| or four or more | 4 |
| Don't know/Can't remember | 8 |

c. In the past seven years, for how long were you in paid work altogether?

ROUND UP TO NEAREST MONTH/YEAR

IF LESS THAN 1 YEAR WRITE IN NO. OF MONTHS: ☐☐

IF 1 YEAR OR MORE WRITE IN NO. OF YEARS: ☐☐

d. And in total, how long have you been unemployed and available for work since 1985?

ROUND UP TO NEAREST MONTH/YEAR

IF LESS THAN 1 YEAR WRITE IN NO. OF MONTHS: ☐☐

IF 1 YEAR OR MORE WRITE IN NO. OF YEARS: ☐☐

---

**IF CURRENTLY WORKING (CODES 01-02 AT Q95a.) OR HAS WORKED IN PAST 7 YEARS (CODES 02-07 AT Q99a.)**

100. **IF CURRENTLY IN WORK, ASK ABOUT CURRENT OR MOST RECENT JOB. USE APPROPRIATE TENSE.**

a. I would like to ask you about your present/(most recent) job. What is (was) the name or title of your job?

b. What kind of work do (did) you do in your job? IF RELEVANT: What are (were) the materials made of?

c. What training or qualifications are (were) needed for your job?

d. Do (did) you supervise or have management responsibility for the work of other people?

| | |
|---|---|
| None | 1 |

IF YES: How many?

| | |
|---|---|
| 1 to 24 | 2 |
| 25 or more | 3 |

e. Are (were) you ... READ OUT ...

| | | |
|---|---|---|
| ... an employee | 1 | ASK Q101 |
| working as a temp for an agency | 2 | |
| or, self-employed? | 3 | GO TO Q102 |

101a. **IF EMPLOYEE OR TEMP (CODE 1 OR 2 AT Q100e.)**

How many people are (were) employed at the place where you work(ed) (from)? Is it ... READ OUT ...

| | |
|---|---|
| None | 1 |
| 1 to 24 | 2 |
| 25 or more | 3 |

b. What does (did) your employer make or do at the place where you usually work(ed) from? _____

OFFICE USE ONLY

SIC ☐☐

**102a.** ALL

Now I would like to ask you about your household.

CODE TYPE OF ACCOMMODATION LIVED IN:

| | |
|---|---|
| Whole house | 01 |
| Bungalow | 02 |
| Purpose built flat, maisonette, bedsitter | 03 |
| Self-contained flat, maisonette, bed-sitter in converted house | 04 — ASK b. |
| Room(s) not self-contained | 05 |
| Residential or Nursing Home - own room | 06 |
| Residential or Nursing Home - shared room | 07 — GO TO Q103 |
| Caravan, mobile home, houseboat | 08 |
| Other (SPECIFY) | 09 |

**b.** IF CODES 01-05 AT a.

Can I check, is this sheltered accommodation?

| | |
|---|---|
| Yes | 1 |
| No | 2 |

**103a.** ALL

In whose name is this accommodation owned or rented?

| | |
|---|---|
| Respondent and/or spouse | 1 — ASK b. |
| Other person (ie. not respondent or spouse) | 2 — ASK c. |

**b.** IF RESPONDENT OR SPOUSE (CODE 1 AT a.)

Do you own or rent this accommodation?
IF RENTED, PROBE: Who from? CODE BELOW

**c.** IF 'OTHER PERSON' (CODE 2 AT a.)

Does ... (PERSON RESPONSIBLE FOR IT) own or rent it?
IF RENTED, PROBE: Who from? CODE BELOW

| | |
|---|---|
| Owned (include buying) | 1 — GO TO Q105 |
| Rented from: local authority/new town | 2 — ASK Q104 |
| - housing association/charitable trust | 3 — ASK Q104 |
| - relative | 4 |
| - private landlord or employer | 5 |
| - Squatting | 6 — GO TO Q105 |
| Other (SPECIFY) | 7 — ASK Q104 |

**104.** IF RENTED OR OTHER (CODES 2-5 OR 7 AT Q103c.)

Is it rented furnished or unfurnished?

| | |
|---|---|
| Furnished | 1 |
| Unfurnished/partly furnished | 2 |

**105a.** ALL

Apart from bedsitting rooms, how many living rooms do you have in this accommodation?

(INCLUDE KITCHEN IF LIVED IN)  ENTER NO. LIVING ROOMS [ ]

OR CODE NONE 00

**b.** How many bedrooms including bed sitting rooms, do you have?  BEDROOMS [ ]

**c.** Do you have the use of a bathroom?

| | |
|---|---|
| Yes | 1 |
| No | 2 |

**d.** Do you have the use of an indoor WC?

| | |
|---|---|
| Yes | 1 |
| No | 2 |

**e.** (Can I just check) does your household share any rooms, including a kitchen, bathroom or WC, with any other household?

| | |
|---|---|
| Yes | 1 |
| No | 2 |

**106.** (Can I just check) does your accommodation have ... READ OUT UNTIL 'YES' ...

CODE ONE ONLY

| | |
|---|---|
| ... a shared garden, | 1 |
| its own garden, | 2 |
| a back yard, | 3 |
| or, none of these? | 4 |

**107.** ALL

Can I check, at present are you ... READ OUT AND CODE FIRST TO APPLY ...

| | |
|---|---|
| ... married and living with your husband/wife, | 1 — GO TO Q109 |
| ... separated, | 2 |
| ... divorced, | 3 — ASK Q108 |
| ... widowed, | 4 |
| ... or single and never been married? | 5 |

**108.** IF NOT MARRIED (CODES 2 TO 5 AT Q107)

Can I check, at present are you living as married?

| | | |
|---|---|---|
| Yes | 1 | GO TO Q109 |
| No | 2 | GO TO Q118 |

**109.** IF MARRIED OR LIVING AS MARRIED (CODE 1 AT Q107 OR CODE 1 AT Q108)

At the present time is your husband/wife/partner in paid work, looking for work, a full-time student or doing something else?

PROBE TO DETERMINE CURRENT STATUS

NOTE: 1) FULL-TIME STUDENT (CODE 09) HAS PRIORITY OVER WORKING.
2) IN WORK (CODES 01 & 02) INCLUDES WORK THROUGH A GOVT. SCHEME

CODE ONE ONLY

| | | |
|---|---|---|
| Work full-time (30+ hrs) | 01 | GO TO Q112 |
| Work part-time (less than 30 hrs) | 02 | |
| Waiting to start a job already obtained | 03 | |
| Unemployed and actively looking for work | 04 | ASK Q110 |
| Unemployed, wanting work but not actively looking | 05 | |
| Out of work as temporarily sick | 06 | |
| Permanently sick or disabled | 07 | GO TO Q113 |
| Wholly retired from work | 08 | |
| In full-time education | 09 | |
| Looking after home or family | 10 | ASK Q110 |
| Other (SPECIFY) | 11 | |

**110.** IF CODES 03-06, 09-11 AT Q109

Has your husband/wife/partner had a paid job lasting a month or more since 1985 (in the last 7 years)?

| | | |
|---|---|---|
| Yes | 1 | ASK Q111 |
| No | 2 | GO TO Q118 |
| Don't know | 8 | |

**111.** IF YES AT Q110

How long is it since he/she was last in paid employment?

CODE ONE ONLY

| | |
|---|---|
| Under 1 year | 1 |
| 1 year less than 4 years | 2 |
| 4 years less than 7 years | 3 |
| Don't know | 8 |

**112a.** IF PARTNER CURRENTLY OR HAS BEEN IN WORK IN LAST 7 YEARS

In the past 7 years, how long has he/she been in paid work altogether?

ROUND UP TO NEAREST MONTH/YEAR

IF LESS THAN ONE YEAR WRITE IN NO. OF MONTHS:

IF ONE YEAR OR MORE WRITE IN NO. OF YEARS:

Don't know 98

**b.** Since 1985 (seven years ago), has your husband/wife/partner been unemployed and available for work for at least a month?

| | | |
|---|---|---|
| Yes | 1 | ASK c. |
| No | 2 | GO TO Q116 |
| Can't say | 8 | |

**c.** IF YES AT b. (CODE 1)

How long in total has he/she been unemployed and available for work since 1985?

ROUND UP TO NEAREST MONTH/YEAR

IF UNDER ONE YEAR WRITE IN NO. OF MONTHS:

IF ONE YEAR OR MORE WRITE IN NO. OF YEARS:

Don't know 98    GO TO Q116

**113a.** IF PARTNER PERMANENTLY SICK OR DISABLED (CODES 07/08 AT Q109)

What age was he/she when he/she became wholly retired (unable to work)?

AGE:

Don't know 98

**b.** So, can I just check, how long ago did he/she retire (become unable to work)?

CODE ONE ONLY

| | | |
|---|---|---|
| Less than 1 year ago | 1 | |
| 1 year, less than 4 years ago | 2 | ASK Q114 |
| 4 years, less than 7 years ago | 3 | |
| 7 years ago or more | 4 | GO TO Q118 |
| Can't say | 8 | |

**114a.** IF LESS THAN SEVEN YEARS AGO (CODES 1 TO 3 AT Q113b.)

Has he/she been unemployed and available for work for at least a month in the last seven years?

| | | |
|---|---|---|
| Yes | 1 | ASK b. |
| No | 2 | GO TO Q115 |
| Don't know | 8 | |

**IF YES AT a.**

b. How long in total before being unable to work (retired) was he/she unemployed and available for work in the past seven years?

ROUND UP TO NEAREST MONTH/ YEAR

IF LESS THAN 1 YEAR WRITE IN NO. OF MONTHS: [ ][ ]

IF 1 YEAR OR MORE WRITE IN NO. OF YEARS: [ ][ ]

---

115. **IF RETIRED/BECAME UNABLE TO WORK LESS THAN 7 YEARS AGO**

Has your husband/wife/partner had a paid job lasting a month or more since 1985 (in the last 7 years)?

| | | |
|---|---|---|
| Yes | 1 | ASK Q116 |
| No | 2 | GO TO Q118 |
| Don't know | 8 | |

---

116. **IF SPOUSE/PARTNER IN WORK OR HAS WORKED IN LAST 7 YEARS**

• ASK ABOUT PRESENT JOB IF IN WORK OR MOST RECENT JOB IF NOT IN WORK

• USE APPROPRIATE TENSE

a. I would like to ask about your husband's/wife's/partner's present (most recent) job? What is (was) the name or title of his/her job?

b. What kind of work does (did) he/she do in that job?
IF RELEVANT: What are (were) the materials made of?

c. What training or qualifications are (were) needed for his/her job?

d. Does (did) he/she supervise or have management responsibility for the work of other people?

| | |
|---|---|
| None | 1 |

IF YES: How many?

| | |
|---|---|
| 1 to 24 | 2 |
| 25 or more | 3 |
| Don't know | 8 |

---

117a. **IF SPOUSE/PARTNER IN WORK OR HAS WORKED IN PAST 7 YEARS**

Is (was) he/she ... READ OUT ...

| | | |
|---|---|---|
| ... an employee, | 1 | ASK b. |
| working as a temp. for an agency, | 2 | |
| or, self-employed? | 3 | GO TO Q118 |
| Don't know | 8 | |

b. IF EMPLOYEE OR TEMP (CODES 1 OR 2 AT a.)

How many people are (were) employed at the place where he/she works(ed)?

Is it ... READ OUT ...

| | |
|---|---|
| ... None | 1 |
| 1 to 24 | 2 |
| or 25 or more? | 3 |
| Can't estimate | 8 |

c. What does (did) his/her employer make or do at the place where he/she usually work(ed) from?

OFFICE USE ONLY

SIC [ ]

---

118a. ALL

SHOW CARD F. I have a card showing various categories of weekly and monthly income. Could you show me in to which category your own personal income comes, that is income after tax but including any benefits, pension or other income you receive? Just tell me the number in the middle of the card that applies.

**INCOME CODE** [ ]

| | |
|---|---|
| Refused | 97 |
| Can't estimate | 98 |

b. SHOW CARD F. And into which category does the total income of your household fall - that is income after tax, but including any benefit, pensions or other income you receive?

**INCOME CODE** [ ]

| | |
|---|---|
| Refused | 97 |
| Can't estimate | 98 |

119a. SHOW CARD G. What is the highest qualification you have obtained, either while at school or gained after you left school?

CODE ONE ONLY

NO QUALIFICATIONS OBTAINED — 00 GO TO Q120

CSE Grades 2-5 / GCSE Grades D-G — 01

CODE QUALIFICATION RESPONDENT THINKS IS HIGHEST. IF TWO OR MORE ARE EQUAL, TAKE MOST USEFUL, OR MOST RECENT OF THESE. IF STILL STUDYING TAKE HIGHEST TO DATE.

CSE Grade 1
GCE 'O' level
GCSE Grades A-C
School Certificate
Scottish SCE/SUPE Ordinary
Scottish School leaving Certifi-
cate (SLC) Lower — 02

City & Guilds Craft/Intermediate/
Ordinary/Part I — 03 ASK b.

GCE 'A' level/'S' level
Higher School Certificate
Matriculation
Scottish SCE/SLC/SUPE Higher — 04

Overseas School Leaving Exam/Certificate — 05

ONC/OND/City & Guilds Advanced/Final level/Part II
or III — 06

HNC/HND/City & Guilds Full Technological Certificate — 07
RSA/Other clerical and commercial — 08

Teachers training qualification — 09
Nursing qualification

Professional qualification (membership awarded by
professional institute) — 10
Degree, including higher degree — 11
Other technical or business qualification/certificate — 12
Other (PLEASE SAY WHAT) — 13

b. IF HAS QUALS (CODES 01-13 AT a.)

Did you obtain this qualification in the last
seven years?

Yes 1 ASK d.
No 2 GO TO Q120

c. Are you qualified as a doctor or nurse or
any other kind of health professional?

Yes 1 ASK d.
No 2 GO TO Q120

d. IF 'YES' (CODE 1 AT c.)

What are you qualified as?

Doctor/dentist 1
Nurse 2
Physiotherapist/Occupational therapist/Radiographer 3
Dietitian 4
Other (SPECIFY) 5

ALL

120. Are you currently enrolled in any course of
study or training?

INCLUDE EVENING CLASSES

Yes 1
No 2

121. Turning now to your father

IF QUERIED, TAKE NATURAL FATHER

a. What was your father's year of birth?

YEAR OF BIRTH: [    ] ASK c.

Don't know 9998 ASK b.
Know nothing about father 9997 GOTO Q122

b. IF DON'T KNOW AT a.

Do you know how old your father was when you
were born?

AGE [    ]

Don't know 98

c. (Can I just check) is your father still alive?

Yes 1 ASK d.
No 2 ASK e.
Don't know 8 GO TO Q122

d. IF STILL ALIVE (CODE 1 AT c.)

How old was your father on his last birthday?

AGE [    ] GO TO Q122

Don't know 98

e. IF NO AT c.

How old was your father when he died?

AGE [    ]

Don't know 98

## 122.

Turning now to your mother

**IF QUERIED, TAKE NATURAL MOTHER**

a. What was your mother's year of birth?

YEAR OF BIRTH: [   ]   ASK c.

Don't know   9998   ASK b.

Know nothing about mother   9997   GO TO Q123

**IF DON'T KNOW AT a.**

b. Do you know how old your mother was when you were born?

AGE [   ]

Don't know   98

c. (Can I just check) is your mother still alive?

(TAKE NATURAL MOTHER)

Yes   1   ASK d.

No   2   ASK e.

Don't know   8   GO TO Q123

**IF STILL ALIVE (CODE 1 AT c.)**

d. How old was your mother on her last birthday?

AGE [   ]

Don't know   98

**IF NO AT c.**

e. How old was your mother when she died?

AGE [   ]

Don't know   98

## 123.

I would now like to ask you about any worrying or disruptive event which might have happened to you during the past few years. Some of these might already have been mentioned, but I would like to ask you a bit more about how they affected you when they happened, and whether they still affect you.

---

## 123. HEALTH

I will begin by asking about health

For each item: No....0 / Yes....1

Columns:
- **How much has this disrupted or changed your everyday life?** — No, not at all...0 / Yes, somewhat...1 / Yes, a great deal...2
- **How much has it caused you worry and stress?** — No, not at all...0 / Yes, somewhat...1 / Yes, a great deal...2
- **Or in the past seven years?** — No...0 / Yes...1
- **Does it still affect your everyday life?** — No, not at all...0 / Yes, somewhat...1 / Yes, a great deal...2
- **Does it still cause you worry and stress?** — No, not at all...0 / Yes, somewhat...1 / Yes, a great deal...2

a) Have you developed or found out you had a serious illness or handicap or has an existing condition got worse in the past year?

b) Have you had a serious accident or injury, or had an operation or spent a period in hospital in the past year?

c) Have you had painful or upsetting treatment of a condition in the past year?

d) What about your family and close friends - have any of them had a serious problem with their health in the past year?

## 124. DEATH

a) Has there been a death of any close family in the past year? Spouse / partner, child, parent, other.

b) Has a close friend or other person who was important to you died in the past year?

## 125. WORK

Now I would like to ask you about work.

a) Have you changed jobs in the past year?

b) Have you lost a job or thought that you would soon lose your job in the past year?

c) Have you had any other crisis or serious disappointments in your work or career in general in the past year?

d) Have you retired in the past year?

e) Has your spouse / partner lost a job, or had a crisis or serious disappointment at work in the past year?

f) Has your spouse / partner retired in the past year?

## 126. HOUSING

Now I would like to ask you about housing

| | | How much has this disrupted or changed your everyday life ? | How much has it caused you worry and stress ? |
|---|---|---|---|
| a) Have you moved house in the past year ? | No.....0 Yes.....1 | No,not at all....0 Yes,somewhat.....1 Yes,a great deal.2 | No,not at all....0 Yes,somewhat.....1 Yes,a great deal.2 → c) |
| b) Did you move away from the area or where most of your friends are ? | No.....0 Yes.....1 | No,not at all....0 Yes,somewhat.....1 Yes,a great deal.2 | No,not at all....0 Yes,somewhat.....1 Yes,a great deal.2 |
| c) Have you had any major worries with your housing in the past year ? | No.....0 Yes.....1 | No,not at all....0 Yes,somewhat.....1 Yes,a great deal.2 | No,not at all....0 Yes,somewhat.....1 Yes,a great deal.2 |
| d) Has a member of your family left home or has a new person moved into your house in the past year ? | No.....0 Yes.....1 | No,not at all....0 Yes,somewhat.....1 Yes,a great deal.2 | No,not at all....0 Yes,somewhat.....1 Yes,a great deal.2 |

## 127. RELATIONSHIPS

| | | How much has this disrupted or changed your everyday life ? | How much has it caused you worry and stress ? | Or in the past seven years ? | Does it still affect your everyday life ? | Does it still cause you worry and stress ? |
|---|---|---|---|---|---|---|
| a) Have you become divorced or lived apart in the past year ? | No.....0 Yes.....1 | No,not at all....0 Yes,somewhat.....1 Yes,a great deal.2 | No,not at all....0 Yes,somewhat.....1 Yes,a great deal.2 | No..........0 Yes..........1 | No,not at all....0 Yes,somewhat.....1 Yes,a great deal.2 | No,not at all....0 Yes,somewhat.....1 Yes,a great deal.2 |
| b) Have you had any serious disagreements with your spouse/ partner or felt betrayed or disappointed by them in the past year ? | No.....0 Yes.....1 | No,not at all....0 Yes,somewhat.....1 Yes,a great deal.2 | No,not at all....0 Yes,somewhat.....1 Yes,a great deal.2 | | | |
| c) In the past year have you had any serious difficulty with any of your children because of their health or behaviour, or for any other reason ? | No.....0 Yes.....1 | No,not at all....0 Yes,somewhat.....1 Yes,a great deal.2 | No,not at all....0 Yes,somewhat.....1 Yes,a great deal.2 | | | |
| d) In the past year have you fallen out or had serious disagreement with a friend or relative or felt betrayed by them ? | No.....0 Yes.....1 | No,not at all....0 Yes,somewhat.....1 Yes,a great deal.2 | No,not at all....0 Yes,somewhat.....1 Yes,a great deal.2 | | | |
| e) Have you lost contact with close family or friends for any other reason in the past year ? | No.....0 Yes.....1 | No,not at all....0 Yes,somewhat.....1 Yes,a great deal.2 | No,not at all....0 Yes,somewhat.....1 Yes,a great deal.2 | | | |

## 128. OTHER

| | | How much has this disrupted or changed your everyday life ? | How much has it caused you worry and stress ? | Or in the past seven years ? | Does it still affect your everyday life ? | Does it still cause you worry and stress ? |
|---|---|---|---|---|---|---|
| a) Have you been assaulted or robbed in the past year ? | No.....0 Yes.....1 | No,not at all....0 Yes,somewhat.....1 Yes,a great deal.2 | No,not at all....0 Yes,somewhat.....1 Yes,a great deal.2 | No..........0 Yes..........1 | No,not at all....0 Yes,somewhat.....1 Yes,a great deal.2 | No,not at all....0 Yes,somewhat.....1 Yes,a great deal.2 |
| b) Have you had any major financial problems in the past year ? | No.....0 Yes.....1 | No,not at all....0 Yes,somewhat.....1 Yes,a great deal.2 | No,not at all....0 Yes,somewhat.....1 Yes,a great deal.2 | No..........0 Yes..........1 | No,not at all....0 Yes,somewhat.....1 Yes,a great deal.2 | No,not at all....0 Yes,somewhat.....1 Yes,a great deal.2 |
| c) Have you had any serious problems with officials or with the Law in the past year ? | No.....0 Yes.....1 | No,not at all....0 Yes,somewhat.....1 Yes,a great deal.2 | No,not at all....0 Yes,somewhat.....1 Yes,a great deal.2 | No..........0 Yes..........1 | No,not at all....0 Yes,somewhat.....1 Yes,a great deal.2 | No,not at all....0 Yes,somewhat.....1 Yes,a great deal.2 |
| d) Have you had any other serious upsets or disappointments in the past year ? If 'Yes' Specify | No.....0 Yes.....1 | No,not at all....0 Yes,somewhat.....1 Yes,a great deal.2 | No,not at all....0 Yes,somewhat.....1 Yes,a great deal.2 | No..........0 Yes..........1 | No,not at all....0 Yes,somewhat.....1 Yes,a great deal.2 | No,not at all....0 Yes,somewhat.....1 Yes,a great deal.2 |

129a. Has anything particularly nice happened to you in the past year?

| | |
|---|---|
| Yes | 1   ASK c. |
| No  | 2   ASK b. |

**IF NO AT a.**

b. Or in the last seven years, has anything particularly nice happened to you?

| | |
|---|---|
| Yes | 1   ASK c. |
| No  | 2   GO TO Q130 |

**IF YES (CODE 1) AT a. OR b.**

c. What particularly nice things have happened to you in the past year (last seven years)? PROBE FULLY. RECORD VERBATIM.

130a. This is the last question. Thank you very much indeed. You have been very helpful.

Some interviews in a survey are checked to make sure that people like yourself are satisfied with the way the interview was carried out. Just in case yours is one of the interviews that is checked it would be helpful if we could have your telephone number?

| | |
|---|---|
| Number given (RECORD ON PAGE 2 OF INTERVIEWER CONTACT FORM) | 1 |
| No telephone access | 2 |
| Number refused | 3 |

b. INTERVIEWER CHECK FRONT PAGE AND CODE:

| | | |
|---|---|---|
| Nurse measured in 1984/85 | A | ASK c. |
| Not measured | B | GO TO Q131 |

**IF NURSE MEASURED IN 1984/85**

c. As on the previous occasion, this research study falls into two parts, the first being the questionnaire you have just answered.

The Cambridge University Medical School very much hope you will also help with the second part - not now but in a week or so's time. The second part would take up less of your time and is quite different. A qualified nurse would contact you and ask your permission to visit you at home in order to take some simple measurements - things like weight and blood pressure, just as before.

What times of day are most convenient for you - obviously it would be sensible if the nurse suggested times that are best for you when she gets in touch. RECORD DETAILS ON PAGE 2 OF INTERVIEWER CONTACT FORM.

**IF MORE INFORMATION WANTED, EXPLAIN:** the researchers want to look at the changes that have occurred in your weight, height and blood pressure in the seven years since you last helped them in the Study.

1991/92

P.1178

# HEALTH AND LIFESTYLE SURVEY

MEASUREMENT PROFORMA – PART 1

NURSE NAME

SERIAL NUMBER

WARD

TIME AT START

1. SEX    Male 1   Female 2

2. AGE: Can I check, what was your age last birthday    YEARS:

3. WEIGHT    Kg

4. CLOTHES WORN    Light 1   Heavy 2

5. HEIGHT    cm:

6a. GIRTH    cm:

b. HIPS    cm:

7. RESPIRATORY FUNCTION    1st attempt   2nd attempt   3rd attempt

a. $FEV_1$

b. PEF

c. FVC

8. DENTAL ROLL    Respondent accepted 1   Respondent did not accept 2

---

131a. TIME AT CLOSE OF INTERVIEW:

b. TOTAL INTERVIEW LENGTH:   IN MINUTES

FOR COMPLETION AFTER INTERVIEW

A. Was there a language problem during this interview? IF YES DESCRIBE:    Yes 1   No 2

B. CODE FROM OBSERVATION ETHNIC GROUP:

- Indian (inc. E. African), Pakistani, Bangladeshi   1
- Black, African, West Indian   2
- Other non-white   3
- White/European   4

C. Is this house/flat situated in a ...

- ... High rise development (THIS CODE TAKES PRIORITY)   1
- In a built up area with no open space adjacent   2
- In a built up area with adjacent open space or large garden   3
- In a country district   4
- Elsewhere (SPECIFY)   5

D. Was anyone else, other than interviewer and respondent present at the interview? IF SO, WHO?

- No   1
- Spouse or partner   2
- Child (children)   3
- Parent(s)   4
- Others   5

E. Date of interview    DAY   MONTH   YEAR

F. INTERVIEWER NUMBER

9. **TIME AFTER LAST CIGARETTE/CIGAR/PIPE**

ENTER:

| HOURS | MINUTES |
|---|---|
| ☐☐ | ☐☐ |

OR CODE

Non-smoker     8888
More than 24 hours ago     7777
Smoking during interview     0000

10a. **MEDICATION:** Today, have you taken any (prescribed) pills etc for hay fever, asthma, high or low blood pressure, angina, etc?

Yes    1   ASK b.
No    2   GO TO Q11

b. **IF YES, LIST ALL MEDICATIONS BELOW AND WHAT THEY ARE PRESCRIBED FOR.**

11. **BLOOD PRESSURE**

| | 1st reading | 2nd reading | 3rd reading | 4th reading |
|---|---|---|---|---|
| a. Systolic | ☐☐ | ☐☐ | ☐☐ | ☐☐ |
| b. Mean | ☐☐ | ☐☐ | ☐☐ | ☐☐ |
| c. Diastolic | ☐☐ | ☐☐ | ☐☐ | ☐☐ |
| d. Heart rate | ☐☐ | ☐☐ | ☐☐ | ☐☐ |

**COMMENTS:**

---

| MEASUREMENT PROFORMA – PART 2 |
|---|

SERIAL NUMBER ☐ ☐ ☐ ☐

|REACTION TIME|

12. **IF RESPONDENT HAS NO USE OF ANY FINGERS, RING CODE** ☐ 1 **AND GO TO PART 3**

a. SWITCH ON. PRESS RESET BUTTON.

I would like to see how quick your reactions are. Put your finger on this key marked 'O' and look at the screen. This is the only key you will need to use. Everytime you see a 'O' on the screen press the key once as quickly as you can. We will start with a practice run to make sure you know what to do. Are you clear about it?

I am going to start the machine now, so look for the 'O's and press firmly as soon as you see one.

b. PRESS START BUTTON

CORRECT ANY ERROR DURING 8 PRACTICE TRIALS

WHEN 'WAIT' INDICATOR APPEARS? SAY:

That was fine. Now we can time your reactions. Everytime you see a 'O' on the screen, press the 'O' key as quickly as you can.

c. PRESS START BUTTON. (20 'O's WILL BE DISPLAYED IN TURN)

WHEN DISPLAY FLASHES:

                            MEAN TIME

* Press Key 1 AND RECORD        ☐☐.☐

                         STANDARD DEVIATION

* Press Key 2 AND RECORD:       ☐☐.☐

d. I am now going to give you a slightly harder test. This time the numbers 1, 2, 3, or 4 will appear on the screen. I want you to press the key that has the same number as that on the screen. If you see a 4 on the screen, press key 4 as quickly as possible. If you see a 1, press key 1, and so on.

Use both hands to do this. Put your 2nd and 3rd fingers of each hand on the four keys (1, 2, 3, and 4). (OTHER FINGERS CAN BE USED IF NECESSARY).

IF RESPONDENT HAS A NON-FUNCTIONAL HAND, RING THIS CODE ☐ 1 AND GO TO PART 3

I am going to start the machine again. Remember to press the same number as the number on the screen. This is another practice run.

e. PRESS START BUTTON

CORRECT ANY ERROR DURING 8 PRACTICE TRIALS

WHEN 'WAIT' INDICATOR APPEARS, SAY:

Now let's do it as a proper test. Everytime you see a number on the screen quickly press the key with the same number. Remember to press firmly.

## MEASUREMENT PROFORMA - PART 3

13a. There is a lot of talk these days about fibre in our food. I am going to read out a list of foods. For each one tell me whether you think it has fibre in it or not. **RING CODES 1, 2 OR 8 BELOW UNDER a.**

| FOOD | a. Does this contain fibre? Yes / No / Don't know | d. RECALL |
|---|---|---|
| Roast meat | 1   2   8 | Roast meat / Meat, Roast beef/lamb/etc   2 / 1 |
| Digestive Biscuits | 1   2   8 | Digestive Biscuits / (Other) Biscuits   2 / 1 |
| Potatoes | 1   2   8 | Potatoes / Other 'potato' answers   2 / 1 |
| Eggs | 1   2   8 | Eggs / Other 'Egg' answers   2 / 1 |
| Orange Juice | 1   2   8 | Orange Juice / (Other) Fruit juice, Orange   2 / 1 |
| Grilled Fish | 1   2   8 | Grilled Fish / Fish, Cooked Fish, etc   2 / 1 |
| Weetabix | 1   2   8 | Weetabix / (Other) Breakfast cereal   2 / 1 |
| White Bread | 1   2   8 | White Bread / Bread/other bread   2 / 1 |
| Cheese | 1   2   8 | Cheese / Other 'cheese' answers   2 / 1 |
| Apples | 1   2   8 | Apples / Other 'apple' answers   2 / 1 |
| | | Other types given not listed originally (SPECIFY) |

b. Which hand do you usually use when writing?    Right 1   Left 2

c. Have you always been right/left handed?    Yes 1   No 2

d. We're often being told things and unless we concentrate they just go in one ear and out the other. As a matter of interest, I wonder how many foods you can remember from the list I read out?

**RING CODES AT d. IN GRID ABOVE FOR 'REMEMBERED FOODS'**

**IF CAN'T REMEMBER ANYTHING, RING THIS CODE:** [ 0 ]

**WHEN EVERYTHING REMEMBERED, SAY** 'That's fine'.

**IF ASKED** 'How am I doing', **SAY** 'Fine, can you remember anything else?'

**IF GAP, COUNT SLOWLY UP TO 10. IF NO MORE RESPONSE SAY**
'Good - now let's do something else'.

---

f. PRESS START BUTTON (40 NUMBERS WILL BE DISPLAYED IN TURN)

WHEN DISPLAY FLASHES:

* PRESS Key 1 AND RECORD    MEAN TIME (CORRECT)   [ __ . __ ]

* PRESS Key 2 AND RECORD:    STANDARD DEVIATION (CORRECT)   [ __ . __ ]

* PRESS Key 0 AND RECORD    NUMBER OF ERRORS   [ __ __ ]

* PRESS Key 3 AND RECORD    MEAN TIME (ERRORS)   [ __ . __ ]

* PRESS Key 4 AND RECORD:    STANDARD DEVIATION (ERRORS)   [ __ . __ ]

SWITCH OFF MACHINE

GO TO PART 3

MEASUREMENT PROFORMA - PART 4

14. ENTER SERIAL NUMBER AT FOOT OF SEPARATE BLOCKS SHEET

GIVE TO RESPONDENT WITH PENCIL AND EXPLAIN WHAT TO DO.

"I want you to do something on your own while I pack my things together. These pictures show piles of blocks. Write in the number of blocks contained in each of these piles."

DO NOT LET RESPONDENT DISCUSS IT WITH ANYONE ELSE.

WHEN DONE, ASK "Please read out the number you have written down for each pile of blocks". ENTER CAREFULLY BELOW. PIN SEPARATE SHEET TO BACK OF THESE PROFORMAS.

a) [ ]

b) [ ]

c) [ ]

d) [ ]

e) [ ]

f) [ ]

SELF-COMPLETION QUESTIONNAIRE

15. ENTER SERIAL NUMBER ON FRONT OF SELF-COMPLETION QUESTIONNAIRE. EXPLAIN THAT RESPONDENT IS ASKED TO DO ON OWN AND POST BACK IN ENVELOPE

GIVE QUESTIONNAIRE AND ENVELOPE. RING CODE BELOW.

| | |
|---|---|
| Self-Completion accepted | 1 |
| Self-completion not accepted | |
| - refusal | 2 |
| - cannot read | 3 |
| - other reason (SPECIFY) | 4 |

16. GP REFERRAL

| | | |
|---|---|---|
| - Referred to GP and wishes GP to be informed | 1 | GP Report Form completed and sent to Cambridge |
| - Referred to GP but does not want GP informed | 2 | |
| - Not referred to GP | 3 | |

NOW COMPLETE:

17. TIME AT END: [ ][ ]

18. LENGTH OF SESSION IN MINUTES: [ ][ ]

19. NURSE:     NAME

NUMBER: [ ][ ][ ]

20. DATE:

[ ][ ] DAY   [ ][ ] MONTH   [ ][ ] YEAR

# INDEX

## Blood pressure

## Body measurement

## Education

## Exercise and leisure

## Health

**Socio-economic group**